The Basics

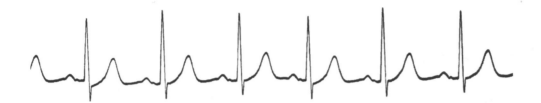

A COMPREHENSIVE OUTLINE OF NURSING SCHOOL CONTENT

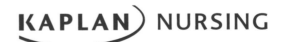 NURSING

Judith A. Burckhardt, Ph.D., R.N.

Joanne Brown, M.S.N., M.P.H., R.N.

Barbara J. Irwin, M.S.N., R.N.

Marlene Redemske, M.S.N., M.A., R.N.

Joseph (Ryan) Goble, M.S.N., R.N.

Pamela Gardner, M.S.N., R.N.

Roberta Harbison, M.S.N., R.N.

Amy Kennedy, M.S.N., R.N.

Contributing Editors

Susan Sanders, D.N.P, R.N., NEA–BC

Vice President, Kaplan Nursing

© 2020 by Kaplan, Inc.

Published by Kaplan Publishing, a division of Kaplan, Inc.
750, Third Avenue
New York, NY 10017

Retail ISBN: 978-1-5062-6289-5
Course ISBN: 978-1-5062-6744-9

10 9 8 7 6 5 4

Kaplan Publishing print books are available at special quantity discounts to use for sales promotions, employee premiums, or educational purposes. For more information or to purchase books, please call the Simon & Schuster special sales department at 866-506-1949.

Table of Contents

Chapter 1: Health Assessment

    Section 1: Health History... 3

    Section 2: Physical Assessment...................................... 5

    Section 3: Mental Status Assessment 17

Chapter 2: Fundamentals of Nursing

    Section 1: Normal Mobility... 21

    Section 2: Altered Functions Related to Immobility 25

    Section 3: Safety 33

    Section 4: Altered Functions Related to Pain........................ 37

    Section 5: Protection from Communicable Diseases 43

    Section 6: Maintenance of Skin Integrity 53

    Section 7: Perioperative Care 63

Chapter 3: Fluid and Electrolyte Balance

    Section 1: Fluid Regulation 73

    Section 2: Electrolyte Imbalances................................... 79

    Section 3: Nursing Measures for Intravenous Therapy 87

Chapter 4: The Cardiovascular System

    Section 1: The Cardiovascular System Overview..................... 103

    Section 2: Alterations in Cardiac Output........................... 109

    Section 3: Vascular Alterations: Hypertension...................... 141

    Section 4: Selected Disorders of Tissue Perfusion 147

    Section 5: Vascular Disorders 153

Chapter 5: The Respiratory System

    Section 1: The Respiratory System Overview........................ 161

    Section 2: Alterations in Airway Clearance and Breathing Patterns ... 165

Chapter 6: Hematological and Immune Disorders

    Section 1: Overview of Hematology................................ 183

    Section 2: Disorders of the Blood 185

    Section 3: The Immune System.................................... 193

Chapter 7: The Gastrointestinal System

    Section 1: Concepts Basic to Nutrition 203

    Section 2: Alterations in Metabolism............................... 225

    Section 3: Selected Disorders 229

    Section 4: Accessory Organs of Digestion (Liver, Gallbladder, Pancreas) 235

    Section 5: The Lower Intestinal Tract.............................. 251

Chapter 8: The Endocrine System

    Section 1: The Endocrine System Overview......................... 269

    Section 2: Endocrine Disorders 271

Chapter 9: The Renal and Urological Systems

    Section 1: The Urinary System Overview 297

    Section 2: Urinary Function... 299

    Section 3: Selected Disorders 307

Chapter 10: The Musculoskeletal System

    Section 1: Alterations in Musculoskeletal Function 319

Chapter 11: Sensory and Neurological Function

    Section 1: Sensation and Perception Functions............................... 343

    Section 2: Alterations in Vision... 377

    Section 3: Alterations in Hearing 387

Chapter 12: Oncology

    Section 1: Cancer... 395

    Section 2: Leukemia... 405

    Section 3: Skin Cancer... 407

    Section 4: Intracranial Tumors 409

    Section 5: Pancreatic Tumors 411

    Section 6: Carcinoma of the Larynx 413

Chapter 13: Maternity and Gynecological Nursing

    Section 1: The Reproductive System....................................... 417

    Section 2: Childbearing—Antepartal Care 435

    Section 3: Labor and Delivery 445

    Section 4: Postpartum 457

    Section 5: The Neonate 461

    Section 6: Childbearing—Maternal Complications 465

    Section 7: Childbearing—Neonatal Complications 473

Chapter 14: Pediatric Nursing

    Section 1: Growth and Development 485

    Section 2: Pediatric Assessment/Wellness 497

    Section 3: Alterations in Pediatric Health 513

Chapter 15: Psychosocial Integrity

    Section 1: Basic Concepts 533

    Section 2: Anxiety 539

    Section 3: Situational Crises... 547

    Section 4: Depressive Disorders 553

    Section 5: Bipolar Disorder 557

    Section 6: Altered Thought Processes...................................... 563

    Section 7: Social Interactions 571

    Section 8: Abuse.. 577

Chapter 16: Pharmacology

    Section 1: Listing of Medications   583

Chapter 17: Terminology

    Section 1: Nursing Abbreviations   669

    Section 2: Medication Terminology   679

    Section 3: Terminology Used for Documentation   681

    Index   687

Chapter 1

HEALTH ASSESSMENT

Sections	**Concepts Covered**
1. Health History	Health Promotion
2. Physical Assessment	Therapeutic Techniques
3. Mental Status Assessment	Ego Integrity/Self Concept
	Intracranial Regulation

HEALTH HISTORY

DEMOGRAPHIC DATA

A. Date

B. Biographical information

C. Client as reliable historian

D. Age, sex, marital status

E. Reason for seeking health care

F. History of present illness/condition

PAST HEALTH HISTORY

A. Past health history
   1. Medical history
   2. Surgical history
   3. Medications
   4. Communicable diseases
   5. Allergies
   6. Injuries/accidents
   7. Disabilities/handicaps
   8. Blood transfusions
   9. Childhood illnesses
   10. Immunizations

B. Family health history
   1. Genogram
   2. Familial/genetic diseases

C. Social history
   1. Alcohol/tobacco/drug use
   2. Travel history
   3. Work environment
   4. Home environment
   5. Hobbies/leisure activities
   6. Stressors
   7. Education
   8. Economic status
   9. Military service
   10. Religion
   11. Culture
   12. Roles/relationships

13. Sexual history

14. Patterns of daily living

D. Health maintenance

1. Sleep

2. Diet

3. Exercise

4. Stress management

5. Safety practices

6. Patterns of health care practices

7. Review of systems

PURPOSE

A. Assess client's current health status

B. Interpret physical data

C. Decide on interventions based on data obtained

PREPARATION

A. Gather equipment
1. Ophthalmoscope
2. Tuning fork
3. Cotton swabs
4. Snellen eye chart
5. Thermometer
6. Penlight
7. Tongue depressor
8. Ruler/tape measure
9. Safety pin
10. Balance scale
11. Gloves
12. Nasal speculum
13. Vaginal speculum

B. Provide for privacy (drape) in quiet, well-lit environment

C. Explain procedure to client

D. Ask client to empty bladder

E. Drape client for privacy

F. Compare findings on one side of body with other side and compare with normal

G. Make use of teaching opportunities (dental care, eye exams, self-exams of breasts or testicles)

H. Use piece of equipment for entire assessment, then return to equipment tray

TECHNIQUES USED IN ORDER PERFORMED, EXCEPT FOR ABDOMINAL ASSESSMENT

A. General assessment
1. Inspection
2. Palpation
3. Percussion
4. Auscultation

B. Abdominal assessment
1. Inspection
2. Auscultation
3. Percussion
4. Palpation

C. Inspection (visually examined)
1. Start with first interaction
2. Provide good lighting
3. Determine
   a. Size
   b. Shape
   c. Color
   d. Texture
   e. Symmetry
   f. Position

D. Palpation (touch)
1. Warm hands
2. Approach slowly and proceed systematically
3. Use fingertips for fine touch (pulses, nodes)
4. Use dorsum of fingers for temperature
5. Use palm or ulnar edge of hand for vibration
6. Start with light palpation, then do deep palpation
7. Use bimanual palpation (both hands) for deep palpation and to assess movable structure (kidney). Place sensing hand lightly on skin surface, place active hand over sensing hand and apply pressure
8. Ballottement—push fluid-filled tissue toward palpating hand so object floats against fingertips
9. Determine
   a. Masses
   b. Pulsation
   c. Organ size
   d. Tenderness or pain
   e. Swelling
   f. Tissue fullness and elasticity
   g. Vibration
   h. Crepitus
   i. Temperature
   j. Texture
   k. Moisture

E. Percussion (tap to produce sound and vibration)
1. Types
   a. Direct—strike body surface with 1 or 2 fingers
   b. Indirect—strike finger or hand placed over body surface
   c. Blunt—use reflex hammer to check deep tendon reflexes; use blunt percussion with fist to assess costovertebral angle (CVA) tenderness

2. Sounds (produced by direct or indirect percussion)

   a. Resonance—moderate to loud, low-pitched (clear, hollow) sound of moderate duration; found with air-filled tissue (normal lung)

   b. Hyperresonance—loud, booming, low-pitched sound of longer duration found with over-inflated, air-filled tissue (pulmonary emphysema); normal in child due to thin chest wall

   c. Tympany—loud, drum-like, high-pitched or musical sound of moderately long duration found with enclosed, air-filled structures (bowel)

   d. Dull—soft, muffled, moderate to high-pitched sound of short duration; found with dense, fluid-filled tissue (liver)

   e. Flat—very soft, high-pitched sound of short duration; found with very dense tissue (bone, muscle)

3. Determine

   a. Location, size, density of masses

   b. Pain in areas up to depth of 3–5 cm (1–2 in)

4. Performed after inspection and palpation, except for abdominal assessment; for abdomen, perform inspection, auscultation, percussion, palpation

F. Auscultation (listen to sounds)

   1. Equipment

      a. Use diaphragm of stethoscope to listen to high-pitched sounds (lung, bowel, heart); place firmly against skin surface to form tight seal (leave ring)

      b. Use bell to listen to soft, low-pitched sounds (heart murmurs); place lightly on skin surface

   2. Listen over bare skin (not through clothing); moisten body hair to prevent crackling sounds

Table 1-1 NORMAL VITAL SIGNS			
AGE	NORMAL RESPIRATORY RATE	NORMAL PULSE RATE	NORMAL BLOOD PRESSURE (BP)
Newborn	30–60 per min	120–140 beats per minute (bpm) May go to 180 when crying	65/41 mm Hg
1-4 years	20–30 per min	70–110 bpm	85/40–93/50 mm Hg
5-12 years	16–22 per min	60–95 bpm	93/53–106/62 mm Hg
Adult	12–20 per min	60–100 bpm	Less than 120/80 mm Hg

Factors influencing respiration: fever, anxiety, medications, disease

Factors influencing BP: disease, medications, anxiety, cardiac output, peripheral resistance, arterial elasticity, blood volume, blood viscosity, age, weight, exercise

Factors influencing pulse rate and rhythm: medications, pathology, exercise, age, gender, temperature, BP, serum electrolytes

Gerontologic considerations: increased systolic blood pressure, possible decrease in diastolic BP, widened pulse pressure

FINDINGS

A. General survey

   1. General appearance

      a. Apparent age

      b. Sex

      c. Racial and ethnic groups

      d. Apparent state of health

      e. Proportionate height and weight

      f. Posture

      g. Gait, movements, range of motion

      h. Suitable clothing

      i. Hygiene

      j. Body and breath odor

      k. Skin color, condition

      l. Presence of assistive device, hearing aid, glasses

   2. General behavior

      a. Signs of distress

      b. Level of consciousness, oriented ×3, mood, speech, thought process appropriate

      c. Level of cooperation, eye contact (culture must be considered)

B. Vital signs (see Table 1-1)

   1. Temperature (see Table 1-2)

      a. Infants—performed axillary, rectally

      b. Intra-auricular probe allows rapid, noninvasive reading when appropriate

      c. Tympanic membrane sensors—positioning is crucial, ear canal must be straightened

   2. Pulse (rate, rhythm)

   3. Respirations (rate, pattern, depth)

      a. Adult—costal (chest movement), regular, expiration slower than inspiration, rate 12–20 respirations/min

Table 1-2 NORMAL BODY TEMPERATURE		
METHOD USED	**FAHRENHEIT**	**CELSIUS**
Oral	98.6°	37.0°
Rectal	99.6°	37.6°
Axillary	97.6°	36.5°
Factors influencing reading: elderly client (normal temperature may be 95-97° F), faulty thermometer, dehydration, environment, infections		

      b. Neonates—diaphragmatic (abdominal movement), irregular, 30–60 respirations/min

      c. Breathing patterns

         1) Abdominal respirations—breathing accomplished by abdominal muscles and diaphragm; may be used to increase effectiveness of ventilatory process in certain conditions

         2) Apnea—temporary cessation of breathing

3) Cheyne-Stokes respirations—periodic breathing characterized by rhythmic waxing and waning of the depth of respirations

4) Dyspnea—difficult, labored, or painful breathing (considered "normal" at certain times, e.g., after extreme physical exertion)

5) Hyperpnea—abnormally deep breathing

6) Hyperventilation—abnormally rapid, deep, and prolonged breathing
   a) Caused by central nervous system disorders, medications that increase sensitivity of respiratory center, or acute anxiety
   b) Produces respiratory alkalosis due to reduction in CO_2

7) Hypoventilation—reduced ventilatory efficiency; produces respiratory acidosis due to elevation in CO_2

8) Kussmaul's respirations (air hunger)—marked increase in depth and rate

9) Orthopnea—inability to breathe except when trunk is in an upright position

10) Paradoxical respirations—breathing pattern in which a lung (or portion of a lung) deflates during inspiration (acts opposite to normal)

11) Periodic breathing—rate, depth, or tidal volume changes markedly from one interval to the next; pattern of change is periodically reproduced

12) Cyanosis—skin appears blue because of an excessive accumulation of unoxygenated hemoglobin in the blood

13) Stridor—harsh, high-pitched sound associated with airway obstruction near larynx

14) Cough
   a) Normal reflex to remove foreign material from the lungs
   b) Normally absent in newborns

4. Blood pressure
   a. Check both arms and compare results (difference 5–10 mm Hg normal)
   b. Pulse pressure is difference between systolic and diastolic readings; normal 30–40 mm Hg
   c. Cover 50% of limb from shoulder to olecranon with cuff; too narrow: abnormally high reading; too wide: abnormally low reading

C. Nutrition status
   1. Height, weight; ideal body weight, men: 106 lb for first 5 ft, then add 6 lb/in; women: 100 lb for first 5 ft, then add 5 lb/in; add 10% for client with larger frame; subtract 10% for client with small frame

D. Skin
   1. Check for pallor on buccal mucosa or conjunctivae, cyanosis on nail beds or oral mucosa, jaundice on sclera
   2. Scars, bruises, lesions
   3. Edema (eyes, sacrum), moisture, hydration
   4. Temperature, texture, turgor (pinch skin, tented 3 seconds or less is normal), check over sternum for elderly

E. Hair
   1. Hirsutism—excess
   2. Alopecia—loss or thinning

F. Nails (indicates respiratory and nutritional status)

1. Color

2. Shape, contour (normal angle of nail bed ≤160°; clubbing: nail bed angle ≥180° due to prolonged decreased oxygenation)

3. Texture, thickness

4. Capillary refill—blanch nail beds of fingers or toes and quickly release pressure; color should quickly return to normal (≤3 seconds)

G. Head

1. Size, shape, symmetry

2. Temporal arteries

3. Cranial nerve function (see Table 1-3)

H. Eyes

1. Ptosis—drooping of upper eyelid

2. Color of sclerae, conjunctivae

3. Pupils: size, shape, equality, reactivity to light and accommodation (PERRLA)

4. Photophobia—light intolerance

5. Nystagmus—abnormal, involuntary, rapid eye movements

6. Strabismus—involuntary drifting of one eye out of alignment with the other eye; "lazy eye"

7. Corneal reflex

8. Visual fields (peripheral vision)

9. Visual acuity—Snellen chart, normal 20/20

10. Ophthalmoscope exam

    a. Red reflex—red glow from light reflected from retina

    b. Fundus

    c. Optic disk (the blind spot)

    d. Macula

11. Gerontologic considerations—sclera yellowish-colored; milky-colored ring around periphery of cornea; decreased corneal reflex; decreased tear secretion; delayed pupil reflex and accommodation; cataracts; presbyopia; increased incidence of "floaters"

I. Ears

1. Pull pinna up and back to examine children's (≥3 years of age) and adults' ears

2. Pull pinna down and back to examine infants' and young children's (less than 3 years of age) ears

3. Tympanic membrane—cone of light at 5 o'clock position right ear, 7 o'clock position left ear

4. Weber test—assesses bone conduction; vibrating tuning fork placed in middle of forehead; normal: hear sound equally in ears

5. Rinne test—compares bone conduction with air conduction; vibrating tuning fork placed on mastoid process, when client no longer hears sound, positioned in front of ear canal; normal: should still be able to hear sound; air conduction greater than bone conduction by 2:1 ratio (positive Rinne test)

J. Nose and sinuses

1. Septum midline

2. Alignment, color, discharge

3. Palpate and percuss sinuses

Table 1-3 CRANIAL NERVES			
(#) NERVE	**FUNCTION**	**NORMAL FINDINGS**	**NURSING CONSIDERATIONS**
(I) Olfactory	Sense of smell	Able to detect various odors in each nostril	Have client smell a nonirritating substance such as coffee or tobacco with eyes closed Test each nostril separately
(II) Optic	Sense of vision	Clear (acute) vision near and distant	Snellen eye chart for far vision Read newspaper for near vision Ophthalmoscopic exam
(III) Oculomotor	Pupil constriction, raising of eyelids	Pupils equal in size and equally reactive to light	Instruct client to look up, down, inward too Observe for symmetry and eye opening Shine penlight into eye as client stares straight ahead Ask client to watch your finger as you move it toward his/her face
(IV) Trochlear	Downward and inward movement of eyes	Able to move eyes down and inward	(See Oculomotor)
(V) Trigeminal	Motor—jaw movement Sensory—sensation on the face and neck	Able to clench and relax jaw Able to differentiate between various stimuli touched to the face and neck	Test with pin and wisp of cotton over all three branches (forehead, cheek, jaw on both sides of face) Ask client to open jaw, bite down, move jaw laterally against pressure Stroke cornea with wisp of cotton
(VI) Abducens	Lateral movement of the eyes	Able to move eyes in all directions	(See Oculomotor)
(VII) Facial	Motor—facial muscle movement Sensory—taste on the anterior two-thirds of the tongue (sweet and salty)	Able to smile, whistle, wrinkle forehead Able to differentiate tastes among various agents	Observe for facial symmetry after asking client to frown, smile, raise eyebrows, close eyelids against resistance, whistle, blow Place sweet, sour, bitter, and salty substances on tongue
(VIII) Acoustic	Sense of hearing and balance	Hearing intact Balance maintained while walking	Test with watch ticking into ear, rubbing fingers together, Rinne, Weber Test posture, standing with eyes closed Otoscopic exam
(IX) Glossopharyngeal	Motor—pharyngeal movement and swallowing Sensory—taste on posterior one-third of tongue (sour and bitter)	Gag reflex intact, able to swallow Able to taste	Place sweet, sour, bitter, and salty substances on tongue Note ability to swallow and manage secretions Stimulate pharyngeal wall to elicit gag reflex
(X) Vagus	Swallowing and speaking	Able to swallow and speak with a smooth voice	Inspect soft palate—instruct to say "ah" Observe uvula for midline position Rate quality of voice
(XI) Spinal accessory	Motor—flexion and rotation of head; shrugging of shoulders	Able to flex and rotate head; able to shrug shoulders	Inspect and palpate sternocleidomastoid and trapezius muscles for size, contour, tone Ask client to move head side to side against resistance and shrug shoulders against resistance
(XII) Hypoglossal	Motor—tongue movements	Can move tongue side to side and stick it out symmetrically and in midline	Inspect tongue in mouth Ask client to stick out tongue and move it quickly side to side Observe midline, symmetry, and rhythmic movement

K. Mouth and pharynx
1. Oral mucosa
2. Teeth (normal: 32)
3. Tongue
4. Hard and soft palate
5. Uvula, midline
6. Tonsils
7. Gag reflex
8. Swallow
9. Taste

L. Neck
1. Range of motion of cervical spine
2. Cervical lymph nodes (normal ≤1 cm round, soft, mobile) non-tender
3. Trachea position
4. Thyroid gland
5. Carotid arteries—check for bruit and thrill
6. Jugular veins

M. Thorax and lungs
1. Alignment of spine
2. Anteroposterior to transverse diameter (normal adult 1:2 to 5:7); 1:1 barrel chest
3. Respiratory excursion
4. Respirations
5. Tactile fremitus—vibration produced when client articulates "99"
6. Diaphragmatic excursion—assesses degree and symmetry of diaphragm movement; percuss from areas of resonance to dullness
7. Breath sounds—bilaterally equal
    a. Normal
        1) Vesicular—soft and low-pitched breezy sounds heard over most of peripheral lung fields; inspiraton ≥ expiration
        2) Bronchovesicular—medium-pitched, moderately loud sounds heard over the mainstem bronchi; inspiration = expiration
        3) Bronchial—loud, coarse, blowing sound heard over the trachea; inspiration ≤ expiration
    b. Adventitious (abnormal); caused by fluid or inflammation
        1) Fine Crackles—crackling or popping sounds commonly heard on late inspiration; atelectatic crackles clear with coughing
        2) Coarse Crackles—harsh, moist popping sounds heard commonly on early inspiration; originate in large bronchus
        3) Sonorous wheeze—low pitched, coarse snoring sounds commonly heard on expiration
        4) Sibilant wheeze—squeaky sounds heard during inspiration and expiration associated with narrowed airways
        5) Pleural friction rub—grating sound or vibration heard during inspiration and expiration

8. Vocal resonance
    a. Bronchophony—say "99" and hear more clearly than normal; loud transmission of voice sounds caused by consolidation of lung
    b. Egophony—say "E" and hear "A" due to distortion caused by consolidation of lung
    c. Whispered pectoriloquy—hear whispered sounds clearly due to dense consolidation of lung

9. Costovertebral angle percussion—kidneys

N. Heart sounds
1. Angle of Louis—manubrialsternal junction at second rib
2. Aortic and pulmonic areas—right and left second intercostal spaces alongside sternum
3. Erb's point—third intercostal space just left of sternum
4. Tricuspid area—fourth or fifth intercostal space at lower left of sternal border
5. Mitral area—fifth intercostal space at left midclavicular line (apex of heart)
6. Point of maximal impulse (PMI)
    a. Impulse of the left ventricle felt most strongly
    b. Adult—left fifth intercostal space in the midclavicular line (8–10 cm to the left of the midsternal line)
    c. Infant—lateral to left nipple; heart failure-displaced down and to left

7. S1 and S2
    a. S1 "lub"—closure of tricuspid and mitral valves; dull quality and low pitch; onset of ventricular systole (contraction); louder at apex; use diaphragm
    b. S2 "dub"—closure of aortic and pulmonic valves; snapping quality; onset of diastole (relaxation of atria, then ventricles); loudest at base; use diaphragm

8. Murmurs—abnormal sounds caused by turbulence within a heart valve; turbulence within a blood vessel is called a bruit; three basic factors result in murmurs:
    a. High rate of blood flow through either a normal or abnormal valve
    b. Blood flow through a sclerosed or abnormal valve, or into a dilated heart chamber or vessel
    c. Blood flow regurgitated backward through an incompetent valve or septal defect

9. Pulse deficit—difference between apical and radial rate
10. Jugular veins—normally distend when client lies flat, but are not visible when the client's head is raised 30 to 45°

O. Peripheral vascular system
1. Pulses
    a. Radial—passes medially across the wrist; felt on radial (or thumb) side of the forearm
    b. Ulnar—passes laterally across the wrist; felt on the ulnar (little finger) side of the wrist
    c. Femoral—passes beneath the inguinal ligament (groin area) into the thigh; felt in groin area
    d. Carotid—pulsations can be felt over medial edge of sternocleidomastoid muscle in neck
    e. Pedal (dorsalis pedis-dorsal artery of the foot)—passes laterally over the foot; felt along top of foot
    f. Posterior tibial—felt on inner side of ankle below medial malleolus
    g. Popliteal—felt in popliteal fossa, the region at the back of the knee
    h. Temporal—felt lateral to eyes
    i. Apical—left at fifth intercostal space at midclavicular line

P. Breasts and axillae
1. Size, shape, symmetry
2. Gynecomastia—breast enlargement in males
3. Nodes—normal: nonpalpable

Q. Abdomen
1. Knees flexed to relax muscles and provide for comfort
2. Inspect and auscultate, then percuss and palpate
3. Symmetry, contour (flat, rounded, protuberant, or scaphoid)
4. Umbilicus
5. Bowel sounds; normal high-pitched gurgles heard with the diaphragm of the stethoscope at 5- to 20-s intervals
   a. Hypoactive: less than 3/min
   b. Hyperactive: loud, frequent
6. Aortic, renal, iliac, femoral arteries auscultated with the bell of the stethoscope
7. Peritoneal friction rub—grating sound varies with respirations; inflammation of liver
8. Liver and spleen size
9. Inguinal lymph nodes
10. Rebound tenderness—inflammation of peritoneum
11. Kidneys
12. Abdominal reflexes

R. Neurological system
1. Deep tendon reflexes (DTRs)—assess sensory and motor pathways; compare bilaterally; 0 (absent) through 4+ (hyperactive) scale
2. Cerebellar function—coordination; point-to-point touching, rapid, alternating movements, gait
3. Mental status (cerebral function) (see Unit 3 of this chapter)
4. Cranial nerve function
5. Motor function
   a. Strength
   b. Tone
6. Sensory function
   a. Touch, tactile localization
   b. Pain
   c. Pressure
   d. Temperature
   e. Vibration
   f. Proprioception (position sense)
   g. Vision
   h. Hearing
   i. Smell
   j. Taste

S. Musculoskeletal system
  1. Muscle tone and strength
  2. Joint movements; crepitus-grating sound abnormal

T. Genitalia
  1. Provide privacy
  2. Use firm, deliberate touch
  3. Male
     a. Penis—foreskin, glans
     b. Hypospadias—meatus located on underside of penile shaft
     c. Epispadias—meatus located on upper side of penile shaft
     d. Scrotum
     e. Inguinal area
  4. Female
     a. Lithotomy position
     b. Cervix
     c. Ovaries
     d. Vaginal canal

U. Anus and rectum
  1. Rectal prolapse—protrusion of rectal mucous membrane through anus
  2. Hemorrhoids—dilated veins
  3. Anal sphincter
  4. Male—prostate gland
  5. Stool—normal color brown; assess for presence of blood

MENTAL STATUS ASSESSMENT Section 3

Done during interview and neurological assessment

DATA GATHERING

A. Observation
1. Gait and posture
2. Mode of dress
3. Involuntary movements
4. Voice (consider language and culture)
5. Affect and speech content
6. Logic, judgment, speech patterns
7. Attention, memory, insight
8. Spatial perception, calculation, abstract reasoning, thought processes and content

GENERAL FINDINGS

A. Note client's ability to wait patiently

B. Posture relaxed, slumped, or stiff

C. Body movement: look for control and symmetry

D. Abnormal: restlessness, tenseness, pacing, slumped posture, slow gait, poor eye contact (culture must be considered), slow movements or speech, and poor personal hygiene may indicate mental illness

E. Communication findings
1. Note client's ability to speak coherently and carry out commands
2. Note client's affect—abnormal findings: blunt, inappropriate, elated, hostile
3. Note presence of aphasia

F. Cognitive findings—client should be able to:
1. Demonstrate orientation to time, place, and person
2. Correctly repeat a series of 5 or 6 numbers
3. Give important facts, such as dates or names, and repeat information given in the previous five minutes during exam
4. Make decision(s) based on sound reasoning
5. Demonstrate a realistic awareness of self
6. Copy simple figures and identify familiar sounds
7. Perform simple calculations
8. Give the meaning of a simple figure of speech, as in "a stitch in time saves nine"
9. Give responses that are based in reality and that are logical, goal-oriented, and clear

10. Abnormal findings
   a. Inability to: recall immediate or long-term information, recognize objects (agnosia), perform purposeful movements (apraxia), calculate (dyscalculia), describe in abstractions, generalize, apply general principles
   b. Impaired judgment
   c. Unrealistic perceptions of self
   d. Illogical thought processes
   e. Blocking
   f. Flight of ideas
   g. Confabulation (making up answers unrelated to facts)
   h. Echolalia (involuntary repetitions of words spoken by another person)
   i. Delusions of grandeur or persecution
   j. Hallucinations, illusions, and delusions

STANDARDIZED INSTRUMENT SCREENING TOOL

A. Mini-Mental State exam (MMSE)
   1. Used to diagnose dementia or delirium
   2. Tests orientation, short-term memory and attention, ability to perform calculations, language, and construction
   3. Cannot be used if client cannot read, write, or speak English

B. Mental Status Exam
   1. Provides a baseline of current cognitive processes
   2. Used frequently to assess changes in the client's stauts

Chapter 2

FUNDAMENTALS OF NURSING

Sections	**Concepts Covered**
1. Normal Mobility	Mobility
2. Altered Functions Related to Immobility	Mobility
3. Safety	Growth and Development
4. Altered Functions Related to Pain	Sensory Perception
5. Protection from Communicable Diseases	Health Promotion
6. Maintenance of Skin Integrity	Skin Integrity
7. Perioperative Care	

NORMAL MOBILITY

NORMAL DEVELOPMENTAL STRUCTURES AND FUNCTIONS—MUSCULOSKELETAL SYSTEM

A. Developmental stages and related functions (see Table 2-1)

B. Joint movement and action (see Table 2-2)

C. General data base
   1. Physical assessment
      a. Body build, height, weight—proportioned within normal limits
      b. Posture, body alignment—erect
      c. Gait, ambulation—smooth
      d. Joints—freely moveable
      e. Skin integrity—intact
      f. Muscle tone, elasticity, strength—adequate

   2. History
      a. Psychosocial assessment
         1) Exercise level
         2) Rest and sleep patterns
         3) Sexual activity
         4) Job-related activity

      b. Health history
         1) Pregnancy
         2) Structural or functional defects of the nervous system
         3) Structural or functional defects of the musculoskeletal system
         4) Diagnostic procedures and medical or surgical treatments that require activity restriction
         5) Conditions or treatments that result in pain
         6) Endocrine disorders that affect rest and activity

D. Potential problems
   1. Joints—contractures and deformities
   2. Body alignment
      a. Poor posture
      b. Lower back pain
      c. Lumbar lordosis—exaggerated concavity in the lumbar region
      d. Kyphosis—exaggerated convexity in the thoracic region
      e. Scoliosis—lateral curvature in a portion of the vertebral column

E. Gerontologic considerations
   1. Bones—less dense; less strong; more brittle; decreased mineralization; elderly females have increased osteoclatic bone resorption; osteoporosis incidence higher in women; high incidence of deformity, pain, stiffness, fractures; increased osteoporosis with smoking, decreased calcium intake, alcohol use, physical inactivity

2. Joints—rigid, fragile cartilage; decreased water content in cartilage; decreased intervertebral disk height; limited or painful stiff movement; crepitation with movement

3. Muscles—loss of muscle mass, tone, agility and strength; slowed reaction time; muscle fatigue; muscle function can be maintained with exercise

Table 2-1 DEVELOPMENTAL STAGES OF THE MUSCULOSKELETAL SYSTEM	
AGE	**NORMAL FINDINGS**
0–1 month (period of involuntary movement)	Full range of motion High degree of muscle tone Moves mostly involuntarily
1–3 months	Turns and raises head and chest when prone Stretches arms Muscles are well flexed
3–6 months	Sits with support Rolls over Shakes objects with two hands Transfers objects from hand to hand
6–9 months	Has erect body posture Sits up Holds a bottle with fingers Feeds self with fingers Grasps with one hand Crawls
9–18 months	Develops lower body control Pulls self up, stands Begins to walk
18 months–4 years	Walks up and down stairs Runs
4–6 years	Hops, skips Dresses self and meets basic needs with direction
6–13 years (period of rapid skeletal growth)	Increases rapidly in height Refines motor skills Likes athletics
Adolescent; 13–18 years (period of awkwardness)	Grows taller in spurts with growth of long bones Epiphyses close Reaches maximum height Feels and looks awkward
Adult	May begin to develop kyphosis, especially women Has more fat deposits
Older adult	Decreases in height due to bone and cartilage calcifications and kyphosis Decreasing muscle mass and bulk Decreasing muscle strength and tone Decreasing motor activity Joint stiffness Decreased range of motion, increased rigidity of neck, shoulders, hips Slowed reflexes and reaction time

Table 2-2	JOINT MOVEMENT AND ACTION
MOVEMENT	**ACTION**
Flexion	Decrease angle of joint, e.g., bending elbow
Extension	Increase angle of joint, e.g., straightening elbow
Hyperextension	Excessively increase angle of joint, e.g., bending the head backward
Abduction	Move body part away from midline of body
Adduction	Move body part toward midline of body
Rotation	Move joint around its central axis
Pronation	Turn wrist so that the palm is down
Supination	Turn wrist so that the palm is up
Dorsiflexion	Point the toes toward the head
Plantarflexion	Point the toes away from the head
Inversion	Rotate the ankle and sole of foot inward
Eversion	Rotate the ankle and sole of foot outward
Radial flexion	Rotate the hand inward at the wrist
Ulnar flexion	Rotate the hand outward at the wrist

MAINTENANCE AND PROMOTION OF NORMAL BODY STRUCTURE AND FUNCTION

A. Rest—basic physiological need
1. Allows body to repair its own damaged cells
2. Enhances removal of waste products from the body
3. Restores tissue to maximum functional ability before another activity is begun

B. Sleep—basic physiological body need, although the purpose and reason for it are unclear; possible theories include:
1. To restore balance among different parts of the central nervous system
2. To mediate stress, anxiety, and tension
3. To help a person cope with daily activities
4. Gerontologic considerations
   a. Older adults do not need more sleep
   b. Hypothalamus changes—decreased stage IV sleep; difficulty getting to sleep, remaining asleep; decreased sleep time; awaken more at night
   c. Contributing factors—depression, heart disease, pain, cognitive dysfunction, sleep apnea, medication
   d. Chronic sleep deprivation—disorientation, increased risk of falls

C. Activity and exercise
1. Activity
   a. Maintains muscle tone and posture
   b. Serves as outlet for tension and anxiety

2. Exercise
   a. Maintains joint mobility and function
   b. Promotes muscle strength
   c. Stimulates circulation
   d. Promotes optimum ventilation
   e. Stimulates appetite
   f. Promotes elimination
   g. Enhances metabolic rate

3. Prevents injury
   a. Motor vehicle accidents—use of seat belts and helmets
   b. Job-related accidents—following safety procedures
   c. Contact sports—proper body conditioning and use of protective devices
   d. Aging—rugs should be secure; stairways lit and clear of debris
   e. Pregnancy—bathtub grips; low-heeled shoes

4. Gerontologic concerns
   a. Assess present activity level, medications that may affect activity, range of motion, muscle strength
   b. Include warm-up and cool-down exercises
   c. Maintain hydration and temperature during exercise
   d. Do 30 minutes activity 5 times a week
   e. Swimming, walking, games, exercise programs

ALTERED FUNCTIONS RELATED TO IMMOBILITY

PREDISPOSING FACTORS

A. Musculoskeletal injuries/trauma

B. Congenital defects affecting the musculoskeletal system

C. Diseases of the musculoskeletal system

D. Therapeutic procedures related to the musculoskeletal system

ADVERSE EFFECTS OF IMMOBILITY

(see Table 2-3)

REHABILITATION PRINCIPLES OF MOBILITY

A. Positioning

    1. Purpose

        a. To prevent contractures

        b. To promote circulation

        c. To promote pulmonary function

        d. To relieve pressure on body parts

        e. To promote pulmonary drainage

    2. Common client positions and their corresponding therapeutic functions (see Table 2-4)

B. Different forms of exercise and their therapeutic functions (see Table 2-5)

C. Ambulation

    1. Use of tilt table

        a. Weight bearing on long bones to prevent decalcification, resulting in weakening of the bone and renal calculi

        b. Stimulate circulation to lower extremities

        c. Use elastic stockings to prevent postural hypotension

        d. Should be done gradually; blood pressure should be checked during the procedure

        e. If blood pressure goes down and dizziness, pallor, diaphoresis, tachycardia, or nausea occurs, stop procedure

Table 2-3 ADVERSE EFFECTS OF IMMOBILITY		
SYSTEM	COMPLICATION	SEQUELAE
Integumentary	Pressure injury Decreases wound healing	Osteomyelitis Tissue maceration Infection
Musculoskeletal	Osteoporosis Decreased muscle mass strength Atrophy Contractures	Pathological fractures Loss of endurance Deformities Decreased stability
Respiratory	Change in lung volume Atelectasis Stasis of secretions	Decreased lung expansion Decreased hemoglobin Respiratory muscle weakness Pneumonia
Cardiovascular	Increased cardiac workload Thrombus formation Orthostatic hypotension	Tachycardia Pulmonary emboli Weakness, faintness, dizziness
Metabolic	Decreased basal metabolic rate Altered nutrient metabolism Hypercalcemia	Decreased cellular activity Weight gain Loss of lean body mass
	Altered nutrient metabolism	Negative nitrogen balance Anorexia, weight loss, debilitation Slow wound healing and tissue growth
	Hypercalcemia	Increased diuresis Increased excretion of electrolytes
Elimination	Constipation Urinary stasis	Fecal impaction Urine retention, urinary infections Renal calculi
Psychosocial	Depression Sensory deprivation Confusion Increased dependence	Insomnia, restlessness

Table 2-4 THERAPEUTIC FUNCTIONS OF CLIENT POSITIONS	
POSITION	FUNCTION
Supine (flat, face up)	Minimizes hip flexion
Side	Allows drainage of oral secretions
Side with leg bent (Sims')	Allows drainage of oral secretions (abdominal tension)
Head elevated (Fowler)	Increased venous return; allows maximal lung expansion
Head and knees elevated slightly	Increased venous return; relieves pressure on lumbosacral area
Elevation of extremity	Increases venous return
Flat on back, thighs flexed, legs abducted (lithotomy)	Exposes perineum
Prone (flat, face down)	Promotes extension of hip joint

Table 2-5 THERAPEUTIC EXERCISES		
EXERCISE	DESCRIPTION	RATIONALE
Passive range of motion	Performed by nurse without assistance from client	Retention of joint range of motion; maintenance of circulation
Active assistive range of motion	Performed by client with assistance of nurse	Measures motion in the joint
Active range of motion	Performed by client without assistance	Maintains joint mobility and increases muscle strength
Active resistive range of motion	Performed by client against manual or mechanical resistance	Provision of resistance to increase muscle power; 5-lb bags/weights may be used
Isometric exercises	Performed by client; alternate contraction and relaxation of muscle without moving joint	Maintains muscle strength when joint is immobilized

2. Transfer activities
   a. Definition—to move a client from one surface to another. (i.e., from a bed to a stretcher)
   b. Basic guidelines
      1) If client has a stronger and a weaker side, move the client toward the stronger side (easier for client to pull the weak side)
      2) Use the larger muscles of the legs to accomplish a move rather than the smaller muscles of the back
      3) Move client with drawsheet; do not slide a client across a surface
      4) Always have an assistant standing by if there is any possibility of a problem in completing a transfer

3. Technique for sitting client at edge of bed
    a. Place hand under knees and shoulders of client
    b. Instruct client to push elbow into bed; at same time lift shoulders and bring legs over edge of bed, or use one leg to move other leg over edge of bed

4. Technique for assisting client to stand
    a. Place client's feet directly under body; client should wear nonskid slippers
    b. Face client and firmly grasp each side of rib cage
    c. Push one knee against one knee of the client
    d. Rock client forward as client comes to a standing position
    e. Ensure that client's knees are "locked" while standing
    f. Give client enough time to balance while standing
    g. Pivot with client to position and transfer client's weight quickly to chair placed on client's stronger side

5. Use of a transfer board

6. Teaching ADL—guidelines
    a. Observe what client can do and allow client to do it
    b. Encourage client to exercise muscles used for activity
    c. Start with gross functional movement before going to finer motions
    d. Extend period of activity as much and as fast as the client can tolerate
    e. There are alternative ways of doing one thing
    f. Give immediate positive feedback after every act of accomplishment

Table 2-6 CRUTCH WALKING GAITS		
GAIT	**DESCRIPTION**	**USES**
Four-point	Slow, safe; right crutch, left foot, left crutch, right foot	Use when weight-bearing is allowed for both legs
Two-point	Faster, safe; right crutch and left foot advance together; left crutch and right foot advance together	Use when weight-bearing is allowed for both legs; less support than four-point gait
Three-point	Faster gait, safe; advance both crutches simultaneously (no weight bearing on affected leg) than advance good leg	Use when weight-bearing is allowed on one leg
Swing-to-swing-through	Fast gait but requires more strength and balance; advance both crutches followed by both legs (or one leg is held up)	Use when partial weight-bearing is allowed on both legs; requires coordination
NOTE: To go up stairs: advance good leg first, followed by crutches and affected leg. To go down stairs: advance crutches with affected leg first, followed by good leg. ("Up with the good, down with the bad.")		

7. Crutch walking
   a. General guidelines
      1) Client should support weight on handpiece, not in axilla—brachial plexus may be damaged, producing "crutch palsy"
      2) Position crutches 8–10 inches to side
      3) Crutches should have rubber tips
   b. Crutch gaits—description and uses (see Table 2-6)

GENERAL NURSING GOALS AND INTERVENTIONS FOR IMMOBILITY

A. Assist with self-care
   1. Assess client's activity level
   2. Encourage motion necessary to improve activity level
   3. Start with simple, gross activity before going to finer motor movements
   4. Increase period of activity as rapidly as client can tolerate
   5. Support client with positive feedback for effort/accomplishments

B. Gerontologic considerations
   1. Assess range of motion, ability to perform ADLs, activity level
   2. Good supportive footwear
   3. Walker or cane as needed
   4. Avoid environmental hazards (steps, throw rugs)
   5. Aerobic exercise
   6. Rise slowly from bed or sitting position

C. Prevent contracture of muscle
   1. Frequent position change and range of motion exercises
   2. Proper body alignment
      a. Use pillows and trochanter rolls
   3. Balanced diet

D. Prevent osteoporosis
   1. Weight-bearing on long bones
   2. Balanced diet

E. Prevent negative nitrogen balance—give high-protein and easily digestible diet in small, frequent feedings

F. Prevent constipation
   1. Ambulation as appropriate
   2. Increase fluid intake
   3. Ensure privacy in use of bedpan or commode
   4. Administer stool softeners, e.g., Colace

G. Prevent urinary stasis

1. Have client void in normal position, if possible
2. Increase fluid intake
3. Low-calcium diet—increase acid-ash residue to acidify urine and prevent formation of calcium stones
4. Evaluate adequacy of urine output

H. Prevent pressure injuries

1. Frequent turning, skin care, keep skin dry
2. Ambulation as feasible
3. Use draw sheet when turning to avoid shearing force
4. Balanced diet with adequate protein, vitamins, and minerals
5. Use air mattress, flotation pads, elbow and heel pads, sheepskin
6. Assist with use of Stryker frame or Circ-O-Lectric bed
7. Gerontologic considerations
   a. Increased risk—poor nutritional status and weight loss, vitamin and protein deficiencies, decreased peripheral sensation, moisture
   b. Identify clients at risk–Braden scale, weight loss greater than total body weight, serum albumin less than 3.5 g/dL, pressure areas
   c. Avoid friction during position change, eliminate moisture, move weight bearing from pressure areas (e.g., heel protectors), include high protein, vitamins, and carbohydrates in diet

I. Prevent thrombus formation

1. Leg exercises—flexion, extension of toes and feet for five minutes every hour
2. Ambulation as appropriate
3. Frequent change of position
4. Avoid "gatching" bed or using pillow to support knee flexion for extended periods
5. Use of TEDs or elastic hose

J. Prevent increase in cardiac workload

1. Use of trapeze to decrease Valsalva maneuver
2. Teach client how to move without holding breath
3. Teach client to rise from bed slowly
4. Increase activity gradually

K. Prevent stasis of respiratory secretions

1. Teach client the importance of turning, coughing, and deep breathing
2. Administer postural drainage as appropriate
3. Teach use of incentive spirometer

L. Prevent depression and boredom

1. Allow visitors, use of radio, television
2. Schedule occupational therapy

M. Usual problems

1. Alterations in comfort

2. Impaired ambulation

3. Inability to perform ADLs

4. Complications of immobility

5. Infection

6. Safety

7. Fatigue

8. Insomnia

SAFETY Section 3

PRIMARY HEALTH CONCERN OF NURSING

A. Second level of Maslow's hierarchy of human needs

1. Besides prevention of injury, includes protection from physical and psychological harm, freedom from pain, and provision of a stable, dependable, orderly, and predictable environment

2. Nursing has primary responsibility for ensuring the safety of clients in health care facilities and influencing the safety of persons in the home, work, and community environments

B. Factors affecting safety

1. Age/development

   a. Children—accidents constitute leading cause of death in all age groups except infancy

      1) Infants—accidents occur primarily in second half of first year

         a) Mouthing any object that they handle

         b) Unsupervised/unrestrained rolling over, crawling, walking can result in falls and enhance accessibility to small objects, electric cords, poisonous substances, etc.

      2) Toddlers—high incidence of accidents

         a) Increasing curiosity; exploring using all senses (especially taste and touch); learning by trial and error

         b) Increasing gross and fine motor activity, climbing, running, grasping, etc.

         c) Totally uncomprehending and fearless of consequences; increasing negativism as part of autonomy

      3) Preschoolers—continued risk

         a) Increasing imitative behavior

         b) Refining fine and gross motor ability without cognitive ability to foresee potential dangers

      4) School-ages—although better muscular control, increased cognitive capacity, and more readiness to respond to rules, there continues to be increased risk of accidents related to identification with "super heroes," increased involvement and competitiveness in sports, and sensitivity to peer pressure

      5) Adolescents—high incidence; caused by motor vehicles, physical awkwardness related to growth changes, conflict over dependence/independence; peer orientation and approval seeking; increasing goal orientation and risk-taking behavior; and inner perception of omnipotence and immortality

   b. Adults—disregard for safety regulations

   c. Elderly—diminished muscular strength and/or coordination, diminished sensory acuity, and impaired balance create special problems

2. Awareness of environment, self, and others

   a. Impacts ability to perceive and react to surroundings/circumstances

       b. Factors that may reduce perceptual awareness and ability to perform ADL

          1) Level of consciousness

          2) Neurological function

          3) Sensory perception

       c. Illness-associated signs and symptoms, treatments, anxiety, and degree of weakness/impaired mobility

       d. Hospitalization

       e. Lack of sleep

       f. Medication(s)

3. Ability to communicate—physical impairment, language barrier, illiteracy

4. Environment

       a. Work place, e.g., hazardous machinery, chemicals, high stress

       b. Residence, e.g., high crime areas, poorly maintained living conditions

       c. Unfamiliar surroundings in which specific safety information is essential, e.g., hospital

       d. Physical and biological dimensions

          1) Space—defined personal areas sufficient for the purpose (play, chores, hobby), with privacy as appropriate

          2) Lighting—natural/artificial appropriate to function (as above) as well as to provide for day-night cycle; night lights in bathroom or bedroom

          3) Temperature and humidity—the very young (especially neonate) and very old are particularly vulnerable to extreme variations

          4) Ventilation

             a) Smoking should not be allowed in any confined areas where susceptible individuals may be affected, e.g., any health care facility

             b) Room or central air conditioners should have high-quality filters that are changed frequently

             c) Steps and hallways; hand rails

          5) Sound—chronic exposure to loud noises can lead to permanent hearing loss, interfere with work performance, precipitate sleep problems and psychological stress

          6) Physical layout

             a) Neatness and cleanliness—clutter may create hazards

             b) Immediate physical environment at home, work, hospital may have to be adapted to the functional ability of the inhabitant

             c) Steps and hallways; hand rails

       e. Community resources

          1) Food and water quality

          2) Waste disposal

          3) Air quality

          4) Traffic management

             a) Child restraint laws

             b) Advocacy situations, e.g., traffic light for areas of high elderly/children populations, gun laws

C. Assessment for individual risk factors at home and in health care facilities (see Table 2-7)

1. History of accidents—if previous incident(s) of accidents, there is increased risk for other mishap(s)

2. Concern for/perception of hazards; cognitive or sensory deficits

3. Evidence of unsafe behaviors—smoking in bed, non-use of seat belts, storage of toxic substances within reach of children

4. Physical/psychological impediments to safe function—level of alertness, mental status, sensory acuity, mobility limitations

Table 2-7 NURSING MANAGEMENT OF THE CHILD AT DIFFERENT DEVELOPMENTAL STAGES

ACTION	RATIONALE
Birth to 6 months	
Keep sharp and hot objects out of child's reach	Has strong grasp reflex
Do not leave unattended; can roll off flat surfaces	Rolls over by about 3 months
Administer unpleasant medications slowly via nipple or syringe	Aspirations can easily occur
6 months to 1 year	
Restrain child adequately	Can resist with entire body, has active cortical control
Enlist aid of parent in doing difficult procedures, if possible	Knows parent as source of comfort and security
1 to 3 years	
Administer medications from a cup	Prefers less dependent behavior
Expect turbulent temperament; tantrums common	Control environment; be consistent in expectations
3 to 6 years	
Take special care to explain all actions in advance	Illness and procedures are seen as punishment, body mutilation is feared
6 to 13 years	
Provide time for child to handle and play with equipment if possible	Interested in learning; industrious
Adolescent	
Noncompliance is the norm; attempt to impose as few orders as possible	Independence is important to their emotional growth

D. Plan/Implementation—requires attention to general principles of safety as well as identification of specific hazards/risks and subsequent measures to prevent injury; includes appropriate anticipatory and responsive client education, and prevention of injury by active/passive identification of hazards such as:

1. Orient new client to the immediate environment—call-bell/signal, bed controls, location of bathroom, operation of overhead and bed lights, schedule of unit activities

2. Maintain the bed in the lowest position except when care is being provided, side rails in raised position when client is in bed

3. Provide adequate help when ambulating client, especially for the first time

4. Ensure client area is free of clutter—mop up or call housekeeping to remove spills

5. Never leave the client in total darkness—use night light when room lights are off

6. Always secure call–bell/signal within the client's reach

7. Encourage the client to wear shoes when ambulating

8. Use brakes when moving the client in or out of wheelchair, commode, bed

9. Label and report malfunction of any equipment immediately

10. Restrain client only as necessary; restraints used only as long as necessary; padded to prevent undue pressure/constriction; checked every 1–2 hours; removed every 2 hours while client is awake; never tied to side rail; health care provider order necessary

11. In case of accident, institute follow-up procedures—document subjective and objective data concerning the incidence of accidents/injury as well as reported/observed use/non-use of identified safety measures; incident report; fall assessment

12. High environmental temperature—2–3 L fluid/day (precautions when heart failure or renal failure present), wear natural fiber clothing, use tepid or cool baths or showers, fan, or air conditioning

13. Low environmental temperature—avoid alcohol, keep room temperature greater than 65°F, eat a nutritious, high protein diet

14. Gerontologic considerations

    a. Risk factors for falls—environment (rugs, clutter, lighting, side rails), medications, sensory deficits, cardiac dysrhythmias, mobility problems, orthostatic hypotension, cognitive impairment, footwear, elimination problems, depression, wandering

    b. Assessment—history of falling, environment, medications, visual acuity, peripheral sensation, muscle strength, range of motion, gait, orthostatic hypotension, cognitive function, heart rate and rhythm, use of assistive devices

    c. Plan/implementation—floor mat or mattress by bed, cleared debris from area, call light within reach, lights in room or bathroom, assistive device within reach, elevated toilet seat, sit on edge of bed before getting up, minimize use of hypnotics and sedatives, wear glasses as needed, wear proper footwear, grab bars in bathroom

ALTERED FUNCTIONS RELATED TO PAIN

CHARACTERISTICS

A. Definition of pain—"whatever the person says it is, and it exists whenever the person says it does"

B. Types (see Table 2-8)

1. Acute: an episode of pain that lasts from a split second to about 6 months; may cause decreased healing, vital sign changes, diaphoresis

2. Chronic: an episode of pain that lasts for 6 months or longer; may cause depression, weight gain, fatigue, immobility

Table 2-8 TYPES OF PAIN		
SYSTEM	**ACUTE PAIN**	**CHRONIC PAIN**
Musculoskeletal	Disrupts sleep	Fatigue
Nutritional	Appetite reduced	Changes in weight
Cardiovascular	Fluid intake reduced Activation of sympathetic nervous system	Stress-induced changes
Psychological	Anxiety present Restlessness Inability to concentrate	Depression Job loss Difficulty in concentration Problems with interpersonal relationships
Digestive	Nausea and vomiting	Constipation, anorexia
Immune		Depresses immune response Delays wound healing

C. Phases of the pain experience (see Table 2-9)

1. Anticipatory (fear, anxiety about impending pain)

2. Sensation of pain (mild, moderate, severe)

3. Pain aftermath (weakness, nausea, sweating)

Table 2-9 RESPONSES TO PAIN STIMULI		
SYSTEM	CHANGE	RESULT
Cardiovascular	Increased blood pressure and heart rate lead to increased blood flow to brain and muscles Rapid, irregular respiration leads to increased O_2 supply to brain and muscles	Enhanced alertness to threats
Neurological	Increased papillary diameter leads to increased eye accommodation to light	Visual perception of threat
Skin integrity	Increased perspiration	Removal of excess body heat
Musculoskeletal	Increased muscle tension or activity leads to neuromuscular responsiveness	Musculoskeletal system ready for rapid motor activity
Psychosocial	Aroused apprehension, irritability, and anxiety Verbalized pain	Enhanced mental alertness to threat Communication of suffering and pleas for help

D. Factors influencing pain experiences
   1. Cultural factors—individual's responses or reactions to pain are generally dependent on what is expected and accepted in client's culture
   2. Past experiences with pain—past experiences with pain generally make the individual more sensitive to the pain experience

E. Gerontologic considerations—chronic pain affects 50–80% older population; common types of pain include low back pain, postfracture pain, joint pain; decreased transmission of pain impulse, decreased pressure sensation may influence pain response; client may not use word *pain*, may have decreased ADLs, social interaction, sleep disturbances, and depression due to pain

SELECTED NURSING DIAGNOSES RELATED TO PAIN

A. Acute or chronic pain
B. Imbalanced nutrition: less than body requirements
C. Social isolation
D. Activity intolerance
E. Readiness for enhanced comfort
F. Ineffective therapeutic regimen management

INTERVENTIONS

A. Pain management
   1. Allow client to use own words in describing pain experience
   2. Use a variety of relief measures
   3. Use measures before pain becomes severe
   4. Include measures that client believes will be effective

5. Consider the client's ability or willingness to participate in pain-relief measures

6. Determine the effectiveness of pain-relief measures according to client's response

7. If pain-relief measure is ineffective the first time, try it one more time before abandoning the measure

8. Be open-minded about what may relieve the pain

9. Use preventive approach in medication administration
   a. If pain is expected to occur throughout most of a 24-hours period, a regular schedule is better than prn
   b. Advantages of preventive approach
      1) Usually can take a smaller dose to alleviate mild pain or prevent occurrence of pain
      2) Pain relief is more complete and client spends fewer hours in pain
      3) Helps prevent addiction
   c. Individualized dosage is important because each person may metabolize and absorb medication differently

B. Nursing goals and interventions
   1. Establish a relationship
      a. Tell client you believe description of pain experience
      b. Listen and allow client to verbalize
   2. Establish a 24-h pain profile
      a. Location and radiation
         1) External
         2) Internal
         3) Both external and internal
         4) Area of body affected
      b. Character and intensity
         1) Acute/chronic
         2) Mild/severe
         3) Allow client to use own words in describing pain
         4) Use same pain scale consistently
            a) Number rating scale (0 to 10)
            b) Visual analogue scale (no pain to unbearable pain)
      c. Onset
         1) Sudden
         2) Insidious
      d. Duration
      e. Precipitating factors/aggravating factors (e.g., What makes pain worse?)
      f. Identify associated manifestations, as well as alleviating or aggravating factors
      g. Relieving factors
   3. Teach client about pain and its relief
      a. Explain quality and location of impending pain (e.g., before uncomfortable procedure)
      b. Help client learn to use slow, rhythmic breathing to promote relaxation
      c. Explain effects of analgesics and benefits of preventive approach
      d. Demonstrate splinting technique, which helps reduce pain perception

4. Reduce anxiety and fears
   a. Give reassurance
   b. Offer distraction
   c. Spend time with client

5. Provide comfort measures
   a. Proper positioning
   b. Cool, well-ventilated, quiet room
   c. PCA (patient-controlled analgesia) pump—a portable device that delivers predetermined dosage of intravenous pain medication (e.g., dose of 1 mg morphine [with a lock-out interval of 5–15 min]; basal rate (e.g., mg/h morphine) and demand dose (varies with medication)
   d. Back rub
   e. Allow for rest
   f. Distraction
   g. Imagery
   h. Relaxation techniques

6. Administer pain medication (see Table 2-10)
   a. Use preventive approach
   b. Monitor therapeutic/toxic dose and adverse effects
   c. Heat/cold application as appropriate
   d. Gerontologic considerations—greater risk of adverse reactions and toxicity, greater risk of drug interaction between analgesics and medications (e.g., analgesics, anti-epileptics, and antidepressants); start with lower dose and increase gradually

7. Refer for alternative methods of pain relief
   a. Anesthesia—block pain pathway
   b. Local nerve block
   c. Neurectomy/sympathectomy
   d. Hypnosis
   e. Acupuncture
   f. Biofeedback
   g. Massage
   h. Exercise/yoga
   i. Transcutaneous electrical nerve stimulation (TENS)
   j. Heat/cold application
   k. Distraction
   l. Relaxation
   m. Herbal remedies
   n. Therapeutic touch; consider cultural factors

Table 2-10 COMMON PAIN MEDICATIONS		
MEDICATION	**ADVERSE EFFECTS**	**NURSING CONSIDERATIONS**
Non Opioid		
Salicylates	Short-term use—GI bleeding, heartburn, occasional nausea Prolonged high dosage—salicylism: metabolic acidosis, respiratory alkalosis, dehydration, fluid and electrolyte imbalance, tinnitus	Observe for bleeding gums, bloody or black stools, bruises Give with milk, water, or food, or use enteric-coated tablets (Ecotrin) to minimize gastric distress Contraindications—GI disorders, severe anemia, vitamin K deficiency
Acetaminophen	Overdosage may be fatal, liver toxicity GI adverse effects are not common	Do not exceed recommended dose
Nonsteroidal anti-inflammatory drugs (NSAIDs): Ibuprofen Naproxen Ketorolac	Headache, dizziness, epigastric distress Peptic ulcer disease GI bleeding Prolonged bleeding Renal impairment	Administer with food Optimal therapeutic response is seen after two weeks of treatment Use cautiously in clients with history of aspirin allergy Ketorolac—dosage decreased in clients ≥ 65 years or clients with impaired renal function; duration of treatment ≤ 5 days Indomethacin
Opioids		
Morphine sulfate Fentanyl	Liver damage Dizziness, weakness Sedation or paradoxic excitement Nausea, flushing and sweating Respiratory depression, decreased cough reflex Constipation, miosis, hypotension	Give in smallest effective dose Observe for development of dependence Encourage respiratory exercises Use cautiously to prevent respiratory depression Monitor vital signs Monitor I and O, bowel pattern Increased constipation in older adults
Codeine	Same as morphine High doses may cause restlessness and excitement Constipation	Less potent and less dependence potential compared to morphine
Methadone	Same as morphine	Observe for dependence, respiratory depression Encourage fluids and high-bulk foods
Hydromorphone	Sedation, hypotension Urine retention	Keep narcotic antagonist (naloxone) available Monitor bowel function
Combination		
Oxycodone and acetaminophen Oxycodone and aspirin	Light-headedness, dizziness, sedation, nausea Constipation, pruritus Increased risk bleeding percodan	Administer with milk after meals (Commonly prescribed as Percocet, an acetaminophen and oxycodone combination)
NOTE: Most narcotic drugs exhibit qualitatively the same actions and adverse effects. They differ primarily in potency, onset, and duration of action. Medications that increase the effects of opioid analgesics include: central nervous system (CNS) depressants (alcohol, barbiturates, sedatives), anticholinergics (atropine, antihistamines, some psychiatric medications), antihypertensive medications, cimetidine.		

PROTECTION FROM COMMUNICABLE DISEASES

ASSESSMENT OF COMMUNICABLE DISEASES

A. General manifestations
1. Localized infections
   a. Inflammation, redness, warmth, swelling, pain/tenderness, loss of function
   b. Drainage—bloody, serous, cloudy, or purulent
   c. Cellulitis—bacterial skin infection with involvement of connective tissue

2. Generalized infections
   a. Weakness, headache, malaise
   b. Fever, increased pulse, change in blood pressure

B. Diagnostic tests
1. WBC (white blood count/leukocytes)
   a. Neutrophils—increased in most bacterial infections; phagocytosis during acute infection
   b. Eosinophils—increased in allergic reactions
   c. Lymphocytes—increased in chickenpox, mumps, measles, infectious mononucleosis, viral hepatitis; important in immune response
   d. Monocytes—increased in tuberculosis, rickettsial diseases, and in convalescent phase of acute infections; immature macrophages
   e. "Shift to left"—increased number immature neutrophils

2. Cultures and antibiotic sensitivity of suspected infectious site
   a. Should be obtained before onset of antibiotic therapy
   b. Specimens must be carefully collected and identified
   c. Preliminary results in 24 hours; final results in 72 hours

3. Highly sensitive C-reactive protein (hsCRP)—marker of inflammation
4. Sedimentation Rate

ANALYSIS OF CARE

A. Infection control in community
1. International—World Health Organization
2. National Centers for Disease Control
3. Local—public health departments
   a. Food and water control laws
   b. Spraying areas for insect control
   c. Immunizations
      1) Inactivated vaccines
      2) Live attenuated vaccines

B. Infection control in hospital

1. Hospital-acquired infections—nearly 2 million (5%) hospital clients acquire an infection in the hospital
   a. Most common infection—urinary tract infection
   b. Most common organism—*Staphylococcus aureus*

2. Prevention of hospital-acquired infections
   a. External environment—handwashing
   b. Internal environment—good nutrition and personal hygiene
   c. Prevention of UTI—strict aseptic technique during instrumentation
   d. Prevention of surgical wound infections—handwashing, surgical asepsis
   e. Prevention of respiratory infections—clean nebulizers
   f. Prevention of bacteremias—excellent sterile technique with intravascular systems

PLAN/IMPLEMENTATION

A. Standard precautions (barrier) used with all clients in all settings

1. Apply to contact with blood, body fluid, nonintact skin, and mucous membranes

2. Handwashing
   a. Done immediately on contact with blood or body fluids
   b. Wash hands before putting on or taking off gloves, between client contacts, between procedures or tasks with same client, or immediately after exposure to blood or bodily fluids

3. Gloves (Personal Protective Equipment)
   a. Use clean, nonsterile gloves when touching blood, body fluids, secretions, excretions, contaminated articles
   b. Put on gloves just before touching mucous membranes or nonintact skin or if gloves torn or heavily soiled
   c. Change gloves between tasks/procedures
   d. Remove gloves promptly after use, before touching items and environmental surfaces

4. Masks, eye protection, face shield (Personal Protective Equipment)
   a. Used to protect mucous membranes of eyes, nose, mouth during procedures and client care activities likely to generate splashes or sprays

5. Gowns (Personal Protective Equipment)
   a. Use clean, nonsterile gowns, to protect skin and prevent soiling of clothing during procedures and client care activities likely to generate splashes and sprays—blood, bodily fluids, or execretions
   b. Remove promptly and wash hands after leaving client's environment

6. Environment control
   a. Do not need to use special dishes, glasses, eating utensils; can use either reusable or disposable
   b. Do not recap used sharps, or bend, break, or remove used needles
   c. Do not manipulate used needle with two hands; use a one-handed scoop technique
   d. Place used sharps in a puncture-resistant container
   e. Use mouthpieces, resuscitation bags, or other devices for mouth-to-mouth resuscitation

7. Client placement
   a. Private room if client has poor hygiene habits, contaminates the environment, or can't assist in maintaining infection control precautions (e.g., infants, children, altered mental status client)
   b. When cohorting (sharing room), consider the epidemiology and mode of transmission of the infecting organism

8. Transport
   a. Use barriers (e.g., mask, impervious dressings)
   b. Notify personnel of impending arrival and precautions needed
   c. Inform client of ways to assist in prevention of transmission

B. Transmission-based precautions—apply to client with documented or suspected infections with highly transmissible or epidemiologically important pathogens; prevent spread of pathogenic organisms
1. Airborne precautions
   a. Used with pathogens smaller than 5 microns that are transmitted by airborne route; droplets or dust particles that remain suspended in the air
   b. Private room with monitored negative air pressure with 6–12 air changes per hour (airborne infection isolation room)
   c. Keep door closed and client in room; susceptible persons should not enter room or wear N-95 HEPA filter
   d. Can cohort or place client with another client with the same organism, but no other organism
   e. Place mask on client if being transported
   f. Tuberculosis—wear fit-test respirator mask
   g. Example of disease in category: measles (rubeola), *M. tuberculosis*, varicella (chicken pox), disseminated zoster (shingles)

2. Droplet precautions
   a. Used with pathogens transmitted by infectious droplets; droplets larger than 5 microns
   b. Involves contact of conjunctiva or mucous membranes of nose or mouth; happens during coughing, sneezing, talking, or during procedures such as suctioning or bronchoscopy
   c. Private room or with client with same infection but no other infection; wear mask if in close contact
   d. Maintain spatial separation of three feet between infected client and vistors or other clients; visitors wear mask if less than three feet
   e. Door may remain open
   f. Place mask on client if being transported
   g. Examples of disease in category: diphtheria, Group A Streptococcus pneumonia, pneumonia or meningitis caused by *N. meningitidis* or *H. influenzae* Type B, Rubella, mumps, pertussis

3. Contact precautions
   a. Needed with client care activities that require physical skin-to-skin contact (e.g., turn clients, bathe clients), or occurs between two clients (e.g., hand contact), or occurs by contact with contaminated inanimate objects in client's environment
   b. Private room or with client with same infection but no other infection
   c. Clean, nonsterile gloves for client contact or contact with potentially contaminated areas
   d. Change gloves after client contact with fecal material or wound drainage
   e. Remove gloves before leaving client's environment and wash hands with antimicrobial agent

f. Wear gown when entering room if clothing will have contact with client, environment surfaces, or if client is incontinent, has diarrhea, an ileostomy, colostomy, or wound drainage

g. Remove PPE before leaving room

h. Use dedicated equipment or clean and disinfect between clients

i. Example of diseases in category: infection caused by multidrug-resistant organisms (e.g., MRSA and Vancomycin-resistent organisms), herpes simplex, herpes zoster, *Clostridioides difficile*, respiratory syncytial virus, pediculosis, scabies, excessive wound drainage, fecal incontinence, discharge that suggests increased potential for environmental contamination, rotavirus, hepatitis type A (diapered or incontinent clients), localized herpes zoster

C. Neutropenic precautions—prevent infection among clients with immunosuppression; absolute neutrophil count ≤ 1000 mm^3

1. Assess skin integrity every 8 hours; auscultate breath sounds, presence of cough, sore throat; check temperature every 4 hours; report if greater than 101°F (38°C); monitor CBC and differential daily

2. Private when possible

3. Thorough hand hygiene before entering client's room

4. Allow no staff with cold or sore throat to care for client

5. No fresh flowers or standing water

6. Clean room daily

7. Low microbial diet; no fresh salads, unpeeled fruits and vegetables

8. Deep breathe every 4 hours

9. Meticulous body hygiene

10. Inspect IV site; meticulous IV site care

Figure 1. Recommended immunization schedule for adults aged 19 years or older by age group, United States, 2018

This figure should be reviewed with the accompanying footnotes. This figure and the footnotes describe indications for which vaccines, if not previously administered, should be administered unless noted otherwise.

Vaccine	19–21 years	22–26 years	27–49 years	50–64 years	≥65 years
Influenza[1]	1 dose annually				
Tdap[2] or Td[2]	1 dose Tdap, then Td booster every 10 yrs				
MMR[3]	1 or 2 doses depending on indication (if born in 1957 or later)				
VAR[4]	2 doses				
RZV[5] (preferred)					2 doses RZV (preferred)
or					or
ZVL[5]					1 dose ZVL
HPV–Female[6]	2 or 3 doses depending on age at series initiation				
HPV–Male[6]	2 or 3 doses depending on age at series initiation				
PCV13[7]					1 dose
PPSV23[7]	1 or 2 doses depending on indication				1 dose
HepA[8]	2 or 3 doses depending on vaccine				
HepB[9]	3 doses				
MenACWY[10]	1 or 2 doses depending on indication, then booster every 5 yrs if risk remains				
MenB[10]	2 or 3 doses depending on vaccine				
Hib[11]	1 or 3 doses depending on indication				

Recommended for adults who meet the age requirement, lack documentation of vaccination, or lack evidence of past infection

Recommended for adults with other indications

No recommendation

Table   2-11

Figure 2. Recommended immunization schedule for adults aged 19 years or older by medical condition and other indications, United States, 2018

This figure should be reviewed with the accompanying footnotes. This figure and the footnotes describe indications for which vaccines, if not previously administered, should be administered unless noted otherwise.

Vaccine	Pregnancy[1-6]	Immuno-compromised (excluding HIV infection)[3-7,11]	HIV infection CD4+ count (cells/μL)[3-7,9-10]		Asplenia, complement deficiencies[7,10,11]	End-stage renal disease, on hemodialysis[7,9]	Heart or lung disease, alcoholism[7]	Chronic liver disease[7-9]	Diabetes[7,9]	Health care personnel[3,4,9]	Men who have sex with men[6,8,9]
			<200	≥200							
Influenza[1]	1 dose annually										
Tdap[2] or Td[2]	1 dose Tdap each pregnancy	1 dose Tdap, then Td booster every 10 yrs									
MMR[3]	contraindicated			1 or 2 doses depending on indication							
VAR[4]	contraindicated			2 doses							
RZV[5] (preferred)					2 doses RZV at age ≥50 yrs (preferred)						
or					or						
ZVL[5]	contraindicated			1 dose ZVL at age ≥60 yrs							
HPV–Female[6]		3 doses through age 26 yrs			2 or 3 doses through age 26 yrs						
HPV–Male[6]		3 doses through age 26 yrs			2 or 3 doses through age 21 yrs						2 or 3 doses through age 26 yrs
PCV13[7]		1 dose									
PPSV23[7]		1, 2, or 3 doses depending on indication									
HepA[8]		2 or 3 doses depending on vaccine									
HepB[9]		3 doses									
MenACWY[10]		1 or 2 doses depending on indication, then booster every 5 yrs if risk remains									
MenB[10]		2 or 3 doses depending on vaccine									
Hib[11]		3 doses HSCT recipients only	1 dose								

Recommended for adults who meet the age requirement, lack documentation of vaccination, or lack evidence of past infection

Recommended for adults with other indications

Contraindicated

No recommendation

Table 2–11 (*Continued*)

Footnotes. Recommended immunization schedule for adults aged 19 years or older, United States, 2018

1. Influenza vaccination
www.cdc.gov/vaccines/hcp/acip-recs/vacc-specific/flu.html

General information
- Administer 1 dose of age-appropriate inactivated influenza vaccine (IIV) or recombinant influenza vaccine (RIV) annually
- Live attenuated influenza vaccine (LAIV) is not recommended for the 2017–2018 influenza season
- A list of currently available influenza vaccines is available at www.cdc.gov/flu/protect/vaccine/vaccines.htm

Special populations
- Administer age-appropriate IIV or RIV to:
  - **Pregnant women**
  - Adults with **hives-only egg allergy**
  - Adults with **egg allergy other than hives** (e.g., angioedema or respiratory distress): Administer IIV or RIV in a medical setting under supervision of a health care provider who can recognize and manage severe allergic conditions

2. Tetanus, diphtheria, and pertussis vaccination
www.cdc.gov/vaccines/hcp/acip-recs/vacc-specific/tdap-td.html

General information
- Administer to adults who previously did not receive a dose of tetanus toxoid, reduced diphtheria toxoid, and acellular pertussis vaccine (Tdap) as an adult or child (routinely recommended at age 11–12 years) 1 dose of Tdap, followed by a dose of tetanus and diphtheria toxoids (Td) booster every 10 years
- Information on the use of Tdap or Td as tetanus prophylaxis in wound management is available at www.cdc.gov/mmwr/preview/mmwrhtml/rr5517a1.htm

Special populations
- **Pregnant women:** Administer 1 dose of Tdap during each pregnancy, preferably in the early part of gestational weeks 27–36

3. Measles, mumps, and rubella vaccination
www.cdc.gov/vaccines/hcp/acip-recs/vacc-specific/mmr.html

General information
- Administer 1 dose of measles, mumps, and rubella vaccine (MMR) to adults with no evidence of immunity to measles, mumps, or rubella
- Evidence of immunity is:
  - Born before 1957 (except for health care personnel, see below)
  - Documentation of receipt of MMR
  - Laboratory evidence of immunity or disease
- Documentation of a health care provider-diagnosed disease without laboratory confirmation is not considered evidence of immunity

Special populations
- **Pregnant women and nonpregnant women of childbearing age** with no evidence of immunity to rubella: Administer 1 dose of MMR (if pregnant, administer MMR after pregnancy and before discharge from health care facility)

- **HIV infection and CD4 cell count ≥200 cells/μL for at least 6 months** and no evidence of immunity to measles, mumps, or rubella: Administer 2 doses of MMR at least 28 days apart
- **Students in postsecondary educational institutions, international travelers,** and **household contacts of immunocompromised persons:** Administer 2 doses of MMR at least 28 days apart (or 1 dose of MMR if previously administered 1 dose of MMR)
- **Health care personnel born in 1957 or later** with no evidence of immunity: Administer 2 doses of MMR at least 28 days apart for measles or mumps, or 1 dose of MMR for rubella (if born before 1957, consider MMR vaccination)
- Adults who **previously received ≤2 doses of mumps-containing vaccine and are identified by public health authority to be at increased risk for mumps in an outbreak:** Administer 1 dose of MMR
- MMR is contraindicated for pregnant women and adults with severe immunodeficiency

4. Varicella vaccination
www.cdc.gov/vaccines/hcp/acip-recs/vacc-specific/varicella.html

General information
- Administer to adults without evidence of immunity to varicella 2 doses of varicella vaccine (VAR) 4–8 weeks apart if previously received no varicella-containing vaccine (if previously received 1 dose of varicella-containing vaccine, administer 1 dose of VAR at least 4 weeks after the first dose)
- Evidence of immunity to varicella is:
  - U.S.-born before 1980 (except for pregnant women and health care personnel, see below)
  - Documentation of receipt of 2 doses of varicella or varicella-containing vaccine at least 4 weeks apart
  - Diagnosis or verification of history of varicella or herpes zoster by a health care provider
  - Laboratory evidence of immunity or disease

Special populations
- Administer 2 doses of VAR 4–8 weeks apart if previously received no varicella-containing vaccine (if previously received 1 dose of varicella-containing vaccine, administer 1 dose of VAR at least 4 weeks after the first dose) to:
  - **Pregnant women without evidence of immunity:** Administer the first of the 2 doses or the second dose after pregnancy and before discharge from health care facility
  - **Health care personnel without evidence of immunity**
- Adults with **HIV infection and CD4 cell count ≥200 cells/μL:** May administer, based on individual clinical decision, 2 doses of VAR 3 months apart
- VAR is contraindicated for pregnant women and adults with severe immunodeficiency

5. Zoster vaccination
www.cdc.gov/vaccines/hcp/acip-recs/vacc-specific/shingles.html

General information
- Administer 2 doses of recombinant zoster vaccine (RZV) 2–6 months apart to adults aged 50 years or older regardless of past episode of herpes zoster or receipt of zoster vaccine live (ZVL)

- Administer 2 doses of RZV 2–6 months apart to adults who previously received ZVL at least 2 months after ZVL
- For adults aged 60 years or older, administer either RZV or ZVL (RZV is preferred)

Special populations
- ZVL is contraindicated for pregnant women and adults with severe immunodeficiency

6. Human papillomavirus vaccination
www.cdc.gov/vaccines/hcp/acip-recs/vacc-specific/hpv.html

General information
- Administer human papillomavirus (HPV) vaccine to **females through age 26 years** and **males through age 21 years** (males aged 22 through 26 years may be vaccinated based on individual clinical decision)
- The number of doses of HPV vaccine to be administered depends on age at initial HPV vaccination
  - **No previous dose of HPV vaccine:** Administer 3-dose series at 0, 1–2, and 6 months (minimum intervals: 4 weeks between doses 1 and 2, 12 weeks between doses 2 and 3, and 5 months between doses 1 and 3; repeat doses if given too soon)
  - **Aged 9–14 years at HPV vaccine series initiation and received 1 dose or 2 doses less than 5 months apart:** Administer 1 dose
  - **Aged 9–14 years at HPV vaccine series initiation and received 2 doses at least 5 months apart:** No additional dose is needed

Special populations
- Adults with **immunocompromising conditions (including HIV infection)** through age 26 years: Administer 3-dose series at 0, 1–2, and 6 months
- **Men who have sex with men** through age 26 years: Administer 2- or 3-dose series depending on age at initial vaccination (see above); if no history of HPV vaccine, administer 3-dose series at 0, 1–2, and 6 months
- **Pregnant women** through age 26 years: HPV vaccination is not recommended during pregnancy, but there is no evidence that the vaccine is harmful and no intervention needed for women who inadvertently receive HPV vaccine while pregnant; delay remaining doses until after pregnancy; pregnancy testing is not needed before vaccination

7. Pneumococcal vaccination
www.cdc.gov/vaccines/hcp/acip-recs/vacc-specific/pneumo.html

General information
- Administer to immunocompetent adults aged 65 years or older 1 dose of 13-valent pneumococcal conjugate vaccine (PCV13), if not previously administered, followed by 1 dose of 23-valent pneumococcal polysaccharide vaccine (PPSV23) at least 1 year after PCV13; if PPSV23 was previously administered but not PCV13, administer PCV13 at least 1 year after PPSV23
- When both PCV13 and PPSV23 are indicated, administer PCV13 first (PCV13 and PPSV23 should not be administered during the same visit); additional information on vaccine timing is available at www.cdc.gov/vaccines/vpd/pneumo/downloads/pneumo-vaccine-timing.pdf

Table 2-11 (*Continued*)

Special populations

- Administer to adults aged 19 through 64 years with the following chronic conditions 1 dose of PPSV23 (at age 65 years or older, administer 1 dose of PCV13, if not previously received, and another dose of PPSV23 at least 1 year after PCV13 and at least 5 years after PPSV23):
  - **Chronic heart disease** (excluding hypertension)
  - **Chronic lung disease**
  - **Chronic liver disease**
  - **Alcoholism**
  - **Diabetes mellitus**
  - **Cigarette smoking**
- Administer to adults aged 19 years or older with the following indications 1 dose of PCV13 followed by 1 dose of PPSV23 at least 8 weeks after PCV13, and a second dose of PPSV23 at least 5 years after the first dose of PPSV23 (if the most recent dose of PPSV23 was administered before age 65 years, at age 65 years or older, administer another dose of PPSV23 at least 5 years after the last dose of PPSV23):
  - **Immunodeficiency disorders** (including B- and T-lymphocyte deficiency, complement deficiencies, and phagocytic disorders)
  - **HIV infection**
  - **Anatomical or functional asplenia** (including sickle cell disease and other hemoglobinopathies)
  - **Chronic renal failure and nephrotic syndrome**
- Administer to adults aged 19 years or older with the following indications 1 dose of PCV13 followed by 1 dose of PPSV23 at least 8 weeks after PCV13 (if the dose of PPSV23 was administered before age 65 years, at age 65 years or older, administer another dose of PPSV23 at least 5 years after the last dose of PPSV23):
  - **Cerebrospinal fluid leak**
  - **Cochlear implant**

8. Hepatitis A vaccination
www.cdc.gov/vaccines/hcp/acip-recs/vacc-specific/hepa.html
General information

- Administer to adults who have a specific risk (see below), or lack a risk factor but want protection, 2-dose series of single antigen hepatitis A vaccine (HepA; Havrix at 0 and 6–12 months or Vaqta at 0 and 6–18 months; minimum interval: 6 months) or a 3-dose series of combined hepatitis A and hepatitis B vaccine (HepA-HepB) at 0, 1, and 6 months; minimum intervals: 4 weeks between first and second doses, 5 months between second and third doses

Special populations

- Administer HepA or HepA-HepB to adults with the following indications:
  - **Travel** to or work in countries with high or intermediate hepatitis A endemicity
  - **Men who have sex with men**
  - **Injection or noninjection drug use**
  - **Work with hepatitis A virus in a research laboratory or with nonhuman primates infected with hepatitis A virus**
  - **Clotting factor disorders**
  - **Chronic liver disease**

- Close, personal **contact with an international adoptee** (e.g., household or regular babysitting) during the first 60 days after arrival in the United States from a country with high or intermediate endemicity (administer the first dose as soon as the adoption is planned)
- Healthy adults **through age 40 years who have recently been exposed to hepatitis A virus**; adults older than age 40 years may receive HepA if hepatitis A immunoglobulin cannot be obtained

9. Hepatitis B vaccination
www.cdc.gov/vaccines/hcp/acip-recs/vacc-specific/hepb.html
General information

- Administer to adults who have a specific risk (see below), or lack a risk factor but want protection, 3-dose series of single antigen hepatitis B vaccine (HepB) or combined hepatitis A and hepatitis B vaccine (HepA-HepB) at 0, 1, and 6 months (minimum intervals: 4 weeks between doses 1 and 2 for HepB and HepA-HepB; between doses 2 and 3, 8 weeks for HepB and 5 months for HepA-HepB)

Special populations

- Administer HepB or HepA-HepB to adults with the following indications:
  - **Chronic liver disease** (e.g., hepatitis C infection, cirrhosis, fatty liver disease, alcoholic liver disease, autoimmune hepatitis, alanine aminotransferase [ALT] or aspartate aminotransferase [AST] level greater than twice the upper limit of normal)
  - **HIV infection**
  - **Percutaneous or mucosal risk of exposure to blood** (e.g., **household contacts** of hepatitis B surface antigen [HBsAg]-positive persons; adults younger than age 60 years with **diabetes mellitus** or aged 60 years or older with diabetes mellitus based on individual clinical decision; adults in predialysis care or receiving **hemodialysis or peritoneal dialysis**; recent or current **injection drug users**; **health care and public safety workers** at risk for exposure to blood or blood-contaminated body fluids)
  - **Sexual exposure risk** (e.g., sex partners of HBsAg-positive persons; sexually active persons not in a mutually monogamous relationship; persons seeking evaluation or treatment for a sexually transmitted infection; and **men who have sex with men** [MSM])
  - Receive care in **settings where a high proportion of adults have risks for hepatitis B infection** (e.g., facilities providing sexually transmitted disease treatment, drug-abuse treatment and prevention services, hemodialysis and end-stage renal disease programs, institutions for developmentally disabled persons, health care settings targeting services to injection drug users or MSM, HIV testing and treatment facilities, and correctional facilities)
  - **Travel** to countries with high or intermediate hepatitis B endemicity

10. Meningococcal vaccination
www.cdc.gov/vaccines/hcp/acip-recs/vacc-specific/mening.html

Special populations: Serogroups A, C, W, and Y meningococcal vaccine (MenACWY)

- Administer 2 doses of MenACWY at least 8 weeks apart and revaccinate with 1 dose of MenACWY every 5 years, if the risk remains, to adults with the following indications:
  - **Anatomical or functional asplenia** (including sickle cell disease and other hemoglobinopathies)
  - **HIV infection**
  - **Persistent complement component deficiency**
  - **Eculizumab use**
- Administer 1 dose of MenACWY and revaccinate with 1 dose of MenACWY every 5 years, if the risk remains, to adults with the following indications:
  - **Travel to or live in countries where meningococcal disease is hyperendemic or epidemic**, including countries in the African meningitis belt or during the Hajj
  - At risk from a **meningococcal disease outbreak attributed to serogroup A, C, W, or Y**
  - **Microbiologists** routinely exposed to *Neisseria meningitidis*
  - **Military recruits**
  - **First-year college students who live in residential housing** (if they did not receive MenACWY at age 16 years or older)

General Information: Serogroup B meningococcal vaccine (MenB)

- May administer, based on individual clinical decision, to young adults and adolescents aged 16–23 years (preferred age is 16–18 years) who are not at increased risk 2-dose series of MenB-4C (Bexsero) at least 1 month apart or 2-dose series of MenB-FHbp (Trumenba) at least 6 months apart
- MenB-4C and MenB-FHbp are not interchangeable

Special populations: MenB

- Administer 2-dose series of MenB-4C at least 1 month apart or 3-dose series of MenB-FHbp at 0, 1–2, and 6 months to adults with the following indications:
  - **Anatomical or functional asplenia** (including sickle cell disease)
  - **Persistent complement component deficiency**
  - **Eculizumab use**
  - At risk from a **meningococcal disease outbreak attributed to serogroup B**
  - **Microbiologists** routinely exposed to *Neisseria meningitidis*

11. *Haemophilus influenzae* type b vaccination
www.cdc.gov/vaccines/hcp/acip-recs/vacc-specific/hib.html

Special populations

- Administer *Haemophilus influenzae* type b vaccine (Hib) to adults with the following indications:
  - **Anatomical or functional asplenia** (including sickle cell disease) or undergoing elective splenectomy: Administer 1 dose if not previously vaccinated (preferably at least 14 days before elective splenectomy)
  - **Hematopoietic stem cell transplant** (HSCT): Administer 3-dose series with doses 4 weeks apart starting 6 to 12 months after successful transplant regardless of Hib vaccination history

Table   2-11 (*Continued***)**

	Table 2-11 SUMMARY OF ADOLESCENT/ADULT IMMUNIZATION RECOMMENDATIONS				
	TETANUS, DIPHTHERIA AND ACELLULAR PERTUSSIS (Td/Tdap)	**INFLUENZA**	**PNEUMOCOCCAL POLYSACCHARIDE (PPSV)**	**MEASLES AND MUMPS**	**SMALL POX**
Indications	All adults Tdap should replace a single dose of Td for adults aged less than 65 years who have not previously received a Tdap dose.	Ages 19–49 for persons with medical/exposure indications Adults 50 years and older Clients with chronic conditions During influenza season for women in 2nd and 3rd trimester of pregnancy Persons traveling to foreign countries Residents of nursing homes, long-term care, assisted-living facilities	Ages 19–64 for persons with medical/exposure indications Adults 65 years and older Alaskan Natives and some Native Americans Residents of nursing homes, long-term care, assisted-living facilities	Adults born after 1957 without proof of vaccine on or after first birthday HIV-infected persons without severe immunosuppression Travelers to foreign countries Persons entering college	First responders
Schedule	Two doses 4–8 wk apart Third dose 6–12 months Booster at 10 years intervals for life Tdap or Td vaccine used as indicated	Annually each fall	One dose Should receive at age 65 if received at least 5 years previously Administered if vaccination status unknown	One dose Two doses if in college, in health care profession, or traveling to foreign country with 2nd dose one month after 1st	One dose
Contra-indications	Severe allergic reaction to previous dose Encephalopathy not due to another cause within 7 days of DTaP	Allergy to eggs		Severe allergic reaction Known severe immunod-eficiency	History of eczema or other skin conditions that disrupt epidermis, pregnancy or breast feeding, or women who wish to conceive 28 days after vaccination Immunosuppression, allergy to small pox vaccine receiving topical ocular steroid medication, moderate-to-severe recurrent illness, being under the age of 18, household contacts with history of eczema
Comments	Precautions: Moderate or severe illness with or without fever			Check pregnancy status of women Should avoid pregnancy for 30 days after vaccination Elevated temperature may be seen for 1–2 weeks Precautions: Recent receipt of antibody-containing blood product Moderate or severe illness with or without fever	Vaccinia can be transmitted from an unhealed vaccination site to other persons by close contact. Wash hands with soapy water immediately after changing bandage; place bandages in sealed plastic bag; cover site with gauze and wear long-sleeved clothing. When performing client care, keep site covered with gauze and a semiper-meable dressing.

Table 2-11 SUMMARY OF ADOLESCENT/ADULT IMMUNIZATION RECOMMENDATIONS (CONTINUED)						
	RUBELLA	HEPATITIS B	POLIOVIRUS: IPV	VARICELLA	HEPATITIS A	HUMAN PAPILLOMA VIRUS VACCINE (HPV)
Indications	Persons (especially women) without proof of vaccine on or after first birthday Health-care personnel at risk of exposure to rubella and who have contact with pregnant clients	Persons at risk to exposure to blood or blood-containing body fluids Clients and staff at institutions for developmentally disabled Hemodialysis clients Recipients of clotting-factor concentrates Household contacts and sex partners of clients with HBV Some international travelers Injecting drug users Men who have sex with men Heterosexuals with multiple sex partners or recent STD Inmates of long-term correctional facilities All unvaccinated adolescents	Travelers to countries where it is epidemic Unvaccinated adults whose children receive IPV	Persons without proof of disease or vaccination or who are seronegative Susceptible adolescents/adults living in house holds with children Susceptible healthcare workers Susceptible family contacts of immunocompromised persons Nonpregnant women of childbearing age International travelers High risk persons: teachers of young children, day care employees, residents and staff in institutional settings, college students, inmates and staff of correctional institutions, military personnel	Travelers to countries with high incidence Men who have sex with men Injecting and illegal drug users Persons with chronic liver disease Persons with clotting factor disorders Food handlers	Children 11 12 years to 26 years (c be given starting at years of ag For adults aged 27 through 4! years, publ health ben of HPV vaccinatio in this age range is minimal
Schedule	One dose	Three doses Second dose 1–2 months after 1st Third 4–6 months after 1st	IPV recommended Two doses at 4-8 wk intervals Third dose 2–12 months after second **OPV no longer recommended in U.S.**	Two doses separated by 4–8 wk	Two doses separated by 6–12 months	Three doses Second dos 2 months after 1st Third dose 6 months after 2nd
Contra-indications	Allergy to neomycin Pregnancy Receipt of immune globulin or blood/ blood products in previous 3–11 months	Severe allergic reaction to vaccine	Severe allergic reaction after previous dose	Severe allergic reaction to vaccine Immunosuppressive therapy or immunodeficiency (including HIV infection) Pregnancy	Severe allergic reaction to vaccine	
Comments	Check pregnancy status of women Should avoid pregnancy for 3 months after vaccination	Precautions: Low birth weight infant Moderate or severe illness with or without fever	Temperature elevation may be seen for 1–2 weeks Precautions: Pregnancy moderate or severe illness with or without fever	Check pregnancy status of women Should avoid pregnancy for 1 month after vaccination Immune globulin or blood/ blood product in previous 11 months Moderate or severe illness with or without fever	Swelling and redness at injection site common Precaution: pregnancy	HPV vaccinatio most effec when give before exposure t any HPV, a in early adolescenc

MAINTENANCE OF SKIN INTEGRITY

OVERVIEW

A. Structure and function of dermal tissue

  1. Structure—largest organ of body
     a. Epidermis—dead squamous cells; no blood supply; outer layer
     b. Dermis—collagen fibers, blood vessels, nerves
     c. Sweat glands
     d. Sebaceous glands
     e. Subcutaneous connective tissue

  2. Functions
     a. Protection against injury
     b. Temperature, water, and electrolyte regulation

B. Assessment of skin integrity

  1. History of infectious disorders
  2. Potential skin trauma (environmental, occupational) or irritants (dyes)
  3. Seasonal (e.g., dry, low humidity, sun)
  4. Medications (corticosteroids)
  5. Chronic diseases (diabetes)
  6. History of allergic reactions
  7. Inspection
     a. Color—red in inflammation
     b. Temperature—hot with inflammation; cool with decreased perfusion
     c. Elasticity—swollen and painful to movement with inflammation

  8. Skin lesions—describe size, shape, location, color, and distribution

C. Plan/Implementation

  1. Diagnostic tests
     a. Skin biopsy
     b. Skin culture

  2. Nursing interventions
     a. Cleansing baths—remove oils, prevent odor, provide medication (see Table 2-12)
     b. Nutrition—deficiencies of nutrients can cause skin disorders, dryness
     c. Promote rest—emotional conditions affect skin
     d. Administer medications (see Table 2-13)

Table 2-12 THERAPEUTIC BATHS		
TYPE	PURPOSE	COMMON USE
Colloidal, e.g., oatmeal, cornstarch	Antipruritic	Chickenpox
Potassium permanganate	Antifungal	Slow-healing ulcers
Burow's solution	Antibacterial	Soaks
Tar preparations	Antipruritic	Psoriasis
Oils, e.g., Alpha-Keri	Antipruritic	Moisturizing

e. Apply dressings
   1) Open wet—antipruritic, vasoconstrictive
      a) Soak nonresidue cloth in tepid solution
      b) Apply for 3–5 min
      c) Reapply repeatedly for 15–20 min
      d) Dry skin
   2) Closed wet—soften keratinized tissue
   3) Wet to damp—debride wounds

f. Promote wound healing (see Table 2-14)

Table 2-13 COMMON SKIN MEDICATIONS		
MEDICATION	ADVERSE REACTIONS	NURSING CONSIDERATIONS
Bacitracin ointment	Nephrotoxicity Ototoxicity	Overgrowth of nonsusceptible organisms can occur
Neosporin cream	Nephrotoxicity Ototoxicity	Allergic dermatitis may occur
Povidone-iodine solution	Irritation	Do not use around eyes May stain skin Do not use full-strength on mucous membranes Allergic dermatitis may occur
Silver sulfadiazine cream	Neutropenia Burning	Use cautiously if sensitive to sulfonamides
Tolnaftate cream	Irritation	Use small amount of medication Use medication for duration prescribed
Nystatin cream	Contact dermatitis	Do not use occlusive dressings

D. Evaluation of skin disorders (see Table 2-15)

   1. Performs appropriate skin care

   2. Adjusts to socialization problems of skin disorders

Table 2-14 GENERAL NURSING MEASURES TO PROMOTE WOUND HEALING	
MEASURE	RATIONALE
Leave dry dressings intact	Prevention of contamination of area
Use sterile dressings and technique for open wounds	Prevention of infection
Observe for fever, elevated WBC count, swelling, redness of wound; wound culture of drainage	Signs of potential wound infection
Elevate extremities	Adequate circulation of WBC, nutrients promote healing
Debride or assist with debriding wound if necessary	Debris may also promote increased inflammation
Frequent dressing changes if drainage copious	Purulent drainage promotes skin breakdown; moisture promotes bacterial growth
Adequate nutrition including protein and vitamin C	Collagen formation requires protein and vitamin C

Table 2-15 SELECTED SKIN DISORDERS		
DISORDER	**ASSESSMENT**	**NURSING CONSIDERATIONS**
Impetigo	Reddish macule becomes honey-colored crusted vesicle, then crust; pruritus Caused by *Staphylococcus, Streptococcus*	Skin isolation: careful handwashing; cover draining lesions; discourage touching lesions Antibiotics—may be topical ointment (Garamycin) and/or PO Loosen scabs with Burow's solution compresses; remove gently Restraints if necessary; mitts for infants to prevent secondary infection Monitor for acute glomerulonephritis (complication of untreated impetigo)
Herpes simplex type I	Pruritic vesicular groupings on nose, lips, and oral mucous membranes Chronically recurrent	Spread by direct contact, handwashing; bland, soft foods; avoid direct contact; administer antivirals (acyclovir, famciclovir, and valacyclovir); topical anesthetics; cold or hot compresses; wash linens and towels in hot water
Herpes zoster (shingles)	Vesicular eruption along nerve distribution Pain, tenderness, and pruritus over affected region Primarily seen on face, thorax, trunk	Caused by reactivation of chickenpox virus (varicella) or decreased immunity Analgesics; compresses; oatmeal baths Systemic corticosteroids to diminish severity Prevent spread—contagious to anyone who has not had chickenpox or who is immunosuppressed; airborne or contact precautions Antivirals: Famciclovir, valacyclovir, acyclovir
Scabies	Minute, reddened, itchy lesions Linear burrowing of a mite at finger webs, wrists, elbows, ankles, penis	Reduce itching—topical antipruritic (calamine lotion/topical steroids), permethrin 5% cream or crotamiton 10% cream Institute skin precautions to prevent spread Scabicide—permethrin or crotamiton lotion; apply lotion (not on face) to cool, dry skin (not after hot shower because of potential for increased absorption); treat all family members (infants upon recommendation of health care provider) Repeat in 7 days Launder all clothing and linen after above treatment The rash and itching may last for 2–3 weeks even though the mite has been destroyed; treat with antipruritic
Pediculosis (lice)	Scalp: white eggs (nits) on hair shafts, with itchy scalp Body: macules and papules Pubis: red macules	Permethrin 1% cream/lotion Kills both lice and nits with one application May suggest to repeat in 7 days—depends on severity
Tinea	Pedis (athlete's foot)—vesicular eruptions in interdigital webs Capitis (ringworm)—breakage and loss of hair; scaly circumscribed red patches on scalp that spread in circular pattern; fluoresces green with Wood's lamp Corporis (ringworm of body)—rings of red scaly areas that spread with central clearing	Antifungal—topical ointment, creams, lotions include ketoconazole, miconazole, terbinafine Keep areas dry and clean Frequent shampooing

DISORDER	ASSESSMENT	NURSING CONSIDERATIONS
Psoriasis	Chronic recurrent thick, itchy, erythematous papules/plaques covered with silvery white scales with symmetrical distribution Commonly on the scalp, knees, sacrum, elbows, and behind ears Elevated sedimentation rate with negative rheumatoid factor	Topical medications: cortisone creams, anthralin, coal tar, moisturizers, creams with vitamins Immuno suppressants: methotrexate or cyclosporine Biological response modifiers: adalimumab, infliximab, etanercept Ultraviolet light (wear goggles to protect eyes) Counseling to support/enhance self-image/self-esteem
Acne vulgaris	Comedones (blackheads/whiteheads), papules, pustules, cysts occurring most often on the face, neck, shoulders, and back	Good hygiene and nutrition PO tetracycline (advise sunscreen with SPF of 15; avoid sun exposure) Antibacterial medications—azelaic acid, clindamycin, erythromycin Isotretinoin–risk of elevated LFTs, dry skin and fetal damage Drying preparations—Benoxyl/vitamin A may cause redness and peeling early in treatment and photosensitivity Ultraviolet light and dermabrasion Monitor for secondary infection Emotional support Isotretinoin (contraindicated with pregnancy)
Eczema (Atropic dermatitis)	Children: rough, dry, erythematous skin lesions that progress to weeping and crusting; distributed on the cheeks, scalp, and extensor surfaces in infants and on flexor surfaces in children Adults: hard, dry, flaking, scaling on face, upper chest, and antecubital and popliteal fossa	Onset usually in infancy around 2–3 mo; often outgrown by 2–3 years May be precursor of adult asthma or hay fever Elimination from diet of common offenders, especially milk, eggs, wheat, citrus fruits, and tomatoes Eliminate clothing that is irritating (rough/wool) or that promotes sweating; cotton clothing is best Avoid soap and prolonged or hot baths/showers, which tend to be drying; may use warm colloid baths (e.g., Aveeno/cornstarch) Lotions to affected areas—Eucerin/Alpha-Keri Keep fingernails short and clean; arm restraints/mittens may be necessary Topical steroids Antihistamines

Table 2-15 SELECTED SKIN DISORDERS *(CONTINUED)*

EFFECTS OF DEVELOPMENT ON SKIN DISORDERS

A. Infant and toddler
1. Diaper dermatitis—usually on convex areas or folds (often due to *Candida albicans*)
2. Seborrheic dermatitis (cradle cap)—crusting of infant's scalp due to hyperactive sebaceous glands caused by maternal hormones
   a. Cleanse with shampoo
   b. Oil scalp and remove crusts

B. School-age
1. Age of communicable diseases
2. See Prevention of Communicable Diseases (e.g., tonsillitis)

C. Adolescent
1. Changes of puberty—sebaceous gland active, eccrine glands functioning, body hair develops
2. Acne develops

D. Elderly
1. Assessment—usual changes
   a. Loss of subcutaneous tissue and melanocytes—skin tears more easily; increased risk ultraviolet damage
   b. Degeneration of collagen and elastic fibers—wrinkling, skin tears more often
   c. Increased capillary fragility; decreased circulation—increased bruising, decreased wound healing
   d. Hormonal changes and decreased immune function—dry and more permeable skin
2. Intervention—Bathe every day or less often; avoid use of strong, scented, or alcohol-based soaps; avoid bath oil in tubs; keep room humidity at 60%

PRIMARY SKIN LESIONS

A. Macule
1. Flat and circumscribed
2. Nonpalpable
3. Smaller than 1 cm
4. Example—freckle, flat nevi, petechiae

B. Papule
1. Solid elevation
2. Palpable
3. Less than 1 cm
4. Example—wart, mole

C. Nodule
1. Elevated solid lesion
2. Deep, may extend into dermis
3. Greater than 1 cm
4. Example—xanthoma, fibroma

D. Wheal

    1. Localized area of edema

    2. Elevated and firm, itchy

    3. Example—mosquito bite, allergic reaction (hive)

E. Vesicle

    1. Elevation of skin filled with clear fluid

    2. Less than 1 cm

    3. Example—blister, herpes simplex, herpes zoster, early chicken pox

F. Pustule

    1. Elevation of skin filled with pus

    2. Example—acne, impetigo

G. Ulcer

    1. Loss of epidermis dermis, subcutaneous tissue

    2. Irregular shape, may bleed

    3. Granulation tissue, slough, necrotic tissue

    4. Example—pressure sores, chancre

H. Atrophy

    1. Thinning of skin, may bleed easily

    2. Example—aging, disuse syndrome

I. Erosion

    1. Loss of epidermis; shallow depression

    2. Moist with no bleeding; heals without scarring

    3. Example—skin trauma

DERMATOLOGICAL DISORDERS

A. Impetigo—highly contagious superficial streptococcal/staphylococcal infection of outer layers of skin

    1. Incubation—1–2 days

    2. Assessment—itchy vesicular lesion progressing to thick honey-colored crust most commonly found around the nose and chin (may also be in axillae and on extremities) and spreads peripherally from initial lesion

    3. Care

        a. Skin isolation; careful handwashing; cover draining lesions; discourage touching lesions

        b. Antibiotics—may be topical ointment (Garamycin, Neosporin) and/or PO; systemic antibiotics if more severe

        c. Loosen scabs with Burow's solution compresses; remove gently

        d. Restraints if necessary; mitts for infants to prevent secondary infection

        e. Monitor for acute glomerulonephritis

B. Herpes simplex type I–"fever blisters," "cold sores," canker sores
1. Assessment
    a. Tingling, pruritic, burning vesicular groupings on nose, lips, and oral mucous membranes that usually ulcerate/crust; chronically recurrent; increases with age and immunosuppression
    b. May develop into herpes gingivostomatitis in children with extremely painful lesions in lips, gums, tongue, and hard palate; causes a foul breath odor and difficulty in and refusal to eat/drink; dehydration is of concern

2. Care
    a. Relieve pain–topical anesthetic
    b. Maintain hydration and nutrition–bland, soft, tepid foods and drink; use a straw
    c. Prevent spread–avoid direct contact; maintain scrupulous handwashing; contagious for 3–5 days; wash linens and towels in hot water
    d. Oral antivirals–acyclovir, famciclovir, or valacyclovir
    e. Cold or hot compresses

C. Herpes zoster (shingles)–acute viral infection of nervous system caused by reactivation of dormant varicella (chickenpox) virus, may be due to decreased immunity
1. Assessment–several days of unilateral pain, followed by painful, itchy, tender vesicular eruptions along peripheral sensory nerve distribution, primarily on face, thorax, trunk; may reoccur

2. Care
    a. Control pain–analgesics; compress; oatmeal baths
    b. Systemic corticosteroids to diminish severity
    c. Prevent spread–contagious to anyone who has not had chickenpox or who is immuno-suppressed; airborne or contact precautions
    d. Antiviral medications–acyclovir, famciclovir, or valacyclovir

D. Scabies–skin disorder caused by mites transmitted via close contact with infested person or clothing/bedding
1. Assessment–intensely itchy (especially at night), red, excoriated, tiny lesions and burrow formation found primarily in the webs of fingers, under the breasts, on groin, knees, and/or elbow surfaces, around the wrists or ankles, not on the face

2. Care
    a. Reduce itching–topical antipruritic (calamine lotion/topical steroids)
    b. Prevent spread
        1) Institute skin precautions
        2) Scabicide–crotamiton lotion or permethrin
            a) Apply lotion (not on face) to cool, dry skin (not after hot shower because of potential for increased absorption); leave on for 8–12 hours, then shower off; crotamiton may be applied at bedtime for two or more consecutive nights; risk for neurotoxicity in children
            b) Treat all family members (infants upon recommendation of health care provider)
        3) Launder all clothing and linen after above treatment; dry in hot dryer
        4) The rash and itching may last for 2–3 wk, even through the mite has been destroyed; treat with antipruritic

E. Pediculosis—parasitic lice infection spread by close contact and shared clothing, brushes/combs, bedding

1. Assessment
   a. Corporis—white eggs (nits) and lice in clothing; seldom on nonhairy skin of body; intensely itchy, erythematous macules on upper back and areas of tight clothing
   b. Capitus—nits resembling dandruff that are difficult to dislodge, cling to hair shafts in occipital region and over ears; severe itching
   c. Pubis—pubic hair infested with crab-shaped lice, intensely itchy, red macules in hairy regions and abdomen

2. Care
   a. Avoid transmission—do not share combs, hats, bedding
   b. Permethrin, may repeat if necessary
   c. Launder all clothing as above; soak personal care items in pediculicide
   d. Comb hair with fine-tooth comb to remove nits

F. Tinea—fungal infection transmitted via person-to-person contact and animals/soil

1. Assessment
   a. Pedis (athlete's foot)—vesicular eruptions in interdigital webs
   b. Capitis (ringworm)—breakage and loss of hair; scaly, circumscribed, red patches on scalp that spread in a circular pattern; fluoresces green with Wood's lamp
   c. Corporis (ringworm of body)—rings of red scaly areas that spread with central clearing

2. Care
   a. Antifungal—topical ointment, creams, lotions
   b. Keep areas dry and clean
   c. Frequent shampooing

G. Psoriasis—chronic dermatitis with familial predisposition; often precipitated by stress, trauma, infection

1. Assessment
   a. Chronic, recurrent, thick, erythematous papules/plaques covered with silvery white scales with symmetrical distribution commonly found on the scalp, knees, sacrum, elbows, and behind ears
   b. May be painful or itchy
   c. Elevated sedimentation rate with negative rheumatoid factor seen with psoriatic arthritis

2. Care
   a. Topical medications: cortisone creams, anthralin, coal tar, moisturizers, creams with vitamins
   b. Immunosuppressants: methotrexate or cyclosporine
   c. Biological response modifiers: adalimumab, infliximab, etanercept
   d. Ultraviolet light—natural/artificial
   e. Counseling to support/enhance self-image/self-esteem

H. Acne vulgaris—chronic skin disorder associated with increased sebum production and inflammation of sebaceous follicles; onset most often at puberty and continues throughout adolescence

1. Assessment—lesions may be comedones (blackheads/whiteheads), papules, pustules, and/or cysts, occurring most often on the face, neck, shoulders, and back

2. Care

   a. Adequate rest, good hygiene and nutrition; eliminate any foods that are associated with increased symptoms

   b. PO tetracycline—advise sunscreen (SPF of at least 15) because of increased sensitivity to sun; do not use in pregnancy/lactation

   c. Drying preparations—Benozyl/vitamin A acid (may be used concurrently with tetracyclines but not applied at same time); may cause redness and peeling early in treatment; may cause photosensitivity

   d. Isotretinoin—risk of elevated LFTs, dry skin, and depression; teratogenic

   e. Ultraviolet light and surgery may be used for cystic/abscessed lesions (dermabrasion)

   f. Monitor for secondary infections

   g. Emotional support—based on growth and developmental characteristics of adolescence; peer group sessions discussing treatment as part of overall self-image enhancement is often helpful

PERIOPERATIVE CARE

A. Assessment

　1. Stress—vasovagal responses

　2. Fears (see Table 2-16)

Table 2-16 FEARS OF SURGERY AT DIFFERENT DEVELOPMENTAL STAGES		
AGE GROUP	**SPECIFIC FEARS**	**NURSING CONSIDERATIONS**
Toddler	Separation	Teach parents to expect regression, e.g., in toilet training and difficult separations
Preschooler	Mutilation	Allow child to play with models of equipment Encourage expression of feelings, e.g., anger
School-age	Loss of control	Explain procedures in simple terms Allow choices when possible
Adolescence	Loss of independence; being different from peers, e.g., alterations in body image	Involve adolescent in procedures and therapies Expect resistance Express understanding of concerns Point out strengths
Elderly	Physical decline Decreased independence Fear of death Fear of nursing home placement	Assess ability to handle physical and emotional stress Assess cognitive function Explain procedures at level appropriate for client Involve caregivers as appropriate

B. Intervention

　1. Teaching (see Tables 2-17 and 2-18)

　　a. Age-appropriate

　　　1) Toddler—simple directions

　　　2) Preschool and school-aged—allow to play with equipment

　　　3) Adolescent—expect resistance

　　b. Family oriented—have parents reinforce teaching

2. Preparation for surgery (see Table 2-19)

Table 2-17 PREOPERATIVE TEACHING GUIDE
Factors for Nurse to Assess Before Teaching
History of illness
Rationale for surgery
Nature of surgery—curative or palliative, minor or major, extent of disfigurement, potential alterations, e.g., ostomies
Factors related to client's readiness for learning—age, mental status, preexisting knowledge about condition, concerns about condition, family's reaction to need for surgery
Content Areas to Cover During Teaching
Elicit client's concerns, e.g., fears about anesthesia
Provide information to clear up misconceptions
Explain preoperative procedures, remove jewelry, nail polish
Lab tests
Skin preparation—cleansing, possibly shaving
Enemas if indicated, e.g., before intestinal surgery
Rationale for withholding food and fluids (NPO)
Preoperative medications, IV line
Teach postoperative procedures—deep breathing, leg exercises, moving in bed, incentive spirometer (sustained maximal inspiration device), equipment to expect postoperatively
Explain importance of reporting pain or discomfort after surgery
Explain what will be done to relieve pain, e.g., changing position, medication
Provide for growth and development needs of children

    a. Preoperative Checklist
       1) Informed consent
       2) Lab tests, chest x-ray, EKG
       3) Skin prep
       4) Bowel prep
       5) IVs
       6) NPO
       7) Preop meds, sedation, antibiotics
       8) Removal of dentures, jewelry, nail polish
       9) Nutrition—may need PN or tube feedings preoperatively

3. Culturally sensitive perioperative care
    a. Assess primary language spoken
    b. Assess feelings regarding surgery and pain
    c. Determine attitudes about pain management
    d. Determine expectations of the intraoperative and postoperative periods
    e. Evaluate client's support system
    f. Assess feelings about self-care
    g. Use professional interpreters
    h. Use pictures or phrase cards with various languages
    i. Provide printed teaching materials in a variety of languages

4. Complementary and Alternative Therapies
    a. Supplements should not be taken near the time of surgery; may interact with anesthesia, may affect coagulation parameters
        1) Echinacea
        2) Ephedra (currently removed from the retail market in the United States)
        3) Garlic
        4) Ginkgo
        5) Ginseng
        6) Kava
        7) St. John's wort
    b. Eliminate all dietary supplements (other than multivitamins) at least 2 to 3 weeks before surgery
    c. May resume the supplements with the advice of the health care provider

INTRAOPERATIVE CARE

A. Assessment (see Table 2-18)
B. Intervention—monitor effects of anesthesia during postinduction; vital signs
    1. Aseptic technique
    2. Appropriate grounding devices
    3. Fluid balance
    4. Sponge/instrument count

Table 2-18 ANESTHESIA		
MEDICATION	**ADVERSE EFFECTS**	**NURSING CONSIDERATIONS**
General anesthesia via inhalation	Respiratory depression, circulatory depression Delirium during induction and recovery Nausea and vomiting, aspiration during induction, myocardial depression, hepatic toxicity	Check history of sensitization Maintain airway Protect and orient client Monitor vital signs, labs Prevent aspiration postop by elevating head of bed, turning head to side (unless contraindicated)
Nitrous oxide	Hypotension, postop nausea and vomiting	Monitor vital signs Adequate oxygenation is essential, especially during emergence
IV thiopental sodium	Respiratory depression, low BP, laryngospasm Poor muscle relaxation, hypotension, irritating to skin and subcutaneous tissue	Monitor vital signs, especially airway, breathing Straps for operative table, proper positioning Protect IV site, check for placement periodically
Spinal anesthesia Saddle	Hypotension, headache	Monitor vital signs Encourage oral fluids
Conduction blocks Epidural Caudal	Hypotension, respiratory depression	Headache not experienced Monitor vital signs
Local anesthesia	Excitability, toxic reactions such as respiratory difficulties, vasoconstriction if substance contains epinephrine	Monitor client Do not use local anesthesia with epinephrine on fingers (circulation is less optimal)
Moderate (conscious) sedation Midazolam Diazepam	Respiratory depression, apnea, hypotension, bradycardia	Never leave client alone Constantly monitor airway, level of consciousness, pulse oximetry, ECG Vital signs every 15–30 min Assess client's ability to maintain patent airway and respond to verbal commands

Table 2-19 PREMEDICATIONS AND POTENTIAL PROBLEMS		
MEDICATIONS	ADVERSE EFFECTS	NURSING CONSIDERATIONS
Morphine	Resiratory depression, gastric irritability	Monitor vital signs, especially respirations; observe for vomiting Side rails elevated to prevent accidents
Promethazine hydrochloride (anxiety, antiemetic)	Hypotension	Monitor vital signs
Atropine sulfate (to decrease secretions and prevent laryngospasm)	Tachycardia	Monitor vital signs Advise client about dry mouth

POSTOPERATIVE CARE

A. Assessment—anesthesia, immobility, and surgery can affect any system in the body and require a full systems assessment

B. Neuropsychosocial
1. Stimulate client postanesthesia
2. Monitor level of consciousness

C. Cardiovascular
1. Generally monitor vital signs q 15 min times 4, q 30 min times 2, q 1 hour times 2, then as needed
2. Monitor I and O
3. Check potassium level
4. Monitor CVP

D. Respiratory
1. Check breath sounds
2. Turn, cough, and deep breathe (unless contraindicated; e.g., brain, spinal, eye surgery)
3. Splint wound
4. Offer pain medication
5. Teach incentive spirometer
6. Get out of bed as soon as possible

E. Gastrointestinal
1. Check bowel sounds in 4 quadrants 5 min each
2. Keep NPO until bowel sounds present
3. Provide good mouth care while NPO
4. Provide antiemetics for nausea and vomiting
5. Check abdomen for distention
6. Check for passage of flatus and stool

F. Genitourinary
1. Monitor I and O
2. Encourage to void
3. Notify health care provider if unable to void within 8 hours
4. Catheterize, if needed

G. Extremities
   1. Check pulses
   2. Assess for color, edema, temperature
   3. Inform client not to cross legs
   4. Keep knee gatch flat
   5. Prohibit pillows behind knee
   6. Apply antiembolic stockings (TED hose) prior to getting out of bed (OOB)
   7. Monitor for calf pain and/or calf swelling
   8. Pneumatic compression device

H. Wounds
   1. Dressing
      a. Document amount and character of drainage
      b. Health care provider changes first postop dressing
      c. Aseptic technique
      d. Note presence of drains

   2. Incision
      a. Assess site: edematous, inflamed, excoriated
      b. Assess drainage: serous, serosanguineous, purulent
      c. Note type of sutures
      d. Note if edges are well approximated
      e. Risk of infection 3–5 days postop
      f. Debride wound, if needed, to reduce inflammation
      g. Change dressing frequently to prevent skin breakdown around site and minimize bacterial growth

I. Drains—to prevent fluids from accumulating in tissues (see Table 2-20)

Table 2-20 SURGICAL DRAINS		
TYPE	DESCRIPTION	NURSING CONSIDERATIONS
Penrose	Simple latex drain	Note location Usually not sutured in place, but layered in gauze dressing Expect drainage on dressing
T-tube	Used after gallbladder surgery Placed in common bile duct to allow passage of bile	Monitor drainage Initially 500–1,000 mL per day Usually bloody for first 2 hours Keep drainage bag below level of gallbladder May be discharged with T-tube in place Teach client about care

Table 2-20 SURGICAL DRAINS *(CONTINUED)*		
TYPE	**DESCRIPTION**	**NURSING CONSIDERATIONS**
Jackson-Pratt	Portable wound self-suction device with reservoir	Monitor amount and character of drainage Notify health care provider if it suddenly increases or becomes bright red
HemoVac	Larger portable wound self-suction device with reservoir Used after mastectomy	Monitor and record amount and character of drainage Notify health care provider if it suddenly increases or becomes bright red Empty when full or every 8 hours Remove plug (maintain sterility), empty contents, place on flat surface, cleanse opening and plug with alcohol sponge, compress evacuator completely to remove air, replace plug, check system for operation

POTENTIAL COMPLICATIONS OF SURGERY

Table 2-21 POTENTIAL COMPLICATIONS OF SURGERY		
COMPLICATION	**ASSESSMENT**	**NURSING CONSIDERATIONS**
Hemorrhage	Decreased BP, increased pulse, cold, clammy skin	Replace blood volume Monitor vital signs
Paralytic ileus	Absent bowel sounds, no flatus or stool	Nasogastric suction IV fluids Decompression tubes
Atelectasis and pneumonia	Dyspnea, cyanosis, cough Tachycardia Elevated temperature Pain on affected side	Experienced second day postop Suctioning Postural drainage Antibiotics Cough and turn
Embolism	Dyspnea, pain, hemoptysis Restlessness ABG—low O_2, high CO_2	Experienced second day postop Oxygen Anticoagulants (heparin) IV fluids
Infection of wound	Elevated WBC and temperature Positive cultures	Experienced 3–5 days postop Antibiotics, aseptic technique Good nutrition
Dehiscence	Separation of wound edges	Experienced 5–6 days postop Low-fowler position, no coughing NPO Notify health care provider
Evisceration	Bowel erupts through surgical site	Experienced 5–6 days postop Low-fowler position, no coughing NPO Cover viscera with sterile saline dressing or wax paper (if at home) Notify health care provider
Psychosis	Inappropriate affect	Therapeutic communication Medication
Cardiovascular compromise	Decreased BP, increased pulse, cold, clammy skin	Treat cause Oxygen IV fluids

Table 2-21 POTENTIAL COMPLICATIONS OF SURGERY *(CONTINUED)*		
COMPLICATION	**ASSESSMENT**	**NURSING CONSIDERATIONS**
Urinary retention	Unable to void after surgery Bladder distention	Experienced 8–12 hours postop Catheterize as needed
Urinary infection	Foul-smelling urine Elevated WBC	Experienced 5–8 days postop Antibiotics Force fluids
Venous thromboembolism	Calf pain and/or calf swelling Ultrasound	Experienced 6–14 days up to 1 year later Anticoagulant therapy

Chapter 3

FLUID AND ELECTROLYTE BALANCE

Sections	Concepts Covered
1. Fluid Regulation	Fluid and Electrolyte Balance
2. Electrolyte Imbalances	Fluid and Electrolyte Balance
3. Nursing Measures for Intravenous Therapy	Fluid and Electrolyte Balance

FLUID VOLUME IMBALANCE

A. Assessment of fluid volume balance (see Table 3-1)

Table 3-1 FLUID VOLUME IMBALANCES		
	DEFICIENT FLUID VOLUME	**EXCESS FLUID VOLUME**
Assessment	Thirst (early sign) Temperature increases Rapid and weak pulse Respirations increase Poor skin turgor—skin cool, moist Hypotension Emaciation, weight loss Dry eye sockets, mouth, and mucous membranes Anxiety, apprehension, exhaustion Urine specific gravity greater than 1.030 Decreased urine output Increased hemoglobin, hemaocrit, Na^+ serum osmolality, BUN Headache, lethargy, confusion, disorientation	No change in temperature Pulse increases slightly and is bounding Respirations increase, shortness of breath, dyspnea, fine crackles Peripheral edema—bloated appearance, weight increase Hypertension May have muffled heart sounds Jugular vein distention Urine specific gravity less than 1.010 Apprehension Increased venous pressure Decreased hematocrit, BUN, hemoglobin, Na^+, serum osmolality
Analysis	Isotonic loss Vomiting Diarrhea GI suction Sweating Decreased intake Hemorrhage Third space shift	Isotonic gain, increase in the interstitial compartment, intravascular compartment, or both CHF Renal failure Cirrhosis of the liver Excessive ingestion of sodium Excessive or too rapid intravenous infusion
Plan/Implementation	Force fluids Provide isotonic IV fluids: Lactated Ringer's or 0.9% NaCl I and O, hourly outputs Daily weights (1 liter fluid = 1 kg or 2.2 lb) Monitor vital signs Check skin turgor Assess urine specific gravity	Administer diuretics Restrict fluids Sodium-restricted diet (average daily diet—6-15 g Na^+) Daily weight Assess breath sounds Check feet/ankle/sacral region for edema Semi-Fowler position if dyspneic

1. Signs and symptoms
2. Diagnostics—central venous pressure (CVP) (right atrial pressure) (see Figure 3-1)
   a. Purpose—measurement of effective blood volume and efficiency of cardiac pumping of the right side of the heart; measures pressure in superior vena cava
      1) Indicates ability of right side of heart to manage a fluid load
      2) Guide to fluid replacement

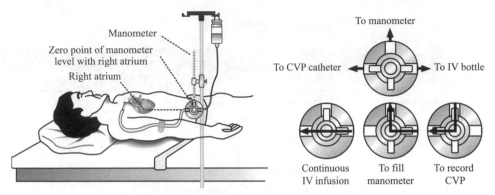

Figure 3-1. CENTRAL VENOUS PRESSURE

   b. Equipment
      1) Central line inserted into superior vena cava
      2) Water manometer with three-way stopcock or transducer
      3) IV fluids
   c. Procedure
      1) Client has catheter in jugular, subclavian, or median antecubital vein
      2) Attach manometer to a three-way stopcock that also connects IV to central catheter inserted into jugular, subclavian, or median cubital vein
      3) Zero on manometer placed at the level of the right atrium at midaxillary line
      4) Measured with client flat in bed
      5) Stopcock opened to the manometer, which allows for filling with IV fluid to level of 18–20 cm
      6) Stopcock turned to allow for fluid in manometer to flow to client
      7) Level of fluid fluctuates with respirations
      8) When level stabilizes, reading is taken at highest level of fluctuation
      9) Return stopcock to proper position and adjust IV flow rate
      10) Normal reading 2–8 mm Hg (3–11 cm of water)
         a) Elevated: greater than 8 mm Hg (11 cm of water) hypervolemia or poor cardiac contractility
         b) Lowered: less than 2 mm Hg (3 cm of water) hypovolemia
      11) Potential complications
         a) Pneumothorax
         b) Air embolism
         c) Infection at insertion site

12) Nursing management

   a) Dry, sterile dressing

   b) Change dressing, IV fluid bag, manometer, and tubing every 24 hours

   c) Instruct client to hold breath (Valsalva maneuver) when tubing changed to prevent air embolism

   d) Check and secure all connections

B. Definition of terms (see Table 3-1)

1. Tonicity—concentration of a substance dissolved in water

2. Isotonic fluids—same concentration as body fluids

3. Hypertonic solution—solute concentration greater than that of body fluids

4. Hypotonic solution—solute concentration less than that of body fluids

5. ECF—extracellular fluid

6. Intake refers to all possible avenues of intake, e.g., oral fluids, food, IV fluids, gavage feedings, irrigations

7. Output refers to all possible avenues of output, e.g., insensible losses, urine, diarrhea, vomitus, sweat, blood, and any drainage

C. Plan/Implementation (see Table 3-1)

1. Fluid deficit

   a. Causes

      1) Vomiting

      2) Diarrhea

      3) GI suction

      4) Sweating and warm weather

      5) Decreased intake; increased caffeine and alcohol intake

      6) Hyperthermia

      7) Diuretics

      8) Elderly—decreased total body water; inability to regulate sodium and water balance; decreased thirst perception

   b. Signs and symptoms

      1) Weight loss

      2) Decreased skin turgor

      3) Oliguria

      4) Concentrated urine

      5) Postural hypotension

      6) Weak, rapid pulse

      7) Increased hematocrit, hemoglobin, BUN, Na^+, serum osmolality

      8) Hyperthermia—increased pulse, decreased blood pressure, disorientation; treatment is fluid replacement

      9) Older adults—orthostatic hypotension, falls, pressure injuries, constipation, dry oral mucous membranes not reliable, vital signs not reliable in early dehydration

    c. Nursing management (see Table 3-2)

       1) Give fluids as appropriate; space fluids over 24 hours

       2) Isotonic IV fluids—lactated Ringer's or 0.9% NaCl

       3) I and O, hourly outputs

       4) Daily weights (1 liter fluid = 1 kg or 2.2 lb)

       5) Monitor vital signs and pulse quality

       6) Check skin turgor

       7) Assess urine specific gravity (should be greater than 1.020)

2. Fluid overload—isotonic gain

    a. Increase in the interstitial compartment, intravascular compartment, or both

    b. Causes

       1) Heart failure

       2) Renal failure (late phase)

       3) Cirrhosis of the liver

       4) Excessive ingestion of sodium

       5) Excessive or too rapid intravenous infusion

    c. Signs and symptoms

       1) Edema

       2) Distended veins

       3) Increased blood pressure

       4) Bounding pulse

       5) Crackles; increased respiratory rate, shallow respirations

       6) Decreased hematocrit and BUN—normal: 10–20 mg/dL (adult); elderly is slightly higher

       7) Weight gain

    d. Nursing management

       1) Administration of diuretics

       2) Restriction of fluids

       3) Sodium-restricted diet (500 mg to 4 g salt diet)

       4) I and O

       5) Daily weight

       6) Assess breath sounds

       7) Check for edema feet/ankle/sacral region

       8) Semi-Fowler position if dyspneic

       9) Skin care

	Table 3-2	INTRAVENOUS FLUIDS
TYPE OF FLUID	**IV FLUID**	**NURSING CONSIDERATIONS FOR IVS**
Isotonic	0.9% NaCl Ringer's solution Lactated Ringer's 5% dextrose in water*	Main purpose—to maintain or restore fluid and electrolyte balance Secondary purpose—to provide a route for medication, nutrition, and blood components Type, amount, and sterility of fluid must be carefully checked
Hypotonic	0.45% NaCl	Macrodrip—delivers 10, 12, or 15 drops per milliliter; should be used if rapid administration is needed
Hypertonic	10–15% dextrose in water 3.0% NaCl Sodium bicarbonate 5%	Microdrip—deliver 60 drops per milliliter; should be used when fluid volume needs to be smaller or more controlled, e.g., clients with compromised renal or cardiac status, clients on "keep-open" rates, pediatric clients Maintain sterile technique Monitor rate of flow; set IV pump properly Assess for infiltration—cool skin, swelling, pain Assess for phlebitis—redness, pain, heat, swelling Change tubing every 72 hours, change bottle every 24 hours
*Becomes hypotonic as dextrose is metabolized		

ELECTROLYTE IMBALANCES

NOTE: Ranges may vary by resource or facility

POTASSIUM IMBALANCES

Main intracellular ion; involved in cardiac rhythm, nerve transmission (normal level 3.5–5 mEq/L [3.5–5 mmol/L])

(see Tables 3-3 and 3-4)

A. Hypokalemia (less than 3.5 mEq/L [3.5 mmol/L])
1. Causes
    a. Vomiting
    b. Gastric suction
    c. Prolonged diarrhea
    d. Diuretics and steroids
    e. Inadequate intake

2. Signs and symptoms
    a. Anorexia, nausea, vomiting
    b. Weak peripheral pulses
    c. Muscle weakness, paresthesias; decreased deep tendon reflexes
    d. Impaired urine concentration
    e. Ventricular dysrhythmias
    f. Potential for digitalis toxicity
    g. Shallow respirations

3. Nursing management
    a. Administration of oral potassium supplements—dilute in juice and give with meals to avoid gastric irritation
    b. Increase dietary intake—raisins, bananas, apricots, oranges, beans, potatoes, carrots, celery
    c. IV supplements—20–40 mEq/L usual concentration; cannot give concentration greater than 1 mEq/10 mL into peripheral IV, or without cardiac monitor; do not exceed 20 mEq/hour infusion rate; stop solution immediately if burning occurs
    d. Assess renal function prior to administration
    e. Risk for digitalis toxicity

B. Hyperkalemia (greater than 5 mEq/L [5 mmol/L])
1. Causes
    a. Renal failure
    b. Use of potassium supplements
    c. Burns
    d. Crushing injuries
    e. Severe infection

    f. Potassium-sparing diuretics

    g. ACE inhibitors

2. Signs and symptoms

    a. EKG changes–peaked T waves, wide QRS complexes

    b. Dysrhythmias, ventricular fibrillation, heart block

    c. Cardiac arrest

    d. Muscle twitching and weakness

    e. Numbness in hands and feet and around mouth

    f. Nausea

    g. Diarrhea

Table 3-3 ELECTROLYTE(S) MODIFIERS

AGENTS	ACTION
Alkalinizing	Release bicarbonate ions in stomach and secrete bicarbonate ions in kidneys
Calcium salts	Provide calcium for bones, teeth, nerve transmission, muscle contraction, normal blood coagulation, cell membrane strength
Hypocalcemic	Decrease blood levels of calcium
Hypophosphatemic	Bind phosphates in GI tract, lowering blood levels; neutralize gastric acid, inactivate pepsin
Magnesium salts	Provide magnesium for nerve conduction and muscle activity and activate enzyme reactions in carbohydrate metabolism
Phosphates	Provide body with phosphorus needed for bone, muscle tissue, metabolism of carbohydrates, fats, proteins, and normal CNS function
Potassium exchange resins	Exchange Na^+ for K^+ in intestines, lowering K^+ levels
Potassium salts	Provide potassium needed for cell growth and normal functioning of cardiac, skeletal, and smooth muscle
Replacement solution	Provide water and Na^+ to maintain acid-base and water balance, maintain osmotic pressure
Urinary acidifiers	Secrete H^+ ions in kidneys, making urine acidic
Urinary alkalinizers	Convert to sodium bicarbonate, making the urine alkaline

3. Nursing management

    a. Restrict dietary potassium and potassium-containing medications or IV solutions

    b. Sodium polystyrene sulfonate–cation-exchange resin (causes diarrhea)

        1) Orally–dilute to make more palatable

        2) Rectally–give in conjunction with sorbitol to avoid fecal impaction

    c. In emergency situation

        1) Calcium gluconate given IV

        2) Sodium bicarbonate given IV

    d. IV administration of regular insulin and dextrose shifts potassium into the cells

    e. Peritoneal or hemodialysis

    f. Diuretics

Table 3-4 ELECTROLYTES AND REPLACEMENT SOLUTIONS		
MEDICATION	**ADVERSE EFFECTS**	**NURSING CONSIDERATIONS**
Calcium carbonate Calcium chloride	Dysrhythmias Constipation	Foods containing oxalic acid (rhubarb, spinach), phytic acid (bran, whole cereals), and phosphorus (milk, dairy products) interfere with absorption Monitor EKG Take 1–1.5 hours pc if GI upset occurs
Magnesium chloride	Weak or absent deep tendon reflexes Hypotension Respiratory paralysis	Respirations should be greater than 16/min before medication given IV Test deep tendon and patellar reflexes before each dose Monitor I and O
Potassium chloride Potassium gluconate	Dysrhythmias, cardiac arrest Abdominal pain Respiratory paralysis	Monitor EKG and serum electrolytes Take with or after meals with full glass of water or fruit juice
Sodium chloride	Pulmonary edema	Monitor serum electrolytes

SODIUM IMBALANCES

Main extracellular ion; responsible for water balance (normal: 135–145 mEq/L [135-145 mmol/L])

A. Hyponatremia (less than 135 mEq/L [135 mmol/L])

1. Causes

   a. Vomiting

   b. Diuretics

   c. Excessive administration of dextrose and water IVs

   d. Burns, wound drainage

   e. Excessive water intake

   f. Syndrome of inappropriate antidiuretic hormone secretion (SIADH)

   g. Elderly—kidneys unable to excrete free water

2. Signs and symptoms

   a. Nausea

   b. Muscle cramps

   c. Confusion

   d. Muscular twitching, coma

   e. Seizures

   f. Headache

   g. Delirium in older adults

3. Nursing management
   a. Oral administration of sodium-rich foods—beef broth, tomato juice
   b. IV lactated Ringer's or high concentrations of NaCl (0.9%)
   c. Water restriction (safer method)
   d. I and O
   e. Daily weight

B. Hypernatremia (greater than 145 mEq/L [145 mmol/L])
   1. Causes
      a. Hypertonic tube feedings without water supplements
      b. Hyperventilation
      c. Diabetes insipidus
      d. Ingestion of OTC medications such as citric acid (1000 mg), aspirin (325 mg), or sodium bicarbonate
      e. Inhaling large amounts of saltwater (near drowning)
      f. Inadequate water ingestion

   2. Signs and symptoms
      a. Elevated temperature
      b. Weakness
      c. Disorientation
      d. Irritability and restlessness
      e. Thirst
      f. Dry, swollen tongue
      g. Sticky mucous membranes
      h. Postural hypotension with ↓ ECF
         Hypertension with normal or ↑ ECF
      i. Tachycardia
      j. Elderly—mental status changes, coma

   3. Nursing management
      a. IV administration of hypotonic solution—0.3% NaCl or 0.45% NaCl; 5% dextrose in water
      b. Offer fluids at regular intervals
      c. Decrease sodium in diet
      d. Daily weight

CALCIUM IMBALANCES

Need for blood clotting, skeletal muscle contraction (normal ionized serum calcium level: 4.6–5.1 mg/dL [1.15 to 1.27 mmol/L]; normal total serum calcium level: 8.2–10.2 mg/dL [2.05-2.55 mmol/L]); regulated by the parathyroid hormone and vitamin D, which facilitates reabsorption of calcium from bone and enhances reabsorption from the GI tract

A. Hypocalcemia (less than 4.6 mg/dL [1.15 mmol/L] {ionized serum calcium} or less than 8.2 mg/dL [2.05 mmol/L] {total serum calcium})

  1. Causes

    a. Hypoparathyroidism

    b. Pancreatitis

    c. Renal failure

    d. Steroids and loop diuretics

    e. Inadequate intake

    f. Post-thyroid surgery

  2. Signs and symptoms

    a. Nervous system becomes increasingly excitable

    b. Tetany

      1) Trousseau's sign—inflate BP cuff on upper arm to 20 mm Hg above systolic pressure, carpal spasms within 2–5 min indicate tetany

      2) Chvostek's sign—tap facial nerve 2 cm anterior to the earlobe just below the zygomatic arch; twitching of facial muscles indicates tetany

    c. Hyperactive reflexes

    d. Confusion

    e. Paresthesias

    f. Irritability

    g. Seizures

  3. Nursing management

    a. Orally—calcium gluconate (less concentrated) or calcium chloride; administer with orange juice to maximize absorption

    b. Parenterally—calcium gluconate

      1) Effect is transitory and additional doses may be necessary

      2) Caution with digitalized clients because both are cardiac depressants

      3) Calcium may cause vessel irritation and should be administered through a long, stable intravenous line

      4) Avoid infiltration because tissue can become necrotic and slough

      5) Administer at a slow rate to avoid high serum concentrations and cardiac depression

      6) Seizure precautions

      7) Maintain airway because laryngeal stridor can occur

      8) Safety needs due to confusion

      9) Increase dietary intake of calcium

      10) Calcium supplements

       11) Regular exercise

       12) Administer phosphate-binding antacids, calcitriol, vitamin D

B. Hypercalcemia (greater than 5.1 mg/dL [1.27 mmol/L] {ionized serum calcium} or greater than 10.2 mg/dL [2.55 mmol/L] {total serum calcium})

  1. Causes

    a. Malignant neoplastic diseases

    b. Hyperparathyroidism

    c. Prolonged immobilization

    d. Excessive intake

    e. Immobility

    f. Excessive intake of calcium carbonate antacids

  2. Signs and symptoms

    a. Lack of coordination

    b. Anorexia, nausea, and vomiting

    c. Confusion, decreased level of consciousness

    d. Personality changes

    e. Dysrhythmias, heart block, cardiac arrest

  3. Nursing management

    a. IV administration of 0.45% NaCl or 0.9% NaCl

    b. Encourage fluids

    c. Furosemide

    d. Calcitonin—decreases calcium level

    e. Mobilizing the client

    f. Dietary calcium restriction

    g. Prevent development of renal calculi

       1) Increase fluid intake

       2) Maintain acidic urine

       3) Prevent urinary tract infection

    h. Injury prevention

    i. Limit intake of calcium carbonate antacids

    j. Surgical intervention may be indicated in hyperparathyroidism (cause of hypercalcemia)

       1) Preoperatively—directed toward preventing dangerously high serum calcium levels

       2) Postoperatively

          a) Observe for signs of hypocalcemia (reverse of preop)

          b) Due to calcium drop postop, large quantities of calcium salts may be required

          c) Encourage early ambulation to aid in recalcification of bones

MAGNESIUM IMBALANCE

Interdependent with calcium (normal: 1.3–2.1 mEq/L) (0.65-1.05 mmol/L)

A. Hypomagnesemia (less than 1.3 mEq/L [0.65 mmol/L])

1. Causes
   a. Alcoholism
   b. GI suction
   c. Diarrhea
   d. Intestinal fistulas
   e. Poorly controlled diabetes mellitus
   f. Malabsorption syndrome

2. Signs and symptoms
   a. Increased neuromuscular irritability
   b. Tremors
   c. Tetany
   d. Hyperactive deep tendon reflexes
   e. Seizures
   f. Dysrhythmias especially if hypokalemia present
   g. Disorientation
   h. Confusion

3. Nursing management
   a. Increased intake of dietary Mg—green vegetables, nuts, bananas, oranges, peanut butter, chocolate
   b. Parenteral administration of supplements—magnesium sulfate
      1) Monitor cardiac rhythm and reflexes to detect depressive effects of magnesium
      2) Keep self-inflating breathing bag, airways, and oxygen at bedside in case of respiratory emergency
      3) Calcium preparations may be given to counteract the potential danger of myocardial dysfunction that may result from magnesium intoxication secondary to rapid infusions
   c. Oral—long-term maintenance with oral magnesium
   d. IV—assess renal function
   e. Monitor for digitalis toxicity
   f. Seizure precautions
   g. Safety measures for confusion
   h. Test ability to swallow before PO fluids/food because of dysphagia

B. Hypermagnesemia (greater than 2.1 mEq/L [1.05mmol/L])—potent vasodilator

1. Causes
   a. Renal failure
   b. Excessive magnesium administration (antacids, cathartics)

2. Signs and symptoms
   a. Depresses the CNS
   b. Depresses cardiac impulse transmission
   c. Cardiac arrest
   d. Facial flushing
   e. Muscle weakness
   f. Absent deep tendon reflexes
   g. Paralysis
   h. Shallow respirations

3. Nursing management
   a. Discontinue oral and IV Mg
   b. Emergency
      1) Support ventilation
      2) IV calcium gluconate
   c. Hemodialysis
   d. Monitor reflexes
   e. Teach regarding over-the-counter medications containing Mg
   f. Monitor respiratory status
   g. Monitor cardiac rhythm; have calcium preparations available to antagonize cardiac depressant

NURSING MEASURES FOR INTRAVENOUS THERAPY

PURPOSE

A. Main—to maintain or restore fluid and electrolyte balance

B. Secondary—to provide a route for medication, nutrition, and blood components

EQUIPMENT

A. Solution

  1. Type, amount, and sterility of fluid must be carefully checked

    a. If sterility is compromised, bacteria will be introduced directly into the bloodstream

    b. Fluid overload is possible

      1) Isotonic

        a) 0.9% NaCl

        b) Ringer's solution

        c) Lactated Ringer's

      2) Hypotonic

        a) 5% dextrose in water (is isotonic but becomes hypotonic when glucose is metabolized)

        b) 0.45% NaCl

      3) Hypertonic

        a) 10–15% dextrose in water

        b) 3% NaCl

        c) Sodium bicarbonate 5%

        d) 5% dextrose in 0.9% saline

B. Equipment

  1. Administration set—plays important role in the amount of fluid the client receives

    a. Macrodrip—can deliver 10, 12, or 15 drops per milliliter; should be used if rapid administration is needed

    b. Microdrip—delivers 60 drops per milliliter; should be used when fluid volume needs to be smaller or more controlled, e.g., clients with compromised renal or cardiac status, clients on "keep-open" rates, and pediatric clients

  2. Cannula, catheter, wing-tipped needle or angiocath

  3. Skin prep, tape, IV, pole, arm board, tourniquet

  4. Controller or pump, if indicated

Table 3-5 CALCULATIONS FOR IV RATE

1) Milliliters per hour:

$$\frac{\text{Total solution}}{\text{Hours to run}} = \text{mL/h}$$

Example: 1000 mL in 8 hours

$$\frac{1000}{8} = 125 \ \text{mL/h}$$

2) Drops per minute:

$$\frac{\text{Total volume} \times \text{Drop factor}}{\text{Time in minutes}} = \text{gtts} \Big/ \text{min}$$

Example: 1000 mL in 8 hours, with a drop factor of 15

$$\frac{1000 \times 15}{8 \times 60} =$$

$$\frac{1000 \times 1}{8 \times 4} =$$

$$\frac{250}{8} =$$

31.25 or 31 gtts / min

PROCEDURE TO BEGIN INTRAVENOUS THERAPY

A. Peripheral IV

1. Location
   a. Condition of vein
   b. Type of fluid/med to be infused
   c. Duration of therapy
   d. Client's age, size, stability
   e. Skill of nurse

2. Insertion of catheter
   a. Explain procedure, check ID
   b. Distend veins by applying tourniquet 4–6" above site, tap on vessel or have client open and close fist, or hang arm over side of bed
   c. Clean site; press applicator against skin and use back-and-forth friction to scrub for at least 30 seconds
   d. Repeat cleaning with povidone-iodine or antiseptic solution
   e. Hold skin taut to stabilize vein
   f. Insert catheter bevel up at 15–20° (direct method—thrust catheter through skin and vein in one smooth motion; indirect method—first pierce skin, then vessel)
   g. Lessen the angle and advance catheter; watch for flashback of blood
   h. Once blood return observed, advance catheter 1/4" and then remove tourniquet
   i. Withdraw needle from catheter; advance catheter up to hub
   j. Secure catheter
   k. Attach IV tubing
   l. Begin IV infusion
   m. Check for infiltration or hematoma

3. Complications
   a. Infiltration—fluid into tissue
      1) Assessment
         a) Edema
         b) Pain
         c) Coolness in area
         d) Decrease in flow rate
      2) Nursing management
         a) Discontinue IV
         b) Apply warm compresses to infiltrated site
         c) Apply sterile dressing
         d) Elevate arm
         e) Start IV at new site proximal to infiltrated site if same extremity used; may use different vein distal to infiltrated site (basilic or cephalic)
   b. Phlebitis—inflammation of vein
      1) Assessment
         a) Reddened, warm area around insertion site or on path of vein
         b) Tenderness
         c) Swelling
      2) Nursing management
         a) Discontinue IV
         b) Apply warm, moist compresses
         c) Restart IV at new site
   c. Thrombophlebitis—inflammation of vein with clot
      1) Assessment
         a) Pain at insertion site or above site
         b) Swelling
         c) Redness and warmth around insertion site or along path of vein
         d) Fever
         e) Leukocytosis

2) Nursing management
   a) Discontinue IV
   b) Apply warm compress
   c) Elevate the extremity
   d) Restart the IV

d. Circulatory Overload
   1) Assessment
      a) Crackles
      b) Dsypnea
      c) Confusion
      d) Seizures

   2) Nursing Care
      a) Reduce IV rate
      b) Assess VS
      c) Assess lab values
      d) Notify health care provider

e. Hematoma
   1) Assessment
      a) Ecchymosis
      b) Immediate swelling at site
      c) Leakage of blood at site

   2) Nursing management
      a) Discontinue IV
      b) Apply pressure with sterile dressing
      c) Apply cool compresses (or ice bag) for 24 hours to site, followed by warm compresses
      d) Restart IV

f. Clotting
   1) Assessment
      a) Decreased IV flow rate or absent flow rate
      b) Backflow of blood into IV tubing

   2) Nursing management
      a) Discontinue IV
      b) Do not irrigate or milk the tubing
      c) Do not increase the IV flow rate or hang the solution higher
      d) Do not aspirate clot from the cannula
      e) Urokinase may be injected into catheter to clear occlusion

FACTORS AFFECTING FLOW RATE

A. Circulatory physiology
  1. Structures
     a. Arteries—originate in the aorta or its branches; transport blood to the systemic circulation

      1) Aorta—assists the flow of blood to the arteries or acts as a reservoir for blood during ejection of the ventricles

      2) Pulmonary artery—originates in the right ventricle and transports unoxygenated blood from the circulation to the lungs to be oxygenated (only artery carrying unoxygenated blood)

  b. Veins—carry unoxygenated blood and body wastes from the systemic circulation to the right atrium by way of the inferior and superior vena cava; valves help to direct the flow of blood toward the heart

  c. Capillaries—small vessels

2. Circulation

  a. Oxygenated blood leaves left ventricle, travels though aorta and arterioles (smaller branches)

  b. Unoxygenated blood returns to the right side of heart by inferior and superior vena cava

  c. Coronary circulation—circulation to the myocardium

  d. Peripheral circulation—circulation through the periphery (extremities)

3. Factors regulating circulation

  a. Nervous system—regulates heart rate, influences arteriolar constriction and blood pressure

     1) Neural reflexes are controlled via the vasomotor center in the medulla oblongata; there are four centers:

       a) Vasoconstrictor center—reduces diameter of blood vessels

       b) Vasodilator center—increases diameter of blood vessels

       c) Cardioaccelerator center—increases heart rate

       d) Cardioinhibitory center—decreases heart rate

     2) The four centers are stimulated or inhibited by the following:

       a) Pressoreceptors (baroreceptors)—specialized nerve endings affected by changes in pressure of blood in arteries

       b) Chemoreceptors—located in the aortic arch and carotid bodies; sensitive to oxygen lack, increased blood carbon dioxide, and decreased pH

       c) Medullary ischemic reflex—produces vasoconstriction of small blood vessels in response to stimulation of the vasoconstrictor center by CO_2 excess and oxygen lack

4. Blood pressure—the pressure exerted by the blood against the walls of vessels

  a. Arterial blood pressure (pressure exerted against arterial wall)

     1) Systolic blood pressure—maximum pressure of blood exerted against the arterial wall when the heart is contracting

     2) Diastolic blood pressure—force of blood exerted against the wall of the artery when the heart is at rest

     3) Pulse pressure—difference between diastolic and systolic blood pressure; normal is 30–40 mm Hg

     4) Circulatory factors influencing arterial pressure

       a) Cardiac output—increase causes increased blood pressure; decrease causes decreased blood pressure

       b) Peripheral resistance (afterload)—narrowed arterioles increase blood pressure; dilated arterioles decrease blood pressure

       c) Arterial elasticity—elastic vessels accommodate to changes in blood flow; rigid sclerotic vessels cause increases in systolic blood pressure and pulse pressure

      d) Blood volume (preload)—decreased blood volume (e.g., due to hemorrhage) results in decreased pressure

      e) Blood viscosity—increased viscosity (e.g., due to overabundance of RBC) results in high pressure; decreased viscosity (e.g., due to anemia) results in lower pressure

   5) Other factors influencing pressure

      a) Age—increases with age

      b) Weight—increases with excess weight

      c) Emotions—increases with release of epinephrine (caused by strong emotion)

      d) Exercise—extreme physical activity increases pressure

CENTRAL VENOUS ACCESS DEVICES (CVAD) (3 TYPES)

A. Peripherally Inserted Central Catheter (PICC)

1. Venipuncture performed above or below antecubital fossa into basilic, cephalic, or axillary veins of dominant arm (encourages blood flow and reduces risk of dependent edema)

2. Tip of catheter is in superior vena cava or brachiocephalic veins

3. May be single, double, or triple lumen

4. May stay in place up to weeks to months

5. Potential complications

   a. Malposition

   b. Dysrhythmias

   c. Nerve or tendon damage

   d. Respiratory distress

   e. Catheter embolism

   f. Thrombophlebitis

6. Nursing management

   a. No blood pressure or phlebotomy affected arm

   b. Change dressing 2–3 times/wk, and when wet or non-occlusive

   c. Flush with saline or heparinized saline according to agency policy

B. Tunneled Central Catheters

1. Increases in size (2 gauges, 2.5 cm in length) 2 hours after insertion, becomes softer

2. Venipuncture 2–3 finger breadths above antecubital fossa or 1 finger breadth below antecubital fossa into cephalic, basilic, or median cubital vein

3. Long-term use; may stay in place for years

4. Catheter may be single or double lumen; examples: Hickman, Groshong, Permacath

5. Complications

   a. Thrombosis

   b. Phlebitis

   c. Air embolism

   d. Infection

   e. Bleeding

   f. Vascular perforation

6. Nursing management

   a. Change dressing 2–3 times/wk, and when wet or non-occlusive

    b. Flush with normal saline alone or with normal saline followed by heparinized saline according to agency policy

    c. Anchor catheter securely

    d. Avoid chemotherapy or parenteral nutrition

C. Non-tunneled Percutaneous Central Catheters

  1. Inserted through subclavian vein; tip in superior vena cava

  2. Non-tunneled central catheters; 7 to 10 inches long

    a. Used for short-term IV therapy

    b. Inserted by health care provider

    c. Triple-lumen central catheter—distal lumen (16 gauge) used to infuse or draw blood samples; middle lumen (18-gauge) used for PN infusion; proximal lumen (18-gauge) used to infuse or draw blood and administer medications

  3. Implanted infusion port

    a. Used for long-term home IV therapy

    b. End of catheter attached to chamber placed in subcutaneous pocket on client's chest wall or forearm

    c. Use Huber needle to access port

    d. Example: Hickman

  4. Insertion

    a. Placed supine in head-low position (dilates vessel and prevents air embolism)

    b. Client turns head away from site during procedure

    c. While catheter is being inserted, client performs Valsalva maneuver

    d. Antibiotic ointment and transparent dressing applied using sterile technique

    e. Verify position of tip of catheter by x-ray

    f. Each lumen secured with Luer-Lok cap and labeled to indicate location (proximal, middle, distal)

  5. Nursing management

    a. Catheter changed according to agency policy

    b. Flush with normal saline alone or with normal saline followed by heparinized saline according to agency policy; flushed also after each infusion, specimen withdrawal, medication administration, or when disconnected

    c. Never use force to flush catheter; if resistance met, notify health care provider

    d. Dressing changes 2–3 times/wk and PRN; place in low-fowler position; nurse and client wear masks; alcohol and then iodine swabs used to clean site

    e. Change IV tubing every 72 to 96 hours according to agency policy

BLOOD TRANSFUSIONS

A. Overview

  1. Purposes

    a. Restore blood volume following hemorrhage, burns, or injuries to blood vessels

    b. Combat shock

    c. Treat severe chronic anemia by increasing the oxygen–carrying capacity of the blood

2. Equipment—blood or blood product, normal saline (0.9% NaCl), tubing with filter, 19-gauge needle for venous access (see Table 3-6)

Table 3-6 BLOOD COMPONENTS		
PRODUCT	ADVERSE REACTIONS	NURSING CONSIDERATIONS
Packed red cells	Reactions less common than with whole blood	Companion solution—0.9% NaCl Use standard blood filter Give over 2–4 hours
Platelets	Some febrile reactions	Companion solution—0.9% NaCl Nonwettable filter Give as quickly as possible, 4 units/hour
Plasma	Circulatory overload risk	Administer with straight line set Give as quickly as possible (coagulation factors become unstable)
Albumin	Circulatory overload risk	Use administration set provided 25% albumin—give at 1 mL/min Give as quickly as possible if client in shock
Prothrombin	Hepatitis risk greater than with whole blood Allergic/febrile reactions	Use straight line set
Factor VIII	Allergic and febrile reactions	Use component drip set or syringe

3. Procedure
   a. Ask client about any allergies or previous blood reactions (see Table 3-8)
   b. Type and cross-match blood—ensures that the donor's blood and recipient's blood are compatible (see Table 3-7)
   c. Check blood for bubbles, dark color, or cloudiness
   d. Change entire IV line for each unit of blood
   e. ID checks by two nurses
      1) Health care provider's order
      2) Hospital ID band name and number
      3) Blood component tag name and number matched to client
      4) Blood type and Rh

Table 3-7 BLOOD GROUP COMPATIBILITY		
BLOOD GROUP	CAN ACT AS DONOR TO	CAN RECEIVE BLOOD FROM
O	O, A, B, AB	O
A	A, AB	O, A
B	B, AB	O, B
AB	AB	O, A, B, AB

Table 3-8 BLOOD TRANSFUSION REACTIONS			
TYPE OF REACTION	**CAUSE**	**SYMPTOMS**	**NURSING CONSIDERATIONS**
Allergic reaction Hypersensitivity	Hypersensitivity to antibodies in donor's blood	Occurs immediately or within 24 hours Mild–urticaria, itching, flushing Anaphylaxis– hypotension, dyspnea, decreased oxygen saturation, flushing	Prevention–premedicate with antihistamines Stop the transfusion Restart the 0.9% NaCl Notify the health care provider Supportive care: diphenhydramine, oxygen, corticosteroids
Acute Intravascular Hemolytic reaction	Incompatibility	Occurs within minutes to 24 hours Nausea, vomiting, pain in lower back, hypotension, increase in pulse rate, decrease in urinary output, hematuria	Stop the transfusion Supportive care: oxygen, diphenhydramine, airway management
Febrile non-hemolytic reaction (most common)	Antibodies to donor platelets or leukocytes	Occurs in minutes to hours Fever, chills, nausea, headache, flushing, tachycardia, palpitations	Stop the transfusion Supportive care Aspirin Seen with clients after multiple transfusions
Sepsis	Contaminated blood products	Occurs within minutes to less than 24 hours Tachycardia, hypotension, fever, chills, shock	Stop the transfusion Obtain blood culture Antibiotics, IV fluids, vasopressors, steroids
Circulatory overload	Large volume over short time	Occurs within minutes to hours–dyspnea, crackles, increased respiratory rate, tachycardia	Monitor clients at high-risk (elderly, heart disease, children) Slow or discontinue transfusion

f. Check baseline vital signs, including temperature

g. Start with normal saline (0.9% NaCl)

h. Run blood slowly for first 15 min

i. Stay with client 15–30 min

j. Recheck vital signs 15 min after infusion started

k. If no untoward effects, increase rate

l. Take vital signs every hour until completed, then hourly for 3 hours

m. Ask client to report itching or flank pain over kidneys

BURN MANAGEMENT

A. Types

1. Thermal—contact with hot substance (solids/liquids/gases)

2. Chemical—contact with strong acids or strong bases; prolonged contact with almost any chemical

   3. Electrical—contact with live current; internal damage may be more severe than expected from external injury

   4. Radiation—exposure to high doses of radioactive material

B. Emergency care—on the scene
   1. Stop the burning process
      a. Thermal—smother; stop, drop, and roll
      b. Chemical—remove clothing and flush/irrigate skin/eyes
      c. Electrical—shut off electrical current or separate person from source with a nonconducting implement

   2. Ensure airway, breathing, and circulation
   3. Immediate wound care; keep client warm and dry; wrap in clean, dry sheet/blanket

C. Assessment
   1. Extent of the burn—"Rule of Nines" (see Figure III-2 for adult; see Figure III-3 for child less than 10 years old; formula is used to determine body surface
   2. Determination of intensity (see Table 3-9)

D. Nursing management (see Table 3-10)
   1. Fluid replacement
      a. Emergent/Resuscitative phase (first 24–48 hours)
         1) IV fluids to replace fluid losses; balanced salt solution (lactated Ringer's) to avoid over/under hydration
            a) Rapid for first 8 hours
            b) More slowly over remaining 16 hours

         2) Plasma to increase blood volume and to increase O_2

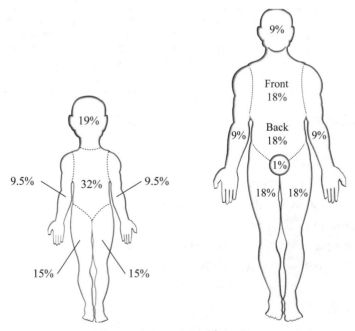

Figure 3-2. CHILD/ADULT

Table 3-9 CLASSIFICATION OF BURNS				
SUPERFICIAL	SUPERFICIAL PARTIAL-THICKNESS	DEEP PARTIAL-THICKNESS	FULL-THICKNESS	DEEP FULL-THICKNESS
Similar to first-degree	Similar to second-degree	Similar to second-degree	Similar to third-degree	Similar to third-degree
Skin pink to red Painful	Skin pink to red Painful	Skin red to white Painful	Skin red, white, brown, black Pain possible	Skin black No pain
Epidermis Sunburn	Epidermis and dermis Scalds, flames	Epidermis and dermis Scalds, flames, tar, grease	All skin layers Prolonged contact with hot objects	All skin layers, possibly muscles and tendon Flames, electricity
Heals in 3 to 5 days	Heals in 2 weeks	Heals in 1 month Possible grafting	Heals in weeks to months	Heals in weeks to months Escharotomy Grafting

2. Acute/Intermediate phase (2–5 days postburn)
   a. Water and electrolytes to maintain Na$^+$ and K$^+$
   b. Packed RBC to maintain O_2 carrying capacity

3. Indwelling catheter to monitor hourly output; should be at least 30 mL/h; weigh daily

4. NG tube to prevent gastric distention, early acute gastric dilation, and paralytic ileus associated with burn shock; monitor bowel sounds; H2 histamine blockers and antacids to prevent a Curling's ulcer

5. Pain medication (morphine)—given IV at first due to impaired circulation and poor absorption from muscles/subcutaneous tissue; monitor VS frequently; analgesic 30 minutes before wound care

6. Tetanus prophylaxis; tetanus immune globulin when history of immunization is questionable

7. Avoidance of hypothermia—warm and humid environment

8. Frequent regular and routine monitoring of VS

9. Clean, safe environment; meticulous hand hygiene; cap, gown, mask, gloves worn by nurse

10. Wound care—early and continuous
    a. Debridement (removal of nonviable tissue)—hydrotherapy is used to loosen dead tissue, 30 minutes maximum; hydrotherapy tank, spray table, tubbing, under as clean conditions as possible (gown, gloves, masks, hat, plastic disposable tub liner)
    b. Escharotomy (incising of leathery covering of dead tissue conducive to bacterial growth)—used to alleviate constriction; minimize infection
    c. Dressing
       1) Wound may be covered or left exposed
       2) Application of topical antibacterial medications
          a) Silver sulfadiazine (Silvadene)—closed method; monitor for hypersensitivity, rash, itching, burning sensation in areas other than burn; decreased WBC
          b) Mafenide (Sulfamylon)—open method; monitor acid/base balance and renal function; remove previously applied cream
          c) Silver nitrate—keep dressings wet with solution to avoid overconcentrations; handle carefully, can leave a gray/black stain
    d. Early excision of burn followed by grafting
       1) Biological (human amniotic membrane, cadaver, allograft)
       2) Synthetic
       3) Autografting when granulation bed is clean and well vascularized
11. Diet—high caloric, high carbohydrate, high protein; may require TPN or tube feeding at first; oral nutrient supplements; vitamins B and C; iron, possibly zinc (excretion of increased zinc may cause loss of taste)
12. Administration of antacid to prevent stress ulcer (Curling's ulcer)
13. Control of itching—a major problem with healing
14. Psychological counseling
15. Prevent contractures—maintain joints in neutral position of extension; shoes to prevent foot drop; splints; active and passive ROM exercises at each dressing change; turn side to side frequently; skin care to prevent breakdown
16. Assist client in coping with immobilization, pain, and isolation
17. Prepare client for discharge—anticipate readmission for release of contractures/cosmetic surgery; proper use of any correctional orthopedic appliances/pressure garments; how to change dressings

Table 3-10 NURSING CARE FOR BURN CLIENT	
GOAL	**NURSING CONSIDERATIONS**
Correct fluid and electrolyte imbalance	First 24–48 hours (emergent/resuscitative phase): • IV fluids balanced salt solution (LR), plasma After calculation of 24-hours replacement: Rapid for first 8 hours, more slowly over remaining 16 hours • 1/2 delivered in first 8 hours, 1/4 over second 8 hours, and 1/4 over third 8 hours 2–5 days after burn (acute/intermediate phase): • Packed RBCs • Indwelling catheter to monitor hourly output; should be at least 30 mL/h • Careful administration of IV fluids; check for signs of fluid overload vs. dehydration • Monitor blood pressure, TPR, wt, serum electrolytes
Promote healing	Cap, gown, mask, gloves worn by nurse Wound care at least once a day Debridement (removal of nonviable tissue)—hydrotherapy is used to loosen dead tissue, 30 min maximum Escharotomy (incising of leathery covering of dead tissue conducive to bacterial growth)—used to alleviate constriction, minimize infection Dressing: careful sterile technique, avoid breaking blisters, wound may be covered or left exposed Application of topical antibacterial medications: Silver sulfadiazine (Silvadene)—closed method; monitor for hypersensitivity, rash, itching, burning sensation in areas other than burn, decreased WBC; Mafenide (Sulfamylon)—open method; monitor acid/base balance and renal function; remove previously applied cream; Silver nitrate—keep dressings wet with solution to avoid over concentrations; handle carefully; can leave a gray/black stain Grafting: biological (human amniotic membrane, cadaver, allograft); autografting when granulation bed is clean and well vascularized Tetanus prophylaxis Avoid hypothermia and add humidity
Support nutrition	High-caloric, high-carbohydrate, high-protein diet; may require TPN or tube feeding; oral nutrient supplements; vitamins B, C, and iron; H2 histamine blockers and antacids to prevent stress ulcer (Curling's ulcer) NG tube to prevent gastric distention, early acute gastric dilation, and paralytic ileus associated with burn shock; monitor bowel sounds
Control pain	Pain medication (morphine)—given IV at first due to impaired circulation and poor absorption Monitor VS frequently; analgesic 30 min before wound care

Table 3-10 NURSING CARE FOR BURN CLIENT *(CONTINUED)*	
GOAL	NURSING CONSIDERATIONS
Prevent complications of immobility	Prevent contractures—maintain joints in neutral position of extension; shoes to prevent foot drop; splints; active and passive ROM exercises at each dressing change; turn side to side frequently; skin care to prevent breakdown
	Stryker frame or Circ-O-Lectric bed may facilitate change of position
	Facial exercises and position that hyperextends neck for burns of face and neck
	Consult with physical therapist
Support client	Counsel client regarding change in body image
	Encourage expression of feelings and demonstrate acceptance of client
	Evaluate client's readiness to see scarred areas, especially facial area
	Assist client's family to adjust to changed appearance
	Consider recommending client for ongoing counseling
	Support developmental needs of children, e.g., sick children need limits on behavior
	Assist client in coping with immobilization, pain, and isolation
	Prepare client for discharge—anticipate readmission for release of contractures/cosmetic surgery; proper use of any correctional orthopedic appliances, pressure garments (used to decrease scarring); how to change dressings

Chapter 4

THE CARDIOVASCULAR SYSTEM

Sections	Concepts Covered
1. The Cardiovascular System Overview	Perfusion
2. Alterations in Cardiac Output	Perfusion, Fluid and Electrolyte Balance
3. Vascular Alterations: Hypertension	Perfusion
4. Selected Disorders of Tissue Perfusion	Perfusion
5. Vascular Disorders	Perfusion

THE CARDIOVASCULAR SYSTEM OVERVIEW

ANATOMY

A. Circulation—functions
1. Delivers oxygen, nutrients, hormones, and antibodies to organs, tissues, and cells
2. Removes end products of metabolism from tissue and cells

B. Heart—functions
1. Pumps oxygenated blood into arterial system to supply capillaries and tissues
2. Pumps oxygen-poor blood from the venous system through the lungs to be reoxygenated

C. Blood vessels (arteries, capillaries, veins)—function is to carry blood to and from the body's tissues and cells

D. Structure of the heart—cone-shaped, hollow, muscular organ located in the mediastinum (space between lungs in the thoracic cavity) (see Figure 4-1)
1. Base directed toward the body's right side
2. Apex directed toward the left, resting on the diaphragm
3. Two-sided double pump
   a. Right side receives deoxygenated blood from the body and pumps it to the lungs
   b. Left side receives oxygenated blood from the lungs and pumps it through the aorta to the body

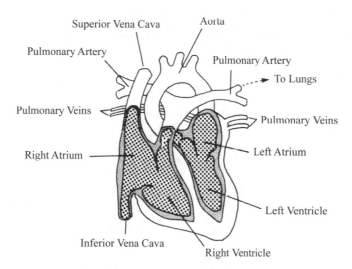

Figure   4-1.   THE HUMAN HEART

4. Pericardium—loose-fitting membrane or fibroserous covering of the heart
5. Cardiac layers
   a. Epicardium—outer layer
   b. Myocardium—middle layer; composed of striated muscle fibers; myocardial fibers stiffen with age
   c. Endocardium—innermost layer; continuous with the blood vessels, lining the heart's cavities and valves

6. Cardiac chambers
   a. Atria (auricles)—two upper "receiving" chambers
      1) Right atrium—receives deoxygenated blood from body via superior and inferior venae cavae and pumps into right ventricle
      2) Left atrium—receives oxygenated blood from lungs and pumps into left ventricle
      3) Interatrial septum separates the atria
      4) Elderly—atrial stretching and distension
   b. Ventricles—two lower "distributing" chambers
      1) Right ventricle—receives blood from right atrium and pumps out to lung via pulmonary artery
      2) Left ventricle (largest, most muscular chamber)—receives oxygenated blood from left atrium and pumps out blood to body
      3) Ventricular septum separates the ventricles

7. Cardiac valves provide for one-way flow of blood
   a. Atrioventricular valves—tricuspid and mitral valves
      1) Tricuspid valve guards opening between right atrium and ventricle (prevents backflow)
      2) Mitral valve guards opening between left atrium and ventricle (prevents backflow)
   b. Semilunar valves—prevent backflow into ventricles
      1) Pulmonary semilunar valve (between pulmonary artery and right ventricle)
      2) Aortic semilunar valve (between aorta and left ventricle)

8. Coronary arteries—disease of these arteries is leading cause of death in the United States (see Figure 4-2)
   a. Left coronary arteries—supply the left ventricle, septum, and apex
   b. Right coronary arteries—supply the right ventricle and the SA node
   c. Elderly—coronary arteries narrow

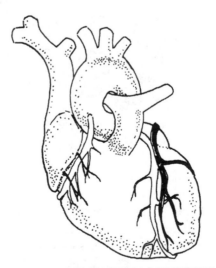

Figure 4-2. CORONARY BLOOD VESSELS

CARDIAC FUNCTION

A. Cardiac contraction

1. Regulation of rate and rhythm—special properties of cardiac muscle

   a. Rhythmicity—rhythm in the formation and conduction of electrical impulses from atria to ventricles

   b. Irritability (excitability)—ability of cardiac muscle cells to respond to stimuli

      1) All or nothing law—irritated muscle responds to stimuli with strongest possible contraction

      2) Adequate oxygen supply, normal neural and hormonal functioning, and balanced diet are essential to maintaining normal function

      3) Drug therapy, infection, lack of oxygen, and disruptions in neural and hormonal balances can increase irritability and result in conduction disturbances

   c. Refractory mechanism—prevents heart muscle from responding to a new stimulus while still in a state of contraction from an earlier stimulus, thereby maintaining rhythm

      1) Absolute refractory period—will not respond to new stimuli of any magnitude

      2) Relative refractory period—muscle begins to be ready for new stimuli; regains irritability

   d. Conductivity—ability of cardiac muscle fibers to transmit electrical impulses

   e. Contractility—shortening of the cardiac muscle fibers in response to a stimulus; occurs rhythmically and is followed by a relaxation period corresponding to the filling and emptying of the cardiac chambers

   f. Automaticity—ability of the heart to beat spontaneously and repetitively without external neurohormonal control; linked to fluid and electrolyte balance rather than to nervous system control

   g. Extensibility (expansibility)—ability of heart muscle to expand (stretch) while the chambers fill with blood between muscle contractions

      1) Starling's Law—the greater the stretch (expansion) of cardiac muscle, the more forceful the contraction of the heart

      2) Overstretched muscle can result in alterations in filling and decrease forcefulness of contraction

B. Cardiac conduction system—composed of modified cardiac muscle cells able to conduct electrical impulses; controlled by autonomic nervous system (ANS); sympathetic branch increases rate while parasympathetic branch slows rate

1. Sinoatrial node (SA node) or pacemaker—site of impulse initiation 60–100/min (see Figure 4-3)

   a. Located at junction of superior vena cava and right atrium

   b. Regulates heart rate, rhythm, and regularity

   c. Other components of conduction pathway have potential to discharge impulses independently; however, the SA node releases impulses more rapidly and therefore assumes control over the process

   d. Elderly—decreased number of SA cells; possible decreased heart rate

2. Atrioventricular node (AV node or AV junction)—(see Figure 4-3)
    a. Located in base of right atrium
    b. Receives impulses from SA node and delays them slightly
    c. Generates impulses when SA node fails (at a rate of approximately 40 to 60 beats per minute)
    d. Elderly—decreased number of AV node cells

3. Bundle of His (Purkinje system)—continuous with AV node; bundle of His also known as AV bundle
    a. Composed of special cardiac muscle fibers that originate in the AV node, then break into left and right bundle branches that extend down the interventricular septum, where they are continuous with Purkinje fibers
    b. Relays impulses from AV node to ventricles
    c. Purkinje fibers enable electrical impulses responsible for myocardial contraction to spread rapidly over all parts of the ventricles
    d. Elderly—decreased number of Purkinje system cells

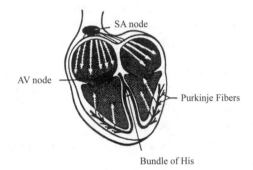

Figure   4-3. SA NODES AND AV NODES

C. Cardiac cycle—equivalent to one complete heartbeat
    1. Two parts
        a. Systole—contraction of (ejection of blood from) both atria and then both ventricles; initiated by release of impulse by SA node
        b. Diastole—relaxation and filling of both atria and then both ventricles

    2. Cardiac output—stroke volume × heart rate
        a. Stroke volume—amount of blood ejected with each beat
        b. Heart rate—number of beats per minute

    3. Cardiac output depends upon
        a. Preload
        b. Afterload
        c. Contractility
        d. Age—decreased beta receptor responsiveness with age; altered autonomic nervous system control

D. Cardiac reserve—ability of the heart to adjust to increased demands from stresses such as exercise, excitement, fever, cold, acceleration, deceleration, or disease states; elderly may have significantly decreased cardiac reserve, especially with decreased blood volume, febrile conditions, infections, cardiac dysrhythmias

VASCULAR SYSTEM

A. Structure

1. Arteries—originate in the aorta or its branches; transport blood to the systemic circulation
   a. Aorta—assists the flow of blood to the arteries or acts as a reservoir for blood during ejection of the ventricles
   b. Pulmonary artery—originates in the right ventricle and transports deoxygenated blood from the circulation to the lungs to be oxygenated (only artery carrying deoxygenated blood)

2. Gerontologic considerations—loss of arterial elasticity, blood vessel lumen narrows

3. Veins
   a. Carry deoxygenated blood and body waste from the systemic circulation to the right atrium by way of the inferior and superior vena cava
   b. Superior vena cava and inferior vena cava—largest veins in the body; bring deoxygenated blood from the upper and lower body to the right atrium
   c. Pulmonary veins—return oxygenated blood from the lungs to the left atrium (only vein carrying oxygenated blood)

4. Capillaries
   a. Arterioles—smallest arteries
   b. Venules—smallest veins

5. Layers
   a. Tunica intima—smooth lining of blood vessel
   b. Tunica media—muscle layer
   c. Tunica adventitia—connective tissue binds vessels to adjacent structures

6. Veins have valves to ensure unidirectional blood flow

B. Function (physiology)

1. Oxygenated blood leaves left ventricle, travels though aorta and arterioles (smaller branches)
2. Deoxygenated blood returns to the right side of heart by inferior and superior venae cavae
3. Coronary circulation—circulation to the myocardium
4. Peripheral circulation—circulation through the periphery (extremities)
   a. Delivers oxygen, nutrients, hormones, and antibodies to organs, tissues, and cells
   b. Removes end products of metabolism from tissues and cells

C. Mechanics

1. Autonomic nervous system—regulates heart rate, influences arteriolar constriction and blood pressure
   a. Neural reflexes are controlled via vasomotor center in the medulla oblongata
   b. Stimulation and inhibition of the circulatory system
      1) Pressoreceptors (baroreceptors)—specialized nerve endings affected by changes in pressure of blood in arteries
      2) Chemoreceptors—located in the aortic arch and carotid bodies; sensitive to lack of oxygen, increased blood CO_2, and decreased pH
      3) Medullary ischemic reflex—produces vasoconstriction of small blood vessels in response to stimulation of the vasoconstrictor center by excess CO_2 and lack of oxygen

    c. Sympathetic branch ("fight or flight")
       1) Increases blood pressure, heart rate, respiratory rate, blood glucose, and blood flow to the muscles of the legs
       2) Inhibits blood flow to the GI tract

    d. Parasympathetic branch ("rest and relax")
       1) Counterbalances the sympathetic branch to maintain blood pressure, heart rate, and respiratory rate within normal limits
       2) Stimulates blood flow to the GI tract

2. Blood pressure—the pressure exerted by the blood against the walls of vessels
    a. Systolic blood pressure—maximum pressure of blood exerted against the arterial wall when the heart is contracting
    b. Diastolic blood pressure—lowest pressure of blood exerted against the wall of the artery when the heart is at rest
    c. Pulse pressure—difference between systolic and diastolic blood pressure

D. Factors affecting cardiovascular performance
1. Cardiac output
    a. Preload—ventricular end-diastolic pressure (VEDP)
       1) Venous return—increased return increases VEDP
       2) End-systolic volume—increased volume increases VEDP
       3) Frank-Starling law of the heart—within a physiologic range of muscle contraction, increased preload will increase cardiac output; excessive preload will decrease cardiac output

    b. Afterload—resistance to ejection of blood from the left ventricle; correlates with aortic systolic pressure; increased afterload increases myocardial oxygen demand
    c. Myocardial contractility—determined by preload, sympathetic nervous stimulation, myocardial oxygen supply
    d. Heart rate—tachycardia or bradycardia decrease cardiac output

ALTERATIONS IN CARDIAC OUTPUT

CARDIOPULMONARY ARREST

A. Assessment—breathless, pulseless, unconscious

B. Analysis

1. Failure to institute ventilation within 4 to 6 minutes will result in cerebral anoxia and brain damage

2. Purpose of cardiopulmonary resuscitation (CPR)—to reestablish CO_2/O_2 exchange and adequate circulation so oxygenated blood can be delivered to vital organs

C. Plan/Implementation

1. Basic Life Support

   a. Recognition
      1) All ages: unresponsive
      2) Adults: no breathing or no normal breathing (e.g., only gasping)
      3) Children and infants: no breathing or only gasping
      4) No pulse palpated within 10 seconds

   b. Activate EMS system

   c. CPR sequence: C-A-B

   d. Compression rate: 100 to 120/minute for all populations

   e. Compression depth
      1) Adults: at least 2 inches (5 cm)
      2) Children: at least ⅓ anterior posterior diameter or about 2 inches (5 cm)
      3) Infants: at least ⅓ anterior posterior diameter or about 1½ inches (4 cm)

   f. Chest wall recoil
      1) Allow complete recoil between compressions
      2) HCPs rotate compressors every 2 minutes, or sooner if fatigued

   g. Compression interruptions
      1) Minimize interruptions in chest compressions
      2) Attempt to limit interruptions to less than 10 seconds

   h. Airway
      1) Head tilt-chin lift
      2) HCP suspected trauma; jaw thrust

   i. Compression-to-ventilation ratio (until advance airway placed)
      1) Adult: 30:2; 1 or 2 rescuers
      2) Children and infants: 30:2 single rescuer; 15:2 2 HCP rescuers

   j. Ventilations when rescuer untrained or trained and not proficient: compressions only

k. Ventilations with advanced airway (HCP)
   1) 1 breath every 6 seconds (10 breaths/minute)
   2) Avoid excessive ventilation; can cause gastric inflation and subsequent regurgitation and aspiration, increased intrathoracic pressure, decreased venous return to the heart, diminished cardiac output, and reduced blood flow to the brain secondary to cerebral vasoconstriction
   3) Asynchronous with chest compressions
   4) Visible chest rise

l. Defibrillation
   1) Attach and use AED as soon as possible for ventricular fibrillation and pulseless ventricular tachycardia
   2) Shock energy for defibrillation: initial dose of 120 to 200 J when using biphasic device; 360 J when using monophasic device
   3) Resume CPR beginning with compressions immediately after each shock

m. Medications
   1) Asystole or pulseless electrical activity (PEA): Epinephrine 1 mg IV or IO every 3 to 5 minutes.
   2) Ventricular fibrillation or pulseless ventricular tachycardia that is unresponsive to defibrillation: Amiodarone 300 mg bolus IV or IO as first dose, 150 mg bolus IV or IO as second dose, if indicated **or** lidocaine 1 to 1.5 mg/kg IV or IO as first dose, 0.5 to 0.75 mg/kg IV or IO as second dose, if indicated

n. Reversible causes
   1) Hypovolemia
   2) Hypoxia
   3) Hydrogen ion (acidosis)
   4) Hypo-/hyperkalemia
   5) Hypothermia
   6) Tension pneumothorax
   7) Tamponade, cardiac
   8) Toxins
   9) Thrombosis, pulmonary
   10) Thrombosis, cardiac

2. Continue CPR until one of the following occurs
   a. Victim responds
   b. Another qualified person takes over
   c. Victim is transferred to an emergency room
   d. Rescuer is physically unable to continue

DISTURBANCES IN CARDIAC OUTPUT

A. Heart disease

B. EKG interpretation (see Figures 4-4 and 4-5)

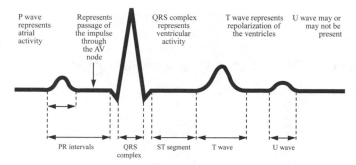

Figure 4-4. COMPONENTS OF AN EKG

1. Determine rate
   a. Count the number of 0.2-s intervals between two R waves, divide by 300
   b. Count the number of R-R intervals in 6 seconds, multiply by 10 (only for regular rhythm)

2. Determine rhythm
   a. Presence or absence of P wave—SA node originated impulse
   b. Measure P-R interval—normal: 0.12–0.20 s
   c. Measure QRS duration—normal: less than 0.12 s
   d. Check P wave, QRS complex, ST segment, and T wave

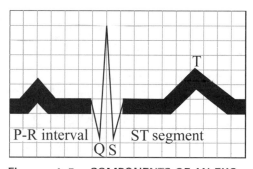

Figure 4-5. COMPONENTS OF AN EKG

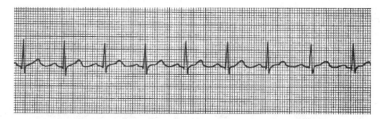

Figure 4-6. RULES FOR NORMAL SINUS RHYTHM

Regularity: The R-R intervals are constant; the rhythm is regular.

Rate: The atrial and ventricular rates are equal; heart rate is between 60 and 100 beats per minute.

P wave: The P waves are uniform. There is one P wave in front of every QRS complex.

PRI: The PR interval measures between 0.12 and 0.20 s.
QRS: The QRS complex measures less than 0.12 s.

Table   4-1   CARDIAC DISORDERS CLASSIFIED BY PHYSIOLOGICAL DISTURBANCE

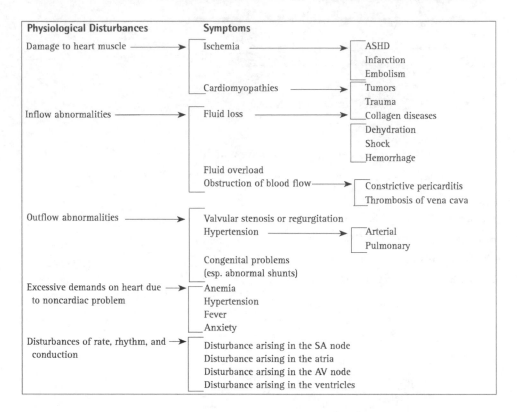

Physiological Disturbances	Symptoms	
Damage to heart muscle	Ischemia	ASHD Infarction Embolism
	Cardiomyopathies	Tumors Trauma
Inflow abnormalities	Fluid loss	Collagen diseases Dehydration Shock Hemorrhage
	Fluid overload	
	Obstruction of blood flow	Constrictive pericarditis Thrombosis of vena cava
Outflow abnormalities	Valvular stenosis or regurgitation	
	Hypertension	Arterial Pulmonary
	Congenital problems (esp. abnormal shunts)	
Excessive demands on heart due to noncardiac problem	Anemia Hypertension Fever Anxiety	
Disturbances of rate, rhythm, and conduction	Disturbance arising in the SA node Disturbance arising in the atria Disturbance arising in the AV node Disturbance arising in the ventricles	

RHYTHM DISTURBANCES (DYSRHYTHMIAS)

(refer to Figures 4-7 through 4-18)

A. Assessment

1. Dizziness, syncope

2. Chest pain, palpitations

3. Nausea, vomiting

4. Dyspnea

5. Abnormal rate—increased, decreased, or irregular

6. Abnormal heart sounds

B. Analysis

1. Caused by interruption in normal conduction process

2. Can occur at any point in the normal conduction pathway

3. Are accompanied by alterations in myocardial tissues, automaticity, regularity, and excitability: these changes can result in hemodynamic alterations affecting the force of contraction and overall cardiac output

4. Types of dysrhythmias

   a. <u>Sinus dysrhythmias</u> —dysrhythmias originate in the SA node and are conducted along the normal conductive pathways

      1) *Tachycardia* —sympathetic nervous system increases the automaticity of the SA node

         a) Heart rate is increased above 100 beats per minute

         b) Causes include pain, exercise, hypoxia, pulmonary embolism, hemorrhage, hyperthyroidism, or fever

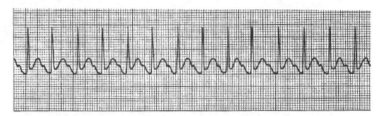

Figure 4-7. RULES FOR SINUS TACHYCARDIA

Regularity:	The R-R intervals are constant; the rhythm is regular.
Rate:	The atrial and ventricular rates are equal; heart rate is greater than 100 beats per minute (usually between 100 and 160 beats per minute).
P wave:	There is a uniform P wave in front of every QRS complex.
PRI:	The PR interval measures between 0.12 and 0.20 s; the PRI measurement is constant across the strip.
QRS:	The QRS complex measures less than 0.12 s.

      2) *Bradycardia* —parasympathetic nervous system (vagal stimulation) causes automaticity of the SA node to be depressed

         a) Heart rate decreased to below 60 beats per minute

         b) Causes—myocardial infarction, the Valsalva maneuver, or vomiting; arteriosclerosis in the carotid sinus area; ischemia of SA node; hypothermia; hyperkalemia; depression or medications such as digitalis and propranolol

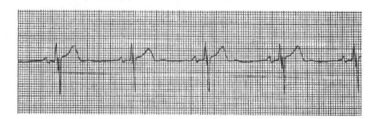

Figure 4-8. RULES FOR SINUS BRADYCARDIA

Regularity:	The R-R intervals are constant; the rhythm is regular.
Rate:	The atrial and ventricular rates are equal; heart rate is less than 60 beats per minute.
P wave:	There is a uniform P wave in front of every QRS complex.
PRI:	The PR interval measures between 0.12 and 0.20 s; the PRI measurement is constant across the strip.
QRS:	The QRS complex measures less than 0.12 s.

b. <u>Atrial dysrhythmias</u> —abnormal electrical activity that results in stimulation outside the SA node but within the atria

1) *Premature atrial contractions (PAC)*

a) Ectopic focus within one of the atria fires prematurely

b) Normal phenomenon in some individuals but may be caused by emotional disturbances, fatigue, tobacco, or caffeine

c) May be early sign of abnormal electrical activity associated with organic heart disease

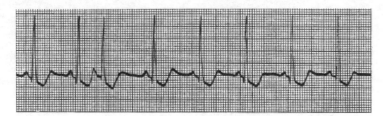

Figure 4-9. RULES FOR PREMATURE ATRIAL CONTRACTION

Regularity: Because this is a single premature ectopic beat, it will interrupt the regularity of the underlying rhythm.

Rate: The overall heart rate will depend on the rate of the underlying rhythm.

P wave: The P wave of the premature beat will have a different morphology than the P waves of the rest of the strip. The ectopic beat will have a P wave, but it can be flattened, notched, or otherwise unusual. It may be hidden within the T wave of the preceding complex.

PRI: The PRI should measure between 0.12 and 0.20 s but can be prolonged; the PRI of the ectopic beat will probably be different from the PRI measurements of the other complexes.

QRS: The QRS complex measurement will be less than 0.12 s.

2) *Paroxysmal atrial tachycardia (PAT)*

a) Rapid rhythmic discharge of impulses originating from an ectopic focus within the atria, followed by a normal ventricular response at a rate of 160 to 250 beats per minute

b) If prolonged, the period of ventricular filling is shortened, stroke volume is reduced, and cardiac output is diminished, possibly resulting in pump failure, hypotension, and additional dysrhythmias

c) Causes—atrial muscle ischemia, rheumatic heart disease, acute myocardial infarction, psychological factors (e.g., anxiety, stress, emotional trauma), decrease in potassium (leads to cardiac irritability), smoking, caffeine, ingestion of large meals

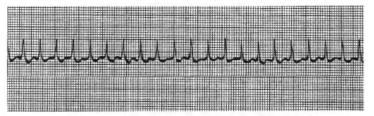

Figure 4-10. RULES FOR ATRIAL TACHYCARDIA

Regularity: The R-R intervals are constant; the rhythm is regular.

Rate: The atrial and ventricular rates are equal; the heart rate is usually 150–250 beats per minute.

P wave: There is one P wave in front of every QRS complex. The configuration of the P wave will be different from that of sinus P waves; they may be flattened or notched. Because of the rapid rate, the P waves can be hidden in the T waves of the preceding beats.

PRI: The PRI is between 0.12 and 0.20 s and constant across the strip. The PRI may be difficult to measure if the P wave is obscured by the T wave.

QRS: The QRS complex measures less than 0.12 s.

3) *Atrial flutter*

a) Arises from an ectopic focus in the atrial wall causing the atrium to contract 250 to 400 times per minute

b) AV node blocks most of the impulse, thereby protecting the ventricles from receiving every impulse

c) Some clients are unaware of this dysrhythmia, whereas others complain of palpitations or fainting

d) Causes—stress, hypoxia, medications, or disorders such as chronic heart disease, hypertension

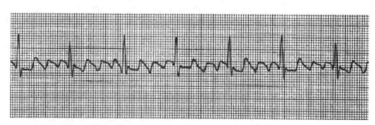

Figure 4–11. **RULES FOR ATRIAL FLUTTER**

Regularity: The atrial rhythm is regular. The ventricular rhythm will be regular if the AV node conducts impulses in a consistent pattern. If the pattern varies, the ventricular rate will be irregular.

Rate: Atrial rate is between 250 and 350 beats per minute. Ventricular rate will depend on the ratio of impulses conducted through to the ventricles.

P wave: When the atria flutter, they produce a series of well-defined P waves. When seen together, these "flutter" waves have a sawtooth appearance.

PRI: Because of the unusual configuration of the P wave (flutter wave) and the proximity of the wave to the QRS complex, it is often impossible to determine a PRI in this dysrhythmia. Therefore, the PRI is not measured in atrial flutter.

QRS: The QRS complex measures less than 0.12 s; measurement can be difficult if one or more flutter waves is concealed within the QRS complex.

4) *Atrial fibrillation*

   a) Most common atrial dysrhythmia arising from several ectopic foci

   b) Client presents with a grossly irregular pulse rate

   c) Confusion, syncope, and dizziness may occur with severe hypoxia; pump failure may result

   d) Causes include chronic lung disease, heart failure, and rheumatic heart disease, hypertension

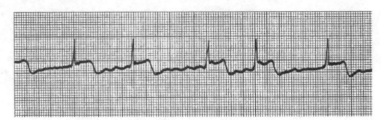

Figure 4-12. RULES FOR FIBRILLATION

Regularity:	The atrial rhythm is unmeasurable; all atrial activity is chaotic. The ventricular rhythm is grossly irregular, having no pattern to its irregularity.
Rate:	The atrial rate cannot be measured because it is so chaotic; research indicates that it exceeds 350 beats per minute. The ventricular rate is significantly slower because the AV node blocks most of the impulses. If the ventricular rate is below 100 beats per minute, the rhythm is said to be "controlled"; if it is over 100 beats per minute, it is considered to have a "rapid ventricular response."
P wave:	In this dysrhythmia the atria are not depolarizing in an effective way; instead, they are fibrillating. Thus, no P wave is produced. All atrial activity is depicted as "fibrillatory" waves, or grossly chaotic undulations of the baseline.
PRI:	Because no P waves are visible, no PRI can be measured.
QRS:	The QRS complex measurement should be less than 0.12 s.

c. <u>Ventricular dysrhythmias</u> —occur when one or more ectopic foci arise within the ventricles

   1) *Premature ventricular contractions (PVC)*

      a) One or more ectopic foci stimulate a premature ventricular response

      b) May decrease the efficiency of the heart's pumping action

      c) Palpitations, a feeling of irregular heartbeat, or a "lump in the throat"

      d) Causes—ischemia due to a myocardial infarction, infection, mechanical damage due to pump failure, deviations in concentrations of electrolytes (e.g., potassium, calcium), nicotine, coffee, tea, alcohol, medications such as digitalis and reserpine, psychogenic factors (stress, anxiety, fatigue), and acute or chronic lung disease

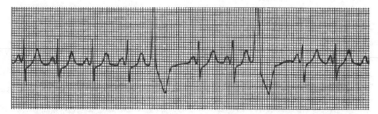

Figure 4-13. RULES FOR PREMATURE VENTRICULAR CONTRACTIONS

Regularity: The underlying rhythm can be regular or irregular. The ectopic PVC will interrupt the regularity of the underlying rhythm (unless the PVC is interpolated).

Rate: The rate will be determined by the underlying rhythm. PVCs are not usually included in the rate determination because they frequently do not produce a pulse.

P wave: The ectopic is not preceded by a P wave. You may see a coincidental P wave near the PVC, but it is dissociated.

PRI: Because the ectopic comes from a lower focus, there will be no PRI.

QRS: The QRS complex will be wide and bizarre, measuring at least 0.12 s. The configuration will differ from the configuration of the underlying QRS complexes. The T wave is frequently in the opposite direction from the QRS complex.

2) *Ventricular tachycardia*
   a) Three or more PVCs occurring in a row
   b) Indicative of severe myocardial irritability
   c) Physical effects include chest pain, dizziness, fainting, occasional collapse

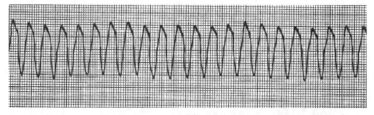

Figure 4-14. RULES FOR VENTRICULAR TACHYCARDIA

Regularity: This rhythm is usually regular, although it can be slightly irregular.

Rate: Atrial rate cannot be determined. The ventricular rate range is 150–250 beats per minute. If the rate is below 150 beats per minute, it is considered a slow VT. If the rate exceeds 250 beats per minute, it's called ventricular flutter.

P wave: None of the QRS complexes will be preceded by P waves. You may see dissociated P waves intermittently across the strip.

PRI: Because the rhythm originates in the ventricles, there will be no PRI.

QRS: The QRS complexes will be wide and bizarre, measuring at least 0.12 s. It is often difficult to differentiate between the QRS and the T wave.

3) *Ventricular fibrillation*

   a) Most serious of all dysrhythmias due to potential cardiac standstill; death will occur if not treated

   b) Several ectopic foci within the ventricles are discharged at a very rapid rate

   c) Causes—acute myocardial infarction, hypertension, rheumatic or arteriosclerotic heart disturbances, hypoxia, accidental electrical shock, and hyperkalemia

   d) Unless blood flow is restored by CPR and the dysrhythmia is interrupted (by defibrillation), death will result within 90 s to 5 min

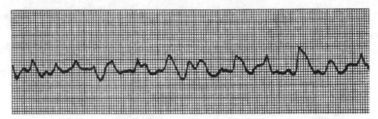

Figure   4–15.   RULES FOR VENTRICULAR FIBRILLATION

Regularity:	There are no waves or complexes that can be analyzed to determine regularity. The baseline is totally chaotic.
Rate:	The rate cannot be determined because there are no discernible waves or complexes to measure.
P wave:	There are no discernible P waves.
PRI:	There is no PRI.
QRS:	There are no discernible QRS complexes. No cardiac output. Clinical death.

d. <u>Heart block</u> —delay in the conduction of impulses within the AV system

   1) *Bundle branch block*

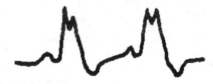

   a) Right or left branches of the bundle of His are blocked, causing the impulses to change their path of conduction or pass through the myocardial tissue

   b) Cause—myocardial ischemia or digitalis toxicosis

   c) Left bundle branch tends to be more serious and may indicate left-sided heart problems

   2) *First-degree AV block* —AV junction conducts all impulses, but duration of AV conduction is prolonged

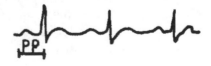

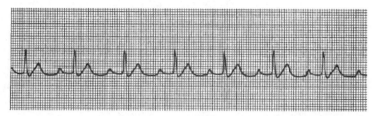

Figure 4-16. RULES FOR FIRST-DEGREE HEART BLOCK

Regularity: This will depend on the regularity of the underlying rhythm.

Rate: The rate will depend on the rate of the underlying rhythm.

P wave: The P waves will be upright and uniform. Each P wave will be followed by a QRS complex.

PRI: The PRI will be constant across the entire strip, but it will always be greater than 0.20 seconds.

QRS: The QRS complex measurement will be less than 0.12 s.

3) *Second-degree AV block* —type I and type II; AV junction conducts only some impulses arising in the atria

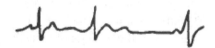

a) Causes—infections, digitalis toxicosis, coronary artery disease

b) Symptoms—slow heart rate, fainting, decreased blood pressure

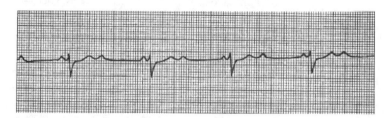

Figure 4-17. RULES FOR CLASSIC SECOND-DEGREE HEART BLOCK

Regularity: If the conduction ratio is consistent, the R-R interval will be constant, and the rhythm will be regular. If the conduction ratio varies, the R-R will be irregular.

Rate: The atrial rate is usually normal. Because many of the atrial impulses are blocked, the ventricular rate will usually be in the bradycardia range, often one-half, one-third, or one-fourth of the atrial rate.

P wave: P waves are upright and uniform. There are always more P waves than QRS complexes.

PRI: The PRI on conducted beats will be constant across the strip, although it might be longer than a normal PRI measurement.

QRS: The QRS complex measurement will be less than 0.12 s.

4) *Third-degree (complete) heart block*
   a) AV junction blocks all impulses to the ventricles, causing the atria and ventricles to dissociate and beat independently (each with its own pacemaker establishing a rate; ventricular rate is low, 20 to 40 beats per minute)
   b) Causes—congenital defects, vascular insuffiency, fibrosis of the myocardial tissue, or myocardial infarction
   c) Symptoms—palpitations, dizziness, syncope, dyspnea, mental confusion, and cyanosis
   d) If not treated immediately, may lead to death

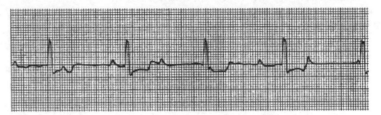

Figure   4-18.   RULES FOR THIRD-DEGREE HEART BLOCK

Regularity: Both the atrial and the ventricular foci are firing regularly; thus the P–P intervals and the R-R intervals are regular.

Rate: The atrial rate will usually be in a normal range. The ventricular rate will be slower. If a junctional focus is controlling the ventricles, the rate will be 40–60 beats per minute. If the focus is ventricular, the rate will be 20–40 beats per minute.

P wave: The P waves are upright and uniform. There are more P waves than QRS complexes.

PRI: Because the block at the AV node is complete, none of the atrial impulses is conducted through to the ventricles. There is no PRI. The P waves have no relationship to the QRS complexes. You may occasionally see a P wave superimposed on the QRS complex.

QRS: If the ventricles are being controlled by a junctional focus, the QRS complex will measure less than 0.12 s. If the focus is ventricular, the QRS will measure 0.12 s or greater.

C. Plan/Implementation
   1. Vital signs
   2. Cardiac monitor—identify any changes in rhythm and rate
   3. Medications
      a. Antidysrhythmic (see Table 4–2)

   4. *Provide or assist with emergency treatment*
      a. Precordial shock—electric current delivered to the heart through either externally placed paddles (closed chest procedure) or paddles applied directly to myocardium during surgery (open chest procedure); used to halt life-threatening and dangerous dysrhythmias
         1) Defibrillation—paddles placed over right sternal border and over the apex of the heart (see Table 4-3)
            a) Used in treatment of ventricular fibrillation
            b) Completely depolarizes all myocardial cells so SA node can be pacemaker
            c) Nursing responsibilities

i.   Start CPR before defibrillation

ii.   Plug in defibrillator and turn on

iii.   Turn on monitor and attach leads to client

iv.   Be sure synchronizer switch is turned off

v.   Apply gel or paste to paddles (rub paddle surfaces together)

Table 4-2 ANTIDYSRHYTHMIC MEDICATION		
MEDICATION	**ADVERSE EFFECTS**	**NURSING CONSIDERATIONS**
Class IA		
Quinidine Procainamide Disopyramine	Hypotension Heart failure	Monitor blood pressure Monitor for widening of the PR, QRS, or QT intervals Toxic effects ,has limited use
Class IB		
Lidocaine	CNS: slurred speech, confusion, drowsiness, confusion, seizures Hypotension and bradycardia	Monitor for CNS adverse effects Monitor BP and heart rate and cardiac rhythm
Class IC		
Flecainide Propafenone hydrochloride	Bradycardia Hypotension Dysrhythmias CNS: anxiety, insomnia, confusion, seizures	Monitor for increasing dysrhythmias Monitor heart rate and blood pressure Monitor for CNS effects
Class II		
Beta Blockers Propranolol Acebutolol Esmolol hydrochloride	Bradycardia and hypotension Bronchospasm Increase in heart failure Fatigue and sleep disturbances	Monitor apical heart rate, cardiac rhythm, and blood pressure Assess for shortness of breath and wheezing Assess for fatigue, sleep disturbances Assess apical heart rate for 1 minute before administration
Class III		
Amiodarone hydrochloride Ibutilide fumarate	Hypotension Bradycardia and atrioventricular block Muscle weakness, tremors Photosensitivity and photophobia Liver toxicity	Continuous monitoring of cardiac rhythm during IV administration Monitor QT interval during IV administration Monitor heart rate, blood pressure during initiation of therapy Instruct client to wear sunglasses and sunscreen
Class IV		
Calcium Channel Blockers Verapamil Diltiazem hydrochloride	Bradycardia Hypotension Dizziness and orthostatic hypotension Heart failure	Monitor apical heart rate and blood pressure Instruct clients about orthostatic precautions Instruct clients to report signs of heart failure to health care provider

       vi.   Select electric charge as ordered—360 joules

      vii.   Position paddles on chest wall; one to right of sternum just below clavicle, the other to the left of the precordium

    viii.   Person with paddles calls "all clear"

      ix.   Push discharge button

       x.   Check carotid pulse

      xi.   Sodium bicarbonate given to treat acidosis

2) Cardioversion (see Table 4-3)
   a) Elective procedure for dysrhythmias such as atrial fibrillation
   b) Nursing responsibilities
      i. Informed consent
      ii. Diazepam or Midazolam IV
      iii. Voltage 25–360 watts/s
      iv. Digoxin withheld for 48 hours prior to procedure
      v. Synchronizer turned on, check at the R wave
      vi. Oxygen discontinued
      vii. Assess airway patency
      viii. Assess vital signs every 15 min for 1 hour; every 30 min for 2 hours; then every 4 hours
   c) Implantable cardioverter–defibrillator available for clients at risk for sudden cardiac death

3) Pacemakers—electronic apparatus used to initiate heartbeat when the SA node is seriously damaged and unable to act as a pacemaker
   a) Types of pacemakers (see Table 4-4)
      i. Internal or implantable—stimulating electrodes placed inside the chest wall
      ii. External—stimulating electrodes placed outside the chest wall
      iii. Temporary—usually external
      iv. Permanent—electrode wire inserted percutaneously and threaded through to the ventricle; battery pack is implanted under skin
   b) Major methods of cardiac pacing
      i. Rate responsiveness pacemaker—allows faster pacing rates to meet increased bodily demands
      ii. Demand pacemakers—fire on demand or when necessary to stimulate ventricular contraction; advantageous for clients who are frequently in normal sinus rhythm but suffer periods of bradycardia or syncope
   c) Technical problems associated with cardiac pacing
      i. Dislodgement and migration of endocardial leads
      ii. Wire breakage
      iii. Cracking of insulation surrounding wires
      iv. Infection of sites surrounding either pacing wires or pulse generator
      v. Battery exhaustion

Table 4-3	DEFIBRILLATION VERSUS CARDIOVERSION	
	DEFIBRILLATION	CARDIOVERSION
Indication	Emergency treatment of ventricular fibrillation	Elective procedure for dysrhythmias such as atrial fibrillation
Action	Completely depolarizes all myocardial cells so SA node can re-establish as pacemaker	Same
Nursing considerations	Start CPR before defibrillation Plug in defibrillator and turn on Turn on monitor and attach leads to client Apply gel or paste to paddles (rub paddle surfaces together) Select electric charge as ordered Paddles placed over right sternal border and over the apex of the heart Person with paddles calls "all clear" Push discharge button Check monitor between shocks for rhythm Don't stop to check pulse after shocks, continue CPR, intubate, start IV Epinephrine given 1 mg IV push every 3-5 min Sodium bicarbonate given to treat acidosis	Informed consent Diazepam or Midazolam IV Digoxin withheld for 48 hours prior to procedure Synchronizer turned on, check at the R wave Oxygen discontinued Assess airway patency Plug in defibrillator and turn on Turn on monitor and attach leads to client Apply gel or paste (rub paddle surfaces together) Voltage 25-360 joules Paddles placed over right sternal border and over the apex of the heart Person with paddles calls "all clear" Push discharge button Check monitor between shocks for rhythm After procedure, assess vital signs every 15 min for 1 hour; every 30 min for 2 hours; then every 4 hours

   d) Nursing responsibilities

      i. Assess for infection

      ii. Monitor heart rate and rhythm

      iii. Provide emotional support

      iv. Teaching

         • Check pulse daily, report any sudden increase or decrease

         • Carry ID card

         • Request hand-scanning at security check points at airports

         • Periodic checking of generator

         • Take frequent rest periods at home and at work

         • Avoid the use of electrocautery devices, ungrounded power tools, large electrical devices

D. Evaluation—client is free from dysrhythmias as evidenced by regular and stable vital signs

Table 4-4 PACEMAKERS			
TYPES	ACTION	COMPLICATIONS	NURSING CONSIDERATIONS
Demand (synchronous; noncompetitive)	Functions when heart rate goes below set rate	Dislodgment and migration of endocardial leads	Assess for infection, bleeding
Fixed rate (asynchronous; competitive)	Stimulates ventricle at preset constant rate	Wire breakage	Monitor heart rate and rhythm; for preset rate pacemakers, client's rate may vary 5 beats above or below set rate
		Cracking of insulation surrounding wires	Provide emotional support
Temporary	Used in emergency situations (after MI with heart block, cardiac arrest with bradycardia)	Infection of sites surrounding either pacing wires or pulse generator	Check pulse daily, report any sudden increase or decrease in rate
	Inserted through peripheral vein, tip of catheter is placed at apex of right ventricle	Interference with pacemaker function by exposure to electro-magnetic fields (old microwave ovens, MRI equipment, metal detectors at airports)	Carry ID card or wear identification
Permanent	Lead is passed into right ventricle, or right atrium and right ventricle, and generator is implanted under skin below clavicle or in abdominal wall	Perforation of myocardium or right ventricle	Request hand scanning at security check points at airports
		Abrupt loss of pacing	Avoid situations involving electro-magnetic fields
			Periodically check generator
			Take frequent rest periods at home and at work
			Wear loose clothing over area of pacemaker
			All electrical equipment used in vicinity of client should be properly grounded
			Immobilize extremity if temporary electrode pacemaker is used to prevent dislodgement
			Document model of pacemaker, date and time of insertion, location of pulse generator, stimulation threshold, pacer rate
			Place cellular phone on side opposite the generator

HEART FAILURE (HF)

Clinical syndrome resulting from structural or functional cardiac disorders that impair the ability of a ventricle to fill or eject blood

A. Assessment—symptoms result from a decrease in cardiac output and involve congestion of either the pulmonary circulatory system, the venous system, or both; almost all manifestations of HF affect tissues and organs that are located away from the heart (e.g., lungs, kidney, brain, liver, and extremities)

1. Left-sided heart failure—develops as a result of left ventricular dysfunction, which causes blood to back up through the left atrium and into the pulmonary veins

   a. Dyspnea—results from pulmonary congestion due to pulmonary engorgement; poor gas exchange because of fluid in the alveoli, resulting in shortness of breath and air hunger

   b. Orthopnea—shortness of breath occurring when the client is in a recumbent position

   c. Paroxysmal nocturnal dyspnea—occurs when client is asleep

    d. Cheyne-Stokes respirations—exact cause in HF unknown; believed that they occur as a result of prolonged circulation time between the pulmonary circulation and the central nervous system, which in turn affects the respiratory center

    e. Pleural effusion and pulmonary edema—results from severe pulmonary congestion, causing distended capillaries, which leak fluid into the interstitial and alveolar spaces of the lungs

    f. Cough and cardiac asthma—cough productive of large amounts of frothy, blood-tinged sputum results from edema fluid trapped within the pulmonary tree, irritating the delicate mucosa of the lungs

    g. Decreased renal function, edema, and weight gain—kidney function is adversely affected by the development of HF, resulting in sodium and water retention; sequence of events leading to edema is as follows:

       1) Decreased cardiac output results in decreased arterial pressure in the kidneys, reducing glomerular filtration and output of sodium chloride and water

       2) Reduced circulating blood volume triggers an increase in aldosterone secretion by the adrenal cortex, thereby increasing the rate of reabsorption of sodium by renal tubules

       3) Increased sodium reabsorption results in increased concentration of extracellular fluid

       4) Increased osmotic pressure causes an increase in the release of antidiuretic hormone (ADH) from the neurosecretory cells of the hypothalamus, resulting in increased tubular reabsorption of water

       5) Final result is edema

    h. Cerebral anoxia—develops because of the decrease in cardiac output to the brain, which causes irritability, restlessness, and a shortened attention span

    i. Fatigue and muscular weakness—decreased cardiac output diminishes oxygen to tissues and decreases the speed with which metabolic wastes are swept up into the circulation for excretion, thereby creating profound exhaustion

    j. S_3 gallop

    k. b-type natriuretic peptide levels increased

    l. Microalbuminuria

    m. Elderly—may have atypical manifestations (e.g., falls, delirium, chronic cough, weight loss)

2. Right-sided heart failure—develops from a diseased right ventricle that causes backward flow to right atrium and venous circulation; almost always follows left-sided failure due to the stress placed on the right ventricle as it attempts to pump blood against resistance into the congested lungs; venous congestion causes peripheral edema and congestion of organs

    a. Liver enlargement and abdominal pain—as the liver becomes congested with venous blood, it enlarges; stretching of the capsule surrounding the liver causes severe discomfort in the right upper quadrant

    b. Anorexia, nausea, and bloating—secondary to venous congestion of the gastrointestinal tract (anorexia and nausea may also result from digitalis toxicity, a common problem because digitalis is a major drug in treating heart failure)

    c. Dependent edema—early signs of right-sided heart failure include edema of ankles and lower extremities, resulting from venous congestion of kidneys producing compensatory vasoconstriction that decreases renal blood flow, impairing sodium excretion

    d. Coolness of extremities—venous congestion throughout the body reduces peripheral blood flow, often causing coolness of extremities and cyanosis of nail beds

    e. Anxiety and fear—most individuals with heart failure feel anxious and depressed about their condition

    f. Weight gain

  3. Advanced heart failure

    a. Weight loss and cachexia—low cardiac output and venous congestion create malnutrition of tissues, although client may appear puffy and bloated due to edema

    b. Shock syndrome—typical clinical picture of shock usually appears during terminal stages of HF

      1) Stupor

      2) Pallor

      3) Rapid, thready pulse

      4) Cold sweats

      5) Restlessness

      6) Profound hypotension

B. Etiology

  1. Conditions that predispose heart to gradual failure

    a. Inflow of blood to the heart is reduced due to hemorrhage or dehydration

    b. Inflow of blood to the heart is increased due to excessive IV fluids or sodium and water retention

    c. Outflow of blood from the heart is obstructed due to damaged valves and narrowed arteries

    d. The heart muscle is damaged from ischemia or inflammatory processes

    e. The metabolic needs of the body are increased as a result of fever or pregnancy

  2. Diseases that lead to heart failure (see Table 4-5)

  3. Factors that may precipitate heart failure in individuals with diseased hearts

    a. Pregnancy and childbirth

    b. Severe tachycardia or bradycardia

    c. Great mental strain

    d. Sudden elevation of the environmental temperature and humidity

  4. Three major mechanisms to compensate for pathological changes in output

    a. Ventricular dilation—increase in the length of muscle fibers, creating an increase in the volume of the heart chambers

      1) According to Starling's law, a stretched muscle contracts more forcefully; therefore, dilation causes an increased systolic output within limits

      2) This compensatory mechanism is limited because if stretched beyond a certain point, muscle fibers cease to increase contractile power of the heart and because a greatly dilated heart requires more oxygen to meet its metabolic needs, resulting, in time, in hypoxia of the heart muscle

    b. Ventricular hypertrophy—increase in diameter of muscle fibers creating a thickening of the walls of the chambers and a corresponding increase in the weight of the heart

      1) Generally follows persistent dilation, further increasing the contractile power of muscle fibers

      2) Limited compensatory mechanism because in time increased muscle mass of heart outgrows coronary blood supply and becomes hypoxic

    c. Tachycardia—least effective compensatory mechanism because when heart rate becomes too rapid, the ventricles are unable to fill adequately, with resultant hypotension and shock

5. Cardiac decompensation occurs when the heart is unable to cope with the work demands placed upon it and thus expends most of its reserve

6. Diagnosing heart failure
   a. Presence of characteristic symptoms
   b. Muffled heart sounds
   c. Abnormal heart sounds (S_3)
   d. Rales (crackles) at the base of the lungs
   e. Hazy lung fields and prominent, distended pulmonary veins on x-ray
   f. Elevated venous pressure
   g. Distended neck veins

Table 4-5 CAUSES OF HEART FAILURE		
DISEASE	**PATHOLOGY**	**RESULT**
Hypertensive disease	Vessels become narrowed; peripheral resistance increases	Cardiac muscle enlarges beyond its oxygen supply
Arteriosclerosis	Degenerative changes in arterial walls cause permanent narrowing of coronary arteries	Cardiac muscle enlarges beyond its oxygen supply
Valvular heart disease	Stenosed valves do not open freely; scarring and retraction of valve leaflets result in incomplete closure	Workload increases until heart fails
Rheumatic heart disease	Infection causes damage to heart valves, making them incompetent or narrowed	Incompetent valves cause blood to regurgitate backward; workload increases until heart fails
Ischemic heart disease	Coronary arteries are sclerosed or thrombosed	Blood supply is insufficient to nourish heart
Constrictive pericarditis	Inflamed pericardial sac becomes scarred and constricted, causing obstruction in blood flow	Fibrotic, thickened, and adherent pericardium encases heart, impairing ability of atria and ventricles to stretch during diastolic filling
Circulatory overload (IV fluid overload; sodium retention; renal shutdown)	Excessive fluid in circulatory system	Overwhelms heart's ability to pump
Pulmonary disease	Damage to arterioles of lungs causes vascular constriction; this increases workload of heart	Right ventricular enlargement and failure
Tachydysrhythmias	Decreases ventricular filling time	Decreased cardiac output

   h. Prolonged circulation time
   i. Reduction in cardiac output
   j. Presence of albuminuria
   k. Elevated BUN
   l. Gerontologic considerations–may see change in grooming habits, change in personality, dizziness or lightheadedness, decreased appetite, gait and balance alterations, malaise, chronic cough, nocturia; manifestations are worse during exacerbation of heart failure

7. Complications of heart failure
   a. Complications of immobility

b. Acute pulmonary edema—medical emergency that may result in death if not treated immediately; results from fluid from circulation pouring into the alveoli, bronchi, and bronchioles

c. Refractory or intractable heart failure—occurs when diet, medications, and treatments fail to alleviate symptoms

C. Nursing management

1. Medications

a. Cardiac glycosides (see Table 4-6)

1) Digitalis (e.g., digoxin)—fundamental medications in the treatment of heart failure, especially when associated with low cardiac output

a) Actions

i. Direct beneficial effect on myocardial contraction

ii. Increases force of systolic contraction

iii. Increases completeness of ventricular emptying

iv. Increases heart's capacity for work

b) Two categories of dosages

i. Rapid digitalization—aimed at administering the drug rapidly to achieve a detectable effect

ii. Gradual digitalization—client placed on a dose designed to replace the digitalis lost by excretion while maintaining "optimal" cardiac functioning

Table 4-6 CARDIAC GLYCOSIDE MEDICATIONS (DIGITALIS)		
MEDICATION	**ADVERSE EFFECTS**	**NURSING CONSIDERATIONS**
Digoxin	Anorexia Nausea Bradycardia Visual disturbances Confusion Abdominal pain	Administer with caution to elderly or clients with renal insufficiency Monitor renal function and electrolytes Instruct clients to eat high-potassium foods Take apical pulse for 1 full minute before administering Notify health care provider if AP less than 60 (adult), less than 90–110 (infants and young children), less than 70 (older children) Rapid digitalization—0.5 to 0.75 mg po, then 0.125 mg - 0.375mg cautiously until adequate effect is noted Gradual digitalization—0.25 to 0.5 mg may increase dosage every 2 weeks until desired clinical effect achieved Digoxin immune fab (Digibind)—used for treatment of life-threatening toxicity Maintenance dose 0.125–0.5 mg IV or PO (average is 0.25 mg) Teach client to check pulse rate and discuss adverse effects Low K^+ increases risk of digitalis toxicity Serum therapeutic blood levels 0.5–2 nanograms/mL Toxic blood levels $\geq$ 2 nanograms/mL
Action	Increases force of myocardial contraction and slows heart rate by stimulating the vagus nerve and blocking the AV node	
Indications	Heart failure, dysrhythmias	

Table 4-6 CARDIAC GLYCOSIDE MEDICATIONS (DIGITALIS) *(CONTINUED)*		
MEDICATION	**ADVERSE EFFECTS**	**NURSING CONSIDERATIONS**
Adverse effects	Tachycardia, bradycardia, heart block Anorexia, nausea, vomiting Halos around dark objects, blurred vision, halo vision Dysrhythmias, heart block	
Nursing considerations	Instruct client to eat high potassium foods Monitor for digitalis toxicity Risk of digitalis toxicity increases if client is hypokalemic	
Herbal interactions	Licorice can potentiate action of digoxin by promoting potassium loss Hawthorn may increase effects of digoxin Ginseng may falsely elevate digoxin levels Ma-huang (ephedra) increases risk of digitalis toxicity	

c) Digitalized state may be maintained even if a maintenance dose is missed

d) Toxicity—the nurse should be aware of and assess for digitalis toxicity; early symptoms include nausea and vomiting followed by anorexia, diarrhea, abdominal pain, confusion, drowsiness, and visual disturbances

e) Dysrhythmias—excessive slowing of pulse (below 60 beats/min]

f) Factors increasing likelihood of toxicity
   i. Problems with renal function causing toxic accumulation of digitalis
   ii. Depletion of potassium sensitizes the myocardium to digitalis and enhances its effect
   iii. Administration of IV calcium presents a danger of digitalis dysrhythmias because digitalis appears to act on the heart by increasing the amount of calcium in the contractile process

g) If toxicity occurs (greater than 2.0 nanograms/mL)
   i. Discontinue the drug and potassium-wasting diuretics
   ii. Monitor serum potassium
   iii. Administer antidysrhythmic drug as needed: lidocaine
   iv. Atropine or electronic pacing for bradycardia or AV block
   v. Severe toxicity: Fab body fragments (Digibind) administered
   vi. Cholestyramine and activated charcoal orally to suppress absorption

h) Client teaching
   i. Understanding of necessity of digitalis, its action, and its adverse effects
   ii. Teach how to check pulse rates to detect changes, therefore minimizing risk of toxicity
   iii. Notify nurse or health care provider concerning untoward adverse effects

    b. Diuretics (see Table 4-7)

       1) Promote physical and mental rest, while observing for complications of bed rest

         a) Reduces heart's workload; reduces preload

         b) Promotes diuresis

         c) Reduces work of respiratory muscles (decreases dyspnea)

         d) Reduces tissues' demands for oxygen (lessens circulatory demands)

         e) Decreases venous return (lessens pulmonary congestion and dyspnea) and preload

         f) Lowers blood pressure (diminishes arterial resistance against which heart must pump) and afterload

         g) Lowers heart rate (prolongs the recovery period of cardiac muscle, thereby resulting in a more efficient cardiac contraction)

         h) Promote comfort and rest (best if taken early to prevent nocturia)

         i) Reduces anxiety

         j) Instruct client to resume activities slowly

    c. Other medications

       1) Angiotensin-converting enzyme inhibitor (ACE) (decreases afterload)

         a) captopril, enalapril, lisinopril

       2) Angiotensin-receptor blockers (ARBs)–decrease afterload

       3) Beta-adrenergic blocking medications (decrease oxygen demand)

         a) Carvedilol

       4) Vasodilators–nitrates, milrinone–decrease preload and afterload

       5) Administer morphine–sedates and decreases afterload

       6) Administer Human B-type Natriuretic Peptides–nesiritide–for acute heart failure

2. Diet

    a. Restricted sodium diet

       1) Normal intake: 1.5-2.3 g/day

       2) Light in sodium diet: 50% less per serving than the usual sodium level

       3) Reduced sodium diet: 25% less sodium per serving than the usual sodium level

       4) Low sodium diet: 0.14 g/day

       5) Very low sodium diet: 0.035 g/day

       6) Sodium-free diet: less than 0.005 g/day

    b. Low calorie, supplemented with vitamins—promotes weight loss, thereby reducing the workload of the heart

    c. Bland, low residue—avoids discomfort from gastric distention and heartburn

    d. Small, frequent feedings to avoid gastric distention, flatulence, and heartburn

3. Record intake and output

4. Weigh daily

5. Good skin care

6. Oxygen therapy

7. Teaching about disease process and medications

MEDICATION	ADVERSE EFFECTS	NURSING CONSIDERATIONS
Table 4-7 DIURETIC MEDICATION		
Thiazide diuretics		
Hydrochlorothiazide Chlorothiazide	Hypokalemia Hyperglycemia Blurred vision Loss of Na^+ Dry mouth Hypotension	Monitor electrolytes, especially potassium I and O Monitor BUN and creatinine Don't give at bedtime Weigh client daily Encourage potassium-containing foods
Potassium-sparing Spironlactone	Hyperkalemia Hyponatremia Hepatic and renal damage Tinnitus Rash	Used with other diuretics Give with meals Avoid salt substitutes containing potassium Monitor I and O
Loop diuretics Furosemide Ethacrynic acid	Hypotension Hypokalemia Hyperglycemia GI upset Weakness	Monitor BP, pulse rate, I and O Monitor potassium Give IV dose over 1-2 minutes → diuresis in 5-10 min After PO dose diuresis in about 30 min Weigh client daily Don't give at bedtime Encourage potassium-containing foods
Ethacrynic acid Bumetanide	Potassium depletion Electrolyte imbalance Hypovolemia Ototoxicity	Supervise ambulation Monitor blood pressure and pulse Observe for signs of electrolyte imbalance
Osmotic diuretic		
Mannitol	Dry mouth Thirst	I and O must be measured Monitor vital signs Monitor for electrolyte imbalance
Other		
Chlorthalidone	Dizziness Aplastic anemia Orthostatic hypotension	Acts like a thiazide diuretic Acts in 2-3 hours, peak 2-6 hours, lasts 2-3 days Administer in AM Monitor output, weight, BP, electrolytes Increase K^+ in diet Monitor glucose levels in diabetic clients Change position slowly
Action	Thiazides—inhibits reabsorption of sodium and chloride in distal renal tubule Loop—inhibits reabsorption of sodium and chloride in loop of Henle and distal renal tubules Potassium-sparing—blocks effect of aldosterone on renal tubules, causing loss of sodium and water and retention of potassium Osmotic—pulls fluid from tissues due to hypertonic effect	

MEDICATION	ADVERSE EFFECTS	NURSING CONSIDERATIONS
	Table 4-7 DIURETIC MEDICATION *(CONTINUED)*	
Indications	Heart failure Hypertension Renal diseases Diabetes insipidus Reduction of osteoporosis in postmenopausal women	
Adverse effects	Dizziness, vertigo Dry mouth Orthostatic hypotension Leukopenia Polyuria, nocturia Photosensitivity Impotence Hypokalemia (except for potassium-sparing) Hyponatremia	
Nursing considerations	Take with food or milk Take in AM Monitor weight and electrolytes Protect skin from the sun Diet high in potassium for loop and thiazide diuretics Limit potassium intake for potassium-sparing diuretics Used as first-line medications for hypertension	
Herbal interactions	Licorice can promote potassium loss, causing hypokalemia Aloe can decrease serum potassium level, causing hypokalemia Gingko may increase blood pressure when taken with thiazide diuretics	

MYOCARDIAL INFARCTION

Formation of localized necrotic areas within the myocardium, usually following the sudden occlusion of a coronary artery and the abrupt cessation of blood and oxygen to the heart muscle

A. Assessment—major symptoms vary, depending on whether pain, shock, or pulmonary edema dominates the clinical picture
   1. Chest pain—severe, crushing, prolonged; unrelieved by rest or nitroglycerin; often radiating to one or both arms, the neck, and back; caused by accumulation of unoxidized metabolites within ischemic part of myocardium affecting nerve endings (see Figure 4-19)

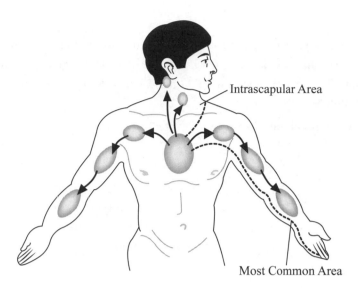

Intrascapular Area

Most Common Area

Figure 4-19. COMMON ISCHEMIC PAIN PATTERN

2. Shock—systolic blood pressure below 80 mm Hg, gray facial color, lethargy, cold diaphoresis, peripheral cyanosis, tachycardia or bradycardia, weak pulse

3. Oliguria—urine output of less than 20 mL/hour, as measured by an indwelling urinary catheter, which is indicative of renal hypoxia

4. Low-grade fever—temperature rises to 100° to 103°F within 24 hours and lasts 3 to 7 days; accompanied by leukocytosis, elevated sedimentation rate, LDH, AST, CK-MB, troponin
   a. Results from destruction of myocardial tissue and accompanying inflammatory process
   b. Fever drops when fibroblasts begin to replace leukocytes and scar tissue starts to form

5. Apprehension—great fear of death; restlessness
   a. Severe pain of a heart attack is terrifying
   b. Restlessness results from shock and pain

6. "Indigestion" or "gas pains around the heart," nausea and vomiting
   a. Client may believe that pain is caused by "indigestion" rather than by heart disease
   b. Nausea and vomiting may result from severe pain or from vasovagal reflexes conducted from the area of damaged myocardium to the gastrointestinal tract

7. Acute pulmonary edema—sense of suffocation, dyspnea, orthopnea, gurgling or bubbling respirations; left ventricle may become severely crippled in pumping action due to infarction, resulting in severe pulmonary congestion accompanied by low cardiac output and shock

8. Dysrhythmias, heart block, asystole

9. Diagnosis
   a. History
   b. EKG changes—ST segment elevation, T wave inversion, Q wave formation
   c. Profound hypotension and shock
   d. Lab findings
      1) WBC—leukocytosis within 2 days, disappears in 1 wk
      2) ESR—elevated

3) Enzymes

    a) CPK (MB isoenzymes)–peaks 18–24 hours; returns to normal 48–72 hours

    b) LDH–may remain elevated 5–7 days; peaks 48–72 hours; not specific for cardiac damage

    c) Myoglobin–begins to rise within 1 hour; peaks in 4–6 hours; returns to normal in less than 24 hours

4) Troponin–peaks in 4–6 hours, remains elevated for up to 2 weeks

B. Etiology

1. Predisposing factors–same as for heart failure

2. Causes

    a. Complete or near complete occlusion of a coronary vessel (most common)

    b. Decreased blood and oxygen supply to the heart muscle; vasospasm

    c. Hypertrophy of the heart muscle from CHF or hypertension

    d. Embolism to a coronary artery

3. Selected nursing diagnoses

    a. Acute pain

    b. Risk for decreased cardiac output

    c. Anxiety/fear

    d. Deficient knowledge (specify)

C. Nursing management

1. Treat acute attack immediately and promptly alleviate symptoms

    a. Provide constant supervision, monitoring, expert nursing care

        1) Provide thrombolytic therapy–streptokinase or tissue-type plasminogen activator (t-PA) to dissolve thrombus in coronary artery within 6 hours of onset

        2) Address client's and family's anxiety

    b. Place client in semi-Fowler position–lowers the diaphragm, thereby increasing lung expansion and promoting better ventilation; decreases venous return to the heart, preventing excessive pooling of blood within pulmonary vessels

    c. Bedrest to decrease stress on the heart; semi-fowler position

    d. Provide oxygen therapy, if necessary, to help relieve dyspnea, chest pain, shock, cyanosis, and pulmonary edema

    e. Monitor vital signs, pain status, lung sounds, level of consciousness, EKG, oxygen saturation

    f. Monitor I and O

        1) Intake–fluid intake should be around 2,000 mL daily; too much may precipitate CHF and too little may precipitate dehydration

        2) Output–urinary catheter, if necessary; oliguria indicates inadequate renal perfusion, and concentrated urine usually indicates dehydration

    g. Carefully monitor IV infusion–vein should be kept open in case emergency IV medications are necessary

2. Administer oxygen

3. Medications (see Table 4-8)

4. Modify lifestyle
   a. Stop smoking
   b. Reduce stress
   c. Decrease caffeine intake
   d. Modify intake of calories, sodium, and fat
   e. Regular physical activity

5. Prevent complications and further attacks
   a. Complications
      1) Dysrhythmias
      2) Shock
      3) CHF
      4) Rupture of heart muscle
      5) Pulmonary embolism
      6) Recurrent MI

6. Teaching
   a. Healing not complete for 6–8 weeks
   b. Medication schedule and adverse effects

Table 4-8 SELECTED CARDIAC MEDICATIONS		
NAME	ACTION	ADVERSE EFFECTS
Propanolol	Beta blocker—blocks sympathetic impulses to heart	Weakness Hypotension Bradycardia Depression Bronchospasm
Nifedipine	Calcium channel blocker—reduces workload of left ventricle; coronary vasodilator	Hypotension; dizziness GI distress Liver dysfunction
Morphine sulfate	Reduces cardiac workload, preload, and afterload pressures Relieves pain, reduces anxiety	Hypotension Respiratory depression Decreased mental acuity

ANGINA PECTORIS

Occurs when oxygen supply to the heart is not sufficient, usually due to atherosclerotic changes in the coronary arteries

A. Assessment
   1. Pain—may radiate down left arm; associated with stress, exertion, or anxiety
   2. Relieved with rest and nitroglycerin
   3. Older adults—may not have typical pain

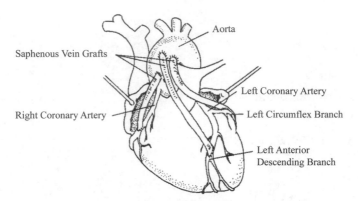

Figure 4-20. CORONARY ARTERY AND HEART

B. Etiology

1. Cause—coronary atherosclerosis

2. Risk factors for coronary artery disease
    a. Nonmodifiable (client has no control)
        1) Increasing age
        2) Family history of coronary heart disease
        3) Men more likely to develop heart disease than are premenopausal women
        4) Race

    b. Modifiable risk factor (client can exercise control)
        1) Elevated serum cholesterol
        2) Cigarette smoking or secondhand exposure
        3) Hypertension
        4) Diabetes mellitus
        5) Physical inactivity
        6) Obesity
        7) Depression or chronic stress
        8) Oral contraceptive use or hormone replacement therapy
        9) Substance abuse—methamphetamines or cocaine

3. Significance—warning sign of ischemia

C. Nursing management

1. Health Promotion
    a. Do not smoke
    b. Follow balanced diet that limits intake of fat and sodium
    c. Check blood pressure and cholesterol regularly
    d. Engage in regular physical activitygoal is reduction of blood pressure and pulse rate upon exertion

2. Medications (see Tables 4-9 through 4-11)

3. Coronary artery bypass surgery
    a. Indications—to increase blood flow to heart muscle in clients with severe angina
    b. Saphenous vein is used for graft; as many as five arteries are bypassed
    c. Preoperative—education and psychological preparation

d. Postoperative
   1) Provide intensive evaluation of organ systems
   2) Provide chest drainage
   3) Pain relief
   4) Be alert to psychological state of disorientation or depression
   5) Provide activity as tolerated with progress as ordered from foot dangling over side of bed, to sitting in chair, to walking in room by third day

e. Provide guidance concerning long-term care and follow-up

f. Percutaneous transluminal coronary angioplasty (PTCA)—balloon-tipped catheter is inserted into diseased coronary artery and pressure applied to stenosed artery; possible stent placement

Table 4-9 ANTIANGINAL MEDICATION		
MEDICATION	**ADVERSE EFFECTS**	**NURSING CONSIDERATIONS**
Nitroglycerin	Flushing Hypotension Headache Tachycardia Dizziness Blurred vision	Avoid alcoholic beverages Sublingual dose may be repeated every 5 min for 3 doses Protect drug from light Should wet tablet with saliva and place under tongue Lie down when taking sublingual nitroglycerin Headache most common adverse effect
Isosorbide	Headache Orthostatic hypotension	Change position slowly Take between meals Don't discontinue abruptly
Beta blockers: Propranolol Metoprolol Atenolol	Bradycardia Hypotension Bronchoconstriction	Should not be given to clients with known or suspected coronary artery spasms Clients who continue to smoke have reduced effectiveness of therapy Clients with asthma may experience bronchospasms Should be used with caution in clients with diabetes mellitus (may mask signs of hypoglycemia) Should be discontinued gradually to prevent rebound angin
Calcium channel blockers: Amlodipine Diltiazem Verapamil	Hypotension	Contraindicated in second- or third-degree heart block, cardiogenic shock, severe bradycardia, heart failure, or hypotension Use cautiously with renal or hepatic impairment Can potentiate the action of digoxin
Angiotensin-converting enzyme inhibitors Captopril	Dry annoying cough Hypotension Hyperkalemia	Diuretics increase effect Avoid high-potassium foods

Table 4-10 ANTICOAGULANT MEDICATIONS		
MEDICATION	**ADVERSE EFFECTS**	**NURSING CONSIDERATIONS**
Action: Inhibits synthesis of clotting factors		
Heparin	Can produce hemorrhage from any body site (10%) Tissue irritation/pain at injection site Anemia Thrombocytopenia Fever Dose dependent on PTT	Monitor therapeutic partial thromboplastin time (PTT) at 1.5–2.5 times the control without signs of hemorrhage Lower limit of normal 20–25 sec; upper limit of normal 32–39 sec For IV administration: use infusion pump, peak 5 minutes, duration 2–6 hours For injection: give deep SQ; never IM (danger of hematoma), onset 20–60 minutes, duration 8–12 hours **Antidote: protamine sulfate within 30 minutes** Can be allergenic
Low-molecular-weight heparin: Enoxaparin	Bleeding Minimal widespread affect Fixed dose	Less allergenic than heparin Must be given deep SQ, never IV or IM Does not require lab test monitoring
Warfarin	Hemorrhage Diarrhea Rash Fever	Monitor therapeutic prothombin time (PT) at 1.5–2.5 times the control, or monitor international normalized ratio (INR) Normal PT 9.5–12 sec; normal INR 2.0–3.5 Onset: 36–72 hours, peak 1.5–3 days, duration: 3–5 days **Antidotes: vitamin K, whole blood, plasma** Teach measures to avoid venous stasis Emphasize importance of regular lab testing Client should avoid foods high in vitamin K: many green vegetables, pork, rice, yogurt, cheeses, fish, milk
Fondaparinux	Hemorrhage Thrombocytopenia	SQ only PT and aPTT aren't suitable monitoring tests
Action: Inhibits activity of clotting		
Dabigatran	Directly inhibits thrombin Used to treat atrial fibrillation Increased risk bleeding age greater than 75, kidney disease, gastrointestinal bleeding, use of NSAIDs	
Action	Note which action each drug uses: Heparin blocks conversion of fibrinogen to fibrin Warfarin interferes with liver synthesis of vitamin K–dependent clotting factors Dabigatran inhibits thrombin	
Indications	For heparin: prophylaxis and treatment of thromboembolic disorders; in very low doses (10–100 units) to maintain patency of IV catheters (heparin flush) For warfarin: management of pulmonary emboli, venous thromboembolism, MI, atrial dysrhythmias, post cardiac valve replacement For Persantine: as an adjunct to coumadin in postop cardiac valve replacement, as an adjunct to aspirin to reduce the risk of repeat stroke or TIAs	

Table 4-10 ANTICOAGULANT MEDICATIONS (CONTINUED)

MEDICATION	ADVERSE EFFECTS	NURSING CONSIDERATIONS
Adverse effects	Nausea Alopecia Urticaria Hemorrhage Bleeding/heparin-induced thrombocytopenia (HIT)	
Nursing considerations	Check for signs of hemorrhage: bleeding gums, nosebleed, unusual bleeding, black/tarry stools, hematuria, fall in hematocrit or blood pressure, guaiac-positive stools Client should avoid IM injections, ASA-containing products, and NSAIDs Client should wear medical information tag Instruct client to use soft toothbrush, electric razor, to report bleeding gums, petechiae or bruising, epistaxis, black tarry stools Monitor platelet counts and signs and symptoms of thrombosis during heparin therapy; if HIT suspected, heparin discontinued and non-heparin anticoagulant (lepirudin) given	
Herbal interactions	Garlic, ginger, ginkgo may increase bleeding when taken with warfarin Large doses of anise may interfere with anticoagulants Ginseng and alfalfa my decrease anticoagulant activity Black haw increases action of anticoagulant Chamomile may interfere with anticoagulants	
Vitamin interaction	Vitamin C may slightly prolong PT Vitamin E will increase warfarin's effect	

Table 4-11 THROMBOLYTIC MEDICATIONS

MEDICATION	ADVERSE EFFECTS	NURSING CONSIDERATIONS (SPECIFIC)
Reteplase Alteplase Tissue plasminogen activator	Bleeding	Tissue plasminogen activator is a naturally occurring enzyme Low allergenic risk but high cost
Anistreplase Streptokinase	Bleeding	Because streptokinase is made from a bacterium, client can have an allergic reaction. Not used if client had recent *Streptococcus* infection or received Streptase in past year
Action	Reteplase and Alteplase break down plasminogen into plasmin, which dissolves the fibrin network of a clot Anistreplase and Streptokinase bind with plasminogen to form a complex that digests fibrin	
Indications	MIs within the first 6 hours after symptoms, limited arterial thrombosis, thrombotic strokes, occluded shunts	
Nursing considerations (general)	Check for signs of bleeding; minimize number of punctures for inserting IVs; avoid IM injections; apply pressure at least twice as long as usual after any puncture	

VASCULAR ALTERATIONS: HYPERTENSION

HYPERTENSION

There are two stages of hypertension, stage 1 and stage 2. Stage 1 hypertension is defined as persistent elevation of the systolic blood pressure between 130-139 mm Hg or the diastolic blood pressure between 80-89 mm Hg. Stage 2 hypertension is defined as a systolic blood pressure of at least 140 mm Hg or a diastolic blood pressure of at least 90 mm Hg.

A. Assessment
   1. May be no symptoms
   2. Headache, dizziness; facial flushing
   3. Anginal pain—insufficient blood flow through coronary arteries to the myocardium
   4. Intermittent claudication—decreased adequacy of blood supply to the legs during periods of activity
   5. Retinal hemorrhages and exudates—damage to arterioles that supply the retina
   6. Severe occipital headaches associated with nausea, vomiting, drowsiness, giddiness, anxiety, and mental impairment due to vessel damage within the brain
   7. Polyuria, nocturia, protein, and RBCs in urine, and diminished ability of kidneys to concentrate urine—hardening of arterioles within the kidney (arteriolar nephrosclerosis)
   8. Dyspnea upon exertion—left-sided heart failure
   9. Edema of the extremities—right-sided heart failure
   10. Client's history should include
       a. Age of onset (all ages, but more common with increasing age)
       b. Family history
       c. History of renal or cardiovascular disease
       d. Recent complaints of dyspnea, fatigue, weakness, anginal-type pain, swelling of feet, or nocturia
       e. Sudden gain or loss of weight
       f. Recent severe headaches or drenching sweats
       g. Personality type
       h. Activity level
       i. Alcohol intake
       j. Diet, including sodium intake
   11. Physical examination should include
       a. Blood pressure reading on both arms in supine and erect positions and on one leg: readings should be taken every one to two hours over an eight-hour period for one to two days (a single blood pressure reading is almost always inaccurate)
       b. Ophthalmoscopic examination for evidence of vascular changes
       c. Examination of the heart and aorta by means of auscultation, EKG readings, and aortography
       d. Palpation of the arteries in the neck, wrists, femoral areas, and feet for evidence of coarctation of the aorta (decreased amplitude of pulses and lower blood pressure in the legs than in the arm)

    e. Neurological examination for signs of cerebral thrombosis or hemorrhage

    f. Gerontologic considerations–high incidence of hypertension; parameters the same as for younger adults; increased systolic blood pressure common; treatment goal is less than 139/89 mm Hg or less than 130/80 mm Hg in diabetic clients; consider effects of antihypertensive medications

12. Laboratory studies–to diagnose type of hypertension present

    a. Urinalysis and urine cultures to determine the presence of protein, RBCs, pus cells, and casts (all indicative of renal disease)

    b. Blood count and sedimentation rate

    c. Serum sodium, potassium, chloride, and carbon dioxide (all indicative of primary aldosteronism)

    d. Urinary catecholamine metabolites (indicative of pheochromocytoma)

    e. Urine 17-ketosteroids and blood corticoids (both indicative of Cushing's disease)

    f. Intravenous pyelogram, urine cultures, radioisotope renogram, renal arteriography, intravenous urograms (all tests for renal disease)

    g. BUN and creatinine

13. If clinical workup indicates no evidence of coarctation of the aorta, adrenal disease, or primary renal disease, then the condition is diagnosed as essential hypertension

B. Etiology

1. Causes

    a. Risk factors

        1) Family history of hypertension

        2) Excessive sodium intake

        3) Excessive intake of calories

        4) Physical inactivity

        5) Excessive alcohol intake

        6) Low potassium intake

        7) Age

    b. Contributing factors–history of renal or cardiovascular disease; stressful lifestyle

    c. Primary (essential or idiopathic)–constitutes 90% of all cases; may be benign (gradual onset and prolonged course) or malignant (abrupt onset and short dramatic course, which is rapidly fatal unless treated)

    d. Secondary–develops as a result of another primary disease of the cardiovascular system, renal system, adrenal glands, or neurological system

2. Cycle of hypertensive cardiovascular disease

    a. Heart meets increased peripheral resistance (increased afterload)

    b. Heart must increase expenditure of energy; increased stretching of muscle fibers

    c. Stretching of muscle fibers results in hypertrophy of the heart and increased oxygen demand

    d. Hypertrophy of the heart may cause coronary insufficiency and result in MI (the enlarged heart muscle has outgrown its blood supply)

    e. If hypertrophied heart maintains cardiac output, left-sided cardiac failure may occur

    f. As diastolic pressure rises, the congestion extends back into the entire pulmonary tree

    g. Increased pressure of blood in arteries, coupled with arteriosclerotic changes (i.e., in kidneys and brain), can cause blood vessels to rupture, producing hemorrhage

    h. Stretching of atrial myocardium may cause atrial fibrillation

  3. Complications

    a. Renal failure

    b. Cerebral vascular accident (CVA)

    c. Transient ischemic attacks (TIAs)

    d. Retinal hemorrhages

C. Plan/Implementation

  1. Medications (see Table 4-12)

  2. Nursing management

    a. Provide a restful, quiet hospital environment

    b. Provide complete explanations of all procedures and diagnostic studies

    c. Listen to the client's fears and worries and offer reassurance

    d. Completely explain dietary restrictions (i.e., salt restriction, low fat)

    e. Document client's blood pressure both standing and lying down

    f. Encourage weight loss if client is obese

    g. Provide moderate salt-restricted diet

    h. Plan program of regular physical exercise

Table 4-12 ANTIHYPERTENSIVE MEDICATIONS		
MEDICATION	**ADVERSE EFFECTS**	**NURSING CONSIDERATIONS**
BETA BLOCKERS		
Atenolol	Bradycardia Hypotension Bronchospasm	Once-a-day dose increases compliance Check apical pulse; if less than 60 bpm, hold drug and call health care provider Don't discontinue abruptly Masks signs of shock and hypoglycemia
Metoprolol	Bradycardia, hypotension Heart failure Depression	Give with meals Teach client to check pulse before each dose; take apical pulse before administration; withhold if pulse is less than 60 bpm
Nadolol	Bradycardia, hypotension Heart failure	Teach client to check pulse before each dose; check apical pulse before administering Withhold if pulse less than 60 bpm Don't discontinue abruptly
Propranolol	Weakness Hypotension Bronchospasm Bradycardia Depression	Blocks sympathetic impulses to heart (beta blocker) Client should take pulse at home before each dose Dosage should be reduced gradually before discontinued
ALPHA BLOCKERS		
Prazosin hydrochloride	Drowsiness, dizziness Weakness Palpitations Nausea	Blocks a mediated vasoconstriction Assess for first-dose syncope Orthostatic hypotension precautions

Table 4-12 ANTIHYPERTENSIVE MEDICATIONS (CONTINUED)

MEDICATION	ADVERSE EFFECTS	NURSING CONSIDERATIONS
ALPHA-2 AGONISTS		
Methyldopa	Drowsiness, dizziness Bradycardia Hemolytic anemia Fever Orthostatic hypotension	Prevent reuptake of norepinephrine Monitor CBC Monitor liver function Take at bedtime to minimize daytime drowsiness Change position slowly
Clonidine	Drowsiness, dizziness Dry mouth, headache Dermatitis Severe rebound hypertension	Don't discontinue abruptly Apply patch to nonhairy area (upper outer arm, anterior chest) Take orthostatic hypotension precautions Older adults—high risk orthostatic hypotension and CNS adverse effects
THIAZIDE DIURETICS		
Hydrochlorthiazide	Hypokalemia Dehydration Postural hypotension	Weigh regularly Monitor for symptoms of hypoklalemia Take postural hypotension precautions
POTASSIUM-SPARING DIURETICS		
Spironolactone	Hyperkalemia GI upset	Weigh regularly Monitor for symptoms of hyperkalemia
VASODILATORS		
Hydralazine	Headache, palpitations Edema Tachycardia and palpitations Lupus erythematosus-like syndrome	Dilates arteriolar smooth muscle Give with meals Observe mental status Check for weight gain, edema
Morphine sulfate	Hypotension Respiratory depression Decreased mental alertness Constipation	Reduces cardiac workload, preload, and afterload pressures Relieves pain, reduces anxiety
CALCIUM CHANNEL BLOCKERS		
Nifedipine Verapamil Diltiazem Amlodipine	Hypotension Dizziness GI distress Liver dysfunction Jitteriness	Reduces workload of left ventricle (calcium channel blocker) Coronary vasodilator Monitor blood pressure during dosage adjustments Assist client with ambulation at start of therapy Nifedipine—high risk hypotension and constipation in older adults
ACE INHIBITORS		
Captopril Enalapril	Dizziness Orthostatic hypertension Persistent cough Hyperkalemia	Blocks conversion of Angiotensin I to Angiotensin II Report swelling of face, lightheadedness
ANGIOTENSIN II RECEPTOR BLOCKER (ARB)		
Losartan	Less likely to cause persistent cough and hyperkalemia than are ACE inhibitors	Prevents binding of angiotensin II with tissue receptor sites Maximal effects require 3 to 6 weeks Can be used in combination with a diuretic for better BP control
Herbal interaction	Ma-huang (ephedra) decreases effect of antihypertensive medications Ephedra increases hypertension when taken with beta blockers Black cohosh increases hypotensive effects of antihypertensives Goldenseal counteracts effects of antihypertensives	

i. Encourage changes in job or domestic settings for clients who live or work under considerable stress

j. Educate client regarding drug therapy
   1) Lie down immediately if faintness, weakness, nausea, or vomiting occurs
   2) Avoid hot baths, excessive amounts of alcohol, and immobility following exercise
   3) Always rise slowly from a lying to a sitting position and from sitting to standing to allow the vascular system to adjust to positional changes
   4) Avoid standing motionless, especially within the first hour or two after receiving medication (standing causes leg vessels to relax, allowing blood to pool within lower extremities)
   5) Use caution when driving an automobile or when operating heavy or dangerous machinery, especially with medications causing sedation
   6) Avoid constipation because it may cause either an increased or irregular absorption of hypotensive medications, which can result in critical hypotensive reactions
   7) Should hypotensive crises occur frequently, wrap legs firmly with elastic bandages when ambulating to promote venous return
   8) Never take a larger dose of drug than prescribed without consulting the health care provider
   9) Always take medication on time and do not skip a dose (noncompliance is common)
   10) Never suddenly discontinue a drug without the health care provider's permission to avoid severe rebound hypertensive reaction
   11) Always report adverse effects to the health care provider; impotence problems warrant change of therapy
   12) Consult with health care provider before taking any prescription or over-the-counter medications
   13) Gerontologic considerations
       a) Blood pressure assessment—inflate cuff pressure to level above disappearance of brachial or radial pulse
       b) Assess for orthostatic blood pressure changes; measure blood pressure in supine, sitting, and standing positions
       c) Elderly may not tolerate systolic blood pressure less than 120 mm Hg
       d) Elderly may have significant drop in blood pressure immediately after meals
       e) Polypharmacy—interaction between NSAIDs and antihypertensive medications

SELECTED DISORDERS OF TISSUE PERFUSION Section 4

SELECTED DISORDERS OF TISSUE PERFUSION

A. Shock—sudden reduction of oxygen and nutrients

1. Assessment—decreased blood volume causes a reduction in venous return, decreased cardiac output, and a decrease in arterial pressure

   a. Tachycardia, weak or absent peripheral pulses

   b. Cyanosis—with severe shock

   c. Decrease in urinary output ranging from oliguria to anuria, increased urine specific gravity

   d. Decrease in body temperature and absence of peripheral pulses due to peripheral vasoconstriction

   e. Anxiety, restlessness, and apprehension due to decreased cerebral tissue perfusion

   f. Respiration may be shallow and rapid; pulse will be weak and thready

   g. Decrease in arterial blood pressure

   h. Dehydration with associated alteration in electrolytes

   i. Nausea, vomiting

   j. In advanced shock, signs of pump failure and renal failure will be present

   k. Cool, clammy skin, decreased capillary refill

   l. Metabolic acidosis

2. Causes

   a. Types and causes of shock

      1) Hypovolemic shock—loss of fluid from circulation

         a) Hemorrhagic shock (external or internal)

         b) Cutaneous shock, e.g., burns resulting in external fluid loss

         c) Diabetic ketoacidosis

         d) Gastrointestinal obstruction, e.g., vomiting and diarrhea

         e) Diabetes insipidus

         f) Excessive use of diuretics

         g) Internal sequestration, e.g., fractures, hemothorax, ascites

      2) Cardiogenic shock—decreased cardiac output

         a) Myocardial infarction

         b) Dysrhythmias

         c) Pump failure

      3) Distributive shock—inadequate vascular tone

    a) Neural-induced loss of vascular tone
  - i. Anesthesia
  - ii. Pain
  - iii. Insulin shock
  - iv. Spinal cord injury

    b) Chemical-induced loss of vascular tone
  - i. Anaphylaxis
  - ii. Toxic shock
  - iii. Capillary leak–burns, decreased serum protein levels

  b. Stages of shock–a dynamic condition in which the client's status is constantly changing
  1) Initial stage–cardiac output is insufficient to supply normal nutritional needs of the body's tissues, but is not low enough to cause serious symptoms
  2) Compensatory stage–cardiac output is further reduced, but due to compensatory vasoconstriction, blood pressure tends to remain within a normal range
     a) Blood flow to the skin and kidneys decreases
     b) Blood flow to central nervous system and myocardium tends to be maintained
     c) A decrease occurs in the blood reservoirs
  3) Progressive stage–unfavorable changes become more and more apparent
     a) Falling blood pressure
     b) Increasing vasoconstriction
     c) Increased heart rate
     d) Oliguria
  4) Irreversible stage–no type of therapy can save the client's life
     a) Myocardial depression
     b) Loss of arteriolar tonus
     c) Infused blood tends to remain in the dilated capillary bed

3. Nursing management
   a. Maintain adequate oxygenation (see Table 4-13)
   b. Increase tissue perfusion
   c. Maintain systolic BP greater than 90 mm Hg
   d. Treat acidosis
   e. Maintain patent airway
      1) If necessary, ensure ventilation by Ambu bag or ventilator assistance
      2) Provide supplemental oxygen to maintain adequate blood PO_2
   f. Indwelling catheter, hourly outputs
   g. Monitor CVP
   h. Monitor vital signs
   i. Assess ABGs
   j. Keep warm (maintain body temperature)
      1) Heat application is contraindicated because it causes peripheral blood vessels to dilate and draws blood back from vital organs
      2) Hypothermia increases blood viscosity and slows blood flow through the microcirculation

METHOD	OXYGEN DELIVERED	NURSING
Nasal cannula or prongs	23–42% at 1–6 L/min	Assess patency of nostril Apply water-soluble jelly to nostrils every 3-4 hours Perform good mouth care
Face mask	40–60% at 6-8 L/min (oxygen flow minimum 5 L)	Remove mask every 1-2 hours Wash, dry, apply lotion to skin Emotional support to decrease feeling of claustrophobia
Partial rebreather mask	50–75% at 8–11 L/min	Adjust oxygen flow to keep reservoir bag two-thirds full during inspiration
Nonrebreather mask	80–100% at 12 L/min	Adjust oxygen flow to keep bag two-thirds full
Venturi mask	24–40% at 4–8 L/min	Provides high humidity and fixed concentrations Keep tubing free of kinks
Tracheostomy collar or T-piece	30–100% at 8–10 L/min	Assess for fine mist Empty condensation from tubing Keep water container full
Oxygen hood	30–100% at 8–10 L/min	Used for infants and young children Provides cooled humid air Check O_2 concentration with O_2 analyzer every 4 hours Refill humidity jar with sterile distilled water Clean humidity jar daily Cover client with light blanket and towel or cap for head Change linen frequently Monitor client's temperature frequently

Table 4-13 OXYGEN ADMINISTRATION

k. Restore fluid volume
   1) Intravenous administration of blood or other appropriate fluids (crystalloids or colloids)
   2) Volume of fluid administered may be pushed until systemic blood pressure, urine volume, and lactate levels return to a relatively normal level or central venous or pulmonary artery pressures, or both, become elevated

l. Medications
   1) Antibiotics—when shock is due to an infection (septic shock), antibiotic therapy should be instituted immediately; blood, urine, sputum, and drainage of any kind should be sent for culture
   2) Medications to vasoconstrict and improve myocardial contractility (e.g., dopamine, norepinephrine, phenylephrine, dobutamine, milrinone)
   3) Medications to maintain adequate urine output, e.g., furosemide
   4) Medication to restore blood pressure (adrenergics/sympathomimetics)
   5) Corticosteroids for septic shock

Table 4-14	EMERGENCY MEDICATIONS FOR SHOCK, CARDIAC ARREST, AND ANAPHYLAXIS	
MEDICATION	**ADVERSE EFFECTS**	**NURSING CONSIDERATIONS**
Norepinephrine	Headache Palpitations Nervousness Epigastric distress Angina, hypertension tissue necrosis with extravasation	Vasoconstrictor to increase blood pressure and cardiac output Reflex bradycardia may occur with rise in BP Client should be attended at all times Monitor urinary output Infuse with dextrose solution, not saline Monitor blood pressure Protect from light
Dopamine	Increased ocular pressure Ectopic beats Nausea Tachycardia, chest pain, dysrhythmias	Low-dose—dilates renal and coronary arteries High-dose—vasoconstrictor, increases myocardial oxygen consumption Headache is an early symptom of drug excess Monitor blood pressure, peripheral pulses, urinary output Use infusion pump
Epinephrine	Nervousness Restlessness Dizziness Local necrosis of skin	Stimulates alpha and beta adrenergic receptors Monitor BP Carefully aspirate syringe before IM and SC doses; inadvertent IV administration can be harmful Always check strength: 1:100 only for inhalation, 1:1,000 for parenteral administration (SC or IM) Ensure adequate hydration
Isoproterenol	Headache Palpitations Tachycardia Changes in BP Angina, bronchial asthma	Stimulates beta 1 and beta 2 adrenergic receptors Used for heart block, ventricular arrhythmias, and bradycardia Bronchodilator used for asthma and bronchospasms Don't give at bedtime interrupts sleep patterns Monitor BP, pulse
Phenylephrine	Palpations Tachycardia Hypertension Dysrhythmia Angina Tissue necrosis with extravasation	Potent alpha 1 agonist Used to treat hypotension

Table 4-14	EMERGENCY MEDICATIONS FOR SHOCK, CARDIAC ARREST, AND ANAPHYLAXIS *(CONTINUED)*	
MEDICATION	**ADVERSE EFFECTS**	**NURSING CONSIDERATIONS**
Dobutamine hydrocholoride	Hypertension PVCs Asthmatic episodes Headache	Stimulates beta 1 receptors Incompatible with alkaline solutions (sodium bicarbonate) Administer through central venous catheter or large peripheral vein using an infusion pump Don't infuse through line with other meds (incompatible) Monitor EKG, BP, I and O, serum potassium
Milrinone	Dysrhythmia Thrombocytopenia Jaundice	Positive inotropic agent Smooth muscle relaxant used to treat severe heart failure
Sodium nitroprusside	Hypotension	Dilates cardiac veins and arteries Decreases preload and afterload Increases myocardial perfusion
Diphenhydramine HCl	Drowsiness Confusion Insomnia Headache Vertigo Photosensitivity	Blocks effects of histamine on bronchioles, GI tract, and blood vessels
Actions	Varies with med	
Indications	Hypovolemic shock Cardiac arrest Anaphylaxis	
Adverse effects	Serious rebound effect may occur Balance between underdosing and overdosing	
Nursing considerations	Monitor vital signs Measure urine output Assess for extravasation Observe extremities for color and perfusion	

PERIPHERAL VASCULAR DISEASE

A. Assessment
   1. General signs and symptoms
      a. Intermittent claudication—severe pain in calf muscle that occurs with walking and is caused by ischemia and a buildup of lactic acid; pain often described as cramping
         1) Exercise increases metabolic needs of tissues
         2) Damaged arteries are unable to dilate and supply tissues with oxygen
      b. Rest pain (pain in extremities occurring when client is resting)—sudden blockage of a vessel by a thrombus reduces blood supply to tissues and produces ischemic pain; pain relieved by dependent position
      c. Coldness and pallor of extremities during elevation
      d. Dependent rubor—tissues of the extremities are reddish blue in color
         1) Indicative of peripheral vessel damage where vessels remain permanently dilated
         2) Develops after prolonged anoxia or exposure to severe cold
      e. Cyanosis of the tissues—occurs when blood contains too little oxygen
      f. Trophic changes—adverse changes in the skin and nails of the extremities result from prolonged ischemia of tissues (loss of lower extremity hair)
      g. Leg ulcers and cellulitis
         1) Venous stasis is a consequence of venous insufficiency
         2) Venous stasis provides a medium for bacterial growth, which results in ulcerations
      h. Gangrenous changes—death and decay of tissues of the extremities result from severe and prolonged ischemia

B. Factors regulating the peripheral vascular system—arteries are contractile in that they can decrease (vasoconstrict) or increase (vasodilate) in response to appropriate stimuli
   1. Arteries have a rich sympathetic nervous system supply
      a. Stimulation causes vasoconstriction
      b. Sympathectomy causes vasodilation
   2. Hormonal and chemical control—3 substances within blood help control the caliber of blood vessels
      a. Epinephrine—constricts superficial blood vessels, but in small doses dilates vessels supplying the muscles, brain, and heart
      b. Norepinephrine—constricts all blood vessels, but particularly affects the peripheral vessels
      c. Angiotensin—constricts arteries
   3. Local regulatory mechanisms—substances that act locally on blood vessels
      a. Histamine—potent vasodilator of small blood vessels, although may also constrict large arteries
      b. Muscle metabolites—strong vasodilators

    c. Acetylcholine—vasodilator whose action is transient and more apparent in the face and upper limbs than in the lower limbs

    d. Serotonin—substance liberated from platelets that sticks to the injured area of a vessel wall: powerful constrictor of cutaneous arterioles but dilates capillaries

C. Peripheral vascular diseases are characterized by disturbances of blood flow through the peripheral vessels, eventually resulting in damage to tissues of the extremities

  1. Adequate blood flow depends on many factors

    a. Efficiency of heart's pumping action

    b. Condition of blood vessels, e.g., patent, dilated, or constricted

    c. Rate of blood flow

    d. Needs of tissues for oxygen and nutrients, as well as for removal of waste products

    e. Nervous system activity

    f. Amount of bloodflow

ARTERIAL PERIPHERAL VASCULAR DISEASE

Arteries must be capable of dilating and constricting normally

A. Assessment

  1. Cool, shiny skin, hair loss

  2. Ulcers, gangrene

  3. Impaired sensation

  4. Intermittent claudication

  5. Decreased peripheral pulses

  6. Diagnostic tests

    a. Angiography (arteriography)—contrast dye is injected into the arteries, and x-ray films are taken of the vascular tree

      1) May indicate abnormalities of blood flow due to arterial obstruction or narrowing

      2) Magnetic resonance angiography—useful for clients with dye allergy

    b. Doppler ultrasound—measures velocity of blood flow through a vessel and emits an audible signal

    c. Duplex imaging—uses Doppler system to map blood throughout artery and gives anatomic and physiological information about the blood vessels

    d. Ankle-brachial index (ABI)—divide ankle blood pressure by brachial blood pressure; normal is greater than or equal to 0.9.

B. Etiology

  1. Types of disease

    a. Arteriosclerosis

    b. Raynaud's disease

    c. Buerger's disease

  2. Predisposing factors

    a. Smoking

    b. Diabetes mellitus

    c. Hyperlipidemia

    d. Hypertension

    e. Obesity

    f. Sedentary lifestyle

    g. Age

C. Nursing management

  1. Check extremities for paleness, coolness, necrosis

  2. Good foot care

    a. Use warm water, dry gently and thoroughly

    b. Use lubricants to keep skin soft

    c. Wear clean cotton socks

  3. Do not cross legs

  4. Regular exercise—promotes collateral circulation

  5. Stop smoking

  6. Lose weight

  7. Interventional radiological procedures

    a. Percutaneous transluminal angioplasty

    b. Laser-assisted angioplasty

    c. Atherectomy catheters

    d. Intravascular stents

  8. Surgical therapy

    a. Arterial bypass with autogenous vein or synthetic graft

    b. Endarterectomy

    c. Patch graft angioplasty

    d. Amputation

  9. Medications

    a. Vasodilators

    b. Anticoagulants

    c. Platelet aggregate inhibitors (e.g., aspirin, clopidrogel)

VENOUS PERIPHERAL VASCULAR DISEASE

Efficiency in returning blood to the heart depends upon competent valves within the veins and adequate pumping action of the muscles surrounding the veins

A. Assessment

  1. Cool, brown skin

  2. Edema

  3. Ulcers

  4. Pain, redness along vein, induration along vein

  5. Normal or decreased pulses

  6. Deep muscle tenderness

  7. Limb may be warmer than opposite limb

  8. Risk for pulmonary embolism

9. Diagnostic tests
   a. Phlebogram (venogram)
   b. Venous pressure measurements—venous occlusion in one leg causes venous pressure to be higher than in unaffected leg
   c. Venous Doppler evaluation, venous duplex ultrasonography
   d. Lung scan and pulmonary arteriogram
   e. D-dimer test—global marker for coagulation

B. Causes
   1. Thrombophlebitis—inflammation of venous wall with clot formation
   2. Predisposing factors
      a. Venous stasis—conditions causing venous stasis include varicose veins, obesity, surgery, pregnancy, prolonged bed rest, and CHF
      b. Hypercoagulability—may be caused by cancer, blood dyscrasias, decreased fibrinolysis, increased clotting factors or increased blood viscosity, oral contraceptives
      c. Injury to the venous wall—may be caused by IV injections, thromboangiitis obliterans (Buerger's disease), fractures and dislocations, chemical injury from sclerosing agents, opaque media for x-ray, certain antibiotics
   3. Age-decreased competency of valves; greater incidence varicose veins; slowed wound healing

C. Nursing management
   1. Ambulation and exercise in bed should be encouraged once anticoagulation therapy is started to decrease venous pressure and promote blood flow by the contraction of muscles compressing the veins
   2. Elevation of legs above the level of the heart facilitates blood flow by force of gravity, thereby preventing venous stasis and formation of new thrombi; also decreases venous pressure, relieving edema and pain
   3. Raise foot of bed rather than using pillows or gatching the bed because these methods often result in elevation of the knee above the foot and interfere with proper flow
   4. Apply intermittent or continuous warm, moist packs—to relieve venospasm, produce analgesia, and hasten resolution of inflammation
   5. Elastic support hose compresses the superficial veins and, with walking, blood flow in the veins is increased and venous pressure is kept to a minimum
   6. Avoid standing and sitting because these increase the hydrostatic pressure in the capillaries, promoting edema
   7. Elastic or compression stockings; 6 to 8 wk
   8. Avoid extremes in temperature
   9. Monitor peripheral pulses
   10. Anticoagulants
   11. Thombolytic therapy—prevents post-phlebitis venous insufficiency; risk of bleeding
   12. Preventive measures
      a. Passive and active range of motion exercises for clients who are postop, postpartum, or on prolonged bed rest
      b. Early ambulation postop and postpartum
      c. Elastic support hose during and after surgery

    d. Deep breathing exercises postop to promote thoracic pumping action

    e. Avoidance of tight clothing

VARICOSE VEINS

Dilated veins caused by incompetent valves

A. Predisposing factors
1. Pregnancy
2. Obesity
3. Heart disease
4. Family history

B. Assessment
1. Pain after prolonged standing
2. Dilated veins
3. Feeling of fullness in legs

C. Nursing management
1. Elevate legs above heart level
2. Knee-length elastic stockings
3. Vein ligation
4. Sclerotherapy—for small or limited number varicosities
5. Radiofrequency energy—shrinks vein
6. Endovenous laser treatment

CHRONIC VENOUS INSUFFICIENCY

A. Predisposing factors—standing for long periods, constrictive clothing, crossed legs, obesity, age
B. Assessment—venous ulcers
C. Nursing management
1. Elevate legs while sleeping and 2–3 times per day
2. Frequent position change
3. Avoid elastic wraps (uneven pressure)
4. Compression stockings—replace every 6 months, remove at night, wash with soap every night, do not put in dryer
5. Wash legs daily with mild soap and water
6. Used mild moisturizers and creams on legs
7. Report skin discoloration, swelling, lesions to health care provider

Chapter 5

THE RESPIRATORY SYSTEM

Sections	Concepts Covered
1. The Respiratory System Overview	Gas Exchange
2. Alterations in Airway Clearance and Breathing Patterns	Gas Exchange

THE RESPIRATORY SYSTEM OVERVIEW

RESPIRATORY SYSTEM

A. Structure

1. Upper respiratory system
   a. Nose—filters, warms, and humidifies inspired air; contains olfactory receptors for sense of smell; older adults have restricted air flow
   b. Sinuses—air-filled cavities provide resonance during speech
   c. Pharynx (throat)—contains adenoids and tonsils; defense mechanisms against infection; gag reflex
   d. Larynx—contains the voice box and epiglottis, which prevents food from entering the trachea; cough reflex

2. Lower respiratory tract
   a. Trachea—smooth, flexible, muscular, tubelike air passage extending from larynx to mainstem bronchi
   b. Mainstem bronchi (right and left)—subdivision of trachea entering lungs
   c. Secondary bronchi—subdivisions of main bronchi branching through each lung field
   d. Bronchioles—smallest subdivisions of bronchi, conducting air from secondary bronchi into alveoli
   e. Alveoli—delicate, thin-walled, minute hollow chambers within the lungs surrounded by networks of capillaries; contain surfactant that keeps alveoli expanded

3. Thoracic cavity—4 subdivisions
   a. Right pulmonary space—contains right lung
   b. Left pulmonary space—contains left lung
   c. Pericardial space—contains heart and pericardial sac
   d. Mediastinal space—center of thoracic cavity, located between pulmonary spaces, containing esophagus, trachea, great blood vessels, and heart
   e. Gerontologic considerations—loss of elastic recoil; increased residual volume; increased use of accessory muscles

4. Lungs—light, spongy, porous, elastic, cone-shaped organs; inflate with inspiration and deflate (but do not completely collapse) with expiration
   a. Base rests on diaphragm
   b. Apex extends above the first rib
   c. Each lung is divided into lobes: the right has 3 lobes; the left has 2

5. Pleurae—two-layered membrane covering each lung and lining the thoracic cavity
   a. Parietal pleura—lines thoracic cavity within each lung chamber
   b. Visceral (pulmonary) pleura—outer covering of the lung within each chamber

6. Pleural space—space between layers containing thin fluid to prevent friction during respiration

7. Diaphragm—muscular partition separating the thoracic and abdominal cavities

B. Function

1. Ventilation—moves air into and out of lungs and along bronchial airways to bring oxygen into the lungs and remove CO_2

   a. Inspiration
      1) Contraction of inspiratory muscles
      2) Enlargement of thoracic cage
      3) Reduction in intrapleural and intrapulmonic pressures
      4) Inflow of air until intrapulmonic pressure equals atmospheric pressure

   b. Expiration
      1) Relaxation of inspiratory muscles
      2) Reduction in size of thoracic cage
      3) Increase in intrapleural and intrapulmonic pressures
      4) Outflow of air until intrapulmonic pressure equals atmospheric pressure
      5) Gerontologic considerations—loss of elastic recoil; increased residual volume; increased use of accessory muscles

   c. Normal breath sounds
      1) Bronchial—high-pitched, loud sounds heard over the trachea
      2) Bronchovesicular—medium-pitched, moderately loud sounds heard over the mainstem bronchi
      3) Vesicular—low-pitched, soft sounds heard over the peripheral lung fields

   d. Normal breathing pattern—eupnea
      1) Rate in adult is 12 to 20 breaths per minute
      2) Smooth with an even respiratory depth
      3) Easy, relaxed; requiring minimal effort
      4) Symmetric chest wall movement
      5) May be abdominal (commonly seen in men) or thoracic (common in women)

2. Effective ventilation—requirements
   a. Patent airway
   b. Elastic, expansive lungs and tracheobronchial tree
   c. Adequate musculoskeletal apparatus of chest wall

C. Mechanics of respiration

1. Lungs and circulation act together to convey respiratory gases between atmospheric air and body tissues; respiration regulated by several components

   a. Muscles—diaphragm and intercostal muscles enhance inspiration and expiration
      1) Inspiration—contraction of diaphragm and intercostal muscles, resulting in downward expansion of the thoracic cavity and elevation of the rib cage
      2) Expiration—passive action involving deflation of lungs, relaxation of thoracic musculature, and reduction in the size of the thoracic cavity
      3) Accessory muscles may be used in pathological states or after exercise when additional expansion is needed; abdominal muscles may be used during coughing

    b. Intrapleural pressure–normally negative (below atmospheric pressures)

       1) Inspiration–reduction in intrapleural and intrapulmonic pressures; air enters the lungs until the intrapulmonic and atmospheric pressures equalize

       2) Expiration–increase in intrapleural and intrapulmonic pressures; gases in the pleural cavity are expelled until intrapulmonic and atmospheric pressures equalize

    c. Lung compliance–when lung compliance is lowered, the respiratory effort is increased

    d. Airway resistance–relationship between airflow and pleural pressure

       1) Highest resistance in the nose

       2) Lowest resistance in the bronchioles

       3) Airway problems (e.g., emphysema) increase airway resistance

2. Four "volumes" affected by ventilation

    a. Tidal volume–normal volume of air inspired and expired with each respiration (breath); the tidal volume has two components:

       1) Dead space–air that fills the bronchial tree

       2) Alveolar ventilation–air entering the alveoli

    b. Inspiratory reserve volume–volume of air that can be inspired above the tidal volume

    c. Expiratory reserve volume–amount of air that is expired forcefully at the end normal tidal volume respiration

    d. Residual volume–amount of air present in the lungs after forceful expiration; decreased in older adults

3. Lung capacity–combination of gas volumes within the lung

    a. Inspiratory capacity–tidal volume plus inspiratory reserve volume (amount of air an individual can breathe in from a resting expiratory level)

    b. Functional residual capacity–expiratory reserve volume plus residual volume (amount of air present in the lungs after normal expiration); increased in older adults

    c. Vital capacity–inspiratory reserve volume plus tidal volume plus expiratory reserve volume (maximum amount of air expelled by the lungs after maximum inspiration); decreased in older adults

    d. Total lung capacity–amount of air contained in the lungs on maximum inspiration

4. Changes anywhere in the pulmonary tracheobronchial tree can affect both pulmonary volume and capacity

5. Alveolar ventilation–membrane allows for easy exchange of gases

    a. Diffusing capacity–volume of gas that diffuses through the membranes each minute for a pressure gradient of 1 mm Hg

    b. Perfusion–amount of blood that supplies the lungs

6. Factors regulating O_2/CO_2 exchange
   a. Respiratory center—located in the medulla oblongata
      1) Stimulated by the concentration of CO_2 in arterial blood; circulating O_2 is less significant
         a) Brain chemoreceptors are stimulated primarily by the amount of hydrogen ions and CO_2 in the cerebrospinal fluid; excess CO_2 and hydrogen ions cause an increase in respiratory rate (loses excess CO_2 and restores blood pH balance)
         b) Respiratory acidosis results from a decrease in pulmonary ventilation, causing a high concentration of CO_2 in the blood that results in accumulation of carbonic acid and hydrogen ions
         c) Respiratory alkalosis occurs when pulmonary ventilation increases and the number of hydrogen ions decreases
   b. Peripheral chemoreceptors—located in the aortic and carotid bodies
      1) Stimulated when O_2 levels drop
      2) Respiratory center responds by stimulating glossopharyngeal, vagus, and phrenic nerve fibers—diaphragm is innervated, and alveolar ventilation and O_2 tension are increased
   c. Gerontologic considerations–diminished response of brain stem to arterial oxygen and carbon dioxide changes; slower change in respiratory rate; decreased effectiveness of respiratory and metabolic compensatory mechanisms

ALTERATIONS IN AIRWAY CLEARANCE AND BREATHING PATTERNS

DEFINITIONS OF BREATHING PATTERNS

A. Abdominal respirations—breathing accomplished by abdominal muscles and diaphragm; may be used to increase effectiveness of ventilatory process in certain conditions; normal in infants and toddlers

B. Apnea—temporary cessation of breathing; may be seen in older adults

C. Cheyne-Stokes respirations—periodic breathing characterized by rhythmic waxing and waning of the depth of respirations; normal in older adults; seen with brain injury and death

D. Dyspnea—difficult, labored, or painful breathing (considered "normal" at certain times, e.g., after extreme physical exertion)

E. Hyperpnea—abnormally deep breathing; may be seen with normal, slow, or increased rate; seen with fever, metabolic acidosis

F. Hyperventilation—abnormally rapid, deep, and prolonged breathing
   1. Caused anxiety, pain, diabetic ketoacidosis, brain injury, stroke
   2. Produces respiratory alkalosis due to reduction in CO_2 tension

G. Hypoventilation—reduced ventilatory efficiency; produces respiratory acidosis due to elevation in CO_2 tension; caused by emphysema, pneumonia, pulmonary edema

H. Kussmaul's respirations (air hunger)—marked increase in depth and rate of breathing; caused by diabetic ketoacidosis or metabolic acidosis

I. Orthopnea—inability to breathe except when trunk is in upright position; caused by severe lung or heart disease

J. Paradoxical respirations—breathing pattern in which a lung (or portion of a lung) deflates during inspiration (acts opposite to normal); caused by severe lung disease or flail chest

K. Periodic breathing—rate, depth, or tidal volume changes markedly from one interval to the next; pattern of change is periodically reproduced

L. Adventitious lung sounds—abnormal breath sounds

Table 5-1 BREATH SOUNDS		
ADVENTITIOUS SOUNDS	**CHARACTERISTICS**	**CLINICAL EXAMPLES**
Fine crackles	Popping sounds; heard mostly on late inspiration and not cleared by coughing; originates in the alveoli; sounds like rubbing hair May clear with coughing	May be heard in pneumonia, heart failure, chronic bronchitis, and asthma
Coarse crackles	Discontinuous popping sounds heard early in inspiration; originate in the large bronchus; sounds are harsh and moist May clear with coughing	May be heard in pneumonia, heart failure, chronic bronchitis, and asthma
Sibilant wheeze	High-pitched, musical sounds similar to a squeak Heard more commonly on expiration, but may be heard on inspiration Auscultated over small airways Does not clear with coughing	Associated with narrowing of the airways, e.g., asthma, bronchospasm
Sonorous wheeze	Low-pitched, coarse, loud, moaning/snoring sounds heard primarily on expiration, but may be present on inspiration, arise from large airways Coughing may clear	Associated with inflammation or partial obstruction of the trachea or bronchi, such as in bronchitis, sputum or foreign body
Stridor	Harsh, high-pitched sounds heard over the trachea	Associated with upper airway (larynx and trachea) inflammation and partial obstruction
Pleural friction rub	A superficial, low-pitched, coarse rubbing or grating sound (sounds like two surfaces rubbing together) Heard throughout inspiration and expiration and not cleared by coughing	Heard in individuals with pleurisy (visceral and parietal pleurae are in contact with each other due to inflammation and edema of the surfaces), pulmonary infarction, lung cancer

UPPER AIRWAY OBSTRUCTION

A. Emergency

    1. Choking

        a. Assessment

            1) Inability to breathe or speak

            2) Cyanosis

            3) Collapse

            4) Death can occur within 4–5 minutes

        b. Analysis and nursing diagnosis—impaired gas exchange related to inadequate airway clearance

c. Nursing management—five and five

    1) Give 5 back blows between should blade with heel of hand

    2) Give 5 abdominal thrusts (Heimlich maneuver)

    3) Alternate between 5 back blows and 5 thrusts until blockage is dislodged

d. Evaluation

    1) Respiratory rate returns to normal

    2) Client is able to speak

B. Intubation (see Figure 5-1 and Table 5-2)

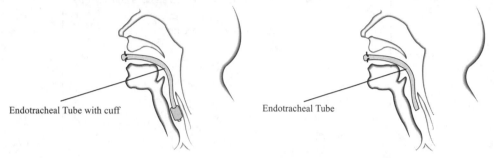

Endotracheal Tube with cuff

Endotracheal Tube

Figure 5-1. ENDOTRACHEAL TUBE

C. Suctioning

1. Assess need for suctioning

2. Wear protective eyewear

3. Hyperoxygenate before and after suctioning—100% oxygen for 3 min, at least 3 deep breaths

4. Explain procedure to client (potentially frightening procedure)

5. Elevate head of bed to semi-Fowler position

6. Lubricate catheter with sterile saline and insert without applying suction

7. Advance catheter about 16–20 cm; client will begin to cough; do not apply suction

8. Withdraw catheter 1–2 cm, apply suction and withdraw catheter with a rotating motion for no more than 10–15 seconds; wall suction set between 80–120 mm Hg

9. Hyperoxygenate for 1–5 min or until client's baseline heart rate and oxygen saturation are reached

10. Repeat procedure after client has rested, up to 3 total suction passes

11. Endotracheal tube or tracheostomy tube suctioned, then mouth is suctioned; provide mouth care

12. Complications

    a. Hypoxia

    b. Bronchospasm

    c. Tissue trauma

    d. Vagal stimulation

    e. Cardiac dysrhythmias

    f. Infection

METHOD	NURSING CONSIDERATIONS
Endotracheal tube—tube passed through the nose or mouth into the trachea	Assess for bilateral breath sounds and bilateral chest excursion Mark tube at level it touches mouth or nose Secure with tape to stabilize Encourage fluids to facilitate removal of secretions
Tracheostomy—surgical incision made into trachea via the throat; tube inserted through incision into the trachea	Cuff is used to prevent aspiration and to facilitate mechanical ventilation Maintain cuff pressure at 20–25 mm Hg (underinflation could lead to aspiration, whereas overinflation could lead to stenosis and scarring of the trachea) Encourage fluids to facilitate removal of secretions Sterile suctioning if necessary Frequent oral hygiene Indications for suctioning tracheostomy – Noisy respirations – Restlessness – Increased pulse – Increased respirations – Presence of mucus in airway

Table 5-2 INTUBATION

D. Tracheostomy care—performed every 8 hours and as needed
   1. Explain procedure
   2. Suction tracheostomy tube
   3. Remove old dressings
   4. Open sterile tracheostomy care kit
   5. Put on sterile gloves
   6. Remove inner cannula (permanent or disposable)
   7. Clean with hydrogen peroxide if permanent inner cannula
   8. Rinse with sterile water, dry
   9. Reinsert into outer cannula
   10. Clean stoma site with hydrogen peroxide and sterile water, then dry
   11. Change ties or velcro tracheostomy tube holders as needed; old ties must remain in place until new ties are secured
   12. Apply new sterile dressing; do not cut gauze pads, use pre-cut gauze
   13. Document site of tracheostomy, type/quantity of secretions, client tolerance of procedure

E. Mechanical ventilation
   1. Ventilator used to overcome dangers of respiratory insufficiency
      a. Forces oxygen into lungs to increase the expiration of CO_2
      b. Allows well-distributed airflow to the alveoli
      c. Client's breathing efforts and energy expenditure are decreased
      d. Improves the effectiveness of coughing and assists with the expulsion of accumulating secretions

2. Nursing responsibilities

    a. Prepare client psychologically for use of ventilator

        1) Inadequately prepared clients may panic and defeat the purpose of the ventilator by "fighting" the machine's cycle and breathing ineffectively

        2) Teach client how the apparatus will help him, what he will feel on the machine, how he can cooperate, and the basic mechanics of the ventilator

    b. Monitor client's response to the ventilator

        1) Assess vital signs at least every 2 hours and prn

        2) Listen to breath sounds (crackles, rhonchi, wheezes, equal breath sounds, decreased or absent breath sounds)

        3) Respiratory monitoring—pulse oximetry

        4) Check ABGs, continuous pulse oximetry monitoring

        5) Provide good oral hygiene at least twice a shift

        6) Perform nasotracheal suctioning as necessary

        7) Assess need for suctioning (tracheal/oral/nasal) of 2 hours and perform as necessary

        8) Check for hypoxia (restlessness, cyanosis, anxiety, tachycardia, increased respiratory rate)

        9) Check neurological status

        10) Check chest for bilateral expansion

        11) Move endotracheal tube to opposite side of mouth every 24 hours to prevent ulcers

        12) Monitor I and O

    c. Create alternative methods of communication with client

    d. Perform and document ventilator checks—care for client first, ventilator second

        1) Check ventilator settings as ordered by health care provider—tidal volume (TV), respiratory rate, pO_2 (fraction of inspired oxygen), mode of ventilation, sigh/button cycle

        2) Check temperature and level of water in humidification system

        3) Drain condensation from tubing away from client

        4) Verify that tracheostomy or endotracheal cuff is inflated to ensure tidal volume

        5) Observe for GI distress

        6) Document observations/procedures in client care record

F. Oxygen administration (see Tables 5-3 and 5-4)

Table 5-3 OXYGEN ADMINISTRATION		
METHOD	**OXYGEN DELIVERED**	**NURSING CONSIDERATIONS**
Nasal cannula or prongs	23–42% at 1–6 L/min	Assess patency of nostril Apply water-soluble jelly to nostrils every 3-4 hours Perform good mouth care
Face mask	40–60% at 6–8 L/min (oxygen flow minimum 5 L)	Remove mask every 1-2 hours Wash, dry, apply lotion to skin Emotional support to decrease feeling of claustrophobia
Partial rebreather mask	50–75% at 8–11 L/min	Adjust oxygen flow to keep reservoir bag two-thirds full during inspiration
Nonrebreather mask	80–100% at 12 L/min	Adjust oxygen flow to keep bag two-thirds full
Venturi mask	24–40% at 4–8 L/min	Provides high humidity and fixed concentrations Keep tubing free of kinks
Tracheostomy collar or T-piece	30–100% at 8–10 L/min	Assess for fine mist Empty condensation from tubing Keep water container full
Oxygen hood	30–100% at 8–10 L/min	Used for neonates Provides cooled humid air Check O_2 concentration with O_2 analyzer every 4 hours Refill humidity jar with sterile distilled water Clean humidity jar daily Cover client with light blanket and towel or cap for head Change linen frequently Monitor client's temperature frequently

Table 5-4 HAZARDS OF OXYGEN ADMINISTRATION	
COMPLICATION	**NURSING CONSIDERATIONS**
Infection	Change masks, tubing, mouthpieces daily
Drying and irritation of mucosa	Administer humidified oxygen
Respiratory depression (CO_2 narcosis)	Monitor respiratory rates frequently Alternate between breathing room air and O_2 at prescribed intervals Administer mixed O_2 (air and O_2) rather than pure O_2 Administer minimal concentrations necessary Periodically inflate the lungs fully
Oxygen toxicity	Premature infants exposed to excessive amounts of O_2 for prolonged periods may develop retinopathy of prematurity (ROP); may result in irreversible blindness from vasoconstriction of the retinal blood vessels Lungs of clients on respirators (children and adults) are most susceptible to pulmonary damage Pulmonary damage includes atelectasis, exudation of protein fluid into alveoli, damage to and proliferation of pulmonary capillaries, and interstitial hemorrhage Early symptoms include cough, nasal congestion, sore throat, reduced vital capacity, and substernal discomfort
Combustion	Be sure electrical plugs and equipment are properly grounded Enforce no-smoking rules Do not use oils on the client or on O_2 equipment

SELECTED PULMONARY DISORDERS

A. Chronic obstructive pulmonary disease (COPD)—term applied to respiratory disorders that involve persistent obstruction of bronchial airflow

1. Assessment
   a. Change in skin color—cyanosis or reddish color
   b. Weakness
   c. Use of accessory muscles of breathing
   d. Weight loss
   e. Dyspnea
   f. Changes in posture—day and hs
   g. Cough
   h. Changes in color, consistency of sputum
   i. Abnormal ABGs—pCO_2, pO_2
   j. Adventitious breath sounds
   k. Changes in sensorium, memory impairment

2. Etiology—group of conditions associated with obstruction of airflow entering or leaving the lungs, due to genetic and environmental causes (e.g., smoking and air pollution)
   a. Risk factors
      1) Smoking tobacco
      2) Passive tobacco smoke
      3) Occupational exposure
      4) Air pollution, coal, gas, asbestos exposure
      5) Genetic abnormalities—alpha 1-antitrypsin deficiency
      6) Older adults—loss of elastic, alveolar collapse

   b. Asthma—chronic disease with episodic attacks of breathlessness
      1) Precipitating factors
         a) Intrinsic—infection in respiratory tract, sensitivity to aspirin and other NSAIDs
         b) Extrinsic—dust, pollen, food
      2) Secondary factors—stress, fatigue, endocrine changes
      3) Status asthmaticus—acute episode of bronchospasm, not relieved by bronchodilatory therapy

   c. Emphysema—overinflation of alveoli, resulting in destruction of alveolar walls; predisposing factors: smoking, chronic infections, and environmental pollution

   d. Chronic bronchitis—inflammation of bronchi with productive cough; predisposing factors: smoking, infections, environmental pollution

   e. Cystic fibrosis—hereditary dysfunction of exocrine glands, causing production of abnormally thick mucous secretions
      1) Causes—sweat gland dysfunction, respiratory dysfunction, GI dysfunction genetic disease
      2) Diagnostic tests
         a) Sweat chloride analysis—elevated levels of sodium and chloride
         b) GI enzyme evaluation—pancreatic enzyme deficiency

3. Nursing management
   a. Assess airway clearance
   b. Listen to breath sounds

    c. Assess vital signs

    d. Administer low-flow oxygen to prevent CO_2 narcosis; monitor response to oxygen therapy

    e. Encourage fluids (6–8 glasses; 3,000 mL/24 hours)

    f. Administer medications–bronchodilators, mucolytics, corticosteroids, anticholinergics, leukotriene inhibitors, influenza and pneumococcal vaccines

    g. Chest physiotherapy–to promote removal of secretions with a minimum expenditure of energy and to decrease the need for deep tracheobronchial suctioning

        1) Breathing exercises

            a) Diaphragmatic or abdominal breathing

                i. Client positioned on back with knees bent

                ii. Place hands on abdomen

                iii. Breathe from abdomen and keep chest still

            b) Pursed lip breathing

                i. Breathe in through nose

                ii. Purse lips and breathe out through mouth

                iii. Exhalation should be twice as long as inspiration

        2) Coughing techniques

            a) Instruct client to lean slightly forward and take several slow, deep breaths through the nose, exhaling slowly through slightly parted or pursed lips

            b) Client should then take another deep breath and cough several times during expiration

            c) Client must be encouraged to cough from deep within the chest and to avoid nonproductive coughing that wastes energy

        3) Postural drainage–uses gravity to facilitate removal of bronchial secretions

            a) Client is placed in a variety of positions to facilitate drainage into larger airways

            b) Secretions may be removed by coughing or suctioning

        4) Percussion and vibration–usually performed during postural drainage to augment the effect of gravity drainage

            a) Percussion–rhythmic striking of chest wall with cupped hands over areas where secretions are retained

            b) Vibration–hand and arm muscles of person doing vibrations are tensed, and a vibrating pressure is applied to the chest as the client exhales

        5) Incentive spirometer–used to maximize inspiration and mobilize secretions

            a) Set incentive spirometer to goal client is to reach or exceed (500 mL often used to start)

            b) Client should do 10 sustained maximal maneuvers per hour and note volume on spirometer

    h. Client teaching

        1) Breathing exercises

        2) Methods of improving breathing effectiveness

        3) Stop smoking

        4) Avoid hot/cold air or allergens

5) Instructions about infection control

    a) Avoid close contact with persons who have respiratory infections or the "flu"

    b) Avoid crowds during times of the year when respiratory infections most commonly occur

    c) Maintain a high resistance with adequate rest, nourishing diet, avoidance of stress, and avoidance of exposure to temperature extremes, dampness, and drafts

    d) Practice frequent, thorough oral hygiene

    e) Advise of prophylactic influenza vaccines

    f) Instruct to observe sputum for indications of infection

Table 5-5 BRONCHODILATORS/MUCOLYTIC MEDICATIONS		
MEDICATION	**ADVERSE EFFECTS**	**NURSING CONSIDERATIONS**
Terbutaline sulfate	Nervousness, tremor Headache Tachycardia Palpitations Fatigue	Short-acting beta agonist most useful when about to enter environment or begin activity likely to induce asthma attack Pulse and blood pressure should be checked before each dose
Ipratropium bromide Tiotropium	Nervousness Tremor Dry mouth Palpitations	Cholinergic antagonist Don't mix in nebulizer with cromolyn sodium Not for acute treatment Teach use of metered dose inhaler: inhale, hold breath, exhale slowly
Albuterol	Tremors Headache Hyperactivity Tachycardia	Short-acting beta agonist most useful when about to enter environment or begin activity likely to induce asthma attack Monitor for toxicity if using tablets and aerosol Teach how to correctly use inhaler
Epinephrine	Cerebral hemorrhage Hypertension Tachycardia	When administered IV, monitor BP, heart rate, EKG If used with steroid inhaler, use bronchodilator first, then wait 5 minutes before using steroid inhaler (opens airway for maximum effectiveness)
Salmeterol	Headache Pharyngitis Nervousness Tremors	Dry powder preparation Not for acute bronchospasm or exacerbations
Montelukast sodium Zafirlukast Zileuton	Headache GI distress	Used for prophylactic and maintenance therapy of asthma Liver tests may be monitored Interacts with theophylline

Table 5-6 BRONCHODILATORS/XANTHINES/RESPIRATORY MEDICATIONS		
MEDICATION	**ADVERSE EFFECTS**	**NURSING CONSIDERATIONS**
Acetylcysteine	Bronchospasm Nausea Vomiting	Mucolytic Administered by nebulization into face mask or mouthpiece Bronchospasm most likely to occur in asthmatics Open vials should be refrigerated and used within 90 hours Clients should clear airway by coughing prior to aerosol

B. Restrictive pulmonary disease
1. Assessment
   a. Dyspnea
   b. Pleuritic pain
   c. Absent or restricted movement on affected side
   d. Decreased or absent breath sounds
   e. Cough
   f. Fever
   g. Hypotension
   h. Cyanosis
   i. Weak, rapid pulse
   j. Anxiety

2. Etiology/Causes—disorders associated with restrictive pulmonary disease
   a. Pleural effusion—collection of fluid in pleural space
      1) Pulmonary congestion so severe that distended capillaries leak fluid into alveolar spaces of the lungs
      2) Large amounts of fluid can lead to collapse of the lung
      3) Causes—infection, toxic chemicals, malignancies

   b. Pneumothorax—(see Figure 5-2): collapse of lung due to air in pleural space caused by:
      1) Thoracentesis—if needle "nicks" lung during procedure
      2) Thoracic surgery—pleural cavity is entered
      3) Accidental injury
      4) Air leak from pulmonary alveoli or erosion of a disease process through the pleura
         a) Spontaneous—without a known cause; common in tall, thin young men
         b) Tension—pressure builds up, shifting of heart and great vessels, compromising circulation and respiratory functions

   c. Hemothorax: collection of blood in the pleural space caused by:
      1) Injury (e.g., pulmonary laceration, puncture by fractured rib)
      2) Chest surgery

   d. Neoplasms

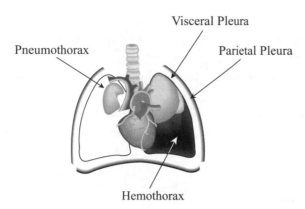

Figure 5-2. PNEUMOTHORAX AND HEMOTHORAX

3. Nursing management
   a. Assess vital signs
   b. Thoracentesis
   c. High-fowler position (head of bed elevated 60–90°)
   d. Oxygen therapy
   e. Chest tubes (see Figures 5-3 and 5-4)

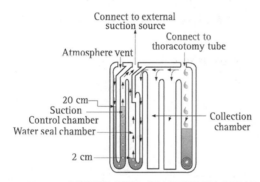

Figure 5-3. WATER SEAL COLLECTION APPARATUS

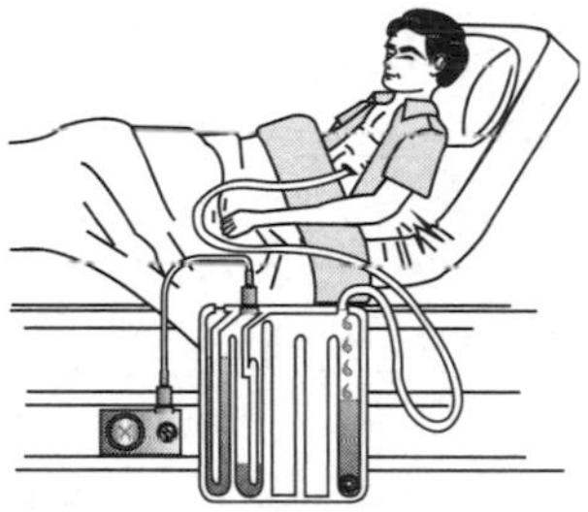

Figure 5-4. PLEUR-EVAC

   f. Procedure
      1) Fill water-seal chamber with sterile water to the 2-cm level (or as required by the manufacturer)
      2) If suction is to be used, fill the suction control chamber with sterile water to the 20-cm level, or as ordered by the health care provider
      3) Encourage the client to change position frequently
      4) The drainage system must be maintained below the level of insertion
      5) Chest tubes are clamped *only momentarily* to check for air leaks and to change the drainage apparatus
      6) Observe for fluctuations of fluid in the water-seal chamber
      7) Gently "milk" tubing in the direction of drainage as needed if agency policy allows
      8) When the health care provider removes the chest tubes, the nurse should instruct the client to do the Valsalva maneuver (forcibly bearing down while holding breath); the chest tube is clamped and quickly removed by the health care provider; an occlusive dressing is applied to the site

g. Complications

1) Observe for constant bubbling in the water-seal chamber; this indicates a leak in the drainage system

2) If the chest tube becomes dislodged, apply an occlusive dressing and notify primary health care provider

3) If the tube becomes disconnected from the drainage system, cut the contaminated tip off the tubing, insert a sterile connector, and reattach to the drainage system; or immerse the end of the chest tube in 2 cm of sterile water until the system can be reestablished

h. Medications

C. Infectious pulmonary disorders

1. Pneumonia

a. Assessment

1) Fever, chills

2) Leukocytosis

3) Cough productive of rusty-colored sputum, green whitish-yellow sputum (depends on organism)

4) Dyspnea, accessory muscle use, upright position

5) Pleuritic pain

6) Tachycardia, crackles, sonorous wheezes, bronchial breath sounds

7) Elevated WBC count, sputum culture and sensitivity, blood culture and sensitivity

b. Etiology

1) Causes include bacteria, fungi, viruses, parasite, chemical

2) Inflammatory process that results in edema of lung tissues and extravasation of fluid into alveoli, causing hypoxia

3) Risk factors

a) Community-acquired pneumonias

i. Older adult

ii. Has not received pneumococcal vaccination

iii. Has not received yearly flu vaccine

iv. Chronic illness

v. Exposed to viral infection or flu

vi. Smokes or drinks alcohol

b) Hospital-acquired pneumonia

i. Older adult

ii. Chronic lung disease

iii. Aspiration

iv. Presence of endotracheal, tracheostomy, or nasogastric tube

v. Mechanical ventilation

vi. Decreased level of consciousness

vii. Immunosuppression (disease or pharmacologic etiology)

c) Older adults—decreased cough effectiveness; decreased immune response; increased risk with decreased mobility and swallowing disorders

   c. Nursing management

      1) Assess vital signs every 4 hours

      2) Cough and breathe deeply every 2 hours

      3) Assess breath sounds and oxygen saturation

      4) Incentive spirometer—5–10 breaths per hour while awake

      5) Encourage fluids to 3,000 mL/24 hours

      6) Suctioning as needed

      7) Oxygen therapy

      8) Semi-Fowler position/bedrest

      9) Teaching: fluid intake and stop smoking

      10) Medications

         a) Mucolytics

         b) Expectorants

         c) Bronchodilators (e.g., beta-2 agonist)—nebulizer or MDI

         d) Antibiotics

2. Croup Syndromes; acute epiglottitis, acute laryngotracheobronchitis, acute laryngitis, respiratory syncytial virus

   a. Assessment

      1) Bark-like cough

      2) Dyspnea

      3) Inspiratory stridor

      4) Cyanosis

   b. Causes

      1) Viral

      2) Medical emergency due to narrowed airway in children

   c. Nursing management

      1) Care at home

         a) Steamy shower

         b) Sudden exposure to cold air

         c) Sleep with cool humidified air

      2) Hospitalization required if:

         a) Increasing respiratory distress

         b) Hypoxia or depressed sensorium

         c) High temperature (102°F)

      3) Nursing care if hospitalized

         a) Maintain airway

         b) Mist tent

         c) Monitor heart and respiratory rate

         d) Oxygen with humidification

         e) IV fluids or oral hydration

         f) Medications—antipyretics, antibiotics, bronchodilators

         g) Position in infant seat or prop with pillow

       h) Calm, quiet environment

       i) Cough and deep breathe at least every 2 hours

3. Tuberculosis (TB)

   a. Assessment

      1) Progressive fatigue, nausea, anorexia, weight loss

      2) Irregular menses

      3) Low-grade fevers over a period of time

      4) Night sweats

      5) Irritability

      6) Cough with mucopurulent sputum, occasionally streaked with blood; chest tightness and a dull, aching chest; dyspnea

      7) Diagnostic procedures

         a) Skin testing (see Table 5-7)

         b) Sputum smear for acid-fast bacilli; induce by respiratory therapy in AM and PM

         c) Chest x-ray—routinely performed on all persons with positive PPD to detect old and new lesions; tubercles may be seen in lungs

         d) Quanti FERON-TB Gold test; results within 24 hours

   b. Etiology

      1) Transmitted by airborne release droplet nuclei; bacillus multiplies in bronchi or alveoli, resulting in pneumonitis; may lie dormant for many years and be reactivated in periods of stress; myobacterium tuberculosis (acid-fast Gram-positive bacillus)

      2) Risk factors

         a) Close contact with someone who has active tuberculosis

         b) Immunocompromised status

         c) IV drug user

         d) Person who lives in institutions

         e) Lower socioeconomic group

         f) Immigrants from countries with high prevalence of tuberculosis (Latin American, Southeast Asia, Africa)

      3) Incidence increasing in immigrant populations, poverty areas, elderly, alcoholics, drug abusers, and persons with AIDS

   c. Nursing management

      1) Notification of state health department; evaluation of contacts

      2) Isoniazid (INH) prophylaxis—not recommended for those individuals greater than 35 years old who are at low risk because of increased risk of associated hepatitis; persons less than 35 get 6–9 months therapy with INH

         a) Household contacts

         b) Recent converters

         c) Persons under age 20 with positive reaction and inactive TB

         d) Susceptible health care workers

         e) Newly infected persons

         f) Significant skin test reactors with abnormal x-ray studies

         g) Significant skin test reactors up to age 35

	Table 5-7 TB SKIN TESTING
TEST	**NURSING CONSIDERATIONS**
Mantoux test	Given intradermally in the forearm
Purified Protein Derivative (PPD)	15 mm or greater induration (hard area under the skin) = significant (positive) reaction for those clients without certain risk factors
	Read in 48–72 hours
	Positive result does not necessarily mean that active disease is present, but indicates exposure to TB or the presence of inactive (dormant) disease
	Greater than 5 mm for clients with AIDS = positive reaction
	TB infection may still be present in elderly or immunocompromised with induration ≤ 10 mm
Multiple puncture test (Tine)	Read test in 48–72 hours
	Vesicle formation = positive reaction
	Screening test only
	Questionable or positive reactions verified by Mantoux test

3) Chemotherapy—to prevent development of resistant strains, two or three medications are usually administered concurrently; frequently a 6- or 9-months regimen of isoniazid and rifampin; ethambutol and streptomycin may be used initially

4) Isolation for 2 to 4 wk (or three negative sputum cultures) after drug therapy is initiated; sent home before this (family already exposed)

5) Teaching
   a) Cover mouth and nose with tissue when coughing, sneezing, laughing; place tissues in plastic bag
   b) Avoid excessive exposure to dust and silicone; wear mask in crowds
   c) Handwashing
   d) Must take full course of medications
   e) Encourage to return to clinic for sputum smears
   f) Good nutrition (increased iron, protein, vitamins B + C)

Table 5-8 ANTITUBERCULAR MEDICATIONS		
MEDICATION	**ADVERSE EFFECTS**	**NURSING CONSIDERATIONS**
First-line Medications		
Isoniazid	Toxic hepatitis Peripheral neuritis Rash Fever	Pyridoxine (B$_6$): 10–50 mg as prophylaxis for neuritis; 50-100 mg as treatment Teach signs of hepatitis Check liver function tests Alcohol increases risk of hepatic complications Therapeutic effects can be expected after 2–3 weeks of therapy Monitor for resolution of symptoms (fever, night sweats, weight loss); hypotension (orthostatic) may occur initially, then resolve; caution client to change position slowly Give before meals Do not combine with Dilantin, causes phenytointoxicity
Ethambutol	Optic neuritis	Use cautiously with renal disease Check visual acuity
Rifampin	Toxic hepatitis Fever	Orange urine, tears, saliva Check liver function tests Can take with food
Streptomycin	Nephrotoxicity VIII nerve damage	Check creatinine and BUN Audiograms if given long-term
Second-line Medications		
Para-amino-salicyclic acid	GI disturbances Hepatotoxicity	Check for ongoing GI adverse effects
Pyrazinamide	Hyperuricemia Anemia Anorexia	Check liver function tests, uric acid, and hematopoietic studies
Action	Inhibits cell wall and protein synthesis of *Mycobacterium tuberculosis*	
Indications	Tuberculosis INH—used to prevent disease in person exposed to organism	
Adverse effects	Toxic hepatitis Optic neuritis Seizures Peripheral neuritis	
Nursing considerations	Used in combination (2 medications or more) Monitor for liver damage and hepatitis With active TB, the client should cover mouth and nose when coughing, confine used tissues to plastic bags, and wear a mask with crowds until three sputum cultures are negative (no longer infectious) In inclient settings, client is placed under airborne precautions and workers wear a N95 or high-efficiency particulate air (HEPA) respirator until the client is no longer infectious	

Chapter 6

HEMATOLOGICAL AND IMMUNE DISORDERS

Sections	**Concepts Covered**
1. Overview of Hematology	Cellular Regulation
2. Disorders of the Blood	Coagulation
3. The Immune System	Immune Response, Immunity, Infection, Inflammation

OVERVIEW OF HEMATOLOGY

PLASMA

A. Albumin—regulates plasma volume; regulates osmotic pressure
B. Serum globulins—transport of lipids, bilirubin; has immune function
C. Fibrinogen—involved in blood coagulation
D. Prothrombin—involved in blood coagulation
E. Plasminogen—involved in blood coagulation

CELLULAR COMPONENTS

A. Produced in bone marrow—hemopoiesis
B. Erythrocytes (RBCs)—transport of oxygen by hemoglobin
C. Leukocytes (WBCs)—protection from infection
D. Thrombocytes (platelets)—involved in coagulation

SIGNS AND SYMPTOMS OF HEMATOLOGIC DISORDERS

A. Chronic fatigue and dyspnea—decrease in erythrocytes (e.g., anemias, leukemias, and hemorrhagic disorders) causes a reduction in the oxygen-carrying capacity of the blood
B. Increased susceptibility to infection—decrease in mature circulating leukocytes
C. Gastrointestinal symptoms—anorexia, weight loss, indigestion, sore mouth and tongue
D. Hemorrhage and bleeding into tissues and joints (hemarthrosis) and from mucous membranes— results from either a decrease in the platelet count or absence of one or more clotting factors
E. Bone pain and deformity—result from hyperactivity of bone marrow or from growth of bone tumors (e.g., multiple myeloma)
F. Jaundice—results from rupture and hemolysis of abnormal erythrocytes, as seen in hemolytic anemias and pernicious anemia, causing the release of large amounts of bilirubin into the circulation
G. Enlarged liver and spleen and hyperplasia of bone marrow—caused by either congestion from overproduction of cells (e.g., polycythemia, leukemia) or excessive demands upon these organs to destroy defective cells (e.g., hemolytic anemias)
H. Mental depression—results from the chronicity of most blood diseases and the fatigue and discomfort characteristic of these disorders
I. Protect the client from chills or burns
  1. Due to poor circulation, anemic clients often report feeling cold—offer warm clothing and blankets
  2. Avoid applying heating pads or hot water bottles to clients with anemia because they burn easily
    a. Skin is poorly supplied with blood and oxygen
    b. Client may be unaware of any burning sensation
J. Isolate client from possible sources of infection—severely anemic clients are typically exhausted and debilitated, consequently develop infections easily

DISORDERS OF THE BLOOD

A. Basic physiological disturbances characterizing hematopoietic disorders
   1. Decrease in number of cells (cytopenia)
      a. Decrease in erythrocytes: anemia
      b. Decrease in leukocytes: leukopenia—associated with increased vulnerability to infection
      c. Decrease in thrombocyte or platelet count: thrombocytopenia—associated with increased risk of hemorrhage

B. Overproduction of either normal or defective cells
   1. Myeloproliferative diseases—malignant overproduction of cells takes place within the bone marrow
      a. Polycythemia—abnormal increase in erythrocyte production
      b. Leukemia—increase in manufacture of abnormal, immature leukocytes
      c. Plasma cell myeloma or multiple myeloma—abnormal malignant proliferation of plasma cells

C. Lymphoproliferative diseases—cellular overproduction occurs within the lymphatic tissues
   1. Hodgkin's lymphoma—malignant proliferation of one form of reticuloentothelial cell within the lymph nodes; lymph nodes contain Reed-Sternberg cells
   2. Non-Hodgkin's lymphoma—all lymphoid cancers that do not contain the Reed-Sternberg cell
   3. Leukemia—overproduction of lymphocytes within the lymph nodes
   4. Lymphosarcoma—abnormal proliferation of lymphocytes or lymphoblasts within the lymph nodes

D. Defects in coagulation mechanism—caused by depletion or absence of one or more clotting factors
   1. Characterized by persistent bleeding and hemorrhage
   2. Includes the hemophilias, hypoprothrombinemia, and disseminated intravascular coagulation

E. Disorders of the spleen
   1. Include enlargement of the spleen (splenomegaly) and splenic rupture (result of accident or trauma)

F. Causative factors
   1. Hemorrhage
   2. Dietary deficiencies
   3. Malabsorptive disorders
   4. Infection
   5. Toxicity of medications
   6. Malignant overproduction of cells
   7. Increased destruction of cells by an overactive spleen
   8. Genetic predisposition
   9. Immunological defects
   10. Older adults—decreased stem cell function; decreased reticulocyte and platelet production (especially during increased demand)

G. Abnormalities of erythrocytes
   1. Two basic pathophysiological developments underlying all erythrocyte disorders

a. A deficient number of circulating red blood cells (anemia) due to one or all of the following:
1) Insufficient erythrocyte production
2) Defective erythrocyte synthesis
3) Increased erythrocyte destruction
4) Increased erythrocyte loss

b. An increased number of circulating red blood cells (polycythemia) due to either
1) A disorder of unknown etiology
2) A compensatory mechanism that develops in response to tissue hypoxia (secondary polycythemia); seen with chronic bronchitis

2. Types of erythrocyte abnormalities
a. Anisocytosis—erythrocytes vary in size from normal
b. Poikilocytosis—abnormally shaped erythrocytes, characteristic of any of the anemias with most bizarre shapes seen in the most severe anemias
c. Microcyte—abnormally small erythrocytes, characteristic of microcytic anemias (e.g., iron deficiency anemia, thalassemia major)
d. Macrocyte—abnormally large erythrocytes, characterized by microcytic anemias (e.g., pernicious anemia, folic acid deficiency anemia)
e. Hypochromic cells—erythrocytes appear pale because of abnormally low hemoglobin content
f. Spherocyte—erythrocytes relatively small and round rather than biconcave in shape, characteristic of thalassemia major or hemoglobin C disease
g. Schistocyte—fragmented erythrocytes with extremely bizarre shapes (e.g., triangles, spirals characteristic of hemolytic anemia)
h. Sickle cell—erythrocytes are crescent- or sickle-shaped due to presence of abnormal hemoglobin (hemoglobin S)

IRON–DEFICIENCY ANEMIA

A decrease in the number of erythrocytes or a reduction in hemoglobin

A. Iron-deficiency anemia—hemoglobin under 13 g/dL (130 g/L) for males; under 12 g/dL (120 g/L) for females
1. Mild
a. Asymptomatic at rest
b. Symptoms usually follow strenuous exertion—palpitations, dyspnea, diaphoresis

2. Moderate
a. Dyspnea
b. Palpitations
c. Diaphoresis
d. Chronic fatigue

3. Severe
a. Pale
b. Exhausted all the time
c. Severe palpitations
d. Sensitivity to cold
e. Loss of appetite

  f. Profound weakness

  g. Dizziness, syncope

  h. Headache

  i. Cardiac complications—CHF, angina pectoris

 4. Diagnostic tests

  a. Total erythrocyte count

  b. Hemoglobin and hematocrit determination; hemoglobin levels decrease after middle age

  c. Plasma ferritin level

  d. ZnPP—heme ratio

  e. Transferrin saturation

 5. Assessment

  a. Presence of symptoms—fatigue, dizziness, headache, "pins and needles" sensation in fingers and toes

  b. Color of urine and stools over past weeks and months (tarry stools and/or brown, hazy, or smoky urine may indicate internal bleeding)

  c. Adequacy of diet

  d. Tolerance of exercise

  e. Medications taken in recent past (increased risk of gastric irritation)

  f. Recent exposure to poisonous substances or insecticides

  g. Whether client is or has been treated for chronic infections, cancer, renal disease, liver disease, bleeding ulcers, or hemorrhoids

  h. Family history—some blood disorders are hereditary (e.g., hereditary spherocytosis), some are linked with race (e.g., sickle cell anemia), and some with ethnicity (e.g., thalassemia major)

  i. Excessive blood loss, (e.g., bleeding due to trauma or cancer)

  j. Deficiencies and abnormalities of erythrocyte production

  k. Dietary deficiencies

  l. Ingestion or absorption of poisons or drugs that suppress the bone marrow

  m. Chronic infections

  n. Genetic abnormalities that result in faulty erythrocyte genesis and/or structure

  o. Excessive destruction of erythrocytes

  p. Gerontologic considerations—iron absorption decreased, iron intake possibly decreased

B. Nursing management

 1. Provide specific treatment

  a. Reverse deficiencies, e.g., iron deficiency anemia is cured with iron preparations and diet

  b. Discontinue any damaging drug or chemical agent

  c. In the case of excessive blood loss, identify cause of bleeding, control bleeding, and administer transfusions as ordered and needed

 2. Encourage frequent rest periods—rest is essential to lower the client's oxygen requirements and reduce strain on the heart and lungs

  a. Plients with mild anemia are rarely hospitalized and are fully ambulatory; should be encouraged to rest and nap frequently, especially if the client experiences dizziness or lightheadedness

  b. Clients with severe anemia are usually hospitalized and placed on bedrest

3. Prevent skin breakdown with frequent turning and positioning
   a. Due to reduction in circulating red blood cells, the tissues of the anemic client do not receive adequate amounts of oxygen
   b. Without proper skin care, hypoxic tissues can cause rapid decubiti formation

4. Provide a diet that is high in protein, iron, and vitamins—these substances are essential to normal erythrocyte formation

5. If anorexia is a problem, serve six small, easily digested meals a day instead of three large meals
   a. Avoid hot, spicy foods if the client suffers from a sore mouth or throat
   b. Provide oral hygiene before and after the client eats
   c. Feed the client if too exhausted to feed self

6. Provide good oral hygiene, especially because these clients often suffer from a sore mouth or tongue
   a. Cleanse the teeth before and after meals with a soft-bristled toothbrush or applicator
   b. Encourage client to rinse mouth every two hours with mouthwash that is cool and slightly alkaline
   c. Lubricate lips frequently with mineral oil or petroleum jelly to prevent dryness or cracking

7. Carefully monitor blood transfusions, if indicated—blood transfusions are valuable in the treatment of anemia due to blood loss

8. Provide oxygen therapy, if indicated
   a. Given to clients with severe anemia due to a greatly reduced capacity of the blood to carry oxygen
   b. Supplemental oxygen helps to prevent tissue hypoxia and lessens the work of the heart as it struggles to compensate for the deficiency of oxygen-carrying hemoglobin

9. Protect the client from chills or burns
   a. Due to poor circulation, anemic clients often complain of feeling cold and being chilled—offer warm clothing and blankets
   b. Avoid applying heating pads or hot water bottles to clients with anemia because they burn easily
      1) Skin is poorly supplied with blood and oxygen, causing tendency to burn
      2) Client may be unaware of any burning sensation

10. Isolate client from possible sources of infection—severely anemic clients are typically exhausted and debilitated, consequently develop infections easily

11. Adminster iron supplements
    a. IM or IV iron dextran: IV route preferred; risk of hypersensitivity reaction; IM route may cause skin staining and pain
    b. Oral iron: administer between meals for better absorption; may give with meals if gastric distress occurs; use straw if liquids used; take oral supplements with ascorbic acid to increase absorption

THALASSEMIA

A. Etiology
   1. Insufficient production of normal hemoglobin
   2. Autosomal recessive genetic disorder

3. Affects ethnic groups with origins near the Mediterranean area

4. Major and minor forms of thalassemia

B. Assessment

1. General symptoms of anemia

2. Thalassemia major: hepatomegaly, splenomegaly, jaundice

3. Growth restriction in children

C. Nursing management

1. Thalassemia major: blood transfusions and chelation therapy

2. Splenectomy

3. Thalassemia minor: generally no treatment, as body adapts to reduction of normal hemoglobin

MEGALOBLASTIC ANEMIAS

A. Etiology

1. Large RBCs; caused by impaired DNA synthesis

2. Folic acid deficiency, vitamin B_{12} deficiency, medications, inborn errors, erythroleukemia

3. Common forms: pernicious anemia (megaloblastic) and folic acid deficiency

4. Pernicious anemia: insidious onset after age 40; high frequency in women

   a. Intrinsic factor no longer secreted by the parietal cells of gastric mucosa

   b. Intrinsic factor necessary for cobalamin (B_{12}) absorption

   c. Autoimmune disease; highest incidence in African Americans and in persons of Scandanavian descent

   d. Also occurs with gastrectomy, bowel resection of the ileum, Crohn's disease

   e. Older adults—insufficient absorption of vitamin B12, decreased vitamin B12 intake

B. Assessment

1. General symptoms of anemia

2. GI manifestations—sore tongue, anorexia, abdominal pain, nausea and vomiting

3. Neuromuscular—paresthesias of hands and feet, ataxia, muscle weakness, impaired thought processes

C. Diagnostic studies

1. Gastric analysis via NG tube

   a. Pentagastrin injected to stimulate gastric juice secretion, and gastric juice withdrawn via tube

   b. Gastric juice with achlorhydria indicates depressed parietal cell function

   c. Schilling test—radioactive cobalamin given to client; cobalamin excreted in urine is measured; small amount excreted if client is unable to absorb cobalamin

D. Nursing management

1. General anemia precautions

2. Protect client from injury due to decreased sensation to temperature and pain

3. Monthly cobalamin injections or cyanocobalamin nasal spray

4. Evaluate family members for pernicious anemia

5. Client is at higher risk for gastric carcinoma; ongoing evaluation

SICKLE CELL DISEASE (SCD)

A. Etiology

1. Family of genetic disorders caused by mutant sickle cell hemoglobin (HbS)

2. Predominant in African Americans and in people of Mediterranean, Caribbean, South and Central American, Arabian, or East Indian ancestry

3. SCD affects 50,000 Americans; incurable

4. Sickle cell anemia is autosomal recessive genetic disorder

5. Sickle cell trait—1/4 of hemoglobin in abnormal "S" form; 3/4 in the normal "A" form

6. Median survival of SCD clients is 40–50 years

B. Assessment

1. Hypoxia changes the RBCs containing HbS from biconcave disk to elongated crescent, or sickle cell

2. Sickle cells clog small capillaries, causing more local hypoxia and more sickling

3. Occluded blood vessels → thrombosis

4. Ischemia and necrosis of infarcted tissue

5. Gradual involvement of all body systems

6. Precipitating factors—viral and bacterial infections, high altitudes, emotional/physical stress, surgery, blood loss, dehydration, cold water

7. Children—impairment of growth and development

8. Symptoms of chronic anemia

9. Hand–foot syndrome—bone infarction causing painful swelling of hands and feet; first symptom of SCD

10. Acute sickle cell crisis

    a. Tissue hypoxia → tissue death, pain, jaundice

    b. Common sites—chest, back, extremities, abdomen

C. Diagnostic studies

1. Hgb level ranges from 7–10 g/dL (70-100 g/L)

2. Peripheral blood smear; sickled cells present

3. Sickle cell preparation

4. Sickledex

D. Complications

1. Heart failure

2. Pulmonary infarction

3. Retinal hemorrhage, scarring, detachment, blindness

4. Renal damage

5. Stroke

6. Leg ulcers

7. Osteoporosis and osteosclerosis

8. Priapism

9. Pneumonia

10. Shock

E. Nursing management

1. Acute crisis—O_2 therapy, rest, fluids, transfusion therapy for aplastic crisis

2. Pain management—narcotic analgesics; client-controlled analgesia (PCA); morphine or hydromorphone

3. Hydroxyurea; antisickling agent lessens the sickling process, decreases incidence of crises; risk of leukemia and bone marrow depression

4. Preventive care—adequate fluid intake, treatment of infections, antibiotics, folic acid,

5. Client education—avoid high altitudes, extreme temperatures, dehydration; promptly treat infection

THROMBOCYTOPENIA

A. Etiology

1. Reduction in platelets to below 150,000 mcL (150×10^9/L)

2. Inherited and acquired disorder

3. May be caused by some foods or medications (chemotherapy or antiseizure medications)

B. Immune thrombocytopenic purpura (ITP)

1. Autoimmune disease seen in children after viral illness; affects adult females between the ages of 20 to 40

2. Platelets destroyed between 1 to 3 days instead of 8 to 10 days

C. Assessment

1. Small, flat, pinpoint red microhemorrhages (petechiae)

2. Numerous petechiae (reddish skin bruise)—purpura; larger lesions—ecchymoses

3. Prolonged bleeding after venipuncture or injection; mucosal bleeding

4. Weakness, fainting, dizziness, tachycardia, abdominal pain, hypotension

D. Diagnostic studies

1. Bleeding time prolonged

2. Activated partial thromboplastin time (APTT)

3. Prothrombin time (PT)/International normalized ratio (INR)

4. Bone marrow aspiration and biopsy

5. Hgb and Hct decreased

6. Antiplatelet antibodies

E. Nursing management

1. Platelet transfusions (ITP) for platelet counts $\leq$ 20,000 mm^3 (20 x $\times$ 10^9/L)

2. IV immunoglobulin (ITP)—IV anti-Rho (D)-raise platelet count

3. Corticosteroids

4. Plasma infusion (TTP)

5. Plasmapheresis and plasma exchange (TTP)

6. Splenectomy for clients not responsive to medical therapy

7. Danazol (Danocrine)—decreases immune response

8. Immunosuppressives, e.g., rituximab, cyclophosphamide, azothioprine

9. Prevent/control hemorrhage

10. Client education
    a. Avoid OTC meds that may cause acquired thrombocytopenia
    b. Avoid Valsalva maneuver; cough, sneeze, and blow nose gently
    c. Avoid any activities that could cause hemorrhage
    d. Report development of new petechiae or nose bleed

HEMOPHILIA

Hereditary bleeding disorder that results from deficiency of or nonfunctioning factor VIII

A. Etiology
1. Hereditary bleeding disorder caused by defective coagulation factor
2. Hemophilia A—factor VIII deficiency; most common
3. Hemophilia B—factor IX deficiency
4. Sex-linked—transmitted to male by female carrier; recessive trait

B. Assessment
1. Spontaneous, easy bruising, subcutaneous hematoma
2. Joint pain with bleeding, hematuria, gingival bleeding, GI bleeding
3. Prolonged internal or external bleeding from mild trauma
4. Pallor, anesthesia from compression caused by hematomas

C. Treatment
1. Transfusions—plasma with factor VIII cryoprecipitate
2. Bedrest
3. Analgesics

D. Diagnostic studies
1. Factor assays—factor VIII, VWF, factor IX
2. Bleeding time
3. Prothrombin time (INR) and thrombin time
4. Platelet count
5. Partial thromboplastin time

E. Nursing management
1. Assess for internal bleeding
2. Analgesics for joint pain, not aspirin
3. Avoid IM injections
4. Stop topical bleeding with pressure or ice
5. Bedrest during bleeding episodes
6. Replacement of deficient clotting factors during acute episodes and prophylactically (cryoprecipitate factor VIII)
7. Client education—prevention of injury; home management; daily oral hygiene

THE IMMUNE SYSTEM Section 3

IMMUNE RESPONSE

A. Functions of the immune system
1. Defense—destruction of viruses, fungi, bacteria
2. Homeostasis—removal of damaged cells
3. Surveillance—removal of mutated cells
4. Altered responses—allergic, autoimmune, immunodeficiency disorders, malignancies

B. Types of acquired specific deficiency
1. Active/natural—contact with antigen (e.g., childhood diseases), develops slowly; protective within weeks; long-term and specific
2. Active/artificial—immunization with antigen (i.e., immunization with live/killed vaccine, toxoid); protective in a few weeks (lasts several years, booster often needed)
3. Passive/natural—transplacental and colostrum transfer; temporary (last months)
4. Passive/artificial—injection of serum from immune human or animal (i.e., human gammaglobulin); immediate immunity (last several weeks)

C. Gerontologic considerations—total WBC count normal in older adults; may see slight drop in neutrophils; decreased T-cell function; decreased primary and secondary humoral antibody response; higher incidence of malignancies; decreased antibody response to immunizations; higher incidence of infections

AIDS

Acquired immune deficiency syndrome

A. Etiology—an RNA virus; replicates inside a living cell, transcribes into DNA, which enters cell nuclei, becoming permanent part of genetic structure
1. Initial infection—viremia
2. Human immunodeficiency virus (HIV) may remain dormant for 8–10 years
3. HIV infects human cells with CD4 receptors on the surfaces—lymphocytes, monocytes/macrophages, astrocytes, oligodendrocytes
4. CD4$^+$ T cells destroyed by HIV

B. Assessment
1. HIV—presence of HIV in the blood
2. AIDS—syndrome with CD4/T-cell counts below 200/µl
3. Diagnostic tests
   a. Positive HIV antibody on enzyme-linked immunosorbent assay (ELISA) and confirmed by Western blot assay or indirect immunofluorescence assay (IFA)—at least 2-months window between infection and detection
   b. Viral load testing, T_4:T_8 ratio, antigen assays
   c. Radioimmunoprecipitation assay (RIPA)

    d. CBC reveals leukopenia with serious lymphopenia, anemia, thrombocytopenia

    e. Home-testing kits on oral secretions

    f. Seroconversion—development of HIV-specific antibodies; flulike syndrome 1–3 wk after injection

    g. Early disease—CD4$^+$ T-cell count drops below 500–600/µl; oral thrush, headache, aseptic meningitis, peripheral neuropathies; cranial nerve palsy

4. Opportunistic infections

    a. *Pneumocystis jiroveci* pneumonia

        1) Gradually worsening chest tightness and shortness of breath

        2) Persistent, dry, nonproductive cough, rales

        3) Dyspnea and tachypnea

        4) Low-grade/high fever

        5) Progressive hypoxemia and cyanosis

    b. *Candida albicans* stomatitis or esophagitis

        1) Changes in taste sensation

        2) Difficulty swallowing

        3) Retrosternal pain

        4) White exudate and inflammation of mouth and back of throat

    c. *Cryptococcus neoformans*—severe, debilitating meningitis

        1) Fever, headache, blurred vision

        2) Nausea and vomiting

        3) Stiff neck, mental status changes, seizures

    d. Cytomegalovirus (CMV)—significant factor in morbidity and mortality

        1) Fever, malaise

        2) Weight loss, fatigue

        3) Lymphadenopathy

        4) Retinochoroiditis characterized by inflammation and hemorrhage

        5) Visual impairment

        6) Colitis, encephalitis, pneumonitis

        7) Adrenalitis, hepatitis, disseminated infection

    e. Kaposi's sarcoma—most common malignancy

        1) Small, purplish-brown, nonpainful, nonpruritic, palpable lesions occurring on any part of the body

        2) Most commonly seen on the skin

        3) Diagnosed by biopsy

5. AIDS—dementia complex (ADC)

    a. Onset of progressive dementia

6. AIDS (acquired syndrome)—a syndrome distinguished by serious deficits in cellular immune function associated with positive HIV; evidenced clinically by development of opportunistic infections (e.g., *Pneumocystis jiroveci* pneumonia, *Candida albicans*, cytomegalovirus), enteric pathogens, and malignancies (most commonly Kaposi's sarcoma)

    a. High-risk groups

        1) Homosexual or bisexual men—especially with multiple partners

2) Intravenous drug abusers

3) Hemophiliacs—via contaminated blood products

4) Blood transfusion recipients prior to 1985

5) Heterosexual partners of infected persons

6) Children of infected women/*in utero* or at birth

    b. Transmission—contaminated blood or body fluids, sharing IV drug needles, sexual contact, transplacental, and possibly through breast milk

    c. Time from exposure to symptom manifestation may be prolonged (8–10 years)

C. Nursing management

  1. Preventive measures

    a. Avoidance of IV drug use (needle-sharing)

    b. Precautions regarding sexual patterns—sex education, condoms, avoid multiple partners

    c. Use of standard precautions—blood/body fluids

  2. Nursing care (see Table 6-1)

    a. No effective cure; antiretroviral medications (see Table 6-2); highly active antiretroviral therapy (HAART)—combination antiretroviral medications

    b. Treatment specific to the presenting condition

      1) Kaposi's sarcoma—local radiation (palliative), single agent/combination chemotherapy

      2) Fungal infections—nystatin swish and swallow, clotrimazole oral solution, amphotericin B with/without flucytosine

      3) Viral infections—acyclovir, ganciclovir

    c. Nutrition—high protein and calories; ketoconazole or fluconazole for candida infections

    d. Symptomatic relief—comfort measures

    e. Maintain confidentiality

    f. Provide support

      1) Client and family coping—identify support systems

      2) Minimize social isolation—no isolation precautions are needed to enter room to talk to client, take VS, administer PO medications

      3) Encourage verbalization of feelings

    g. Client/family discharge teaching

      1) Behaviors to prevent transmission—safe sex, not sharing toothbrushes, razors, and other potentially blood-contaminated objects

      2) Measures to prevent infection—good nutrition, hygiene, rest, skin and mouth care, avoid crowds; avoid raw fruits and vegetables, undercooked meat and eggs, use pepper and paprika immediately before eating

Table 6-1 NURSING CARE OF A CLIENT WITH ACQUIRED IMMUNE DEFICIENCY SYNDROME

PROBLEM	NURSING CONSIDERATIONS
Fatigue	Provide restful environment Assist with personal care Monitor tolerance for visitors
Pain	Give meds as appropriate Assess level of pain Comfort measures Analgesia
Disease susceptibility	Implement infection control precautions Handwashing or alcohol-based rubs on entering and leaving room Monitor for oral infections and meningitis Give antibiotics as ordered No fresh flowers or plants Low bacteria diet
Respiratory distress	Monitor vital signs, chest sounds Give bronchodilators and antibiotics as ordered Suction and maintain O$_2$ as prescribed Monitor for symptoms of secondary infections
Anxiety, depression	Use tact, sensitivity in gathering personal data Encourage expression of feelings Respect client's own limit in ability to discuss problems Guided imagery
Anorexia, diarrhea	Monitor weight Encourage nutritional supplements Assess hydration Give antidiarrheal medication–diphenoxylate Diet–less roughage, spicy foods Monitor perineal area for irritation

Table 6-2 ANTIRETROVIRAL MEDICATIONS

TYPE	MEDICATION NAME
Nucleoside Reverse Transcriptase Inhibitors (NRTIs)	Zidovudine Didanosine Stavudine Lamivudine Combivir (lamivudine and zidovudine combination)
Non-nucleoside reverse transcriptase inhibitors (NNRTIs)	Nevirapine Delavirdine Efavirenz
Protease inhibitors (PIs)	Saquinovir Indinavir Ritonivir Nelfinavir
Fusion inhibitors	Enfurivitide
Integrase strand transfer inhibitor	Raltegravir

IMMUNE RESPONSE

A. Hypersensitivity response
1. Type I: IgE–mediated hypersensitivity reactions–reaction to environmental allergens; rapid
2. Type II: Tissue-specific hypersensitivity reactions–(cytoxic reactions)–hemolytic anemias, hemolytic blood transfusion reaction
3. Type III: Immune complex reactions–systemic lupus erythematosus, rheumatoid arthritis
4. Type IV: Delayed hypersensitivity reactions–positive PPD, tissue transplant rejection; hypersensitivity reaction delayed or absent in older adults

B. Nursing management
1. Careful health history to determine allergies and triggers
2. Teach avoidance of allergens, triggers
3. Antihistamines, adrenalin, corticosteroids, antipruritic medications, cell-stabilizing medications (Cromolyn), immunotherapy

C. Other autoimmune diseases
1. Multiple sclerosis
2. Guillain-Barré syndrome
3. Vasculitis
4. Type 1 diabetes mellitus
5. Ulcerative colitis
6. Glomerulonephritis
7. Sjögren's syndrome
8. Systemic lupus erythematosus (SLE)
9. Rheumatoid arthritis
10. Graves' disease
11. Myasthenia gravis

D. Gerontologic considerations–decreased stem cell function; decreased reticulocyte and platelet production, especially during increased demand (acute or chronic illness)

GLOSSARY OF TERMS

1. AIDS (acquired immune deficiency syndrome)–a profound defect in the immune system that strikes previously healthy individuals who have no known cause for the immunosuppression
2. Antibodies–a collection of protein molecules manufactured by B lymphocytes in response to the presence of specific antigens
3. Antigens–specific substances that induce the development of an immune response
4. Contact transmission–direct, indirect, or droplet contact of an infectious agent to a host
5. Cytomegalovirus (CMV)–one of the herpes-type viruses, commonly found in AIDS clients and also in well homosexuals. Recent evidence, based on new genetic engineering techniques, suggests that CMV and the cells of Kaposi's sarcoma have many genes in common.

6. Epstein-Barr virus (EBV)—linked with Burkitt's lymphoma, a cancer common in children in East Africa, and with nasopharyngeal cancer, a common cancer in China. It is also the cause of infectious mononucleosis, common in adolescents and young adults. EBV is in the herpesvirus family.

7. Hepatitis viruses—occur in several classes. Type A is usually transmitted by the fecal-oral route and causes an illness that is often subclinical in the young and more severe in the elderly. Type B causes more severe illness and is associated with liver cancer. Type B can be transmitted by blood transfusions, from mother to newborn, or through saliva, breast milk, or genital secretions. Hepatitis C is transmitted blood to blood. Hepatitis D occurs only with hepatitis B. Hepatitis E—fecal contamination of food and water; not common in U.S.

8. Herpesviruses—five major types in humans: herpes simplex virus type 1 (HSV-1), 2 (HSV-2), varicella zoster virus (VZV), cytomegalovirus (CMV), and Epstein-Barr Virus (EBV). Each type of virus induces a different spectrum of human diseases; e.g., HSV-2 has a strong association with cervical carcinoma; EBV has a strong association with Burkitt's lymphoma (prevalent in African children), nasopharyngeal carcinoma (NPC; common in China), and infectious mononucleosis; CMV is associated with Kaposi's sarcoma.

9. Immune system—equips an individual to defend against infection. A contemporary definition of the term *immunity* emphasizes the ability to recognize materials or agents as foreign to oneself and to neutralize, eliminate, or metabolize them with or without injury to the host's tissues.

10. Incubation period—the time between infection by a disease-causing organism and the onset of overt symptoms of the disease

11. Infection—presence in the body of a pathogen

12. Interferon—a protein substance thought to be produced or released by cells after viral infection or by other stimuli

13. Lymphadenopathy—an abnormal condition of the lymph nodes and glands, in which the nodes enlarge, grow and swell, and become palpable

14. Lymph nodes—oval structures distributed throughout the body; through them pass the lymphocytes. When enlarged, the lymph nodes become palpable, a useful diagnostic sign of infection. Lymph nodes function as a filter of foreign material and also aid in the circulation of lymphocytes.

15. Lymphocytes—originate in the bone marrow, pass through the bloodstream, and enter other organs (such as the thymus or the gut), where they become modified to T or B lymphocytes

16. Macrophages—cells found in the bloodstream as part of the body's immune system. These cells act by surrounding a foreign particle, virus, or bacterial cell and destroying it—literally "eating" it; T lymphoctyes "present" antigen to macrophages. There is evidence that macrophages activate lymphoctyes as well by producing factors that affect lymphocyte function.

17. Opportunistic infections—various infectious organisms, mostly viruses, fungi, and parasites, which take the "opportunity" to infect a host whose immune system is deficient and thus cannot fend off the disease caused by the agent; *candida albicans, pneumocystis jiroveci* pneumonia (PCP), toxoplasmosis, histoplasmosis

18. Pathogen—microorganism or substance that is capable of producing diseases

19. *Pneumocystis carinii* pneumonia (PCP)—a form of pneumonia caused by a protozoan parasite. It usually does not cause an infection in a host with an intact immune system.

20. Retroviruses—viruses that are known to cause cancer in animals. Recently, genes from these viruses have been found to be very similar to oncogenes or so-called cancer genes found in human and other cells.

21. Slow virus infections—a group of infections caused by viruses. The incubation periods are very long, and the clinical expressions of disease are relatively slow in progression.

22. Spleen—has both nonimmunologic and immunologic functions. It removes worn-out cells from the circulatory system and is a "graveyard" for red blood cells, reintroducing iron from hemoglobin after red cell death. Like the lymph nodes, the spleen produces lymphoctyes and is important early in life. Removal of the spleen has been shown to be associated with overwhelming bacterial infections in infants, children, and young adults.

23. T_4:T_8 ratio (T-helper to T-suppressor ratio)—T_4 is a way of quantifying T-helper cells and T_8 is for quantifying T-suppressor cells. In many immunosuppressed states, the ratio of T_4:T_8 is less than 1:6; in normal states the ratio is above 1:6.

24. T-helper cells—one of the subpopulations of T lymphoctyes that aid in the cytotoxic or killing function of T lymphoctytes. In AIDS clients there is a lowering in the number of T-helper cells and an inverted ratio of helper:suppressor T cells.

25. Thymus—responsible for the development of lymphoctyes. The name *T lymphoctyes* shows that these lymphoctyes are thymus-derived.

26. T lymphocytes—arise in the bone marrow and differentiate or mature in the thymus gland. The mature T cell has cytotoxic properties and can destroy "target" cells. To aid in this killing function, there are T-helper cells. A second subpopulation of T cells are the T-suppressor cells, which have the opposite effect.

27. Varicella-zoster virus (VZV)—the causative agent for both varicella (chickenpox) and herpes zoster.

Table 6-3 HEMATOPOIETIC AND IMMUNOSTIMULANT MEDICATIONS	
MEDICATION	**INDICATION FOR USE**
Epoetin alfa	Treatment of erythrocytopenia Stimulates production of RBC Used in chronic renal failure and with clients undergoing anticancer chemotherapy
Filgrastim	Treatment of severe neutropenia Prevention of infection in clients with cancer chemotherapy-induced neutropenia and in clients undergoing bone marrow transplantation
Pegfilgrastim	Prevention of infection in clients with cancer chemotherapy-induced neutropenia
Sargramostim	Promotion of bone marrow function after bone marrow transplant
Oprelvekin	Prevention of severe thrombocytopenia associated with anticancer chemotherapy

Table 6-4 IMMUNOSUPPRESSANT MEDICATIONS	
MEDICATION	INDICATIONS FOR USE
Azathioprine	Prevent renal transplant rejection Treat severe rheumatoid arthritis not responsive to other treatments
Cyclosporine	Prevent rejection of solid organ (heart, kidney, liver) transplants Prevent graft-versus-host disease in bone marrow transplant
Tacrolimus Etanercept	Prevent liver, kidney, and heart transplant rejection Rheumatoid arthritis treatment (acts to reduce the immune response resulting in inflammation and pain)
Infliximab	Treatment of Crohn's disease (inflammatory bowel disease thought to have autoimmune origins) Treatment of rheumatoid arthritis
Methotrexate	Treatment of severe rheumatoid arthritis unresponsive to other treatments
Prednisone Prednisolone	Autoimmune disease
Basiliximab	Post transplant surgery

Chapter 7

THE GASTROINTESTINAL SYSTEM

Sections	Concepts Covered
1. Concepts Basic to Nutrition	Nutrition
2. Alterations in Metabolism	Metabolism, Elimination
3. Selected Disorders	Metabolism, Elimination, Client Education: Providing
4. Accessory Organs of Digestion (Liver, Gallbladder, Pancreas)	Metabolism, Nutrition, Elimination
5. The Lower Intestinal Tract	Nutrition, Elimination

SUMMARY OF DIGESTION

A. Digestive system (see Figure 7-1)

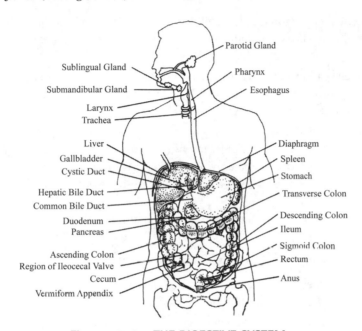

Sublingual Gland
Submandibular Gland
Larynx
Trachea
Liver
Gallbladder
Cystic Duct
Hepatic Bile Duct
Common Bile Duct
Duodenum
Pancreas
Ascending Colon
Region of Ileocecal Valve
Cecum
Vermiform Appendix

Parotid Gland
Pharynx
Esophagus
Diaphragm
Spleen
Stomach
Transverse Colon
Descending Colon
Ileum
Sigmoid Colon
Rectum
Anus

Figure 7-1. THE DIGESTIVE SYSTEM

1. Alimentary canal—consists of oral cavity, pharynx, esophagus, stomach, small intestine, large intestine, rectum; some nutrients are actively absorbed (requiring energy) and some are passively absorbed; older adults—loss of teeth and enamel; increased risk of cavities; increased risk of periodontal disease

2. Secretory glands—glands such as gastric glands line the stomach; others, such as the pancreas and liver, lie outside the stomach and secrete substances via ducts to the intestinal tract; decreased bicarbonate, mucous, and intrinsic factor in older adults

3. Sphincters
   a. Esophageal—between esophagus and stomach; dilation of lower esophagus in older adults; increased risk GERD
   b. Pyloric—between stomach and small intestine
   c. Ileocecal—between small intestine and large intestine
   d. Anal—controls passage of fluids and fecal material

B. Digestive processes
1. Mechanical—food is broken down by teeth, tongue, and peristaltic contractions of stomach and small intestine; sphincters, such as the pyloric sphincter between stomach and duodenum, control the rate of passage of food through the alimentary canal

2. Chemical
   a. Salivary glands—produce saliva, which lubricates food and begins starch digestion
   b. Esophagus—conducts food to stomach via peristaltic waves; decreased motility in older adults
   c. Stomach—gastric glands produce hydrochloric acid and the enzymes pepsin and rennin
      1) Pepsin—digests proteins into shorter polypeptides
      2) Rennin—curdles milk, which delays its passage through the stomach; enzyme is primarily found in mammalian infants
      3) Intrinsic factor—increased absorption of vitamin B12; decreased in older adults
   d. Liver—produces bile, which is stored in the gallbladder before release into the small intestine; bile emulsifies fats into smaller components that are easier to absorb; decreased size older adults
   e. Pancreas—produces enzymes such as lipase (for fat digestion), amylase (for starch digestion), trypsin, and chymotrypsin (for protein digestion); older adults have pancreatic atrophy and fibrosis, decreased production of proteolytic enzymes
   f. Small intestine—the secretory cells in the walls of the intestine produce lipase (for fat digestion), aminopeptidases (for polypeptide digestion), and disaccharidases (for maltose, sucrose, and lactose digestion); absorption is facilitated by out-pocketings in the intestinal wall, called villi, which increase the surface area; decreased absorption of proteins, fats, minerals, vitamins, and carbohydrates in older adults
      1) Duodenum—10 to 12 in long in adult; upper part of small intestine
      2) Jejunum—8 ft long in adult; middle portion of small intestine
      3) Ileum—11 ft long in adult; lower portion of small intestine
   g. Large intestine—site of water resorption; slowed peristalsis in older adults; risk for decreased fiber intake, immobility and medications may contribute
   h. Rectum—transient storage of feces prior to elimination through the anus

C. Gastrointestinal hormones
   1. Gastrin
      a. Secreted in response to mechanical distention
      b. Inhibited by acid
      c. Stimulates production of gastric acid and pepsin
      d. Increases gut motility

   2. Cholecystokinin
      a. Secreted by cells in the duodenum and jejunum
      b. Secreted in response to presence of the digested fat and protein
      c. Causes the gallbladder to contract, forcing bile into the duodenum for fat absorption

   3. Secretin
      a. Produced by the duodenum
      b. Secreted in response to the presence of free fatty acids in the intestine
      c. Stimulates the production of pancreatic juice

   4. Enterogastrone
      a. Hormone of the small intestine
      b. Secreted in response to the presence of acid in the duodenum
      c. Inhibits the secretion of gastric acid

D. Properties of the gastric mucosa
1. Turnover of gastric mucosa—cells replaced every 3 d; cells continually desquamate into the lumen; decreased new cell formation in older adults
2. Permeability of gastric mucosa—unaffected by osmotic gradients, unlike the remainder of the GI tract; pure water is not absorbed, nor is water lost to the lumen if hypertonic solutions are drunk; the duodenum is highly permeable; all fluids are brought to isotonicity
3. Gastric mucosal barrier—impermeable to (and therefore not digested by) secreted acid
    a. Possible causes of barrier breakdown
        1) Salicylates—aspirin and salicylic acid
        2) Ethanol
        3) Bile acids regurgitated from the duodenum
        4) Injuries or infections
        5) Decreased bicarbonate and mucous in older adults
    b. Consequences of barrier breakdown—acid reaches the mucosa, leading to mucosal injury and bleeding or ulcers
        1) Acid stimulates increased motility of the stomach by direct stimulation of intrinsic plexus; the strong contractions cause pain
        2) Acid penetrating the mucosa permits histamine release, leading to edema of the mucosa as the interstitial spaces fill with fluid

E. Rate and quantity of gastric secretion
1. Rate of acid secretion rises to a maximum in the second half-hour after eating
2. Total amount of acid secreted is proportional to the amount of protein ingested
3. Gerontologic considerations—gastric atrophy and decreased intrinsic factor production; increased risk vitamin B12 deficiency

F. Malfunctions involving gastric secretion
1. Loss of gastric juice (e.g., vomiting) leads to metabolic alkalosis—for each H^+ lost, one HCO_3 is retained
2. Mucosal atrophy (may involve autoimmunity to parietal cells)—no acid or pepsinogen secretion; possible lack of intrinsic factor for B_{12} absorption in the terminal ileum; pernicious anemia develops after approximately three years

G. Mechanics of gastric digestion
1. Reception of food—vagally mediated relaxation of the stomach occurs as food distends the esophagus, resulting in little increase in pressure
2. Mixing of chyme—peristaltic waves over the antrum (moving toward the pyloric sphincter) mix food and gastric secretions thoroughly
3. Vomiting—forceful expulsion of stomach contents
4. Gerontologic considerations—decreased gastric motility, volume, blood flow; stomach distension and feeling of fullness may contribute to appetite loss and weight loss

SOCIOCULTURAL INFLUENCES ON NUTRITIONAL INTAKE

*Note: not every member of a culture chooses to follow all of its traditions.

A. Orthodox Jewish
   1. Dietary laws based on biblical and rabbinical regulations
   2. Laws pertain to selection, preparation, and service of food
   3. Laws
      a. Milk/milk products never eaten at same meal as meat (milk may not be taken until 6 hours after eating meat)
      b. Two meals contain dairy products and one meal contains meat
      c. Separate utensils are used for meat and milk dishes
      d. Meat must be kosher (drained of blood)
      e. Prohibited foods
         1) Pork
         2) Diseased animals or animals who die a natural death
         3) Birds of prey
         4) Fish without fins or scales (shellfish—oysters, crab, lobster)

B. Muslim
   1. Dietary laws based on Islamic teachings in Quran
   2. Laws
      a. Fermented fruits and vegetables prohibited
      b. Pork prohibited
      c. Alcohol prohibited
      d. Foods with special value: figs, olives, dates, honey, milk, buttermilk
      e. Humane slaughter of animals for meat
   3. 30-day period of daylight fasting required during Ramadan

C. Hispanic
   1. Basic foods: dried beans, chili peppers, corn
   2. Small amounts of meat and eggs

D. Puerto Rican
   1. Starchy vegetables and fruits (plantain and green bananas)
   2. Large amounts of rice and beans
   3. Coffee main beverage

E. Native American
   1. Food has religious and social significance
   2. Diet includes meat, bread (tortillas, blue corn bread), eggs, vegetables (corn, potatoes, green beans, tomatoes), fruit
   3. Frying common method of food preparation

F. African American
   1. Minimal milk in diet
   2. Leafy greens (turnips, collards, and mustard)
   3. Pork common

G. French American
   1. Foods are strong-flavored and spicy
   2. Frequently contains seafood (crawfish)
   3. Food preparation starts with a roux made from heated oil and flour; vegetables and seafood added

H. Chinese
   1. Freshest food available cooked at a high temperature in a wok with a small amount of fat and liquid
   2. Meat in small amounts
   3. Eggs and soybean products used for protein

I. Japanese
   1. Rice is basic food
   2. Soy sauce is used for seasoning
   3. Tea is main beverage
   4. Seafood frequently used (sometimes raw fish—sushi)

J. Southeast Asian
   1. Rice is basic food, eaten in separate rice bowl
   2. Soups
   3. Fresh fruits and vegetables frequently part of diet
   4. Stir-frying in wok is common method of food preparation

K. Italian
   1. Bread and pasta are basic foods
   2. Cheese frequently used in cooking
   3. Food seasoned with spices, wine, garlic, herbs, olive oil

L. Greek
   1. Bread is served with every meal
   2. Cheese (feta) used for cooking
   3. Lamb and fish frequent
   4. Eggs in main dish, but not breakfast food
   5. Fruit for dessert

BASIC CONCEPTS OF NUTRITIONAL SCIENCE

A. Five axioms of food adequacy
   1. No single food can provide all that is needed for growth and development
   2. The storage and handling of food affect its nutritional value
   3. All nutritional requirements for a well-balanced diet can be met by food
   4. Nutrients required by humans are similar for all people, but amount varies by activity, age, and size
   5. No one food substance operates alone in metabolism

B. Carbohydrates
   1. Functions
      a. Provide energy, 4 kcal/g
      b. Regulate some aspects of protein metabolism

2. Classification
    a. Monosaccharides
        1) Simplest form of carbohydrate
        2) Glucose, fructose, and galactose
    b. Disaccharides
        1) Double sugars made up of two monosaccharides
        2) Sucrose, lactose, and maltose
    c. Polysaccharides—complex carbohydrates made up of more than two monosaccharides
    d. Fiber—multiple polysaccharides plus nondigestible substances, such as wheat bran and cereals

C. Fats
    1. Function—storage form of energy; 9 kcal/g
    2. Classifications
        a. Simple lipids—triglycerides; main form of fat in diet
        b. Compound lipids—phospholipids, glycolipids, and lipoproteins; combinations of fat with other compounds
        c. Derived lipids—digestive products of fats
            1) Glycerol—water-soluble base of triglycerides, metabolically available to form glucose
            2) Steroids—fat-related substances that contain sterols, bile acids, sex hormones, hormones of the adrenal cortex, and vitamin D
            3) Fatty acids—key refined forms of fat
                a) Saturated—primarily from animal sources; mostly solids at room temperature
                b) Polyunsaturated—mostly from plant sources; liquids at room temperature
                c) Essential—needed in diet, body does not manufacture it
                d) Nonessential—not needed in diet; body manufactures it

D. Proteins
    1. Function—to build tissue; 4 kcal/g; contains amino acids
    2. Classifications
        a. Essential amino acids—structural units of protein that body cannot manufacture
        b. Nonessential amino acids—structural units of protein that body can manufacture
        c. Polypeptides—long chains of amino acids

E. Vitamins
    1. Classification
        a. Fat soluble—vitamins A, D, E, and K
        b. Water soluble—vitamin C and B complex

    2. Characteristics
        a. Not a carbohydrate, fat, protein, or mineral
        b. Not manufactured by the body; a necessary dietary substance

    3. Fat-soluble vitamins
        a. Vitamin A

1) Source
   a) Derived from beta carotene
   b) Carotene-containing foods are most important: liver, butter, milk and cheese, and egg yolk; yellow, orange, and some green vegetables (yellow and orange colors are due in large part to carotene content)

2) Deficiency symptoms (hypovitaminosis A)
   a) Eyes: night blindness, corneal desiccation and ulceration, xerophthalmia
   b) Bronchorespiratory epithelium changes from mucus secretion to keratinization
   c) Keratinization and xerosis of the skin
   d) Genitourinary calculi
   e) Sweat gland atrophy
   f) Increased cerebrospinal fluid pressure and pseudotumor cerebri
   g) Impaired smell and taste secondary to keratinization
   h) Defective remodeling of bone
   i) Degeneration of testes and gonadal resorption
   j) Deficiency enhances carcinogenicity in lab animals

3) Toxicity (hypervitaminosis A)
   a) Acute toxicity
      i. CNS—lethargy, headache, and papilledema
      ii. Skin—dry and pruritic skin, desquamation, and erythema
      iii. GI—fatty liver, hepatic cirrhosis, and portal hypertension
      iv. Myalgia—gingivitis and cheilosis
      v. Tender hypcrostoses
      vi. Hypercalcemia, hypoprothrombinemia
   b) Pharmacokinetics
      i. Well absorbed from GI tract
      ii. Absorption mediated by a protein carrier—retino/carrier protein
      iii. Mostly stored in liver

4) Therapeutic uses of vitamin A
   a) Used to treat deficiency symptoms in cases of true deficiency, protein malnutrition (kwashiorkor), or malabsorptive syndromes (steatorrhea, hepatic cirrhosis, postgastrectomy)
   b) Dermatologic disease
      i. Acne vulgaris
      ii. Psoriasis
      iii. Ichthyosis

b. Vitamin D
   1) Source
      a) Primary—sunlight's irradiation of body cholesterol
      b) Secondary—fish oils, fortified dairy products

   2) Deficiency symptoms
      a) Rickets

    i. Uncalcified areas of bone are softened

    ii. Causes deformities of bones from physiological and gravitational stresses on soft sections of bone

  b) Growth restriction and weakness in infants and children

 3) Toxicity symptoms

  a) Hypercalcemia—weakness, vomiting, diarrhea, electrocardiographic changes

  b) Demineralization of bones

  c) Renal calculi and metastatic calcifications of soft tissues

 4) Pharmacokinetics—necessary for absorption of calcium and phosphorus

c. Vitamin E

 1) Chemically functions most clearly as an antioxidant

 2) The most important lipid-soluble antioxidant in the cell

 3) Reduces harmful free radicals to harmless metabolites

 4) Deficiency symptoms

  a) Loss of deep tendon reflexes

  b) Changes in balance and coordination

  c) Muscle weakness, visual disturbances

 5) Pharmacokinetics—absorbed predominantly via lymphatics

d. Vitamin K

 1) Source

  a) Chloroplasts of most plant species

  b) Synthesized by many intestinal bacteria

 2) Physiological function

  a) Functions as an essential cofactor for calcium binding in the clotting cascade

  b) Gamma carboxylation occurs in synthesis of prothrombin, proconvertin, Stuart factor, and plasma thromboplastin component or Christmas factor; also called factors II, VII, IX, and X, respectively

 3) Deficiency symptoms—bleeding tendency

 4) Toxicity

  a) Acute intravenous vitamin K toxicity causes chest pain, flushing, and occasionally death

  b) Large parenteral doses may cause anemia, hepatic and renal damage, and hemolysis, particularly in clients with glucose-6-phosphate deficiency

 5) Pharmacokinetics—most commonly given intramuscularly and absorbed via lymphatics

 6) Therapeutic uses

  a) Given for inadequate intake, e.g., hypoprothrombinemia of the newborn

  b) Given for inadequate absorption, e.g., biliary obstruction or malabsorption syndromes

  c) Given for inadequate utilization, e.g., chronic liver disease

4. Water-soluble vitamins—general characteristics

a. Thiamin (B_1)

 1) Sources—quantities in common foods are less than for vitamins A or C

  a) Beef, liver, whole grains, legumes are good sources

  b) Eggs, fish are fair sources

2) Deficiency symptoms—beriberi
   a) Gastrointestinal—indigestion, appetite loss
   b) Nervous system—nerve irritation and deadening sensations
   c) Cardiovascular—cardiac failure, edema

3) Toxicity—shock

4) Therapeutic uses
   a) During times of high energy requirements such as postsurgery
   b) During pregnancy and lactation
   c) During growth spurts
   d) In chronic alcoholism

b. Riboflavin (B$_2$)
   1) Sources
      a) Milk is most important source
      b) Organ meats
      c) Enriched foods

   2) Deficiency symptoms—tissue inflammation
      a) Wound aggravation—poor healing
      b) Glossitis of the tongue
      c) Cheilosis of the mouth

   3) Toxicity—not common

   4) Therapeutic uses
      a) After surgery, trauma, and burns
      b) Growth periods

c. Niacin
   1) Sources
      a) Meat
      b) Peanuts, beans

   2) Deficiency symptoms—pellagra
      a) Weakness
      b) Lassitude
      c) Loss of appetite

   3) Toxicity
      a) Vasodilation
      b) Flushing

   4) Therapeutic uses
      a) Surgery, trauma, burns
      b) Hypermetabolic states

        d. Pyridoxine (B_6)

             1) Sources—widespread in foods

                a) Yeast, liver, and kidney are good sources

                b) Egg yolks are fair sources

             2) Deficiency symptoms—not common

                a) Anemia—hypochromic

                b) CNS disturbances—seizures

             3) Toxicity—peripheral neuropathy

             4) Therapeutic uses

                a) Need greater in high-protein diets and during isoniazid (INH) therapy

                b) Greater requirement during oral contraceptive use and early pregnancy

        e. Folic acid and cyanocobalamin (B_{12})

             1) Sources—liver and kidney are best

             2) Deficiency symptoms—anemias

                a) Folic acid—megaloblastic anemia (large, immature red blood cells)

                b) B_{12}—pernicious anemia (intrinsic factor needed for intestinal absorption of B_{12})

             3) Toxicity—not common

             4) Therapeutic uses

                a) Intestinal sprue

                b) Mixed anemias

        f. Vitamin C

             1) Sources—citrus fruit and tomatoes

             2) Deficiency symptoms—scurvy

                a) Sore gums

                b) Hemorrhages

                c) Anemia

             3) Toxicity—oxalate hypersensitivity

             4) Therapeutic uses

                a) Postsurgical healing

                b) Fevers and infections

                c) Stress

                d) Growth

F. Minerals

    1. Classification

        a. Major minerals—Ca, Mg, Na, K, P, S, Cl (present in relatively large amounts)

        b. Trace minerals—Fe, Cu, I, Mn, Co, Zn, Mo (present in small amounts)

    2. Characteristics

        a. Regulates activities of many enzymes

        b. Varying amounts required; e.g., calcium is 2% of body weight, whereas iron is only 3 g in whole body

Table 7-1 MINERALS			
MINERAL	**PRIMARY FUNCTION(S)**	**PRIMARY SOURCE(S)**	**DEFICIENCY SYMPTOM(S)**
Calcium	Bone formation Muscle contraction Thrombus formation	Milk products Green leafy vegetables Eggs	Rickets Porous bones Tetany
Phosphorus	Bone formation Cell permeability	Milk, eggs Nuts	Rickets
Fluoride	Dental health	Water supply	Dental caries
Iodine	Thyroid hormone synthesis	Seafood Iodized salt	Goiter
Sodium	Osmotic pressure Acid-base balance Nerve irritability	Table salt Canned vegetables Milk, cured meats Processed foods	Fluid and electrolyte imbalance
Potassium	Water balance in cells Protein synthesis Heart contractility	Grains, meats Vegetables	Dysrhythmias Fluid and electrolyte imbalance
Iron	Hemoglobin synthesis	Liver, oysters Leafy vegetables Apricots	Anemia Lethargy

    c. Maintains acid–base balance and osmotic pressure

    d. Facilitates membrane transfer of essential nutrients; maintains nerve and muscle irritability

  3. Summary of major minerals (see Table 7-1)

G. Nursing management

  1. General diet (see Table 7-2)

  2. My Food Plate—recommendations by the U.S. Department of Agriculture for servings of daily food for Americans (see Figure 7-2 and Table 7-2)

    a. To reduce all-cause mortality, older adults should consume oral protein and energy supplements

  3. General guidelines for herbal and dietary supplements

    a. Supplements do not compensate for an inadequate diet

    b. Recommended daily amounts (RDA) should not be exceeded due to the potential for toxicity

    c. Multivitamin-mineral products recommended for certain age or gender groups contain different amounts of some minerals

    d. Iron supplements beyond those contained in multivitamin-mineral combinations are intended for short-term or special-need (e.g., pregnancy) use and should not be taken for longer periods of time due to the potential for toxicity

    e. Most adolescent and adult females consume calcium 1,000 to 1,300 mg daily

    f. Supplementing with selenium as an antioxidant and zinc to prevent colds and promote wound healing is not proven

4. Common therapeutic diets (see Table 7-3)

5. Herbals used to lower cholesterol

   a. Flax or flax seed

      1) Decreases the absorption of other medications

   b. Garlic

      1) Increases the effects of anticoagulants

      2) Increases the hypoglycemic effects of insulin

   c. Green tea

      1) Produces a stimulant effect when the tea contains caffeine

   d. Soy

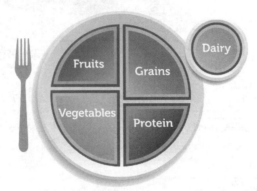

Figure 7-2. CHOOSEMYPLATE.GOV

Table 7-2 MY FOOD PLATE		
GROUP	**FOOD EXAMPLES**	**RECOMMENDED DAILY INTAKE**
Grains	Bread, cereals, cooked cereals, popcorn, pasta, rice, tortillas Half of all grains should be whole grains	Children—3–5 ounce equivalents Teens—5–7 ounce equivalents Young adults—6–8 ounce equivalents Adults—6–7 ounce equivalents Older adults—5–6 ounce equivalents
Vegetables	Dark green vegetables (broccoli, spinach, greens, leafy vegetables), orange vegetables (carrots, pumpkin, sweet potatoes), dried beans and peas (split peas, pinto, kidney, black, soy [tofu]), starchy vegetables (corn, peas, white potatoes)	Children—1–1½ cups Teens—2–3 cups Young adults—2½–3 cups Adults—2½–3 cups Older adults—2–2½ cups
Fruits	Apple, bananas, strawberries, blueberries, orange, melons, dried fruits, fruit juices	Children—1–1½ cups Teens—1½–2 cups Young adults—2 cups Adults—1½–2 cups Older adults—1½–2 cups
Oils	Nuts, butter, margarine, cooking oils, salad dressings	Children—3–4 teaspoons Teens—5–6 teaspoons Young adults—6–7 teaspoons Adults—5–6 teaspoons Older adults—5–6 teaspoons
Milk	Milk, yogurt, cheese, puddings	Children—2 cups Teens—3 cups Young adults—3 cups Adults—3 cups Older adults—3 cups
Meat and beans	Meat, poultry, fish, dry beans, eggs, peanut butter, nuts, seeds	Children—2–4 ounce equivalents Teens—5–6 ounce equivalents Young adults—5½–6½ ounce equivalents Adults—5–6 ounce equivalents Older adults—5–5½ ounce equivalents

Table 7-3 COMMON THERAPEUTIC DIETS		
Clear Liquid Diet	**Full Liquid Diet**	**Low-Fat, Cholesterol-Restricted Diet**
Sample meal items: Gelatin dessert, popsicle, tea with lemon, ginger ale, bouillon, fruit juice without pulp	Sample meal items: Milkshakes, soups, custard; all clear liquids	Sample meal items: Fruit, vegetables, cereals, lean meat
Common medical problems: Postoperative; acute vomiting or diarrhea	Common medical problems: GI upset (diet progression after surgery)	Common medical problems: Atherosclerosis
Purpose: To maintain fluid balance	Purpose: Nutrition without chewing	Purpose: To reduce calories from fat and minimize cholesterol intake
Not allowed: Fruit juices with pulp, milk	Not allowed: Jam, fruit, solid foods, nuts	Not allowed: Marbled meats, avocados, milk, bacon, egg yolks, butter
Sodium-Restricted Diet	**High-Roughage, High-Fiber Diet**	**Low-Residue Diet**
Sample meal items: Cold baked chicken, lettuce with sliced tomatoes, applesauce	Sample meal items: Cracked wheat bread, minestrone soup, apple, Brussels sprouts	Sample meal items: Roast lamb, buttered rice, sponge cake, "white" processed foods
Common medical problems: Heart failure, hypertension, cirrhosis	Common medical problems: Constipation, large bowel disorders	Common medical problems: Temporary GI/elimination problems (e.g., lower bowel surgery)
Purpose: To lower body water and promote excretion	Purpose: To maximize bulk in stools	Purpose: To minimize intestinal activity
Not allowed: Preserved meats, cheese, fried foods, cottage cheese, canned foods, added salt	Not allowed: White bread, pies and cakes from white flour, "white" processed foods	Not allowed: Whole wheat, corn, bran
High-Protein Diet	**Kidney Diet**	**Low-Phenylalanine Diet**
Sample meal items: 30 grams powdered skim milk and 1 egg in 100 mL water *or* Roast beef sandwich and skim milk	Sample meal items: Unsalted vegetables, white rice, canned fruits, sweets	Sample meal items: Fats, fruits, jams, low-phenylalanine milk
Common medical problems: Burns, infection, hyperthyroidism	Common medical problems: Chronic renal failure	Common medical problems: Phenylketonuria (PKU)
Purpose: To reestablish anabolism to raise albumin levels	Purpose: To keep protein, potassium, and sodium low	Purpose: Low-protein diet to prevent brain damage from imbalance of amino acids
Not allowed: Soft drinks, "junk" food	Not allowed: Beans, cereals, citrus fruits	Not allowed: Meat, eggs, beans, bread

NUTRITIONAL ASSESSMENT

A. Clinical signs of nutritional status (see Table 7-4)

Table 7-4 PHYSICAL SIGNS OF ADEQUATE NUTRITIONAL STATUS	
BODY AREA	**NORMAL APPEARANCE**
Hair	Shiny, firm, intact scalp without areas of pigmentation
Teeth	Evenly spaced, straight, no cavities, shiny
Tongue	Deep red in color
Gums	Firm, without redness, even-colored
Skin	Smooth, moist, even shading
Nails	Firm, without ridges
Extremities	Full range of motion
Abdomen	Flat, nontender
Legs	Good color
Skeleton	No malformations
Weight	Normal for height
Posture	Erect
Muscles	Firm
GI	Good appetite and digestion
Vitality	Good endurance, good sleep pattern

B. Health factors
1. Weight—recent gain or loss of 10% is significant
2. Medications—use of antacids, laxatives, diuretics, digitalis, oral contraceptives
3. Illness—cancer, radiation therapy, surgery, GI disease, endocrine disorders, heart disease

NUTRITIONAL PARAMETERS

A. Caloric requirement—a calorie is a measurement unit of energy; person's height and weight, as well as level of activity, determine energy need; average adult requires anywhere from 1,500 kcal to 3,000 kcal/d

B. Fluid requirement—average fluid requirement for normal healthy adult is approximately 1,800–2,500 mL/d

C. Nutrient requirements
1. Carbohydrates—first substance utilized for energy production in starvation; only source of energy production for the brain
2. Fats—second source of energy production utilized by the body in starvation; its waste products are ketone bodies, which can create an acidic environment in the blood
3. Proteins—last energy source utilized in starvation; depletion of protein leads to muscle wasting as well as loss of pressure in the vascular space; low albumin level in the blood indicates protein malnutrition

D. Diagnostic tests
1. Blood (see Table 7-5)

2. Urine
   a. Urinalysis—an elevated level of ketone bodies indicates altered fat metabolism
      1) Schilling test—diagnoses vitamin B_{12} deficiency (pernicious anemia); radioactive vitamin B_{12} is administered to the client; low value excreted in urine indicates pernicious anemia (normal is greater than 10% of dose excreted in 24 hours)

Table 7-5	BLOOD TESTS (RANGES MAY VARY BY RESOURCE AND FACILITY)	
BLOOD TEST	**CONVENTIONAL VALUES**	**SI VALUES**
Serum albumin	3.5–5.0 g/dL	35–50 g/L
Prealbumin	19.5–35.8 mg/dL	195–358 mg/L
Lymphocyte count	20–40% of total white cells	0.2–0.4 of total white cells
Hemoglobin 　Male 　Female 　Children (3-12 (years)	 13 –18 g/dL 12–16g/dL 11 - 12.5 g/dL	 130-180 g/L 120-160 g/L 110 - 125 g/L
Hematocrit 　Male 　Female 　Children (3-12 years)	 42–52% 35–47% 35–45%	 0.42–0.52 0.35–0.47 0.35–0.45
Glucose tolerance test	1 hour—190 mg/100 mL 2 hours—140 mg/mL 3 hours—125 mg/mL	1 hour—10.5 mmol//L 2 hours—7.7 mmol/L 3 hours—6.9 mmol/L
Total cholesterol	150–200 mg/dL	3.9–5.2 mmol/L
Low-density lipoproteins (LDL), mg/100 mL	Less than 160 (no CAD and less than 2 risk factors) Less than 130 (no CAD 2 or more risk factors) Less than 100 if CAD present	Less than 160 (no CAD and less than 2 risk factors) Less than 130 (no CAD 2 or more risk factors) Less than 100 if CAD present

3. Gastric aspirate
   a. pH—measures acid/alkaline range; generally overly acidic environment can lead to ulcerative activity; gastric pH of 1–4 indicates proper placement of NG tube
   b. Guaiac—tests for presence of blood in aspirate; normally, blood absent

4. Stool
   a. Fecal occult blood test (FOBT)—tests for presence of blood; normally, blood absent
   b. Stool for quantitative analysis—reviewed for color, consistency, and amount
   c. Stool for presence of *Clostridioides difficile* infection

5. Special procedures
   a. Upper GI series (barium swallow)
      1) Definition—ingestion of barium sulfate to determine patency and size of esophagus, size and condition of gastric walls, patency of pyloric valve, and rate of passage to small bowel or into small bowel
      2) Preparation

        a) Maintain NPO after midnight; avoid opoids and anticholinergic medications

        b) Inform client that stool will be light-colored after procedure

    3) Post-test—encourage fluids and/or laxative to prevent constipation

  b. Endoscopy

    1) Definition—visualization of esophagus and/or stomach and/or duodenum by means of a lighted, flexible fiberoptic tube introduced through the mouth to the stomach or from rectum through intestines to determine presence of ulcerations or tumors or to obtain tissue or fluid samples

    2) Preparation

        a) Verify that informed consent from client has been obtained

        b) Maintain NPO before procedure (at least 8 hours)

        c) Teach client about numbness in throat due to local anesthetic applied to posterior pharynx by spray or gargle; conscious sedation used

    3) Postprocedure nursing care

        a) Maintain NPO until gag reflex returns

        b) Observe for vomiting of blood, respiratory distress, aspiration

        c) Inform client to expect sore throat for 3 to 4 days after procedure

  c. Gastric analysis

    1) Definition—aspiration of gastric contents to evaluate for presence of abnormal constituents such as blood, abnormal bacteria, abnormal pH, or malignant cells

    2) Preparation—client must be NPO before test; NG tube is passed; contents aspirated and sent for evaluation

    3) Pentagastrin is sometimes used to stimulate hydrochloric acid secretion

  d. Lower GI series (barium enema)

    1) Definition—instillation of barium into colon via rectum for fluoroscopy x-rays to view tumors, polyps, strictures, ulcerations, inflammation, or obstructions of colon

    2) Preparation

        a) Low-residue diet for 1–2 days

        b) Clear liquid diet and laxative evening before test

        c) Cleansing enemas until clear morning of test

    3) Postprocedure nursing care

        a) Cleansing enemas after exam to remove barium and prevent impaction; laxatives adminstered

        b) X-rays may be repeated after all barium is expelled

E. Nursing management

  1. Weight for height tables—ideal body weight at specific heights

  2. Exchange lists

    a. Six classifications; client is given number of allowances

    b. Foods on each list nearly equal in carbohydrates, protein, fat, and calories

  3. Evaluation methods—24-h food recall or 3-d food diary

ALTERNATIVE TECHNIQUES

A. Enteral nutrition—liquid delivered to stomach, distal duodenum, or proximal jejunum via a nasogastric, percutaneous endoscopic gastrostomy (PEG) or percutaneous endoscopic jejunostomy (PEJ) tube (see Table 7-6)

1. Definition—providing nourishment via a tube due to inability of GI tract use

2. Basic principles

   a. Tube must be in proper position before infusion of food or aspiration into lungs can result

   b. Feeding must be administered at room or body temperature at a controlled rate or diarrhea may result

3. Nursing management of tube feeding

   a. Insert tube through the nose to the stomach

      1) X-ray verification most reliable method

      2) Aspirate gastric or duodenal contents for pH testing

         a) pH 0–4 indicates gastric placement

         b) pH greater than 4 usually indicates placement in intestine

         c) pH greater than or equal to 5.5 indicates placement in lungs

      3) Observe color—gastric aspirate usually cloudy and green but may also be off-white, tan, bloody, or brown

   b. Verify placement of tube before administering feeding

      1) X-ray verification most reliable method

      2) Aspirate gastric or duodenal contents for pH testing

         a) pH 0–4 indicates gastric placement

         b) pH greater than or equal to 6 indicates placement in lungs or intestines

      3) Observe color—gastric aspirate usually cloudy and green but may be off-white, tan, bloody, or brown

   c. Aspirate for gastric contents; if more than 50–100 mL residual, hold feeding

   d. Control rate of feeding administration—use enteral pump or count drops in gravity administration

   e. Flush tube with water or normal saline after feeding and before and after medications are administered through the tube

Table 7-6 CONDITIONS REQUIRING ENTERAL FEEDING	
CONDITION	**CAUSE**
Preoperative need for nutritional support	Inadequate intake preoperatively, resulting in poor nutritional state
Gastrointestinal problems	Fistula, short-bowel syndrome, Crohn's disease, ulcerative colitis, nonspecific maldigestion or malabsorption
Oncology therapy	Radiation, chemotherapy
Alcoholism, chronic depression, eating disorders	Chronic illness, psychiatric, or neurologic disorder
Head and neck disorders or surgery	Disease or trauma

4. Complications of enteral feeding (see Table 7-7)

Table 7-7 COMPLICATIONS OF ENTERAL FEEDINGS	
COMPLICATION	**NURSING CONSIDERATIONS**
Mechanical tube displacement	Replace tube
Aspiration	Elevate head of bed, check residual before feeding for intermittent; check residual every 4 hours for continuous. If excess residual present, stop for 1 hour and recheck residual.
Gastrointestinal cramping, vomiting, diarrhea	Decrease feeding rate Change formula Administer at room temperature
Metabolic hyperglycemia	Monitor glucose, serum osmolality Monitor glucose, give insulin if needed Reduce infusion rate
Dehydration	Flush tube with water or normal saline according to hospital policy
Formula-drug interactions	Check compatibility Flush tubing prior to and after medication

B. Parenteral nutrition (see Figure 7-3)

1. Definition—liquid concentrate of hypertonic glucose, amino acids, electrolytes, vitamins, and minerals, given to selected clients to provide nutrition when enteral feeding is not possible or desirable

2. Basic principles

   a. Concentrated solution must be infused in large vessel; rapid dilution is mandatory to prevent complications of high osmolarity

   b. Client must be carefully monitored for signs of complications; infection and hyperglycemia are common; fluid volume overload possible

3. Nursing management

   a. Do not infuse solution until placement of tube is verified as correct by x-ray

   b. Use aseptic technique when changing dressing or handling infusion bottle; use filter

   c. Infuse solution by pump at constant rate to prevent abrupt change in infusion rate

      1) Increased rate results in hyperosmolar state

      2) Slowed rate results in "rebound" hypoglycemia due to delayed pancreatic reaction to change in insulin requirements

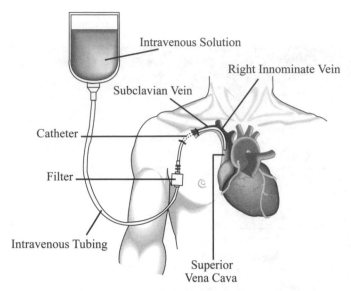

Intravenous Solution

Right Innominate Vein

Subclavian Vein

Catheter

Filter

Intravenous Tubing

Superior
Vena Cava

Figure 7-3. PARENTERAL NUTRITION (PN)

4. Types of solutions
   a. PN—amino acid-dextrose formulas; 2–3 L of solution given over 24 hours; 500 mL of 10% fat emulsions (Intralipid) given with PN over 6 hours 1–3 times/wk; fine bacterial filter used
   b. TNA (total nutrient admixture)—amino acid-dextrose-lipid, "3-in-1" formula; 1 L solution given over 24 hours
   c. Lipids—provides fatty acids

5. Methods of administration
   a. Peripheral—used for peripheral parenteral nutrition to supplement oral intake; should not administer dextrose concentrations above 10% due to irritation of vessel walls; usually used for less than 2 wk
   b. Central—catheter inserted into subclavian vein
      1) Peripherally inserted central catheters (PICC)—catheter threaded through basilic or cephalic vein to superior vena cava; dextrose solution greater than or equal to 10%; duration less than or equal to 4 wks.
      2) Percutaneous central catheters through subclavian vein
      3) Triple-lumen central catheter often used; distal lumen (16-gauge) used to infuse or draw blood samples, middle lumen (18-gauge) used for PN infusion, proximal lumen (18-gauge) used to infuse or draw blood and administer medications; duration less than or equal to 4 wks
      4) If single-lumen catheter used, cannot use to administer medications (may be incompatible) or give blood (RBCs coat catheter lumen); medications and blood must be given through peripheral IV line, not piggybacked to the PN IV line
   c. Atrial
      1) Right atrial catheters—Hickman/Biovac and Groshong
      2) Subcutaneous port—Huber needle used to access port through skin

6. Nursing management
   a. Initial rate of infusion 50 mL/h and gradually increased (100–125 mL/h) as client's fluid and electrolyte tolerance permits
   b. Infuse solution by pump at constant rate to prevent abrupt change in infusion rate
      1) Increased rate results in hyperosmolar state (headache, nausea, fever, chills, malaise)
      2) Slowed rate results in "rebound" hypoglycemia caused by delayed pancreatic reaction to change in insulin requirements; do not discontinue suddenly
   c. Client must be carefully monitored for signs of complications; infection and hyperglycemia are common (see Table 7-8)
   d. Change IV tubing and filter every 24 hours
   e. Keep solutions refrigerated until needed; allow to warm to room temperature before use
   f. If new solution unavailable, use 10% dextrose and water solution until available

Table 7-8 COMPLICATIONS OF PN	
COMPLICATION	NURSING CONSIDERATIONS
Infection/Sepsis	Maintain closed intravenous systems with filter
	No blood drawn or medications given through PN line
	Dry sterile occlusive dressing applied to site
Pneumothorax because of line placement	PN to be started only after chest x-ray validates correct placement
	Monitor breath sounds and for presence of shortness of breath
Hyperglycemia	Monitor glucose level and serum osmolality
Hyperosmolar coma	Administer insulin according to sliding scale insulin
Hypoglycemia	Hang 10% dextrose solution if PN discontinued suddenly
Fluid overload	Monitor breath sounds, weight and peripheral perfusion
	Do not "catch up" if PN behind
Air embolism	Monitor for respiratory distress
	Valsalva maneuver during tubing and cap change

7. Monitor daily weight, glucose, temperatures, I and O; check BUN, electrolytes (calcium, magnesium) three times a week; check CBC, platelets, prothrombin time, liver function studies (AST, ALT), prealbumin serum albumin once per week
8. Do not increase flow rate if PN behind scheduled administration time
9. Discontinuation
   a. Gradually tapered to allow client to adjust to decreased levels of glucose
   b. After discontinuation, isotonic glucose solution administered to prevent rebound hypoglycemia (weakness, faintness, diaphoresis, shakiness, confusion, tachycardia)

ALTERATIONS IN METABOLISM

A. Alterations in protein metabolism (see Table 7-9)

Table 7-9 ALTERATIONS IN PROTEIN METABOLISM		
DISORDER	**ASSESSMENT**	**NURSING CONSIDERATIONS**
Phenylketonuria (PKU)—inborn error of phenylalanine utilization	High blood phenylalanine that leads to intellectual delay	Specially prepared milk substitutes for infants (Lofenalac) Low-protein diet for children (no meat, dairy products, eggs, NutraSweet)
Gout—inborn error of purine metabolism	High uric acid level that leads to progressive joint deterioration	Low-purine diet (no fish or organ meats)
Celiac disease (sprue)—inborn error of wheat and rye metabolism	Intestinal malabsorption that leads to malnutrition Diarrhea Failure to thrive	Gluten-free diet (no wheat, oats, rye, barley)
Kidney failure	Increased protein and albumin losses in urine leads to protein deficiency	High-calorie, low-protein diet, as allowed by kidney function
Protein allergy	Diarrhea that leads to malnutrition and water loss	Change dietary protein source

B. Alterations in fat metabolism (see Table 7-10)

Table 7-10 ALTERATIONS IN FAT METABOLISM		
DISORDER	**ASSESSMENT**	**NURSING CONSIDERATIONS**
Hepatobiliary disease	Decreased bile leads to fat malabsorption	Low-fat, high-protein diet Vitamins
Cystic fibrosis	Absence of pancreatic enzymes leads to malabsorption of fat (and fat-soluble vitamins), weight loss Infection and lung disease lead to increased need for calories and protein	Pancreatic enzyme replacement (Cotazym pancrelipase) before or with meals High-protein diet High-calorie diet in advanced stages
Atherosclerosis (thickening and hardening of the arteries)	Associated with high blood cholesterol and triglyceride levels	Low-saturated-fat diet Cholesterol-lowering medications given before meals

IMPAIRED ABSORPTION OF NUTRIENTS

A. Infections of the GI tract

1. Assessment

   a. Definition—acute illness caused by ingested food or water contaminated by toxins or parasites

   b. Signs and symptoms

      1) Headache

      2) Abdominal discomfort, anorexia

      3) Watery diarrhea, nausea, vomiting

      4) Low-grade fever

   c. Predisposing conditions—ingestion of contaminated food/liquid

2. Types of infection (see Table 7-11)

3. Nursing management

   a. Prevention

      1) Good sanitation

      2) Good hygiene measures (e.g., handwashing)

      3) Proper food preparation (e.g., thorough cooking); heat canned foods 10–20 min; inspect cans for gas bubbles

      4) Proper food storage

   b. Treatment

      1) Maintain fluid and electrolytes; oral rehydration preferred (infants 1 to 3 tsp every 10–15 min)

      2) Monitor vital signs

      3) Medication: antibiotics, antispasmodics as ordered

      4) Maintain respiratory status—botulism can require tracheostomy, respiratory support

Table 7-11 COMMON INFECTIONS OF THE GASTROINTESTINAL TRACT		
PARASITE OR BACTERIUM	SOURCE	NURSING CONSIDERATIONS
Enterotoxigenic *E. coli*	Undercooked beef	Causes rapid, severe dehydration, cook beef until meat no longer pink and juices run clear
Salmonella	Poultry, eggs	Causes gastroenteritis, systemic infection
Campylobacter	Poultry, beef, pork	Cook and store food at appropriate temperatures
Giardia lamblia	Protozoan, contaminated water	Treated with metronidazole, good personal hygiene
Shigella	Fecal contamination	Affects pediatric population, antimicrobial therapy
Clostridioides difficile	Fecal contamination	Greater risk in older adults. Often preceded by antibiotic therapy

Table 7-12 SELECTED ANTIEMETIC MEDICATIONS		
MEDICATION	**ADVERSE EFFECTS**	**NURSING CONSIDERATIONS**
Prochlorperazine	Drowsiness Orthostatic hypotension Diplopia, photosensitivity	Check CBC and liver function with prolonged use
Ondansetron	Headache, sedation Diarrhea, constipation Transient elevations in liver enzymes	New class of antiemetics—serotonin receptor antagonist Administer 30 min prior to chemotherapy
Metoclopramide	Restlessness, anxiety, drowsiness Extrapyramidal symptoms Dystonic reactions	Monitor BP Avoid activities requiring mental alertness Take before meals Used with tube feeding to decrease residual and risk of aspiration Administer 30 min prior to chemotherapy
Meclizine	Drowsiness, dry mouth Blurred vision Excitation, restlessness	Contraindicated with glaucoma Avoid activities requiring mental alertness
Dimenhydrinate	Drowsiness Palpitations, hypotension Blurred vision	Avoid activities requiring mental alertness
Promethazine	Drowsiness Dizziness Constipation Urinary retention Dry mouth	Administer PO, IM, rectal suppository Report excessive sedation Avoid alcohol, other CNS depressants
Ginger	Minor heartburn	May increase risk of bleeding if taken with anticoagulants, antiplatelet, or thrombolytic medications Instruct to stop medication if easy bruising or other signs of bleeding noted; report to health care provider

B. Vomiting

1. Characteristics—color, amount, quality, odor

2. Predisposing factors
   a. Health history—medication adverse effects, GI tract and neurological conditions
   b. Emotional factors—stress can precipitate vomiting

3. Diagnostic Studies
   a. Gastroscopy—direct visualization of gastric mucosa through a lighted endoscope
   b. Barium swallow radiologic study—client swallows a radiopaque liquid

4. Nursing management
   a. Antiemetics—medications that relieve vomiting (see Table 7-12)
   b. Replace lost fluids and electrolytes; oral rehydration preferred
   c. Control odors

SELECTED DISORDERS

HIATAL HERNIA

A. Definition—opening in diaphragm through which the esophagus passes and becomes enlarged, and part of the upper stomach comes up into the lower portion of the thorax

B. Etiology
1. Structural—weakening of diaphragm
2. Increased abdominal pressure—obesity, pregnancy, heavy lifting
3. Gerontologic considerations—weakened diaphragm, kyphosis, medications (calcium channel blockers, nitrates)

C. Clinical manifestations
1. Often no symptoms
2. Feeling of fullness in chest with pain when lying down
3. Client complains of chest pain, heartburn, belching, dysphagia

D. Treatment
1. Antacids (with limitations)
2. H_2 receptor blockers (e.g., cimetidine, ranitidine)
3. Cryoprotective medications (e.g., sucralfate)
4. Proton pump inhibitors (e.g., omeprazole)
5. Surgery to tighten cardiac sphincter (valvuloplasty or antireflux procedure)

E. Dietary
1. Small, frequent meals; avoid caffeine, chocolate, alcohol, fatty foods, NSAIDs

F. Nursing management: client teaching—do not lie down for at least 1 hour after meals; elevate head of bed when sleeping

GASTRITIS

A. Definition—inflammation of stomach, which may be acute or chronic

B. Clinical manifestations—uncomfortable feeling in abdomen, headache, anorexia, nausea, vomiting (possibly bloody), hiccuping

C. Cause—*H. pylori*, NSAIDs, alcohol, radiation therapy, atrophic gastritis in elderly

D. Nursing management
1. Nothing by mouth, slowly progressing to bland diet
2. Antacids often relieve pain
3. Referral to appropriate agency if alcohol abuse is verified
4. Medications—H_2 receptor blockers, proton pump inhibitors, cryoprotective medications, antibiotics

PEPTIC ULCER DISEASE

(see Figure 7-4)

A. Definition—excavation formed in the mucosal wall, caused by erosion that may extend to muscle layers or through the muscle to the peritoneum (see Table 7-13)

B. Assessment—sites

C. Risk factors

1. *H. pylori* infection
2. Acute responses to medical or surgical stressors
3. Psychological stress
4. Gerontologic considerations—increased use of NSAIDs

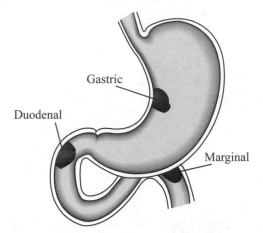

Figure 7-4. SITES FOR ULCERS

Table 7-13 DUODENAL VERSUS GASTRIC ULCER		
	CHRONIC DUODENAL ULCER	**CHRONIC GASTRIC ULCER**
Age	30–60 years	50 years and older
Sex	Male-female ratio: 3:1	Male-female ratio: 1:1
Risk factors	Blood group type O, COPD, chronic renal failure, alcohol, smoking, cirrhosis, stress	Gastritis, alcohol, smoking, NSAIDs, stress
Gastric secretion	Hypersecretion	Normal to hyposecretion
Pain	2–3 hours after meal; nighttime, often in early sleeping hours Food intake relieves pain Older adults—pain may not be first symptom	½–1 hour after meal or when fasting Relieved by vomiting Ingestion of food does not help Older adults—pain may not be first symptom
Vomiting	Rare	Frequent
Hemorrhage	Less likely	More likely
Malignancy	Rare	Occasionally

D. Nursing management—nonsurgical
1. Diet
   a. Avoid oversecretion and hypermotility in the gastrointestinal tract
   b. Eat three meals per day; small, frequent feedings not necessary if taking antacids or histamine blocker
   c. Avoid coffee, alcohol, highly seasoned foods, milk and cream, extremes in food temperature
2. Reduce stress
3. Medications (see Table 7-14)
   a. Antacids: administer 1 hour before or after meals; antacids decrease absorption of other medications
   b. Histamine receptor site antagonist (e.g., cimetidine, ranitidine); administer with meals
   c. Sucralfate; give one hour before meals
   d. Proton pump inhibitors
   e. Antibiotic therapy for *H. pylori* (e.g., metronidazole, tetracycline)
4. Complications
   a. Perforation
   b. Hemorrhage
   c. Peridontitis

E. Surgical intervention (see Figure 7-5)
1. Diagnostic work—upper GI series, endoscopy, CT scan, esophagogastroduodenoscopy (EGD)
2. Minimally invasive surgery by laparaoscopy
3. Gastrectomy—removal of stomach and attachment to upper portion of duodenum
4. Pyloroplasty
5. Vagotomy—cutting the vagus nerve (decreases HCl secretion)
6. Billroth I—partial removal (distal 1/3–1/2) of stomach, anastomosis with duodenum
7. Billroth II—removal of distal segment of stomach and antrum, anastomosis with jejunum

Table 7-14 GI MEDICATIONS		
MEDICATION	ADVERSE EFFECTS	NURSING CONSIDERATIONS
Antacids		
Aluminum hydroxide gel Calcium carbonate Aluminum hydroxide and magnesium trisilicate	Constipation that may lead to impaction Phosphate depletion (aluminum-only products)	Monitor bowel pattern Compounds contain sodium; check if client is on sodium-restricted diet Aluminum and magnesium antacid compounds interfere with tetracycline absorption Calcium compounds can cause hypercalcemia and hypersecretion of gastric acid, causing acid rebound Encourage fluids Monitor for signs of phosphate deficiency—malaise, weakness, tremors, bone pain Shake well

Table 7-14 GI MEDICATIONS *(CONTINUED)*		
MEDICATION	**ADVERSE EFFECTS**	**NURSING CONSIDERATIONS**
Magnesium hydroxide	None at normal dose Excessive dose can produce nausea, vomiting, and diarrhea	Store at room temperature with tight lid to prevent absorption of CO_2 Prolonged and frequent use of cathartic dose can lead to dependence Administer with caution to clients with renal disease
Magnesium trisilicate in combination with aluminum hydroxide	(See aluminum hydroxide gel and magnesium hydroxide, above)	(See aluminum hydroxide gel and magnesium hydroxide, above) Careful use advised for kidney dysfunction
Aluminum hydroxide and magnesium hydroxide combined	Slight laxative effect	Encourage fluid intake
Cytoprotective		
Sucralfate	Constipation Dizziness	Take medication 1 hour before each meal Should not be taken with antacids or H_2 blockers
H2-antagonists		
Cimetidine Ranitidine Famotidine	Diarrhea Confusion and dizziness (esp. in elderly with large doses) Headache	Bedtime dose suppresses nocturnal acid production Compliance may increase with single-dose regimen Avoid antacids within 1 hour of dose Dysrhythmias Cimetidine—high risk of confusion in older adults
Proton Pump Inhibitor		
Omeprazole Lansoprazole Rabeprazole Esomeprazole Pantoprazole	Dizziness Diarrhea	Typically administered 30 to 60 minutes before breakfast Do not crush sustained-release capsule; contents may be sprinkled on food or instilled with fluid in NG tube
Anti Ulcer		
Sucralfate	Nausea Vomiting Decreased absorption of some medication	Shake well before pouring Give on an empty stomach Give 1–2 hours beofre meals
Prostaglandin analogs		
Misoprostol	Abdominal pain Diarrhea (13%) Miscarriage	Notify health care provider if diarrhea more than 1 week or severe abdominal pain or black, tarry stools
Nursing considerations	Other medications may be prescribed, included antacids (time administration to avoid canceling med effect) and antimicrobials to eradicate *H. pylori* infections Client should avoid smoking, alcohol, ASA, and caffeine, all of which increase stomach acid	

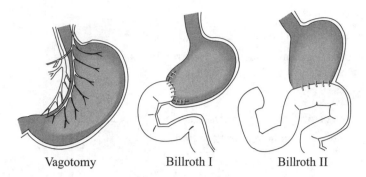

Vagotomy   Billroth I   Billroth II

Figure 7-5. COMMON SURGERIES FOR ULCERS

F. Nursing management—surgical
1. Postoperative
   a. Assess vital signs
   b. Inspect dressings
   c. Observe nasogastric drainage for volume and blood
   d. Provide gastric decompression as ordered
      1) Levin tube—single lumen at low suction
      2) Salem sump—double lumen for drainage
         a) Prevent irritation to nostril
         b) Lubricate tube around nares with water soluble jelly
         c) Control excessive nasal secretions

2. B_{12} via parenteral route (required for life)
3. Encourage deep breathing
4. Observe for peristalsis
   a. Listen for bowel sounds
   b. Record passage of flatus or stool

5. Teach preventive measures for "dumping syndrome" (rapid passage of food to stomach, causing diaphoresis, diarrhea, hypotension); usually occurs 10–15 minutes after eating
   a. Restrict fluids with meals
   b. Avoid stress after eating
   c. Eat smaller, frequent meals
   d. Lie down after eating

PYLORIC STENOSIS IN ADULTS

A. Definition—in adults, narrowing or obstruction of the pyloric sphincter caused by scarring from healing ulcers
B. Assessment
1. Vomiting
2. Epigastric fullness
3. Anorexia
4. Weight loss
5. Constipation

C. Surgical intervention

1. Pyloroplasty—incision through circular muscles of the pylorus

2. Vagotomy and gastroenterostomy—establishes gastric drainage, involves severing of vagus nerve

D. Nursing management

1. Perioperative

   a. Correct fluid and electrolyte abnormalities—alkalosis, hypokalemia

   b. Gastric decompression or small frequent feedings

2. Postoperative

   a. Observe for signs of dumping syndrome, gastritis, and esophagitis (adults)

   b. Check incision; provide fluids

ACCESSORY ORGANS OF DIGESTION (LIVER, GALLBLADDER, PANCREAS)

OVERVIEW OF ACCESSORY ORGANS

(See Figure 7-6)

A. Liver

1. Anatomy
   a. Gland located in right upper quadrant of abdomen below diaphragm
   b. Arterial blood brought to liver by hepatic artery
   c. Filtered blood returns to body via hepatic vein
   d. Blood from the stomach, spleen, pancreas, and intestine is brought to liver for filtration via the portal vein
   e. Older adults—decreased liver size

2. Functions
   a. Manufacture and secrete bile
      1) Bilirubin—from hemoglobin released by red blood cells at end of their life cycle
      2) Bile salts
      3) Cholesterol
      4) Color—greenish or brownish yellow
      5) Bile aids in digestion and leaves liver via channels that form the hepatic duct
   b. Manufacture of fibrinogen and prothrombin
   c. Manufacture of heparin
   d. Aids in destruction of aging red blood cells
   e. Manufacture of vitamin A
   f. Storage of vitamins A, B, D, iron, copper
   g. Metabolism of carbohydrates, fats, proteins
   h. Manufacture of immunoglobulins
   i. Metabolism of drugs, alcohol, and hormones
   j. Regulation of blood volume by storing up to 400 mL of blood
   k. Older adults—decreased enzymatic reactions; decreased metabolism of medications and hormones

B. Biliary tract

1. Common bile duct
   a. Anatomy—composed of cystic duct from the gallbladder and hepatic duct from the liver; leads to duodenum
   b. Function—transport bile from liver and gallbladder to duodenum when food is present in small intestine

2. Cystic duct
   a. Anatomy—leads from gallbladder to the common bile duct
   b. Function—passageway for bile to and from gallbladder

        1) When duodenum is empty, sphincter closes, causing bile from the liver to flow through the cystic duct into the gallbladder

        2) During digestion, sphincter opens as the gallbladder contracts, forcing bile through the cystic duct to the common bile duct into the duodenum

    3. Gallbladder

      a. Anatomy—sac located under the right side of liver

      b. Function—storage and concentration of bile; stimulated to contract by cholecystokinin (a hormone secreted by the small intestine in response to the presence of fat)

C. Pancreas

  1. Anatomy

    a. Gland located behind stomach on left side of abdomen

    b. Composed of lobes, lobules, and ducts

    c. Pancreatic duct joins with the common bile duct at the duodenum

    d. Contains the islets of Langerhans—specialized cells that produce insulin and glucagon

  2. Functions—digestive and exocrine gland functions

    a. Manufacture and release (via pancreatic duct) of pancreatic enzymes to aid digestion

      1) Amylase—helps break down carbohydrates

      2) Lipase—helps break down fats

      3) Trypsin—helps break down protein

    b. Production and release of insulin and glucagon directly into the bloodstream

      1) Alpha cells synthesize glucagon

      2) Beta cells synthesize insulin

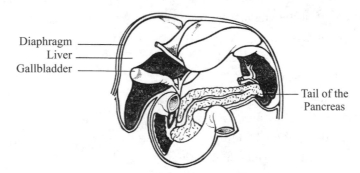

Figure 7-6. LIVER, GALLBLADDER, AND PANCREAS

DIAGNOSTIC TESTING

A. Liver function studies

  1. Liver function test—over 70% of the parenchyma of the liver may be damaged before liver function tests become abnormal (see Table 7-15)

B. Radiographic

  1. Abdominal x-rays—show enlargement or displacement of organs

  2. Cholangiogram—x-ray permitting visualization of bile ducts after IV injection of dye

  3. Liver scan—scanning of liver with radioisotopic-sensitive device after IV injection of radioisotopes; to detect cysts or masses in the liver

Table 7-15 LIVER FUNCTION TESTS			
TEST	**PURPOSE**	**PREPARATION/TESTING** CONVENTIONAL UNITS (SI UNITS)	**POST-TEST NURSING CARE**
Pigment studies	Parameters of hepatic ability to conjugate and excrete bilirubin Abnormal in liver and gallbladder disorders, e.g., with jaundice Direct bilirubin increases in obstruction	Fast 4 hours Normal Serum bilirubin, direct 0.1–0.4 mg/dL (1.7–3.7 mcmol/L) Serum bilirubin, total 0.3–1.0 mg/dL (5–17 mcmol/L) Urine bilirubin, total 0	Over 70% of the parenchyma of the liver may be damaged before liver function tests become abnormal
Protein studies Serum albumin	Proteins are produced by the liver Levels may diminish in hepatic disease Severely decreased serum albumin results in generalized edema	Normal 3.5–5.5 g/dL (35–55 g/L)	None
Coagulation studies Prothrombin time (PT) or International normalized ratio (INR) Partial thromboplastin time (PTT)	May be prolonged in hepatic disease In liver disease, PTT prolonged due to lack of vitamin K	Normal PT 9.0–12.0 seconds PTT 20–39 seconds	Put specimen in ice Apply pressure to site for 5 min (15 min if on anticoagulants)
Liver enzymes	With damaged liver cells, enzymes are released into bloodstream	Normal AST 10–40 units/L ALT 10–40 units/L LDH less than 176 units/L	None
Blood ammonia (Arterial)	Liver converts ammonia to urea With liver disease, ammonia levels rise	Normal 15–45 mcg/dL (11–32 mcmol/L)	None
Abdominal x-ray	To determine gross liver size	None	None
Liver/spleen scan	To demonstrate size, shape of liver, visualize scar tissue, cysts, or tumors; radioactive isotope injected intravenously	Client is not a source of radioactivity	None
Cholecystogram and cholangiography (percutaneous, surgical, or magnetic resonance)	For gallbladder and bile duct visualization; radiopaque material injected directly into biliary tree; determines filling of hepatic and biliary ducts	Question client about seafood (iodine) allergy Fat-free dinner evening before exam Ingestion of dye in tablet form (Telepaque tablets—check history of allergies to iodine) evening before NPO after dye ingestion X-rays followed by ingestion of high-fat meal followed by further x-rays	None

	Table 7-15 LIVER FUNCTION TESTS *(CONTINUED)*		
TEST	PURPOSE	PREPARATION/TESTING CONVENTIONAL UNITS (SI UNITS)	POST-TEST NURSING CARE
Celiac axis arteriography	For liver and pancreas visualization; uses contrast medium of organic iodine	Question client about seafood (iodine) allergy prior to radiopaque dye administration; anaphylaxis possible	None
Splenoportogram (splenic portal venography)	To determine adequacy of portal blood flow; uses contrast medium of organic iodine	Question client about seafood (iodine) allergy prior to radiopaque dye administration; anaphylaxis possible	None
Liver biopsy	Sampling of tissue by percutaneous needle aspiration	Administer vitamin K IM to decrease chance of hemorrhage Informed consent NPO morning of exam (6 hours) Sedative administration just before exam Ask client to hold breath for 5–10 seconds during insertion Performed at bedside, supine position, lateral with upper arms elevated	Position on right side for 1–2 hours and gradually elevate HOB, 30° 1st 2 hours, 45° 2nd 2 hours Maintain bedrest for 24 hours Frequently check vital signs to detect hemorrhage and shock; check clotting time, platelets, hematocrit Expect mild local pain radiating to right shoulder Report complaints of severe abdominal pain immediately— may be indication of perforation of bile duct and peritonitis
Bilirubin	Detect presence of bilirubin due to hemolytic or liver disease	Total bilirubin 0.3–1.0 mg d/L (5–17 mcmol/L) Direct (conjugated) bilirubin 0.1–0.4 mg/dL (1.7–3.7 mcmol/L) Indirect (unconjugated) bilirubin 0.1–0.4 mg/dL (3.4–11.2 mcmol/L)	None

C. Ultrasound

D. Liver biopsy

1. Client preparation

   a. Obtain vital signs and weight

   b. Done at bedside—client in supine position or lateral with upper arms elevated

   c. Empty bladder prior to procedure to avoid accidental perforation

   d. Administer vitamin K IM to decrease chance of hemorrhage; check clotting time

   e. NPO morning of procedure (6 hours before)

   f. Sedative administration just prior to procedure; teach client about holding breath for 5-10 s during procedure

2. Nursing management

   a. Check vital signs frequently for hemorrhage and/or infection; weigh client

   b. Assess dressing and insertion site

   c. Report elevated temperature and/or abdominal pain to health care provider

E. Paracentesis

1. Needle aspiration of abnormal fluid accumulated in abdominal cavity (ascites) for analysis or as therapeutic measure

2. Client preparation

   a. Obtain vital signs and weight

   b. Done at bedside—client typically placed in supine position with HOB slightly elevated

   c. Empty bladder prior to procedure to avoid accidental perforation

3. Nursing management

   a. Check vital signs frequently for hemorrhage and/or infection; weigh client

   b. Assess dressing and insertion site

   c. Report elevated temperature and/or abdominal pain to health care provider

   d. Maintain bedrest according to agency policy

SELECTED DISORDERS OF THE DIGESTIVE ACCESSORY ORGANS

A. Liver disorders

1. Cirrhosis

   a. Definition—group of chronic diseases in which liver tissue is gradually replaced by scar tissue; results in gradual loss of liver function

   b. Assessment

      1) Alcoholic cirrhosis—result of alcoholism and poor nutrition

      2) Biliary cirrhosis—result of chronic biliary obstruction and infection

      3) Postnecrotic cirrhosis—result of a previous viral hepatitis

      4) Older adults—hepatitis C, obesity, chronic alcohol use

      5) Complications

         a) Portal hypertension—elevated blood pressure throughout entire portal venous system

         b) Esophageal varices

            i. Dilated tortuous veins usually found in the submucosa of the lower esophagus

            ii. Hemorrhage from rupture leading cause of death in clients with cirrhosis

   iii. Ascites

   iv. Bleeding disorders

 c. Surgical intervention—cirrhosis/bleeding esophageal varices

  1) Shunts to relieve portal hypertension—last resort intervention for portal hypertension and esophageal varices

   a) Portacaval—blood diverted from portal circulation to vena cava

   b) Splenorenal—blood diverted from splenic vein to left renal artery

   c) Transjugular intrahepatic portosystemic shunt (TIPS)

  2) Liver transplant

  3) Transjugular intrahepatic portosystemic shunt (TIPS)—for clients who have not responded to any other nonsurgical management

 d. Surgical/nonsurgical intervention—bleeding esophageal varices

  1) Insertion of Sengstaken-Blakemore tube with three openings (see Figure 7-7)

   a) Gastric balloon—inflation lumen

   b) Esophageal balloon—inflation lumen

   c) Gastric aspiration lumen

  2) Minnesota tube

   a) Similar to Sengstaken-Blakemore tube but has four lumens

   b) Fourth lumen allows for aspiration of secretions that collect above the esophageal balloon

  3) Injection sclerotherapy—endoscopic injection of a chemical into the esophagus; causes varices to become fibrotic

  4) Endoscopic variceal ligation

  5) Administration of desmopressin acetate—temporarily lowers portal pressure

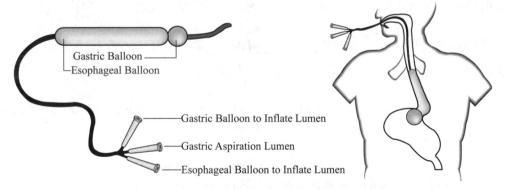

Figure 7-7. SENGSTAKEN-BLAKEMORE TUBE

  6) Shunting procedure—transjugular intrahepatic portosystemic shunt (TIPS)

 e. History

  1) Digestive disturbances

   a) Indigestion

   b) Flatulence

   c) Anorexia

   d) Nausea and vomiting

    2) Circulatory
        a) Esophageal varices
        b) Hematemesis
        c) Hemorrhage
        d) Ascites
        e) Hemorrhoids
        f) Increased bleeding tendencies
        g) Edema in extremities

    3) Biliary
        a) Jaundice
        b) Pruritus
        c) Dark urine
        d) Clay-colored stools

    4) Hepatorenal failure
    5) Hepatic failure

  f. Nursing management
    1) Provide appropriate nutrition
        a) Early stages—high protein, high carbohydrates
        b) Advanced stages—fiber, protein, fat, and sodium restrictions
        c) Small, frequent feedings
        d) Fluid restriction
        e) No alcohol

    2) Maintain skin integrity
        a) Avoid strong soaps
        b) Alleviate dry, itching skin

    3) Promote rest
    4) Reduce exposure to infection
    5) Reduce ascites
        a) Sodium/fluid restrictions
        b) Medications—diuretics
        c) Paracentesis

    6) Monitor fluid/electrolyte balance
    7) Lactulose—decreases serum ammonia levels

2. Jaundice
  a. Definition—condition in which all tissues including skin and sclera are yellow or greenish-yellow because of an increased concentration of bilirubin in the blood
  b. Causes
    1) Hemolytic (prehepatic)—caused by destruction of great number of blood cells, causing a high concentration of bilirubin, exceeding the liver's ability to excrete it
        a) Hemolytic transfusion reactions
        b) Autoimmune hemolytic anemia
        c) Erythroblastosis fetalis

2) Intrahepatic—due to inability of normal amounts of bilirubin to be excreted by a diseased liver

    a) Cirrhosis

    b) Hepatitis

3) Obstructive (post hepatic)—due to intrahepatic or extrahepatic obstruction interfering with bile flow

    a) Cholelithiasis

    b) Tumors

    c) Adverse effect of medications—e.g., phenothiazine derivative, sulfonamides

c. History and assessment

    1) Yellowish or greenish-yellow discoloration of skin and sclera

    2) Dark-colored urine

    3) Clay-colored stools

    4) Pruritus

d. Nursing management

    1) Treatment of underlying cause

    2) Relief of pruritus

        a) Medications—e.g., antihistamines, topical steroids

        b) Diversionary activities

        c) Corn starch, baking soda, oatmeal bath

        d) Keep nails trimmed and clean

3. Hepatitis (see Table 7-16)

    a. Assessment

        1) Fatigue

        2) Jaundice (icterus), yellow sclera

        3) Anorexia, right upper quadrant (RUQ) pain and tenderness, malaise

        4) Clay-colored stools, tea-colored urine

        5) Pruritus—accumulation of bile salts under the skin

        6) Liver function studies; elevated ALT, AST, alkaline phosphatase (ALP)

        7) Prolonged PT

        8) Percutaneous liver biopsy

        9) Antibodies to specific virus; (e.g., anti-HAV)

    b. Nursing management

        1) Frequent rest periods

        2) Appropriate transmission-based precautions

            a) HAV—enteric precautions

            b) HBV, HCV—blood and body fluids precautions

        3) Diet low in fat, high in calories, carbohydrates, and protein; no alcoholic beverages

        4) For pruritus—calamine, short clean nails, antihistamines

5) Medications
  a) Vitamin K
  b) Antiviral medications—interferon and lamivadine
  c) Post exposure hepatitis B vaccine

6) Teach client and family
  a) Avoid alcohol and potentially hepatotoxic prescription/OTC medications (particularly acetaminophen and sedatives)
  b) Balance rest and activity periods
  c) Techniques to prevent spread
  d) Cannot give blood donation
  e) Instruct to note and report recurrence of signs and symptoms

Table 7-16 CLASSIFICATIONS OF HEPATITIS				
TYPE	HIGH RISK GROUP	INCUBATION	TRANSMISSION	NURSING CONSIDERATIONS
Hepatitis A (HAV)	Young children Institutions for custodial care International travelers to developing countries	15–50 days	Common in fall, early winter Fecal-oral Shellfish from contaminated water Poor sanitation Contaminated food handlers Oral-anal sexual activity	Survives on hands Diagnostic tests—Cultured in stool and detected in serum before onset of disease Prevention—improved sanitation; Hepatitis A vaccine Treated with gamma globulin early postexposure No preparation of food
Hepatitis B (HBV)	Immigrants from areas of HBV endemicity Drug addicts Fetuses from infected mothers Homosexually active men Clients on dialysis Male prisoners Transfusion recipients Health care workers	28–160 days	Blood and body fluids Parenteral drug abuse Sexual contact Hemodialysis Accidental contaminated needle exposure Maternal-fetal route	Diagnostic tests—Hepatitis B surface antigen, anti-HBc, anti-HBe Treatment—Hepatitis B vaccine (Heptavax-B, Recombivax HB), Hepatitis B immune globulin (HBIg) postexposure; interferon alpha-2b; lamivudir Chronic carriers—frequent; potential for chronicity 5-10% Complications: cirrhosis; liver cancer
Hepatitis C (HCV)	Persons receiving frequent blood transfusions International travelers Hemophilia clients	15–160 days	Contact with blood and body fluids IV drug users	May be asymptomatic Complications: cirrhosis; liver cancer Great potential for chronicity
Delta or Hepatitis D (HDV)	Drug addicts Concurrent HBV infection	28–160 days	Coinfects with Hepatitis B Close personal contact Parenteral transmission	Diagnostic test—HD Ag in serum

Table 7-16 CLASSIFICATIONS OF HEPATITIS *(CONTINUED)*				
TYPE	**HIGH RISK GROUP**	**INCUBATION**	**TRANSMISSION**	**NURSING CONSIDERATIONS**
Hepatitis E	Persons living in underdeveloped countries	28–35 days	Oral-fecal Contaminated water	Resembles Hepetitis A Does not become chronic Usually seen in young adults Seen in travelers from Asia, Africa, Mexico
Toxic Hepatitis	Elderly (increased use of prescription and over-the-counter medications, decreased liver metabolism) Drug-induced (INH, diuretics, tetracycline, carbon tetrachloride, acetaminophen, ETOH) Alcohol		Noninfectious inflammation of liver	Removal of causative substance Check level of consciousness Encourage fluids

B. Biliary disorders

   1. Cholecystitis

      a. Definition—inflammation of gallbladder

      b. Causes—bacterial invasion via blood, lymph, or bile ducts

      c. Risk factors

         1) Cholelithiasis

         2) Obesity

         3) Sedentary lifestyle

         4) Women affected more than men

         5) Highest incidence age 50–60 years

      d. Assessment

         1) Intolerance to fatty foods

         2) Indigestion

         3) Nausea, vomiting, flatulence

         4) Severe pain in upper right quadrant of abdomen radiating to back and right shoulder

         5) Elevated temperature

         6) Leukocytosis

         7) Dark urine, clay-colored stools

      e. Nursing management

         1) Antibiotics

         2) NPO until acute symptoms subside

         3) Gastric decompression

         4) Analgesics

         5) Weight-reduction diet if needed

         6) Avoidance of fatty, fried foods

2. Laparoscopic cholecystectomy
   a. Laparoscope attached to a video camera visualizes the gallbladder through a small, 10-mm puncture at the umbilicus
   b. A laser is used to dissect the gallbladder away from the liver bed
   c. Laparoscopic forceps extract the gallbladder through puncture site

3. Surgical management of the client with biliary disease
   a. Types of surgery
      1) Cholecystectomy—removal of gallbladder; a Penrose drain may be inserted through the incision to promote drainage into dressings
      2) Cholecystostomy—opening of gallbladder to remove stones, bile, or pus (decompression); a tube (cholecystostomy tube) is sutured into the gallbladder for drainage
      3) Choledochostomy—opening into the common bile duct to remove obstructing stones; a drainage tube (T-tube) is inserted into the duct and connected to drainage
      4) Extracorporeal shock wave lithotripsy—shock wave therapy to destroy stones in the biliary system
         a) Strong analgesics and sedation used before procedure
         b) Treatment followed with oral dissolution therapy

   b. Preoperative care
      1) Routine preop care
      2) Nutritional supplements of glucose and protein hydrolysates to aid in wound healing and prevent liver damage
      3) NG tube insertion before surgery

   c. Postoperative care
      1) Routine postop care to prevent respiratory, circulatory, and fluid electrolyte complications
      2) Promotion of drainage from cholecystostomy or T-tube until normal bile flow is reestablished
         a) Semi-Fowler position
         b) Prevent kinking or twisting of tubes
         c) Position drainage bottle as ordered (usually kept on bed at or below level as gallbladder)
         d) Observe and record amount and character of drainage (expect 500–1,000 mL/d at first)
      3) Check orders regarding clamping of T-tube before/after meals
      4) Check orders regarding fluid replacement of drainage
      5) Provide low-fat, high-carbohydrate, high-protein diet
      6) Note color changes of skin, sclera, and stool as indicators of improved bile flow after T-tube removal
         a) Jaundice should lessen
         b) Stool should slowly progress from light to dark color
      7) Protect skin around incision from drainage and leakage
         a) Apply coat of zinc oxide or petroleum jelly
         b) Change dressing frequently
         c) If drainage amount remains large, record finding (may indicate fistula)

8) Provide pain medication as needed

   a) Position frequently for comfort

   b) Evaluate pain intensity; may indicate other problems, e.g., infection, urinary retention, gas in intestines

9) Monitor signs for K^+ and Na^+ alterations; check serum electrolytes

4. Cholelithiasis

  a. Definition—presence of stones in the gallbladder; cholesterol stones or pigment stones

  b. Causes—an increased concentration and precipitation of bile substances (cholesterol, bile acids, bile pigments)

    1) Metabolic factors—an increased serum cholesterol

      a) Obesity

      b) Pregnancy

      c) Diabetes

      d) Hypothyroidism

    2) Biliary stasis

    3) Biliary system inflammation and cirrhosis of liver

  c. Assessment

    1) Belching immediately following a meal; flatulence

    2) Indigestion following rich, fatty foods

    3) Severe right upper quadrant abdominal pain radiating to back and right shoulder (biliary colic); rebound tenderness

    4) Nausea and vomiting

    5) Biliary colic—severe pain, tachycardia, diaphoresis

  d. Nursing management

    1) Relief of pain—analgesics; meperidine avoided

    2) Anticholinergics—dicyclomine

    3) Control of nausea and vomiting

    4) Gastric decompression

    5) Monitor for dehydration

5. Biliary carcinoma

  a. Risk factors—chronic cholelithiasis

  b. Cause—unknown

  c. Signs and symptoms

    1) Jaundice (advanced disease)

    2) Same as cholelithiasis

  d. Management—cholecystectomy, radiation therapy, chemotherapy

6. Biliary atresia

  a. Definition—congenital absence of bile ducts

  b. Cause—unknown

  c. Assessment

    1) Jaundice of progressive intensity starting at age 2–3 wk

    2) Dark urine

        3) Clay-colored stools

        4) Decreased nutritional fat absorption

        5) Vitamin A, D, E, K (fat-soluble) deficiencies

        6) Low prothrombin level and easy bleeding

        7) Lethargy and slow movement

    d. Nursing management

        1) Reconstructive surgery to create pathway for bile flow into intestines

        2) Poor prognosis—only small percentage of infants can tolerate the surgery

C. Pancreatic disorders

  1. Acute pancreatitis

    a. Definition—inflammatory condition of the pancreas in which pancreatic function can be restored

    b. Etiology

        1) Possible factors: tumors, cysts, abscesses, penetrating ulcers, infections, drug toxicities, heredity, neurogenic and emotional factors, alcoholism, trauma to abdomen

        2) Theory—"autodigestion" of the pancreas by its own enzymes

    c. Assessment

        1) Nausea and vomiting; vomiting does not relieve pain or nausea; may occur after heavy meal or alcohol ingestion

        2) Fluid/electrolyte imbalance

        3) Abdominal and back pain major symptom; pain increased after meals and is unrelieved with antacids

        4) Fever

        5) Jaundice

        6) Hyperglycemia

        7) Weight loss

        8) Ascites

        9) Increased serum amylase and lipase, elevated urine amylase, decreased serum calcium, elevated bilirubin

    d. Nursing management

        1) NPO

        2) Gastric decompression

        3) Antacids and proton pump inhibitors

        4) Analgesics (meperidine contraindicated)

        5) Treating fluid/electrolyte imbalance

        6) Monitor for signs of infection

        7) Monitor for shock, renal failure

        8) Monitor for hyperglycemia

        9) TPN

        10) Long-term treatment includes avoidance of alcohol; low-fat, bland diet; and small, frequent meals

2. Chronic pancreatitis
   a. Definition—chronic fibrosis of the pancreas with obstruction of pancreatic ducts and destruction of pancreatic secreting cells
   b. Causes and risk factors
      1) Develops after repeated episodes of alcohol-induced acute pancreatitis
      2) Associated with chronic obstruction of bile duct
   c. Assessment
      1) Severe upper abdominal and back pain difficult to relieve; pain flares up
      2) Nausea and vomiting
      3) Jaundice
      4) Dark urine
      5) Fever
      6) Diarrhea and steatorrhea
      7) Weight loss and muscle wasting
      8) Diabetes mellitus (polyuria, polydipsia, polyphagia)
   d. Nursing management
      1) Analgesics—opoid and non-opoid analgesics
      2) Medications to decrease gastric acid—H_2 receptor blockers, proton pump inhibitors, or octreotide
      3) Bland, low-fat diet
      4) Six small feedings daily—increased caloric intake
      5) Treatment of exocrine insufficiency—medications containing amylase, lipase, and trypsin to aid digestion, e.g., pancrelipase
      6) Monitor signs and symptoms of diabetes mellitus; possible oral hypoglycemics or insulin
      7) Avoid alcohol

3. Pancreatic cancer
   a. Assessment
      1) Pain is absent in early stages
      2) Pain (abdominal: vague, dull)
      3) Anorexia and fatigue
      4) Weight loss
      5) Nausea, vomiting, flatulence
      6) Jaundice (initial sign, but disease may be advanced)
      7) Clay-colored stools
      8) Dark urine; frothy urine
      9) GI bleeding
      10) Ascites
   b. Nursing management
      1) High-calorie, bland, low-fat diet
      2) Avoid alcohol
      3) Anticholinergics
      4) Chemotherapy—combination of medications
      5) Radiation therapy (external beam or radioactive iodine implantation)

6) Stent placement for obstruction

7) Surgery (Whipple procedure)—removal of head of pancreas, distal portion of common bile duct, the duodenum, and part of the stomach or minimally invasive surgery via laparaoscopy

8) Postop nursing management

   a) Monitor for peritonitis, hemorrhage, thrombophlebitis, diabetes or hypoglycemia

   b) Monitor for intestinal obstruction, paralytic (adynamic) ileus

   c) Monitor for shock, pancreatitis, hepatic failure

THE LOWER INTESTINAL TRACT

ASSESSMENT OF ELIMINATION FUNCTION

A. Anatomy
1. Cecum—first portion; pouch-like structure in lower right quadrant; receives chyme from ileum
2. Colon
   a. Ascending colon—up right side of abdomen
   b. Transverse colon—across abdomen
   c. Descending colon—down left side of abdomen
   d. Sigmoid colon—lower portion of descending colon; contains feces ready for excretion, empties into rectum
   e. Rectum—end portion of large intestine; 7 in long; usually empty except during and immediately before defecation; decreased rectal sensation in older adults
   f. Anal canal—1 in long; has internal and external sphincter

B. Process
1. Waste products are moved along GI tract by muscular contractions called peristalsis
2. Peristalsis is stimulated by presence of bulk in intestine
3. Consistency of stool affected by length of time in large intestine and amount of water reabsorbed
4. Anatomical process
   a. Reflex action
      1) Internal anal sphincter is under autonomic nervous system control
      2) When rectum is full, parasympathetic nerves are stimulated, causing internal anal sphincter to relax
   b. Voluntary action—external anal sphincter is under cerebral cortex control

DIAGNOSTIC TESTS

A. Diagnostic tests of stool—test for presence of fat, pus, pathogens, parasites, occult blood
B. Endoscopy—direct visualization via hollow tube with illuminated fiberoptiscope
1. Proctosigmoidoscopy (sigmoidoscopy)
   a. Definition—visualization of sigmoid colon or rectum and anal canal
   b. Client preparation
      1) Laxative night before exam and enema or suppository morning of procedure
      2) Clear liquid diet 12–24 h before exam (per health care provider order); clear liquids restricted 2-4 h before procedure
   c. Postoperative nursing care—allow client to rest; observe for hemorrhage, perforation; some flatulence and gas pain expected
2. Colonoscopy
   a. Definition—visualization of entire large intestine to assess for cancer, polyps, strictures, ulcers
   b. Client preparation
      1) Clear liquid diet 12–24 hours before exam (per health care provider order); clear liquids restricted 2-4 h before procedure

2) Cathartic in evening, evening before exam

3) Enema evening before exam (electrolyte-balanced solution may be given to induce diarrhea)

4) Enema or suppositories may be required

   c. Nursing management

     1) Allow rest

     2) Observe for passage of blood and abdominal pain—signs of perforation; instruct client to report immediately

C. Barium enema—instillation of barium (radiopaque substance) into colon via rectum for fluoroscopy x-rays

   1. Purpose—viewing tumors, polyps, strictures, ulcerations, inflammation, or obstructions of colon

   2. Client preparation to clear large intestine of most fecal material

     a. Liquid diet and laxative night before exam

     b. Enema on morning of exam

   3. Nursing management

     a. Cleansing enemas or laxative to remove barium to prevent impaction

     b. X-rays may be repeated after all barium is expelled

     c. Instruct client that white-colored stools are expected

NURSING IMPLICATIONS

A. Promotion of normal elimination

   1. Teach client to respond to urge to defecate

   2. Provide facilities, privacy, and sufficient time

   3. Fluids—encourage adequate intake; 8 or more glasses of fluid daily

   4. Encourage consumption of fiber—fruits, vegetables, grains

   5. Activity—encourage exercise and ambulation to maintain muscle tone

   6. Emotional state—teach client that stress affects autonomic nervous system, which controls peristalsis

B. Nutritional alterations

   1. Encourage high-fiber diet

     a. Fruits and vegetables

     b. Bran

     c. Whole-wheat flours and cereals

   2. Diet must be of adequate quantity of food to provide stimulus for peristalsis

C. Decompression of the intestinal tract

   1. Definition—removal of air and fluids from intestines via tube inserted through nose or mouth and attached to suction

   2. Purpose

     a. Drain fluids and gas due to obstruction

     b. Deflate bowel before or after intestinal surgery

     c. Drain fluids and gas due to paralytic ileus

3. Types
    a. Salem sump, Levin and Anderson tubes
        1) Attached to low suction
        2) Levin to low intermittent suction
    b. Miller-Abbott tube (NI)—for obstruction of small intestine
        1) Double-lumen tube—one lumen leads to balloon; other lumen has openings all along tube for drainage
            a) When irrigating, be sure to use lumen marked "suction"
            b) The balloon is inflated with mercury after tube is inserted; clamp the lumen to the balloon and label with "Do Not Touch"
    c. Cantor tube (NI)
        1) Single lumen
        2) Balloon is filled with mercury to provide weight for positioning before insertion

4. Insertion of NI tubes
    a. Mechanical passage into stomach same as NG tube
    b. Passage of tube along intestines is aided by gravity, weight of mercury, and peristalsis
    c. After tube is in stomach, have client lie on right side, then on back (in Fowler position), and then on left side to use gravity to position tube
    d. Position of tube is ascertained by x-ray—do not tape tube to face but coil loosely on bed
    e. Position of tube and absence of telescoping of bowel from weight of tube is ascertained daily by x-ray

5. Nursing management
    a. Measure drainage q shift
    b. Maintain liquid diet
    c. Irrigate as ordered—if unable to aspirate returns, record fluid instilled to be subtracted from total drainage output
    d. General care of client with NG tube
    e. Report signs of return of peristalsis, e.g., bowel sounds, flatus

D. Bowel surgery
1. Overview—purposes of bowel surgery
    a. Removal of diseased portion of bowel
    b. Creation of an outlet for passage of stool when there is an obstruction or need for bowel rest

2. Assessment
    a. Resection and anastomosis (also called partial or hemicolectomy)—diseased portion of bowel is removed and remaining ends are joined together
    b. Temporary cecostomy—opening into cecum (lower right quadrant of abdomen); catheter is inserted into bowel to provide temporary outlet for feces
    c. Abdominoperineal resection
        1) Abdominal incision through which the proximal end of the sigmoid colon is brought out to provide permanent colostomy
        2) Perineal incision through which the anus, the rectum, and the distal portion of the sigmoid are removed

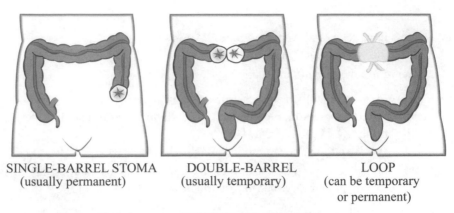

SINGLE-BARREL STOMA (usually permanent) DOUBLE-BARREL (usually temporary) LOOP (can be temporary or permanent)

Figure 7-8. TYPES OF COLOSTOMIES

d. Intestinal ostomies for fecal diversion (see Figure 7-8)

1) Sigmoid colostomy—characteristics

a) Proximal portion of sigmoid colon brought out through abdominal wall to form stoma

b) Distal portion of colon is removed

c) Stoma is located in the lower left quadrant

d) Feces are formed

e) Permanent colostomy—usually done for cancer of the rectum

f) Drainage may be regulated by irrigation, and ostomy appliance may eventually not be needed

2) Transverse loop colostomy

a) Loop is created by bringing a section of transverse colon out through an abdominal incision

b) Support ring is slid under the protruding bowel section to prevent the bowel from sliding back into the abdomen

c) Anterior wall of the bowel loop is cut open while the posterior wall remains intact

d) Single stoma with a proximal opening leading to the ascending colon and a distal opening leading to the descending colon

e) Stoma is located in the upper abdomen

f) Feces are soft

g) Temporary colostomy—divert feces from injured or diseased section of bowel

h) Skin breakdown may be a problem

i) When healing has occurred, the anterior wall of the bowel loop is sutured, and the bowel section is reinserted into the abdomen

3) Transverse double-barrel colostomy—usually temporary

a) Same as single barrel, with two distinct stomas on the abdomen

b) May be permanent colostomy if the distal portion of the colon is later removed

4) Ascending colostomy

a) Portion of the ascending colon is brought out to abdomen to form stoma

b) Stoma location is right upper quadrant

c) All portions of the colon distal to the stoma are removed

d) Permanent colostomy

   e) Feces are liquid to soft

   f) Skin breakdown is common

  5) Ileostomy

   a) Portion of the ileum brought to abdomen to create stoma

   b) All portions of the large intestine are removed

   c) Permanent ostomy; pouch must be worn at all times

   d) Usually done for ulcerative colitis or Crohn's disease

   e) Stoma is located in the right lower quadrant

   f) Drainage is liquid or semi-liquid

   g) Skin breakdown and fluid/electrolyte imbalance occur easily

   h) Continent ileostomy (Kock pouch)—intraabdominal reservoir with valve formed in distal ileum; pouch is reservoir for fecal material and cleaned at regular intervals by catheter insertion

3. Preop nursing management

 a. Psychological support and explanations

 b. Medications—antibiotics before surgery

 c. Diet—high calorie, high protein, high carbohydrates, low residue week before; full liquid diet 24–48 hours before; NPO after midnight

 d. Elimination—laxatives, enemas evening before and morning of surgery

 e. Activity—assist prn; client will be weakened from extensive prep procedures

 f. Monitor for fluid/electrolyte imbalance

 g. Place tube prior to surgery—NG or intestinal

 h. Have enterostomal health care provider see client for optimum placement of stoma

4. Postop nursing management

 a. NG or intestinal decompression until peristalsis returns—maintain NPO status

 b. Clear liquids progressing to solid, low-residue diet for 6–8 weeks

 c. Monitor I and 0 and fluid/electrolyte balance

 d. Observe and record condition of stoma

  1) First few days appears beefy red and swollen

  2) Gradually, swelling recedes and color is pink or red

  3) Notify health care provider immediately if stoma is dark blue, blackish, or purple—indicates insufficient blood supply

 e. Observe and record description of any drainage from stoma (see Figure 7-9)

  1) Usually just mucus or serosanguineous fluid for first 1–2 days

  2) Fecal drainage begins 3–6 days postop

 f. Care of peristomal skin, emptying and changing appliance, irrigation (unless ascending cholecystomy or ileostomy)

 g. Promote positive adjustment to ostomy

  1) Encourage client to look at stoma

  2) Encourage early participation in ostomy care

  3) Reinforce positive aspects of colostomy

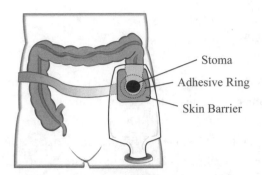

Figure 7-9. COLOSTOMY APPLIANCE

5. Nursing management
   a. Skin care
      1) Influencing factors
         a) Composition, quantity, consistency of drainage
         b) Medications
         c) Location of stoma
         d) Frequency in removal of appliance adhesive
      2) Principles of skin protection
         a) Use skin sealant under all tapes
         b) Use skin barrier to protect skin immediately surrounding the stoma
         c) Cleanse skin gently and pat dry; do not rub
         d) Change appliance immediately when seal breaks; use pouch deodorants
   b. Colostomy irrigations for sigmoid colostomy
      1) Purpose—to stimulate emptying of colon at scheduled times
      2) Usually begins 5–7 days postop
      3) If distal loop of transverse colostomy is irrigated, mucus may be seen in drainage from rectum or through stoma
      4) Ileostomies and ascending colostomies are not irrigated—drainage is liquid
      5) 500–1,000 mL of tepid water used for solution
      6) Special irrigating sleeve and cone are used
      7) Insert catheter 8 cm
      8) Hang irrigating container at shoulder height
      9) Stop procedure if client complains of cramps or if water is forcefully returning around cone or catheter
      10) Time required for return flow varies from 15–45 min
      11) When possible, client should be sitting upright on toilet for procedure
   c. Diet
      1) Usually not restricted after first 6 wk with colostomy
      2) Ileostomy clients remain on low-residue diet—avoid foods that cause diarrhea or constipation in the client
   d. Activity—optimal recovery within 3 mo; no restrictions
   e. Sexuality—no physical interference with ability, conception, pregnancy, or delivery

SELECTED BOWEL DISORDERS

A. Constipation

1. Definition—passage of dry, hard, difficult-to-evacuate stools
2. Causes
   a. Paralytic ileus (absence of peristalsis) resulting from trauma to intestinal nerve endings during abdominal surgery
   b. Atrophy or decreased muscle strength—part of aging process or overuse of laxatives
   c. Decreased level of activity and exercise, causing decreased muscle strength and tone
   d. Inadequate or poor choices of food intake
   e. Older adults—medications (opiates), decreased intake of fluids and fiber, decreased activity level
3. Nursing management
   a. Administration of laxatives (see Table 7-17)
   b. Administration of enemas
      1) Types
         a) Oil retention—softens feces
         b) Soapsuds—irritates colon, causing reflex evacuation, volume expander
         c) Tapwater—softens feces, stimulating evacuation
      2) Procedure
         a) Position on left side
         b) Use tepid solution
         c) Hold irrigation set no more than 18 in above rectum
         d) Insert tube no more than 4 in
         e) Ask client to retain fluid for 5–10 minutes
         f) Do not administer in presence of abdominal pain, nausea, vomiting, or suspected appendicitis
   c. Provide client education regarding promotion of normal elimination
      1) Sit or squat during defecation
      2) Gastrocolic reflex—try to have bowel movement after meals or after warm drink
      3) Avoid routine use of laxatives or enemas
      4) Gerontologic considerations—assess medication use, determine fluid and fiber intake, encourage increased fluid and fiber intake (bran, fruits, vegetables, nuts), avoid routine laxative and enema use

Table 7-17 LAXATIVES AND STOOL SOFTENER MEDICATIONS		
MEDICATION	**ADVERSE EFFECTS**	**NURSING CONSIDERATIONS**
Stimulant		
Bisacodyl	Mild cramps, rash, nausea, diarrhea	Tablets should not be taken with milk or antacids (causes dissolution of enteric coating and loss of cathartic action) Can cause gastric irritation Effects in 6–12 hours
Lubricant		
Mineral oil	Pruritus ani, anorexia, nausea	Administer in upright position Prolonged use can cause fat-soluble vitamin malabsorption Softens stool
Emolliant		
Docusate	Few adverse effects Abdominal cramps	Contraindicated in atonic bowel, nausea, vomiting, GI pain Softens stool Effects in 1–3 days
Osmotic		
Magnesium hydroxide Polyethylene glycol and electrolytes	Hypermagnesemia, dehydration Nausea and bloating	Na^+ salts can exacerbate heart failure Large-volume product—allow time to consume it safely
Bulk forming		
Psyllium hydrophilic mucilloid	Obstruction of GI tract	Take with a full glass of water; do not take dry Report abdominal distention or unusual amount of flatulence
Action	Bulk-forming—absorbs water into stool mass, making stool bulky, thus stimulating peristalsis Lubricants—coat surface of stool and soften fecal mass, allowing for easier passage Osmotic agents and saline laxatives—draw water from plasma by osmosis, increasing bulk of fecal mass, thus promoting peristalsis Stimulants—stimulate peristalsis when they come in contact with intestinal mucosa Stool softeners—soften fecal mass	
Indications	Constipation Preparation for procedures or surgery	
Adverse effects	Diarrhea Dependence	
Nursing considerations	Contraindicated for clients with abdominal pain, nausea and vomiting, fever (acute abdomen) Chronic use may cause hypokalemia	

B. Diarrhea
1. Definition—passage of an increased number of loose stools
2. Causes
   a. Systemic diseases—e.g., uremia, hyperthyroidism
   b. Conditions causing parasympathetic nervous system stimulation—e.g., prolonged stress
   c. Dietary changes in infants
   d. Conditions directly affecting the GI tract, e.g., food allergies, poisoning, or abuse of cathartics
3. Nursing management
   a. Perineal care—prevention of skin breakdown around anus
   b. Prevent dehydration and electrolyte imbalance, especially in infants and the elderly
   c. Prevent metabolic acidosis, especially in infants
   d. Administration of antidiarrheal medications (see Table 7-18)

C. Malabsorption syndrome
1. Definition—group of conditions caused by inadequate absorption of nutrients from the small intestine, resulting in abnormal digestion
2. Causes
   a. Tropical sprue
   b. Gastric resection/bowel resection
   c. Antibiotics
   d. Massive bowel resection
   e. Parasitic infections
   f. Overgrowth of bacteria in small intestine
   g. Radiation injury to mucosa of small intestine
   h. Enteritis
3. Assessment
   a. Steatorrhea—excessive fat in stool
   b. Light yellow to gray, greasy, soft stool
   c. Weight loss, anemia, fatigue
   d. Anorexia
   e. Vitamin deficiency
4. Nursing management
   a. Nutritional support
      1) Enteral feedings
      2) Total parenteral nutrition (PN)
   b. Skin care
   c. Observe for vitamin and mineral deficiencies
   d. Monitor for pulse irregularities, edema

Table 7-18 ANTIDIARRHEAL MEDICATIONS		
MEDICATION	ADVERSE EFFECTS	NURSING CONSIDERATIONS
Bismuth subsalicylate	Darkening of stools and tongue Constipation	Give 2 hours before or 3 hours after other meds to prevent impaired absorption Encourage fluids Take after each loose stool until diarrhea controlled Notify health care provider if diarrhea not controlled in 48 hours Absorbs irritants and soothes intestinal muscle Do not administer for more than 2 days in presence of fever or in client less than 3 years of age Monitor for salicylate toxicity Use cautiously if already taking aspirin Avoid use before x-rays (is radiopaque)
Diphenoxylate hydrochloride and atropine sulfate	Sedation Dizziness Tachycardia Dry mouth Paralytic ileus	Onset 45–60 min Monitor fluid and electrolytes Increases intestinal tone and decreases peristalsis May potentiate action of barbituates, depressants
Opium alkaloids Loperamide	Narcotic dependence, nausea Drowsiness Constipation	Acts on smooth muscle to increase tone Administer with glass of water Discontinue as soon as stools are controlled Monitor children closely for CNS effects
Action	Absorb water, gas, toxins, irritants, and nutrients in bowel; slow peristalsis; increases tone of smooth muscles and sphincters	
Indications	Diarrhea	
Adverse effects	Constipation, fecal impaction; anticholinergic effects	
Nursing considerations	Not used with abdominal pain of unknown origin; monitor for urinary retention	

D. Adult celiac disease (nontropical sprue)
1. Definition—an intolerance to gluten, a protein found in wheat and rye flour
2. Causes
   a. Hypersensitivity response
   b. Hereditary tendency
   c. History of childhood celiac disease
3. Assessment
   a. Same as malabsorption syndrome
   b. Onset usually age 30–60
4. Nursing management
   a. Gluten-free diet
   b. Substitute cornmeal and rice for wheat, rye, oats, barley

E. Appendicitis (inflammation of appendix)

1. Cause—occlusion of lumen of appendix from infection, strictures, or fecal masses
2. Assessment
   a. Abdominal pain in right lower quadrant (McBurney's point)
   b. Anorexia
   c. Nausea and vomiting
   d. Diarrhea or constipation
   e. Rigid abdomen, muscle guarding
   f. Increased temperature
   g. Leukocytosis (WBC 15,000–20,000 cells/mm^3)
   h. Highest incidence 10–30 years of age

3. Nursing management
   a. No heating pads, enemas, or laxatives preop
   b. Maintain NPO status until blood count reports received
   c. No analgesics until cause of pain is determined
   d. Ice bag to abdomen to alleviate pain
   e. Observe for signs and symptoms of peritonitis
   f. Sudden absence of pain can indicate appendix has ruptured

4. Surgical removal of appendix (appendectomy)

F. Peritonitis (inflammation of peritoneal membrane covering abdominal organs)

1. Causes
   a. Ruptured appendix
   b. Perforated ulcer
   c. Bowel perforation
   d. Pelvic inflammatory disease (PID)
   e. Bladder perforation
   f. Traumatic rupture of liver or spleen

2. Assessment
   a. Severe abdominal pain
   b. Abdominal rigidity; decreased bowel sounds
   c. Nausea
   d. Vomiting
   e. Increased temperature
   f. Leukocytosis
   g. Shock: weakness, pallor, diaphoresis
   h. Paralytic ileus
   i. Symptoms may be masked in elderly persons or those receiving corticosteroids

3. Nursing management
   a. Antibiotics and intravenous fluids, as ordered
   b. Gastric decompression; monitor NG drainage
   c. NPO
   d. Reestablish fluid/electrolyte balance; monitor serum electrolyte levels

4. Surgery to alleviate cause—closure of abnormal opening into abdomen and drainage of fluid

G. Meckel's diverticulum—a congenital sac or pouch in the ileum
   1. Assessment
      a. Usually asymptomatic: may cause problems in childhood
      b. Signs and symptoms of appendicitis if diverticulum becomes inflamed from infection

   2. Nursing management
      a. Antibiotics
      b. Rest
      c. Warm application to abdomen
      d. Antispasmodics

   3. Surgical (if symptomatic)—removal of the diverticulum

H. Ileitis (acute Crohn's disease)
   1. Definition—inflammatory condition of intestine
   2. Assessment—same as appendicitis
   3. Nursing management
      a. Nutrition—high-protein, high-calorie, low-fat, and low-fiber diet
      b. Medications—antibiotics, antidiarrheals
      c. Management of client with diarrhea

I. Crohn's disease (regional enteritis, ileitis, or enterocolitis) (see Table 7-19)
   1. Definition—inflammatory condition of any area of large or small intestine, usually ileum and ascending colon
   2. Assessment—characterized by exacerbations and remissions
      a. Severe abdominal pain and cramping in lower-right quadrant of abdomen
      b. Chronic diarrhea
      c. Mucus, pus, fat in stools
      d. Fatigue
      e. Increased temperature
      f. Decreased weight
      g. Highest incidence ages 20–30 and 50–80 years
      h. Diagnostic tests—upper GI series, barium enema, colonoscopy

   3. Nursing management
      a. Diet—high protein, high calorie, low fat, and low fiber; PN used for bowel rest
      b. Medications—analgesics, anticholinergics, antibiotics, corticosteroids, immune modulators, salicydate containing compounds
      c. Maintenance of fluid/electrolyte balance

   4. Surgical intervention—hemicolectomy or ileostomy

J. Ulcerative colitis (see Table 7-19)

1. Definition—inflammatory condition of the colon characterized by eroded areas of the mucous membrane and tissues beneath it

2. Assessment

    a. Diarrhea—10–20 stools per day

    b. Blood, pus, mucus in stool; pain

    c. Fecal incontinence

    d. Dehydration

    e. Weight loss

    f. Weakness, cachexia

    g. Metabolic acidosis

    h. Exacerbations and remissions

    i. Highest incidence age 30–50 years

    j. High correlation to personality traits of perfectionism, rigidity, dependence, insecurity

Table 7-19 CROHN'S DISEASE VERSUS ULCERATIVE COLITIS		
	CROHN'S DISEASE REGIONAL ENTERITIS	ULCERATIVE COLITIS
Assessment		
Usual age of onset	20–30 and 50–80 years	Young adult to middle age (30–50)
Fatty stool (steatorrhea)	Frequent	Absent
Malignancy results	Rare	10–15%
Rectal bleeding	Occasional: mucus, pus, fat in stool	Common; blood, pus, mucus in stool
Abdominal pain	After meals	Predefecation
Diarrhea	Diarrhea rare; 5–6 unformed stools per day	10–20 liquid stools per day; often bloody
Nutritional deficit, weight loss, anemia, dehydration	Common	Common
Fever	Present	Present
Anal abscess	Common	Common
Fistula and anorectal fissure fistula	Common	Rare

Table 7-19 CROHN'S DISEASE VERSUS ULCERATIVE COLITIS *(CONTINUED)*		
	CROHN'S DISEASE REGIONAL ENTERITIS	**ULCERATIVE COLITIS**
Diagnosis		
Level of involvement	Ileum, right colon	Rectum, left colon
Inflammation	Noncontinuous segment	Continuous segment
Course of disease	Prolonged, variable	Remissions and relapses
	Complications–bowel abscess, fistula formation, intestinal obstruction	Complications–hemorrhage, abscess formation, arthritis, uveitis
Nursing considerations	High-protein, high-calorie, low-fat, and low-fiber diet	
	May require PN to rest bowel	
	Analgesics, anticholinergics, sulfonamides, corticosteriods, antidiarrheals, and antiperistaltics	
	Maintain fluid/electrolyte balance	
	Monitor electrolytes	
	Promote rest, relieve anxiety	
	Ileostomy in severe cases	

3. Nursing management
   a. Management of client with diarrhea
   b. Reduce inflammation–steroids
   c. Maintain nutrition–low-residue, high-protein, high-calorie diet
   d. Maintain fluid/electrolyte balance; monitor electrolyte levels
   e. Promote rest and relieve anxiety

4. Surgical intervention–ileostomy

K. Diverticular disease
   1. Definition–infection, inflammation, or obstruction of diverticuli (sacs or pouches in the intestinal wall), causing the client to become symptomatic
   2. Assessment
      a. Colicky pain in left-lower quadrant of abdomen; pain described as cramping
      b. Fever, increased WBC
      c. Constipation, diarrhea, vomiting; constipation may alternate with diarrhea
      d. Decreased bowel sounds
   3. Nursing management
      a. Analgesics
      b. Anticholinergics
      c. Antibiotics–broad-spectrum
      d. No laxatives or enemas
      e. Clear liquid diet or NPO to rest bowel
      f. High fiber diet; there is no evidence based studies to suggest the avoidance of nuts, seeds or popcorn, however certain clients may have food triggers (that trigger an attack) so these foods should be avoided
   4. Surgical intervention–colon resection with or without colostomy

L. Intestinal obstruction

  1. Types

    a. Mechanical—physical blockage of passage through intestines

      1) Strangulated hernia

      2) Tumors

      3) Adhesions

      4) Fecal impaction

      5) Strictures

        a) Radiation

        b) Congenital

      6) Intussusception (telescoping of bowel within itself)

      7) Volvulus—twisting of bowel

    b. Nonmechanical (paralytic ileus)—no mechanical blockage, absence of peristalsis

      1) Abdominal trauma/surgery

      2) Spinal injuries

      3) Peritonitis

      4) Wound dehiscence (breakdown)

  2. Assessment

    a. High-pitched bowel sound above area of obstruction, decreased or absent bowel sounds below the area of obstruction

    b. Abdominal pain and distention; pain often described as "colicky"

    c. Obstipation (absence of stools or gas)

    d. Nausea and vomiting

  3. Nursing management

    a. NG or intestinal decompression

    b. NPO

    c. Fluid/electrolyte replacement; monitor electrolyte levels

    d. Assist with ADL

    e. Good oral and skin care

    f. Fowler position to facilitate breathing

    g. Measure abdominal girth

    h. Analgesics

M. Abdominal hernias

1. Definition—protrusion of an organ through the wall of the cavity in which it is normally contained

2. Types

   a. Inguinal—protrusion of intestine through abdominal ring into inguinal canal

   b. Femoral—protrusion of intestine into femoral canal

   c. Umbilical—protrusion of intestine through umbilical ring

   d. Ventral or incisional—protrusion through site of an old surgical incision

   e. Reducible—the protruding structure can be replaced by manipulation into the abdominal cavity

   f. Irreducible—the protruding structure cannot be replaced by manipulation

   g. Incarcerated—intestinal flow is completely obstructed

   h. Strangulated—blood flow to the intestines, as well as intestinal flow, is completely obstructed

3. Assessment

   a. Lump at site of hernia

   b. Lump may disappear in reclining position and reappear on standing/coughing

   c. Strangulated hernia—severe abdominal pain, nausea and vomiting, distention, intestinal obstruction

4. Nursing management—herniorrhaphy

   a. Preop nursing management

      1) Assess respiratory system for potential causes of increased intraabdominal pressure—may cause interference with postop healing

      2) Surgery is postponed until respiratory conditions are controlled

   b. Postop nursing management

      1) Relieve urinary retention

      2) Prevent paroxysmal coughing

      3) Provide scrotal support

      4) Provide ice packs for swollen scrotum

      5) Advise no pulling, pushing, heavy lifting for 6 wk

      6) Inform client that sexual function is not affected

      7) Instruct client that ecchymosis will fade in a few days

Chapter 8

THE ENDOCRINE SYSTEM

Sections	Concepts Covered
1. The Endocrine System Overview	Metabolism, Cellular Regulation
2. Endocrine Disorders	Metabolism, Client Education: Providing

THE ENDOCRINE SYSTEM OVERVIEW Section 1

OVERVIEW

A. Chemical communication and coordination system that enables reproductive growth and development and regulation of energy
1. Maintains internal homeostasis of body
2. Coordinates response to external and internal environmental changes

B. Composed of glands/glandular tissue
1. Secrete, store, and synthesize chemical messengers (hormones) that travel to target cells throughout the body
2. Include: hypothalamus, pituitary, thyroid, parathyroids, adrenals, pancreas, ovaries, testes, pineal, and thymus
3. Major hormones are amines, peptides, and steroids
4. Important functions include: reproduction, stress response, electrolyte balance, energy metabolism, growth, maturation, and aging (see Table 8-1)

Table 8-1 IMPORTANT FUNCTIONS OF THE ENDOCRINE SYSTEM		
GLAND/HORMONE	TARGET TISSUE	FUNCTION

Thyroid
 	
   Thyroxine (T_4)
 	
   Triiodothyronine (T_3)
 	
   Calcitonin
	All body tissue
	
	Bone
		Regulation of metabolic rate of all cells and processes of cell growth, tissue differentiation
		
		Regulates calcium and phosphorus blood levels

Parathyroids Parathyroid hormone (PTH)	Bone, intestines, kidneys	Regulates calcium and phosphorus blood levels (bone demineralization and intestinal absorption)

Adrenal medulla
 	
   Epinephrine
 	
   Norepinephrine
	Sympathetic effectors	Enhances and prolongs effects of sympathetic nervous system
		
		Response to stress

Adrenal cortex
 	
   Corticosteroids
 	
   Androgens
 	
   Estrogen
 	
   Mineralocorticoids
	All body tissue
	
	Sex organs
	
	Kidney
		Metabolism; stress response
		
		Masculinization
		
		Growth and sexual activity in women
		
		Regulates sodium/potassium balance, water balance

Pancreas
 	
   Islets of Langerhans
 	
   Insulin (beta cells)
 	
   Glucagon (alpha cells)
 	
   Somatostatin
	
	General
	
	General
	
	General
	
	Pancreas
		Promotes movement of glucose out of blood into cells
		
		Promotes movement of glucose from storage into blood
		
		Inhibits insulin and glucagon secretion

Women—ovaries
 	
   Estrogen
 	
   Progesterone
	Reproductive system—breast
	Reproductive system
		Development of secondary sex characteristics, oogenesis, preparation of uterus for fertilization and fetal development; bone growth
		Maintains lining of uterus necessary for successful pregnancy

Men—testes	Reproductive system	Stimulates development of secondary sex characteristics, spermatogenesis

DIABETES MELLITUS

(See Table 8-2)

A. Overview—diabetes mellitus is defined as a genetically heterogeneous group of disorders characterized by glucose intolerance

Table 8-2 ALTERATIONS IN GLUCOSE METABOLISM	
TYPE	**NURSING CONSIDERATIONS**
Type 1 diabetes	Acute onset before age 30 Insulin-producing pancreatic beta cells destroyed by autoimmune process Requires insulin injection Ketosis prone
Type 2 diabetes	Usually older than 30 and obese Decreased sensitivity to insulin (insulin resistance) or decreased insulin production Ketosis rare Treated with diet and exercise Supplemented with oral hypoglycemic medications
Others: Gestational diabetes Impaired fasting glucose	Onset during pregnancy, second or third trimester High-risk pregnancy Fasting plasma glucose of ≥100 mg/dL (≥ 5.6 mmol/L) and less than126 mg/dL (less than 7 mmol/L); risk factor for future diabetes risk

B. Risk factors for type 2 diabetes
1. Parents or siblings with diabetes
2. Obesity (20% or more above ideal body weight)
3. African American, Hispanic, Native American, or Asian American
4. Older than 45 years
5. Previously impaired glucose tolerance
6. Hypertension

C. Diagnostic tests
1. Blood glucose monitoring—presence of sugar in the urine is a sign of diabetes that calls for an immediate blood glucose test; normal range in fasting blood is 70-99 mg/dL (3.89–5.49 mmol/L); older adults may normally have higher glucose levels
2. Oral glucose tolerance test—blood samples are drawn at 1-, 2-, and 3-h intervals after glucose ingestion
   a. Fasting glucose greater than 125 mg/dL (6.9 mmol/L) and 2-h glucose greater than 190 mg/dL (5 mmol/L) on two occasions are diagnostic of diabetes; may see increased fasting glucose in older adults

b. Preparation—usually NPO after midnight (10–12-h fast); client sometimes ingests high-carbohydrate diet for 3 days preceding test

c. Fasting blood sample taken

d. Glucose load (about 75 g/300 mL of flavored beverage) is given

e. Specimens are drawn at 1, 2, and 3 hours after glucose ingestion

3. Urine ketones indicate that diabetic control has deteriorated; body has started to break down stored fat for energy

4. Special considerations—medications, illness, and stress will affect testing

5. Glycosylated hemoglobin (HbA1c)—blood sample can be taken without fasting

    a. Measures control over last 3 months; not affected by carbohydrate intake or exercise

    b. Normal is 4–6%

D. Nursing management

1. Dietary management

    a. Provide all essential food constituents—lower lipid levels if elevated

    b. Achieve and maintain ideal weight

    c. Meet energy needs

    d. Achieve normal range glucose levels

    e. Review food exchange method of meal and snack planning with client/family; foods on list in specified amounts contain equal number of calories and grams of protein, fat, and carbohydrate

2. Proper management of insulin regimen—insulin is secreted by beta cells of the islets of Langerhans and works to lower blood glucose by facilitating uptake and the utilization of glucose by muscle and fat cells and by decreasing the release of glucose from the liver; injection sites must be rotated (see Table 8-3)

3. Oral hypoglycemic medications appear to work by improving both tissue responsiveness to insulin and/or the ability of the pancreatic cells to secrete insulin (see Table 8-4)

4. Prevention and early detection

    a. Signs and symptoms of hypoglycemia (insulin reaction)

        1) Irritability, confusion, tremors, blurring of vision, coma, seizures

        2) Hypotension, tachycardia

        3) Skin cool and clammy, diaphoresis

    b. Treatment of hypoglycemia

        1) Liquids containing sugar if conscious; commercially prepared glucose tablets ideal

        2) Dextrose 50% IV if unconscious, glucagon

    c. Signs and symptoms of hyperglycemia/diabetic ketoacidosis (DKA)

        1) Headache, drowsiness, stupor, coma

        2) Hypotension, tachycardia

        3) Skin warm and dry, dry mucous membranes, elevated temperature

        4) Polyuria progressing to oliguria, polydipsia, polyphagia

        5) Kussmaul's respirations (rapid and deep)

        6) Fruity odor to breath

    d. Treatment of hyperglycemia (DKA)

        1) Normal saline or 0.45% NaCl (DKA)

        2) Regular insulin

3) Potassium as soon as urine output is satisfactory (DKA)

4) Determine and address cause

5) Client education

6) Exercise regimen

Table 8-3 ANTIDIABETIC MEDICATIONS: INSULIN					
INSULIN TYPES	ONSET OF ACTION; (MINS)	PEAK ACTION	DURATION OF ACTION	TIME OF ADVERSE REACTION	CHARACTERISTICS
Rapid-acting					
Lispro Aspart Glulisine	15–30 15–30 10–15	0.5–1.5 hours 1–3 hours 1–1.5 hours	3–5 hours 3–5 hours 3–5 hours	Mid-morning: trembling, weakness	Client should eat within 5–15 min after injection; also used in insulin pumps
Short-acting					
Regular	30–60 min	1–5 hours	6–10 hours	Mid-morning, mid-afternoon: weakness, fatigue	Clear solution; given 20–30 min before meal; can be alone or with other insulins
Intermediate-acting					
NPH	1–2 hours	4–12 hours	16 hours	Early evening: weakness, fatigue	White and cloudy solution; can be given after meals
Very long-acting					
Glargine Insulin detemir	3–4 hours	Continuous (no peak)	24 hours		Maintains blood glucose levels regardless of meals; cannot be mixed with other insulins; given at bedtime
Action	Reduces blood glucose levels by increasing glucose transport across cell membranes; enhances conversion of glucose to glycogen				
Indications	Type 1 diabetes; type 2 diabetes not responding to oral hypoglycemic medications; gestational diabetes not responding to diet				
Adverse effects	Hypoglycemia				
Nursing considerations	Teach client to rotate sites to prevent lipohypertrophy, fibrofatty masses at injection sites; do not inject into these masses Only regular insulin can be given IV; all can be given SQ				
Herbal interactions	Bee pollen, glucosamine may increase blood glucose Basil, bay leaf, chromium, echinacea, garlic, ginseng may decrease blood glucose Ginkgo biloba might interfere with the management of diabetes mellitus. If taking ginkgo, closely monitor blood gluose levels.				

Table 8-4 ORAL HYPOGLYCEMIC MEDICATIONS		
MEDICATION	ADVERSE EFFECTS	NURSING CONSIDERATIONS
ORAL		
Sulfonylureas		
Glimepiride Glipizide Glyburide	GI symptoms and dermatologic reactions	Only used if some pancreas beta-cell function Stimulates release of insulin from pancreas Many medications can potentiate or interfere with actions Take with food if GI upset occurs
Biguanides		
Metformin	Nausea Diarrhea Abdominal discomfort	No effect on pancreatic beta cells; decreases glucose production by liver Not given if renal impairment Can cause lactic acidosis Avoid alcohol Do not give with alpha-glucodiase inhibitors
Alpha-glucosidase inhibitors		
Acarbose Miglitol	Abdominal discomfort Diarrhea Flatulence	Delays digestion of carbohydrates Must be taken immediately before a meal Can be taken alone or with other medications
Thiazolidinediones		
Rosiglitazone Pioglitazone	Infection Headache Pain Rare cases of liver failure	Decreases insulin resistance and inhibits gluconeogenesis Regularly scheduled liver-function studies Can cause resumption of ovulation in perimenopause
Glitinides		
Repaglinide	Hypoglycemia GI disturbances URIs Back pain Headache	Increases pancreatic insulin release Medication should not be taken if meal skipped
Gliptins		
Linagliptin Sitagliptin	Upper respiratory infections Hypoglycemia	Enhances action of incretin hormones
INJECTED		
Incretin mimetics		
Exenatide	GI upset Hypoglycemia Pancreatitis	Interacts with many medications Administer 1 hour before meals
Amylin Mimetics		
Pramlintide	Hypoglycemia Nausea Injection site reaction	Delays gastric emptying Suppresses glucogon secretion
Indications	Type 2 diabetes	
Nursing considerations	Monitor serum glucose levels Avoid alcohol Teaching for disease: dietary control, symptoms of hypoglycemia and hyperglycemia Good skin care	
Herbal interactions	Bee pollen, ginkgo biloba, glucosamine may increase blood glucose Basil, bay leaf, chromium, echinacea, garlic, ginseng may decrease blood glucose	

ACROMEGALY

(See Table 8-5)

A. Definition—hypersecretion of growth hormone; often caused by pituitary adenoma

B. Assessment

1. Enlarged flat bones and terminal portions of long bones; lower jaw and forehead protrude
2. Poor coordination
3. Muscle weakness and atrophy
4. Lethargy
5. Arthralgias and arthritis
6. Changes in visual fields
7. Deep voice and enlarged tongue
8. Emotional instability
9. Sexual abnormalities
10. Hypertension and heart failure
11. Impaired glucose tolerance and diabetes mellitus

C. Diagnosis—growth hormone measured in blood plasma, MRI, increased IGF-1 levels

D. Nursing management

1. Monitor blood sugar level
2. Provide emotional support
3. Administer medications—dopamine agonists (e.g., cabergoline), growth receptor antagonists (e.g., pegvisomant), somastatin analogues (e.g., octreotide)
4. Monitor for adverse effects of radiation therapy
5. Surgery best approach to cure: hypophysectomy (transsphenoidal)
    a. Monitor neurologic status and vision
    b. "Mustache" dressing under nose
    c. Instruct client to report post nasal drip
    d. Monitor for halo sign—clear drainage surrounded by yellow or slight serosanguinous drainage (indicates CSF leak)
    e. Instruct client to avoid coughing, sneezing, blowing nose, bending forward (increases intracranial pressure) and to avoid brushing teeth for 2 weeks
    f. Monitor for meningitis—photophobia, neck stiffness, headache
    g. Administer hormonal replacement as needed—gonadal hormones, cortisol and thyroid

HYPOPITUITARISM

(See Table 8-5)

A. Definition—hyposecretion of growth hormone

B. Assessment

1. Height is below normal
2. Proportion of weight to height is normal
3. Bone and tooth development are retarded
4. Sexual maturity is delayed
5. Features are delicate

C. Diagnosis—growth hormone measured in blood plasma; decreased in hypopituitarism

D. Nursing management

1. Monitor growth and development
2. Provide emotional support
3. Assess body image
4. Refer for psychological counseling as needed
5. Monitor medications
   a. Hormone replacement therapy
   b. Thyroid hormone replacement
   c. Testosterone therapy (males)

Table 8-5 PITUITARY DISORDERS		
	HYPOPITUITARISM (DWARFISM)	**ACROMEGALY**
Assessment	Height below normal, body proportions normal, bone/tooth development retarded, sexual maturity delayed, skin fine, features delicate	Body size enlarged, coordination poor, flat bones enlarged, sexual abnormalities, deep voice, skin thick and soft, visual field changes
Diagnosis	Hyposecretion of growth hormone; occurs before maturity Etiology unclear; predisposition—pituitary tumors, idiopathic hyperplasia Treatment: hormone replacement (human growth hormone, thyroid growth hormone, testosterone) Complication: diabetes	Hypersecretion of growth hormone occurs after maturity Etiology: unclear Diagnosis: growth hormone measured in blood plasma Treatment: external irradiation of tumor, atrium-90 implant transnasally, hypophysectomy (removal of pituitary or portion of it with hormone replacement)
Potential nursing diagnosis	Self-esteem disturbance Risk for sexual dysfunction	Body image disturbance Nutrition, altered Chronic pain Risk for sexual dysfuction

Plan/Implementation	Monitor growth and development
	Provide emotional support
	Assess body image
	Refer for psychological counseling as needed
	Monitor medications
	Hormone replacement therapy
	Thyroid hormone replacement
	Testosterone therapy
	Human chorionic gonadotropin (hCG) injections
		Monitor blood sugar level
		Provide emotional support
		Provide safety due to poor coordination and vision
		Administer dopamine agonists; somatostatin analogs; growth hormone receptor blockers
		Provide care during radiation therapy
		Provide posthypophysectomy care:
		  Elevate head
		  Check neurological status and nasal drainage
		  Monitor BP frequently
		  Observe for hormonal deficiencies (thyroid, glucocorticoid)
		  Observe for hypoglycemia
		  Monitor intake and output
		  Provide cortisone replacement before and after surgery
		Avoid coughing
		Avoid toothbrushing for 2 weeks

DIABETES INSIPIDUS

(See Table 8-6)

A. Definition—deficiency of antidiuretic hormone (ADH)

B. Assessment (see Table 8-6)

1. Excessive urine output, dilute urine

2. Severe dehydration, hypotension, tachycardia, decreased pedal pulse strength

3. Excessive thirst

4. Anorexia

5. Weight loss

6. Mental status changes—irritability, decreased alertness, lethargy, possible coma

7. Poor skin turgor, dry mucous membranes

C. Diagnostic tests

1. Low urine specific gravity (normal for adult 1.010–1.030)

2. Clinical manifestations—especially frequent urination

3. Urinary osmolality below plasma level

4. Increased hemoglobin, hematocrit, BUN

D. Nursing management

1. Monitor fluids and electrolytes
   a. Record intake and output
   b. Urine specific gravity
   c. Skin condition
   d. Weight
   e. Blood pressure, pulse, temperature

2. Administer prescribed medications (hormone replacement)—observe for expected therapeutic effects
   a. Desmopressin acetate (DDAVP) nasal spray
   b. Desmopressin by subcutaneous or intravascular injection (see Table 8-7)

3. Prevent constipation—laxatives and stool softeners

4. Provide skin care

5. Client teaching
   a. How to measure intake and output and signs of early dehydration
   b. Expected responses from medications, e.g., decreased thirst and urination
   c. Lifelong replacement may be needed

PHEOCHROMOCYTOMA

A. Definition—hypersecretion of catecholamines (epinephrine and norepinephrine) due to secreting tumors of the adrenal medulla; tumor can also occur anywhere, from neck to pelvis along course of sympathetic nerve chain; caused by tumor in adrenal medulla

B. Assessment

1. Intermittent hypertension lasting several minutes to several hours; episodes precipitated by increased abdominal pressure (Valsalva maneuver, abdominal palpation)

2. Increased heart rate; palpitations during hypertensive episodes

3. Nausea and vomiting; weight loss

4. Hyperglycemia, glucosuria, polyuria

5. Diaphoresis, pallor

6. Tremor, nervousness during hypertensive episodes

7. Pounding headache during hypertensive episodes

8. Weakness during hypertensive episodes

9. Visual disturbances during hypertensive episodes

10. Pain during hypertensive episodes

C. Diagnostic tests

1. Histamine test, provocative test—causes rise in blood pressure (rarely done)

    a. Normally causes drop in blood pressure, but in this disease, a rise occurs

    b. Given subcutaneously if blood pressure not higher than 170/110 mm Hg

    c. If blood pressure over 170/110 mm Hg, Regitine test done

Table 8-6 ADH DISORDERS		
	DIABETES INSIPIDUS (DECREASED ADH)	**SIADH—SYNDROME OF INAPPROPRIATE ANTIDIURETIC HORMONE SECRETION (INCREASED ADH)**
Assessment	Excessive urine output Chronic, severe dehydration Excessive thirst Anorexia, weight loss Weakness Constipation	Anorexia, nausea, vomiting Lethargy Headaches Change in level of consciousness Decreased deep tendon reflexes Tachycardia Increased circulating blood volume Decreased urinary output

Diagnosis	Head trauma
	Brain tumor
	Meningitis Encephalitis
	Deficiency of ADH
	Diagnosis tests:
	  Low urine specific gravity
	  Urinary osmolality below plasma level
	  High serum sodium
		Small cell carcinoma of lung
		Pneumonia Positive-pressure ventilation
		Brain tumors
		Head trauma
		Stroke
		Meningitis
		Encephalitis
		Feedback mechanism that regulates ADH does not function properly; ADH is released even when plasma hypo-osmolality is present
		Diagnostic tests:
		Serum sodium decreased, plasma osmolality decreased
		Increased urine specific gravity

Nursing considerations	Record intake and output Monitor urine specific gravity, skin condition, weight, blood pressure, pulse, temperature Administer desmopressin acetate	Restrict water intake (500–600 mL/24 hours) Administer diuretics to promote excretion of water Hypertonic saline (3% NaCl) IV Administer demeclocycline Weigh daily I and O Monitor serum Na^+ levels Assess LOC

Table 8-7	DIABETES INSIPIDUS MEDICATIONS	
MEDICATION	ADVERSE EFFECTS	NURSING CONSIDER-ATIONS
Desmopressin nasal spray SQ IV	Excess—smooth muscle contraction, especially arterioles and capillaries Water intoxication Other—hypersensitivity, hypertension, nausea	Antidiuretic hormone Increases water retention by kidney Used to treat diabetes insipidus

2. Regitine test (rarely done)
   a. At least 3 days prior to test, should not receive any sedatives, antihypertensives (especially reserpine), or narcotics—may cause false positive reactions
   b. Phentolamine given IV—adrenergic blocking agent neutralizes epinephrine and causes drop in blood pressure
   c. Decrease in blood pressure of at least 35 mm Hg systolic and 25 mm Hg diastolic within 3–5 minutes considered positive for tumor
   d. Drop in blood pressure lasts 10 min
   e. Vasopressors should be readily available

3. Urinary VMA test
   a. 24-h urine for vanillylmandelic acid—breakdown product of catecholamine metabolism
   b. Normal results: 1–5 mg; positive for tumor if significantly higher
   c. Foods affecting VMA excretion excluded 3 days before test:
      1) Coffee
      2) Tea
      3) Bananas
      4) Vanilla
      5) Chocolate
   d. All medications/drugs discontinued during test
   e. Urine collected on ice or refrigeration and preservative needed

4. Clonidine suppression test—clonidine levels not decreased

D. Nursing management
   1. Promote comfort
      a. Avoid physical and emotional stress
      b. Monitor blood pressure in sitting and lying positions
      c. Frequent bathing but avoid chilling
      d. Administer analgesics for pain, sedatives and tranquilizers for rest and relaxation

   2. Provide appropriate nutrition
      a. Increase calorie, vitamin and mineral intake because of increased metabolic demand (compatible with hyperglycemia and weight loss)
      b. Avoid coffee, tea, cola, and other stimulating foods, foods containing tyramine

3. Limit activity

4. Administer adrenergic blocking medications (e.g., phenoxybenzamine)

5. Administer apresoline for hypertensive crisis

6. Promote safety

    a. Assist with self-care

    b. Eliminate unnecessary equipment and material from client's immediate vicinity

    c. Recruit help and assistance of significant other

    d. Allow time to verbalize concerns to decrease nervousness and tremors

7. Provide postsurgical care—adrenalectomy or medullectomy

ADDISON'S DISEASE (ADRENAL INSUFFICIENCY)

(See Table 8-10)

A. Definition—adrenocortical hypofunction due to insufficient secretion from adrenal cortex

B. Assessment

1. Fatigue and weakness

2. Dehydration

3. Alopecia

4. "Tan" skin

5. Depression

6. Emaciation, weight loss

7. Immune deficiency

8. Fluid and electrolyte imbalance

9. Pathological fractures

C. Diagnostic tests

1. Skull films, CT, MRI

2. Hyperkalemia and hyponatremia

3. Plasma cortisol decreased

4. Urinary 17-hydroxycorticosteriods and 17-ketosteroids decreased

5. ACTH stimulation test

D. Nursing management

1. Teach appropriate diet—high protein, high carbohydrate, high sodium, low potassium

2. Provide emotional support

3. Prevent complications

    a. Wear Medic-Alert bracelet

    b. Protect from infection

    c. Monitor for hypoglycemia, hyponatremia

4. Avoid factors that precipitate Addisonian crisis (adrenal crisis)

    a. Physical stress

    b. Psychological stress

    c. Inadequate steroid replacement

5. Assist with treatment of Addisonian crisis (precipitated by physical or emotional stress, sudden withdrawl of hormones)

   a. Observe for clinical manifestations
   1) Nausea and vomiting
   2) Abdominal pain
   3) Fever
   4) Extreme weakness
   5) Severe hypoglycemia, hyperkalemia and dehydration (develop rapidly)
   6) Blood pressure falls, leading to shock and coma; death results if not promptly treated

   b. Provide treatment and nursing care
   1) Administer hydrocortisone or dexamethasone (see Table 8-11)
   2) Carefully monitor IV infusion of 0.9% NaCl or D5W/NaCl
   3) Administer IV glucose, glucagon
   4) Administer insulin with dextrose in normal saline; administer potassium binding and excreting resin (e.g., Kayexalate)
   5) Monitor vital signs, ECG, serum potassium, serum glucose
   6) Assist with 24-h urine collection for 17-hydroxycorticosteroids; refrigeration of urine during collection is necessary

   c. Administer hormonal replacement—may be lifelong

CUSHING'S DISEASE (CORTISOL EXCESS)

(See Table 8-10)

A. Definition—increased secretion of cortisol from three main causes:
   1. Hyperplasia of adrenocortical tissue due to pituitary dysfunction
   2. Adrenocortical hyperplasia from a separate neoplasm secreting ACTH
   3. Primary adrenocortical hyperplasia from an adrenal tumor

B. Assessment
   1. Muscle wasting
   2. Weakness
   3. Osteoporosis
   4. Edema
   5. Purple striations on skin
   6. Truncal obesity
   7. Mood swings
   8. Poor resistance to infections
   9. Blood sugar imbalance
   10. Hypertension
   11. Buffalo hump

C. Diagnostic tests
   1. Skull films, CT, MRI
   2. Blood sugar analysis
   3. Hypokalemia and hypernatremia
   4. Plasma cortisol level increased
   5. Urinary 17-hydroxycorticosteroids and 17-ketosteroid levels increased

Table 8-8 GLUCOCORTICOID MEDICATIONS

MEDICATION	ADVERSE EFFECTS	NURSING CONSIDERATIONS
Short acting Cortisone acetate Hydrocortisone **Intermediate acting** Methylprednisolone Prednisone **Long acting** Betamethasone Dexamethasone	Increases susceptibility to infection May mask symptoms of infection Edema, changes in appetite Euphoria, insomnia Delayed wound healing Hypokalemia, hypocalcemia Hyperglycemia Osteoporosis, fractures Peptic ulcer, gastric hemorrhage Psychosis	Prevents/suppresses cell-mediated immune reactors Used for adrenal insufficiency Overdosage produces Cushing's syndrome Abrupt withdrawal of drug may cause headache, nausea and vomiting, and papilledema (Addisonian crisis) Give single dose before 9 AM Give multiple doses at evenly spaced intervals Infection may produce few symptoms due to anti-inflammatory action Stress (surgery, illness, psychic) may lead to increased need for steroids Nightmares are often the first indication of the onset of steroid psychosis Check weight, BP, electrolytes, I and O, weight Used cautiously with history of TB (may reactivate disease) May decrease effects of oral hypoglycemics, insulin, diuretics, K$^+$ supplements Assess children for growth restriction Protect from pathological fractures Administer with antacids Do not stop abruptly Solu-Medrol also used for arthritis, asthma, allergic reactions, cerebral edema Decadron also used for allergic disorders, cerebral edema, asthmatic attack, shock
Action	Stimulates formation of glucose (gluconeogenesis) and decreases use of glucose by body cells; increases formation and storage of fat in muscle tissue; alters normal immune response	
Indications	Addison's disease Crohn's disease COPD Lupus erythematosus Leukemias, lymphomas, myelomas Head trauma, tumors to prevent/treat cerebral edema	
Adverse effects	Psychoses, depression Weight gain Hypokalemia, hypocalcemia Stunted growth in children Petechiae Buffalo hump	
Nursing considerations	Monitor fluid and electrolyte balance Don't discontinue abruptly Monitor for signs of infection	
Herbal interactions	Enna, celery seed, juniper may decrease serum potassium; when taken with corticosteroids, may increase hypoglycemia Ginseng taken with corticosteroids may cause insomnia Echinacea may counteract effects of corticosteroids Licorice potentiates effect of corticosteroids	

Table 8-9	MINERALOCORTICOID MEDICATIONS	
MEDICATION	**ADVERSE EFFECTS**	**NURSING CONSIDERATIONS**
Fludrocortisone acetate	Hypertension, edema due to sodium retention Muscle weakness and dysrhythmia due to hypokalemia	Give PO dose with food Check BP, electrolytes, I and O, weight Give low-sodium, high-protein, high-potassium diet May decrease effects of oral hypoglycemics, insulin, diuretics, K^+ supplements
Action	Increases sodium reabsorption, potassium and hydrogen excretion in the distal convoluted tubules of the nephron	
Indications	Adrenal insufficiency	
Adverse effects	Sodium and water retention Hypokalemia	
Nursing considerations	Monitor BP and serum electrolytes Daily weight, report sudden weight gain to health care provider Used with cortisone or hydrocortisone in adrenal insufficiency	

D. Nursing management

1. Provide emotional support—assure the client that most physical changes are reversible with treatment

2. Teach appropriate diet—high protein, low carbohydrate, low sodium, high potassium, low calorie; fluid restriction

3. Prevent complications
   a. Use careful technique to prevent infection
   b. Assist with ambulation
   c. Eliminate environmental hazards for pathological fractures
   d. Observe for hyperactivity and GI bleeding, fluid volume overload

4. Administer aminoglutethimide or metyrapone to decrease cortisol production

5. Provide post-adrenalectomy care
   a. Flank incision—painful breathing, so encourage coughing and deep breathing
   b. Hormone imbalance likely
      1) Monitor for shock
      2) Monitor for hypertension
      3) Administer cortisol as ordered
   c. Monitor urine output
   d. Anticipate slow recovery from anesthesia in obese client
   e. Anticipate slow wound healing
   f. Monitor glucose level
   g. Ensure client safety to decrease risk of fractures
   h. Teach low-sodium, high-potassium diet
   i. Provide long-term hormone therapy because of cortical and mineralocorticoiol deficiency

        1) Given in schedule to mimic diurnal rhythm, with 2/3 dosage in early morning and 1/3 dosage in late afternoon

        2) Dose should meet needs of stress

6. Avoid factors that precipitate Addisonian crisis
   a. Physical stress
   b. Psychological stress
   c. Inadequate steroid replacement

7. Observe for clinical manifestations of Addisonian crisis
   a. Nausea and vomiting
   b. Abdominal pain
   c. Fever
   d. Extreme weakness
   e. Severe hypoglycemia and dehydration develop rapidly
   f. Blood pressure falls, leading to shock and coma; death results if not promptly treated

8. Treatment of Addisonian crisis
   a. Monitor hydrocortisone therapy (see Table 8-11)
   b. Carefully monitor IV infusion of NaCl
   c. Administer vasopressors
   d. Ensure absolute rest
   e. Monitor vital signs

Table 8-10 ADRENAL DISORDERS		
	ADDISON'S DISEASE	**CUSHING'S SYNDROME**
Assessment	Fatigue, weakness, dehydration, ↓ BP, hyperpigmentation, ↓ resistance to stress, alopecia Weight loss, pathological fractures Depression, lethargy, emotional liability	Fatigue, weakness, osteoporosis, muscle wasting, cramps, edema, ↑ BP, purple skin striations, hirsutism, emaciation, depression, decreased resistance to infection, moon face, buffalo hump, obesity (trunk), mood swings, masculinization in females, blood sugar imbalance

Diagnosis	Hyposecretion of adrenal hormones (mineralocorticoids, glucocorticoids, androgens)
	
	Pathophysiology:
	
	  ↓ Na^+ dehydration
	
	  ↓ Blood volume + shock
	
	  ↑ K^+ metabolic acidosis + arrhythmias
	
	  ↓ Blood sugar + insulin shock
	
	Diagnostic tests:
	
	  CT and MRI
	
	  Hyperkalemia and hyponatremia
	
	  ↓ Plasma cortisol
	
	  ↓ Urinary 17-hydroxycorticosteroids and 17-ketosteroids
	
	  ACTH stimulation test
	
	Treatment: hormone replacement
		Hypersecretion of adrenal hormones (mineralocorticoids, glucocorticoids, androgens)
		
		Pathophysiology:
		
		  ↑ Na^+ ↑ blood volume + ↑ BP
		
		  ↓ K^+ metabolic alkalosis + shock
		
		  ↑ Blood sugar + ketoacidosis
		
		Diagnostic tests:
		
		  Skull films
		
		  Blood sugar analysis
		
		  Hypokalemia and hypernatremia
		
		  ↑ Plasma cortisol level
		
		  ↑ Urinary 17-hydroxycorticosteroids and 17-ketosteroids
		
		Treatment: hypophysectomy, adrenalectomy

Table 8-11 ADRENAL DISORDER MEDICATIONS		
MEDICATION	**ADVERSE EFFECTS**	**NURSING CONSIDERATIONS**
Cortisone acetate Hydrocortisone Prednisone	Hyperglycemia, gastric and duodenal ulcers, muscle wasting, fluid retention, K^+ excretion, striae, acne, hirsutism, hypopigmentation, cataracts, osteoporosis Centripetal fat buildup, moon face, buffalo hump Adverse effects occur after prolonged therapy	Overdosage produces Cushing's syndrome Abrupt withdrawal of drug may cause headache, nausea and vomiting, and papilledema Give oral replacement preparation 2/3 in AM; 1/3 in PM Monitor labs, BP, physical exam Infection may produce few symptoms due to anti-inflammatory action Stress (surgery, illness, psychic) may lead to increased need for steroids Nightmares are often the first indication of the onset of steroid psychosis
Dexamethasone	Euphoria, insomnia Peptic ulcer, delayed wound healing	Effects of local injections persist for approximately 24 hours Check weight, BP, electrolytes Check for depression Give PO dose with food

HYPOTHYROIDISM (MYXEDEMA)

(See Table 8-12)

A. Definition—insufficient secretion of thyroid hormone

B. Assessment
   1. Early hypothyroidism—cold intolerance, lethargy, tiredness, slightly decreased temperature, constipation, weight gain
   2. Myxedema—periorbital and peripheral edema, thick speech, hoarseness, alopecia, bradycardia

C. Nursing management
   1. Provide appropriate pacing of activities
      a. Allow client extra time to think, speak, act
      b. Teaching should be done slowly and in simple terms

   2. Promote comfort, rest, and sleep
      a. Frequent rest periods between activities
      b. Maintain room temperature at approximately 75°F
      c. Provide client with extra clothing and bedding

   3. Maintain skin integrity—restrict use of soaps and apply lanolin or creams to skin
      a. Teach appropriate diet
         1) High protein, low calorie
         2) Small, frequent feedings

      b. Prevent constipation—high-fiber, high-cellulose foods

    c. Increase fluid intake

    d. Cathartics or stool softeners as ordered

4. Provide emotional support to client

    a. Explain to client that symptoms are reversible with treatment

    b. Explain to family that client's behavior is part of the condition and will change when treatment begins

5. Administer drug replacement therapy

    a. Dessicated thyroid hormone

    b. Levothyroxine (Synthroid); dose gradually increased and adjusted

    c. Liothyronine sodium (Cytomel)

6. Administer sedatives carefully—risk of respiratory depression

7. Instruct client about causes of myxedema coma (acute illness, surgery, chemotherapy, discontinuation of medication)

HYPERTHYROIDISM (GRAVES' DISEASE)

(See Table 8-12)

A. Definition—oversecretion of thyroid hormone

B. Assessment

    1. Increased physical activity

    2. Tachycardia

    3. Increased sensitivity to heat

    4. Fine, soft hair

    5. Enlarged thyroid

    6. Nervous, jittery, irritable, talkative

    7. Exophthalmos

    8. Weight loss

C. Treatment

    1. Antithyroid medications (e.g., propylthiouracil, methimazole)

    2. Irradiation (^{131}I PO)—short term

    3. Thyroidectomy—usually subtotal resection

D. Nursing management

    1. Promote comfort, rest, and sleep

        a. Limit activities to quiet ones (e.g., reading, knitting)

        b. Provide for frequent rest

        c. Restrict visitors and control choice of roommates

        d. Keep room cool; advise light, cool clothing

        e. Avoid stimulants (e.g., coffee)

    2. Provide emotional support

        a. Accept behavior

        b. Use calm, unhurried manner when caring for client

        c. Interpret behavior to family

3. Administer antithyroid medication (see Table 8-13)

4. Provide post-thyroidectomy care
   a. Prevent strain on suture line
      1) Low or semi-Fowler position
      2) Support head, neck, and shoulders to prevent flexion or hyperextension; elevate head of bed 30°
      3) Tracheostomy set and suction supplies at bedside

   b. Give fluids as tolerated

   c. Check Chvostek's and Trousseau's signs
      1) Chvostek's sign
         a) An abnormal spasm of the facial muscles elicited by light tapping on the cheek of a client with hypocalcemia
         b) Surgical removal of the thyroid gland can damage or remove the parathyroid glands (because they are embedded in the posterior thyroid gland)
         c) Parathyroidectomy causes hypocalcemia and produces symptoms of tetany, including Chvostek's sign

      2) Trousseau's sign
         a) Involuntary flexion of the wrist caused by inflating a blood pressure cuff above the systolic pressure on the upper arm
         b) Occurs in clients with hypocalcemia or hypomagnesemia

      3) Have IV calcium gluconate or calcium chloride available

   d. Offer throat lozenges, analgesics, cold steam inhalations for sore throat

   e. Adjust diet to new metabolic needs

Table 8-12 THYROID DISORDERS		
	MYXEDEMA/HYPOTHYROIDISM	GRAVES' DISEASE/HYPERTHYROIDISM
Assessment	Diagnostic tests: $\downarrow$ BMR (basal metabolic rate) $\downarrow$ T3 $\downarrow$ T4 $\uparrow$ TSH Decreased activity level Sensitivity to cold Potential alteration in skin integrity Decreased perception of stimuli Obesity, weight gain Potential for respiratory difficulty Constipation Alopecia Bradycardia Dry skin and hair Decreased ability to perspire Reproductive problems	Diagnostic tests: $\uparrow$ BMR $\uparrow$ T3 $\uparrow$ T4 High titer anti-thyroid antibodies Hyperactivity Sensitivity to heat Rest and sleep deprivation Increased perception of stimuli Weight loss Potential for respiratory difficulty Diarrhea Tachycardia Exophthalmus Frequent mood swings Nervous, jittery Fine, soft hair
Analysis	Hyposecretion of thyroid hormone Slowed physical and mental functions	Hypersecretion of thyroid hormone Accelerated physical and mental functions
Predisposing factors	Inflammation of thyroid Iatrogenic—thyroidectomy, irradiation, overtreatment with antithyroids Pituitary deficiencies Iodine deficiency Idiopathic Older adults—atrophy, fibrosis	Thyroid-secreting tumors Iatrogenic–overtreatment for hypothyroid Pituitary hyperactivity Severe stress, e.g., pregnancy
Treatment and management	Hormone replacement (Synthroid, Levothyroid)	Antithyroid medications (SSKI methimazole, propylthiouracil) Irradiation (^{131}I) Surgery
Potential nursing diagnosis	Disturbed body image Imbalanced nutrition: more than body requirements Activity intolerance Constipation Hypothermia Deficient knowledge Decreased cardiac output	Activity intolerance Altered body temperature Social interaction, impaired Imbalanced nutrition: less than body requirements Hyperthermia Fatigue Risk for impaired tissue integrity

5. Observe for complications

   a. Laryngeal nerve injury—detected by hoarseness

   b. Thyrotoxic Crisis (abrupt onset of HF, pulmonary edema, delirium, increased temperature and increased pulse, systolic hypertension, altered clotting, seizures, abdominal pain, diarrhea); treatment—hypothermia blanket, O_2, D_5W, potassium iodine, propylthiouracil (PTU), digitalis, propranolol, hydrocortisone, acetaminophen

   c. Hemorrhage; check back of neck and upper chest for bleeding

   d. Respiratory obstruction

   e. Tetany (decreased calcium from parathyroid involvement)—check Chvostek's and Trousseau's signs; have IV calcium gluconate or IV calcium chloride available

Table 8-13 HYPERTHYROIDISM AND HYPOTHYROIDISM MEDICATIONS		
MEDICATION	ADVERSE EFFECTS	NURSING CONSIDERATIONS
Hyperthyroidism Medications		
Carbimazole Methimazole Propylthiouracil	Leukopenia Fever Rash Sore throat Jaundice	Inhibits synthesis of thyroid hormone by thyroid gland Check CBC and hepatic function Report fever, sore throat to health care provider
Lugol's iodine solution Potassium iodide	Nausea, vomiting, metallic taste Rash	Iodine preparation Used 2 wk prior to surgery; decreases vascularity, decreases hormone release Only effective for a short period Give after meals Dilute in water, milk, or fruit juice Stains teeth Give through straw
Radioactive iodine (^{131}I)	Feeling of fullness in neck Metallic taste Leukemia	Destroys thyroid tissue Contraindicated for women of childbearing age Fast overnight before administration Urine, saliva, vomit radioactive 3 days Use full radiation precautions Encourage fluids
Hypothyroidism Medication		
Levothyroxine	Nervousness, tremors Insomnia Tachycardia, palpitations Dysrhythmias, angina	Tell client to report chest pain, palpitations, sweating, nervousness, shortness of breath to health care provider

HYPOPARATHYROIDISM

A. Decreased secretion of parathyroid hormone; causes low serum calcium levels (hypocalcemia); may be due to neck surgery; possible decreased calcium absorption in older adults

B. Assessment

1. Tetany, hyperactive deep tendon reflexes

2. Muscular irritability (paresthesias of lips, hands, feet)

3. Carpopedal spasm

4. Tremor, seizures

5. Dysphagia

6. Disorientation and confusion

7. Laryngeal spasm

8. Personality changes

9. Weakness and muscle cramps

10. Tachycardia and dysrhythmias; decreased cardiac output

11. Positive Chvostek's sign

12. Positive Trousseau's sign

C. Diagnostic tests

1. Serum calcium

2. Serum phosphorus

3. X-ray—bones appear dense

4. Sulkowitch test—test urine for calcium

D. Nursing management

1. Emergency Rx—calcium chloride, calcium gluconate, calcium gluceptate; infuse slowly to prevent hypotension and cardiac arrest

2. Replacement therapy

a. Vitamin D—calcitriol, ergocalciferol

b. Elemental calcium as lactate, gluconate, or carbonate—1.5 to 3 g/day

3. Observe for tetany

4. Administer appropriate diet—low phosphorus, high calcium (green leafy vegetables, soybeans, tofu)

HYPERPARATHYROIDISM

A. Oversecretion of parathyroid hormone; causes elevated serum calcium levels (hypercalcemia); may be due to benign tumor, vitamin D deficiency, long term kidney disease

B. Assessment (see Table 8-14)

C. Diagnostic tests

1. Serum calcium— greater than or equal to 10 mg/dL

2. Serum phosphorus— less than or equal to 4.5 mg/dL

3. X-ray—bones appear porous

4. Sulkowitch test—calcium in urine

5. Parathyroid hormone levels

6. Dual-energy x-ray absorptiometry (DEXA) scan—bone loss

Table 8-14 PARATHYROID DISORDERS		
	HYPOPARATHYROIDISM	HYPERPARATHYROIDISM
Assessment	Tetany Muscular irritability (cramps, spasms) Carpopedal spasm, clonic convulsions Dysphagia Paresthesia, laryngeal spasm Anxiety, depression, irritability Tachycardia + Chvostek's sign + Trousseau's sign	Fatigue, muscle weakness Cardiac dysrhythmias Emotional irritability Renal calculi Back and joint pain, pathological fractures Pancreatitis, peptic ulcer
Diagnosis	Decreased secretion of parathyroid hormone Introgenic–post thyroidectomy Hypomagnesemia Diagnostic tests: Serum calcium ↓ Serum phosphorus ↑ ↓ parathyroid hormone (PTH) X-ray–bones appear dense	Oversecretion of parathyroid hormone Benign parathyroid tumor Parathyroid carcinoma Neck trauma Neck radiation Diagnostic tests: ↑ Serum calcium ↓ Serum phosphorus X-ray–bones appear porous ↑ serum parathyroid hormone
Potential nursing diagnosis	Risk for injury Deficient knowledge	Risk for injury Impaired urinary elimination Nutrition: less than body requirements Constipation
Plan/Implementation	Emergency treatment–calcium chloride or gluconate over 10–15 minutes Calcitriol 0.5–2 mg daily for acute hypocalcemia Ergocalciferol 50,000–400,000 units daily Observe for tetany Low-phosphorus, high-calcium diet	Relieve pain Prevent formation of renal calculi increase fluid intake Offer acid-ash juices (improves solubility of calcium) Administer appropriate diet Prevent fractures Safety precautions Monitor potassium levels (counteracts effect of calcium on cardiac muscles) Provide postparathyroidectomy care (essentially same as for thyroidectomy) IV furosemide and saline promote calcium excretion IV phosphorus is used only for rapid lowering of calcium level Surgery–parathyroidectomy

D. Treatment
1. IV furosemide and saline promote calcium excretion
2. IV phosphorus is used only for rapid lowering of calcium level
3. Biphosphonates (e.g., alendronate) increase bone density and decrease calcium levels
4. Surgery—parathyroidectomy

E. Nursing management
1. Relieve pain
2. Prevent formation of renal calculi: increase fluid intake
3. Offer acid-ash juices (improves solubility of calcium)
4. Administer appropriate diet
5. Prevent fractures
6. Promote body alignment
7. Safety precautions
8. Monitor potassium levels (counteracts effect of calcium on cardiac muscles)
9. Provide post parathyroidectomy care (essentially same as for thyroidectomy)

Chapter 9

THE RENAL AND UROLOGICAL SYSTEMS

Sections	Concepts Covered
1. The Urinary System Overview	Acid-Base Balance, Fluid and Electrolyte Balance
2. Urinary Function	Acid-Base Balance, Fluid and Electrolyte Balance
3. Selected Disorders	Acid-Base Balance, Fluid and Electrolyte Balance, Elimination

OVERVIEW OF THE URINARY SYSTEM

(See Figure 9-1)

A. Kidneys

   1. Anatomy

      a. Bean-shaped, paired organs

      b. Left kidney larger and higher

      c. Positioned adjacent to vertebral column

      d. Two layers—outer cortex, inner medulla

      e. Functional unit—nephron (see Figure 9-2)

         1) Glomerulus—removes filtrate from blood

         2) Bowman's capsule—filtrate passes through to tubule

         3) Tubule

            a) Proximal convoluted tubule

            b) Loop of Henle

            c) Distal convoluted tubule

            d) Collecting tubule

      f. Gerontologic concerns—decreased kidney size; decreased tone and elasticity of bladder, ureters, urethra; decreased bladder capacity

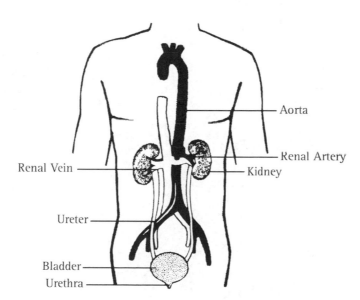

Figure 9-1. URINARY SYSTEM

2. Physiology
   a. Elimination of waste products
   b. Fluid and electrolyte balance regulator
   c. Production of blood cells
   d. Hormonal control of blood pressure

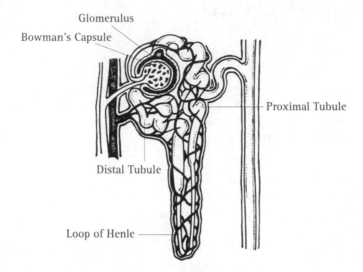

Figure 9-2. NEPHRON

   e. Gerontologic concerns—glomerular sclerosis and decreased renal perfusion; decreased ability to concentrate urine

B. Ureters
   1. Anatomy—hollow tubes, about 12 inches long
   2. Physiology—propel urine to bladder from kidneys

C. Bladder
   1. Hollow, muscular organ
   2. Lies within pelvic cavity
   3. Normal capacity—500 mL
   4. Contracts under voluntary and involuntary control
   5. Nerve supply—parasympathetic and sympathetic

OVERVIEW OF URINARY FUNCTION

A. Urine production
1. Glomerular filtration—begins in afferent arteriole, then to glomerular capillaries, then to glomerulus
2. Tubular reabsorption—ultrafiltrate passes through remainder of nephron

B. Characteristics of urine
1. Color—yellow
2. Consistency—clear, transparent
3. Specific gravity—1.010–1.025
4. pH—4.5–8
5. 24-hours production—1,000–2,000 mL

C. Serum changes
1. BUN (normal 10–20 mg/dL (3.6–7.1 mmol/L); greater than 60 yo 8–20 mg/dL)
2. Creatinine (normal 0.7–1.4 mg/dL) (62–124 µmol/L)

D. Diagnostic studies of the urinary system (see Table 9-1)

E. Promotion of normal urinary function
1. Adults
   a. Adequate hydration
   b. Activity (maintenance of muscle tone)
   c. Regular voiding habits

2. Children
   a. Proper toilet training
      1) 2 1/2 to 3 1/2 years old—bladder reflex control
      2) 3 years old—regular voiding habits
      3) 4 years old—independent bathroom activity
      4) 5 years old (approximate)—nighttime control
   b. Enuresis—lack of nighttime bladder control in school-aged child

Table 9-1 DIAGNOSTIC STUDIES OF THE URINARY SYSTEM		
TEST	CLIENT PREPARATION AND PROCEDURE	NURSING CONSIDERATIONS
Urinalysis Urine culture	Advise client to save first AM urine specimen Cleanse external meatus with povidone-iodine or soap and water prior to test	Overnight urine specimen is more concentrated Obtain midstream specimen Normal—less than 100,000 colonies/mL
Cystometrogram— test of muscle tone	Prepare client for Foley catheter Instillation of saline may cause feeling of pressure in bladder during test Client should report bladder sensations during test	Advise client to report any post-test symptoms
Creatinine clearance	24-hour urine collection	Blood drawn for creatinine level at end of urine collection Normal—women: 75–115 mL/min Men: 85–125 mL/min
Cystoscopy—direct visualization by cystoscope inserted into bladder	Bowel preparation Teach client to deep-breathe to decrease discomfort NPO if general anesthesia used	Post-test nursing care: Monitor character and volume of urine Check for abdominal distention, frequency, fever Check for bleeding Provide antimicrobial prophylaxis
Cystourethrogram—x-ray study of bladder and urethra	Explain procedure to client: catheter inserted into urethra, radiopaque dye injected, client voids, x-rays taken during voiding	Post-test nursing care: Advise client to report any symptoms
Intravenous pyelogram—provides x-ray visualization of kidneys, ureters, and bladder	Bowel preparation NPO after midnight Check for allergies Burning may occur during injection of radiopaque dye into vein X-rays are taken at intervals after dye	Postprocedure x-rays usually done Client should be alert to signs of dye reaction: edema, itching, wheezing, dyspnea
Renal scan—evaluation of kidneys	Radioactive isotope injected IV Radioactivity measured by radioactivity counter Fluids forced before procedure	No Post-test care required
Ultrasound—images of renal structures obtained by sound waves	Noninvasive procedure; no preparation; requires full bladder	No preparation or post-test care required
Renal biopsy—kidney tissue obtained by needle aspiration for pathological evaluation	X-ray taken prior to procedure Skin is marked to indicate lower pole of kidney (fewer blood vessels) Position: prone and bent at diaphragm Client instructed to hold breath during needle insertion	Post-test nursing care: Pressure applied to site for 20 min; check vital signs every 15 min for 1 hour Pressure dressing applied; position on affected side for 30–60 min Client kept flat in bed Bed rest for 6–8 hours Intake 3,000 mL/day Observe for hematuria and site bleeding

MANAGEMENT OF URINARY RETENTION

A. Clinical manifestations
1. Voiding at frequent intervals in small amounts
2. Suprapubic discomfort and bladder distention
3. Appropriate hydration with no urinary output for more than 6 hours
4. Specific gravity is elevated

B. Causes
1. Functional—neurogenic bladder
2. Mechanical—stricture, calculi, trauma

C. Predisposing factors
1. Bedrest
2. Tumors
3. Prostatic hypertrophy
4. Decreased bladder tone—postoperative, neurological
5. Bladder or urethral cancer
6. Postop effects
7. Calculi
8. Medications—nephrotoxicity

D. Complications
1. Rupture of bladder
2. Infection
3. Uremia

E. Nursing care
1. Stimulate voiding, e.g., running water
2. Pouring tepid water over perineum
3. Positioning
4. Catheterization—temporary, may be emergency

F. Surgical Intervention (see Table 9-2)
1. Suprapubic cystostomy—opening into bladder, drainage via catheter through abdominal wall
2. Surgery for kidney stones

Table 9-2 URINARY DIVERSION		
NAME	PROCEDURE	NURSING CONSIDERATIONS
Nephrostomy	Flank incision and insertion of nephrostomy tube into renal pelvis	Penrose drain Surgical dressing
Ureterosigmoidostomy	Ureters detached from bladder and anastomosed to sigmoid colon	Urine and stool are evacuated through anus Encourage voiding via rectum every 2–4 hours; no enemas or cathartics Monitor complications—fluid and electrolyte imbalance, pyelonephritis, obstruction
Cutaneous ureterostomy	Single- or double-barreled stoma, formed from ureter(s) excised from bladder and brought out through the skin into the abdominal wall	Stoma usually constructed on right side of abdomen below waist Extensive nursing intervention required for alteration in body image
Ileal conduit	Portion of terminal ileum is used as a conduit; ureters are replanted into ileal segment; distal end is brought out through skin and forms a stoma	Most common urinary diversion Check for obstruction (occurs at the anastomosis) Postop mucus threads normal
Kock pouch, continent ileal conduit	Ureters are transplanted to an isolated segment of ileum (pouch) with a one-way valve; urine is drained by a catheter	Urine collects in pouch until drained by catheter Valve prevents leakage of urine Drainage of urine by catheter is under control of client Pouch must be drained at regular intervals

CARE OF URINARY DRAINAGE SYSTEMS

A. Urinary catheters (see Table 9-3)

1. To facilitate healing of portion of urinary tract
2. To empty bladder contents, e.g., postoperatively or spinal cord injuries
3. To promote continence
4. To facilitate measurement of urine output

Table 9-3 URINARY CATHETERS		
TYPE	**CHARACTERISTICS**	**COMMENTS**
Bladder drainage system	Double lumen with inflatable balloon toward tip	Indwelling for urinary drainage
Nephrostomy	Placed on temporary basis	Used as nephrostomy tube– anchored in renal pelvis through flank incision
Suprapubic	Placed in bladder via abdominal incision Dressing over site	Used in conjunction with urethral drainage
Straight	Intermittent	Used for neurogenic bladder; bladder outlet obstruction in men; postop after surgical problems in reproductive organs

B. Procedure for catheterization

1. Female
   a. Explain procedure to client
   b. Assemble equipment
   c. Client should be placed in dorsal recumbent position or in Sims' position
   d. Drape client with sterile drapes, using sterile technique
   e. Apply sterile gloves
   f. Lubricate catheter tip and place in sterile catheter tray
   g. Separate labia with thumb and forefinger and wipe from the meatus toward the rectum with sterile cleansing swab and discard
   h. Insert catheter 2–3 in into the urethra; insert catheter an additional inch after urine begins to flow to ensure balloon portion of catheter is in the bladder
   i. Inflate balloon
   j. Gently apply traction to the catheter
   k. Tape drainage tubing to client's thigh

2. Male
   a. If uncircumcised, retract the foreskin to expose urinary meatus
   b. Cleanse glans and meatus with sterile cleansing swabs in circular motion
   c. Hold penis perpendicular to the body; insert catheter into urethra 6–7 in
   d. Replace the foreskin
   e. Inflate balloon

      f. Gently apply traction to the catheter until resistance is felt, indicating the catheter is at the base of the bladder

      g. Tape drainage tubing to client's thigh

  3. Principles of drainage system care

      a. Catheter should not be disconnected from drainage system except to perform ordered irrigations

      b. Urine samples should be obtained from drainage port with a small-bore needle, using sterile technique; clamp tubing below port

      c. Drainage bags should not be elevated above level of cavity being drained (to prevent reflux)

      d. Avoid kinks in tubing

      e. Avoid removing more than 1000 mL at one time; if more urine in bladder, clamp after 1000 mL, wait 15–30 min, then continue

      f. Coil excess tubing on bed

  4. Catheter irrigation

      a. Purpose—prevent obstruction of flow and catheter

      b. Procedure—urethral catheter irrigation

          1) Use closed sysytem; if frequent irrigation is required replace single lumen catheter with multi-lumen catheter

          2) Draw up required solution

          3) Clamp catheter just below port (specimen or irrigation)

          4) Thoroughly clean injection port

          5) Insert syringe into port

          6) Slowly and evenly inject solution into catheter and bladder

          7) Withdraw syringe, cleanse port, remove clamp

          8) Note drainage and document procedure including resistance to flush, client comfort, drainage returned

  5. Nursing management

      a. Use aseptic technique on insertion

      b. Do not disturb integrity of closed drainage system

      c. Check for kinks

      d. Keep urine collection bag below the level of the urinary bladder

      e. Monitor intake and output; minimum urinary drainage catheter output should be 30 mL/h

      f. Monitor for signs and symptoms of infection (foul-smelling urine with pus, blood, or mucus streaks)

      g. Adhere to special precautions for type of catheter used

          1) Ureterostomy tube—never irrigate

          2) Nephrostomy tube—never clamp

      h. Clamp indwelling catheters intermittently prior to removal to improve bladder tone

C. Promotion of normal urinary function

  1. Adequate hydration

  2. Activity (maintenance of muscle tone)

  3. Regular voiding habits

INCONTINENCE

A. Definition—involuntary loss of bladder control due to infection, neurogenic bladder, sphincter weakness, or reduced muscle tone

B. Types

1. Urge incontinence—Strong and sudden urge to void; unknown cause

2. Stress incontinence—occurs with physical exertion such as lifting, sneezing; common in women after childbirth

3. Overflow incontinence—constant dribbling of urine; diabetic neuropathy, prostatic hyperplasia, uterine prolapse

4. Reflex incontinence—large amount of urine retained; central nervous system disease (CVA, MS)

C. Intervention—short term; varies according to type

1. Scheduling, bladder retraining, prompted voiding

2. Pelvic exercises

3. Surgical approaches

4. Condom catheters, incontinence pads

5. Avoid delay in assisting client to bathroom

SURGERY FOR URINARY DIVERSION FOLLOWING SURGERY FOR BLADDER CANCER OR URETHRAL CANCER

(See Figure 9-3 and Table 9-2)

A. Ureterosigmoidostomy—ureters are attached to the sigmoid colon to allow drainage into rectum and elimination control by anus; not as commonly used

B. Cutaneous ureterostomy—one or both ureters are brought to the skin surface to form a stoma to drain urine

C. Ileal conduit—both ureters are attached to a segment of ileum, which is brought to the surface of the lower abdomen to form a stoma to drain urine; most commonly used urinary diversion

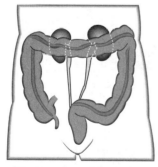
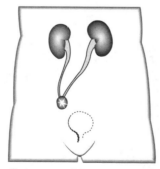
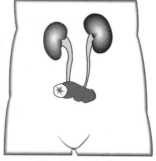
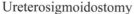

Ureterosigmoidostomy   Cutaneous Ureterostomy   Ileal Conduit

Figure   9-3.   **TYPES OF URINARY DIVERSIONS**

SELECTED DISORDERS OF THE URINARY SYSTEM

A. Cystitis
1. Definition—inflammation of the bladder; may be infectious (bacteria, virus, fungal) or noninfectious (irritation)
2. Assessment
   a. Signs and symptoms
      1) Urgency
      2) Frequency
      3) Burning during urination (dysuria)
      4) Cloudy, foul smelling urine
   b. Predisposing factors
      1) Female more prone
      2) Catheterization, instrumentation
      3) Hospital-acquired infections (e.g., *E. coli)*
3. Nursing management
   a. Encourage/Increase fluids to 3,000 mL/d
   b. Urine for culture and sensitivity (C and S)
   c. Antibiotic therapy (e.g., trimethoprim/sulfamethoxazole) or antifungals (e.g., ketoconazole)
   d. Urinary antiseptics (e.g., nitrofurantoin)
   e. Bladder analgesics (e.g., phenazopyridine)
   f. Encourage drinking cranberry juice to maintain acid urine
   g. Discourage caffeine, carbonated beverages, tomatoes
   h. Teach females to void following intercourse
   i. Clean properly after defecation (front to back)

B. Pyelonephritis—inflammation of the kidney
1. History
   a. Pregnancy
   b. Urinary obstruction
   c. Metabolic disorder (e.g., diabetes mellitus, hypertension)
   d. Trauma
   e. Tumor
   f. Urinary tract infection
2. Assessment
   a. Chills
   b. Fever
   c. General malaise
   d. Urinary frequency, dysuria

  e. Flank pain

  f. Costovertebral angle (CVA) tenderness

 3. Nursing management

  a. Serial urine culture—usually caused by *E. coli*

  b. Periodic blood tests

  c. Bedrest during acute phase

  d. Antibiotic therapy, antiseptics, analgesics

  e. Encourage fluid intake 3000 mL/day

C. Urinary Tract Calculi

 1. Definition—mineral crystallization formed around organic matter

  a. Urolithiasis—urinary stones

  b. Nephrolithiasis—kidney stones

 2. History

  a. UTI, dehydration

  b. Hypercalcemia or increased uric acid

  c. Urinary stasis

  d. Obstruction

 3. Assessment

  a. Pain (renal colic)

   1) Location depends on location of stone

   2) Radiates from flank to abdomen, labia, or scrotum

  b. Nausea, vomiting

  c. Hematuria, WBCs and bacteria in urine

  d. Diaphoresis

  e. Low-grade fever and chills

  f. Diagnostic tests—IVP, CT, MRI, cystoscopy, KUB

 4. Nursing management

  a. Monitor I and 0

  b. Force fluids

  c. Strain urine and check pH of urine

  d. Monitor temperature

  e. Pain management—NSAIDs, oxybutynin, propantheline, opioids

  f. Diet for prevention depends on identified stone from urinary tract

   1) Low in oxalate—spinach, black tea, rhubarb for calcium oxalate stones

   2) Low in protein—to prevent cystine stones, calcium phosphate

   3) Low in sodium—sodium increases calcium in urine

   4) Low in purines to prevent uric acid stones

 5. Medical management

  a. Lithotripsy

   1) Laser lithotripsy and extracorporeal shock-wave lithotripsy most common

   2) Laser probes or high-energy acoustic shock waves shatter the stones

  b. Surgery—stent placement, nephrolithotomy, nephrostomy, retrograde ureteroscopy

D. Hydronephrosis —kidney pelvis dilation, leading to tissue destruction and renal failure

1. Assessment

   a. Pain

     1) Dull flank

     2) Stabbing in flank or abdomen radiating to genitalia

   b. Nausea, vomiting

   c. Signs and symptoms of UTI

   d. Abdominal muscle spasms

2. Nursing management

   a. Bedrest

   b. Antibiotic therapy

   c. Catheterization

   d. Force fluids to 3,000 mL/d

   e. Urinary diversion

   f. Surgical correction

   g. Strain all urine

E. Benign prostatic hyperplasia (BPH)

1. Definition—prostate gland enlargement

2. History

   a. Retention

   b. Hesitancy, frequency, urgency, dysuria

   c. Nocturia

   d. Hematuria before of after voiding

   e. Urinary stream alterations; dilated ureter

   f. Dribbling

3. Diagnostic tests—BUN, prostatic-specific antigen (PSA), ultrasound, biopsy

4. Management

   a. Urinary antiseptics

   b. 5-alpha reductase inhibitor (e.g., finasteride)

   c. Alpha-blocking medications (e.g., tamsulosin)

   d. Saw palmetto or lycopene

   e. Suprapubic cystostomy—to empty bladder

   f. Surgery—three common approaches to prostate gland removal

     1) Transurethral resection of prostate (TURP)

     2) Suprapubic resection (incision through bladder)

     3) Retropubic resection (incision through abdomen)

   g. Postop care of TURP

     1) Assess for shock and hemorrhage—check dressing and drainage: urine may be bright red for 12 hours; monitor vital signs

     2) I and O—after catheter removed, expect dribbling and urinary leakage around wound

     3) Avoid long periods of sitting and strenuous activity until danger of bleeding is over

F. Nephrosis (nephrotic syndrome)—idiopathic syndrome characterized by proteinuria and hypoalbuminemia

1. Definition
   a. Congenital nephrotic syndrome
   b. Secondary nephrotic syndrome—occurs after known glomerular disease
   c. Idiopathic nephrotic syndrome—most common

2. Assessment
   a. Edema
   b. Pallor
   c. Lethargy
   d. Oliguria
   e. Dark, frothy urine
   f. Decreased serum protein, increased serum cholesterol and plasma lipids

3. Nursing management
   a. Steroid and antibiotic therapy; monitor for infection
   b. Bedrest
   c. Fluid restriction, I and O
   d. High-protein, low-sodium, high-caloric diet

G. Acute kidney injury

1. Definition—a rapid loss of renal function due to damage to the kidney.

2. History
   a. Prerenal injury
      1) Circulating volume depletion
      2) Vascular obstruction
      3) Vascular resistance
   b. Intra-renal failure
      1) Acute tubular necrosis (ATN) from nephrotoxic medications or transfusion reaction
      2) Trauma
      3) Glomerulonephritis
      4) Severe muscle exertion
      5) Genetic conditions—polycystic kidney disease
   c. Postrenal failure—obstruction of urine outflow from the kidney; reflux of urine from the bladder back into the kidneys; tumors or renal calculi

3. Assessment
   a. Oliguric phase
      1) Urinary output 0.5 mL/kg/hr
      2) Nausea, vomiting
      3) Irritability
      4) Drowsiness, confusion, coma
      5) Restlessness, twitching, seizures
      6) Increased serum K^+, BUN, creatinine
      7) Increased Ca^+, Na^+, pH, CO_2

8) Anemia

9) Pulmonary edema, CHF

10) Hypertension

11) Albuminuria

b. Diuretic or recovery phase
1) Urinary output 4–5 L/d
2) Increased serum BUN
3) Na^+ and K^+ loss in urine
4) Increased mental and physical activity

4. Nursing management
a. Oliguric and anuric phases—protein sparing diet, restrict fluids, observe for hyponatremia and hypokalemia, dialyze as ordered, prevent infection
b. Diuretic phase—monitor I and O, observe for electrolyte imbalance, provide adequate nutrition, prevent infection

H. Chronic kidney disease
1. Definition—ongoing deterioration of kidney function, resulting in uremia
2. History
a. Hypertension
b. Diabetes mellitus
c. Lupus erythematosus
d. Sickle cell disease
e. Chronic glomerulonephritis
f. Repeated pyelonephritis
g. Polycystic kidney disease
h. Nephrotoxins

3. Assessment
a. Anemia
b. Acidosis
c. Azotemia
d. Fluid retention
e. Urinary output alterations

4. Nursing management
a. Antihypertensives
b. Fluid and sodium restrictions
c. Adherence to diet
d. Monitor I and O
e. Skin care
f. Dialysis—movement of fluid and particles across a semipermeable membrane

I. Kidney transplantation (see Table 9-4 and Figure 9-4)
1. Donor selection
a. Major requirement is histocompatibility

2. Pretransplantation donor—specific transfusions

a. Desensitizes recipient to donor's tissue

b. Identifies unfavorable response to donated organ by recipient

3. Nursing management—preop

a. Explain surgical procedure and follow-up care to client

b. Show client where the donated kidney will be located (iliac fossa on opposite side of body from which the kidney was taken)

Table 9-4	HEMODIALYSIS AND PERITONEAL DIALYSIS	
	HEMODIALYSIS	PERITONEAL DIALYSIS
Circulatory access	Subclavian catheter AV fistula, AV graft	Catheter in peritoneal cavity (Tenckoff, Gore-Tex)
Dialysis bath	Electrolyte solution similar to that of normal plasma	Similar to hemodialysis
Dialyzer	Artificial kidney machine with semipermeable membrane	Peritoneum is dialyzing membrane
Procedure	Blood shunted through dialyzer for 3–5 hours, 2–3 times/wk	Weigh client before and after dialysis Repeated cycles can be continuous Catheter is cleansed and attached to line leading to peritoneal cavity Dialysate infused into peritoneal cavity to prescribed volume Dialysate is then drained from abdomen after prescribed amount of time

Complications	Hemorrhage
	Hepatitis
	Nausea and vomiting
	Disequilibrium syndrome (headache, mental confusion)
	Muscle cramps
	Air embolism
	Sepsis
		Protein loss
		Peritonitis
		  Cloudy outflow, bleeding
		  Fever
		  Abdominal tenderness, lower back problems
		  Nausea and vomiting
		  Exit site infection
		  Hypotension and hypovolemia

Nursing considerations	Check "thrill" and bruit every 8 hours Don't use extremity for BP or to obtain blood specimens Monitor BP, apical pulse, temperature, respirations, breath sounds, weight Monitor for hemorrhage during dialysis and 1 hour after procedure	Constipation may cause problems with infusion and outflow; high-fiber diet, stool softener If problems with outflow, reposition (supine or low-Fowler side client to side) Monitor BP, apical pulse, temperature, respirations, breath sounds, weight Clean catheter insertion site and apply sterile dressing

c. Emphasize need for continued dialysis postop

d. Use of immunosuppressive medications

e. Need for infection prevention

f. Pain management

g. Pulmonary hygiene

h. Maintaining integrity of vascular access

i. Tubings and dressings, locations and purposes

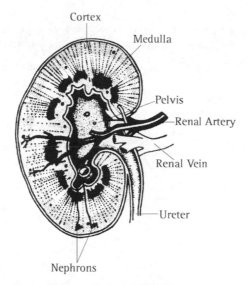

Figure 9-4. KIDNEY

4. Nursing management—postop

a. Monitor vital signs

b. Monitor I and O—expect scant urine production for weeks postop

c. Vascular access care

d. Observe for:

1) Hemorrhage

2) Shock

3) Rejection

a) Rejection—Acute (days to months; decreased urine output, increased BUN and creatinine, fever, tenderness and swelling over graft site); chronic (months to years; gradual decrease in renal function, protcinuria, gradual increase in BUN and creatinine)

4) Infection

5) Pulmonary complications

6) Adverse effects of immunosuppressive and steroid therapies

e. Daily weights

f. Catheter care

g. Psychological support for donor and recipient

OVERVIEW OF DIURETICS

Table 9-5 DIURETIC MEDICATIONS		
MEDICATION	**ADVERSE EFFECTS**	**NURSING CONSIDERATIONS**
Thiazide diuretics Hydrochlorothiazide Chlorothiazide	Hypokalemia Hyperglycemia Blurred vision Loss of Na^+ Dry mouth Hypotension	Monitor electrolytes, especially potassium I and O Monitor BUN and creatinine Don't give at hs Weigh client daily Encourage potassium-containing foods
Potassium-sparing Spironolactone	Hyperkalemia Hyponatremia Hepatic and renal damage Tinnitus Rash	Used with other diuretics Give with meals Avoid salt substitutes containing potassium Monitor I and O
Loop diuretics Furosemide Ethacrynic acid	Hypotension Hypokalemia Hyperglycemia GI upset Weakness	Monitor BP, pulse rate, I and O Monitor potassium Give IV dose over 1–2 minutes → diuresis in 5–10 min After PO dose diuresis in about 30 min Weigh client daily Don't give at hs Encourage potassium-containing foods
Bumetanide	Potassium depletion Electrolyte imbalance Hypovolemia Ototoxicity	Supervise ambulation Monitor blood pressure and pulse Observe for signs of electrolyte imbalance
Osmotic diuretic Mannitol	Dry mouth Thirst	I and O must be measured Monitor vital signs Monitor for electrolyte imbalance
Thiazide-like Chlorthalidone	Dizziness Aplastic anemia Orthostatic hypotension	Acts like a thiazide diuretic Acts in 2–3 hours, peak 2–6 hours, lasts 2–3 days Administer in AM Monitor output, weight, BP, electrolytes Increase K^+ in diet Monitor glucose levels in diabetic clients Change position slowly

Table 9-5 DIURETIC MEDICATIONS *(CONTINUED)*		
MEDICATION	**ADVERSE EFFECTS**	**NURSING CONSIDERATIONS**
Action	Thiazides—inhibits reabsorption of sodium and chloride in distal renal tubule	
	Loop—inhibits reabsorption of sodium and chloride in loop of Henle and distal renal tubules	
	Potassium-sparing—blocks effect of aldosterone on renal tubules, causing loss of sodium and water and retention of potassium	
	Osmotic—pulls fluid from tissues due to hypertonic effect	
Indications	Heart failure	
	Hypertension	
	Renal diseases	
	Diabetes insipidus	
	Reduction of osteoporosis in postmenopausal women	
Adverse effects	Dizziness, vertigo	
	Dry mouth	
	Orthostatic hypotension	
	Leukopenia	
	Polyuria, nocturia	
	Photosensitivity	
	Impotence	
	Hypocalcemia (except for potassium-sparing)	
	Hyponatremia	
Nursing considerations	Take with food or milk	
	Take in AM	
	Monitor weight and electrolytes	
	Protect skin from the sun	
	Diet high in potassium for loop and thiazide diuretics	
	Limit potassium intake for potassium-sparing diuretics	
	Used as first-line drugs for hypertension	
Herbal interaction	Licorice can promote potassium loss, causing hypokalemia	
	Aloe can decrease serum potassium level, causing hypokalemia	
	Gingko may increase blood pressure when taken with thiazide diuretics	

Table 9-6 MEN'S HEALTH MEDICATIONS		
MEDICATION	DVERSE EFFECTS	NURSING CONSIDERATIONS
Alpha 1-adrenergic blockers		
Terazosin	Dizziness Headache Weakness Nasal congestion Orthostatic hypotension	Used to decrease urinary urgency, hesitancy, nocturia in prostatic hyperplasia Caution to change position slowly Avoid alcohol, CNS depressant, hot showers due to orthostatic hypotension Requires titration Administer at bedtime due to risk orthostatic hypotension Effects may not be noted for 4 weeks
Tamsulosin	Dizziness Headache	Used to decrease urinary urgency, hesitancy, nocturia in prostatic hyperplasia Caution to change position slowly Administer 30 min. after same meal each day
5-alpha-reductase inhibitor		
Finasteride	Decreased libido Impotence	Used to treat benign prostatic hyperplasia by slowing prostatic growth May decrease serum PSA levels 6–12 months therapy required to determine if medication effective May cause harm to male fetus. Pregnant women should not be exposed to semen of partner taking finasteride or they should not handle crushed medication Monitor liver function tests
Dutasteride	Decreased libido Impotence	Used to treat benign prostatic hyperplasia by slowing prostatic growth May cause harm to male fetus. Pregnant women should not be exposed to semen of partner taking finasteride or they should not handle crushed medication Monitor liver function
Anti-impotence		
Sildenafil Vardenafil Tadalafil	Headache Flushing Dyspepsia Nasal congestion Mild visual disturbance	Enhances blood flow to the corpus cavernosum to ensure erection to allow sexual intercourse Should not take with nitrates in any form due to dramatic decrease in blood pressure Usually taken 1 hour before sexual activity (sildenafil, vardenafil) Tadalafil has longer duration of action (up to 36 hours) Should not take more than one time per day Notify health care provider if erection lasts longer than 4 hours
Saw palmetto	Urinary antiseptic used to treat PBH; may cause false-negative PSA test result	

Chapter 10

THE MUSCULOSKELETAL SYSTEM

Section	Concepts Covered
1. Alterations in Musculoskeletal Function	Mobility, Skin Integrity, Comfort, Client Education: Providing

ALTERATIONS IN MUSCULOSKELETAL FUNCTION

LOW BACK PAIN

A. Predisposition
   1. Herniated intervertebral disk (most commonly affecting L4–L5 or L5-S1 interspaces (see Figure 10-1)
   2. Fracture of the spine
   3. Spine dislocation
   4. Osteoarthritis
   5. Scoliosis
   6. Tension
   7. Poor posture and/or body mechanics
   8. Lack of muscle tone
   9. Degenerative disk disease
   10. Obesity
   11. Spinal stenosis—narrowing of spinal canal; osteoarthritis most common cause; compression of nerve roots and disk herniation

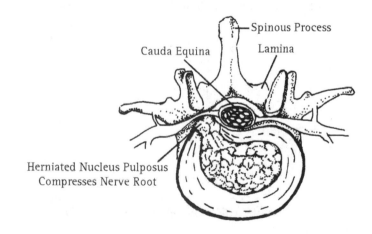

Figure 10-1. HERNIATED INTERVERTEBRAL DISK

B. Diagnostic procedure
   1. Myelography (not commonly done)
   2. MRI, CT scan
   3. Electromyogram (EMG)
   4. Diskogram

C. Assessment
   1. Pain—may be continuous
   2. Depressed or absent Achilles tendon reflex; positive straight-leg raise test; numbness and parethesias of leg

3. Guarded movement

4. Decreased ROM of spine

5. Diagnostic studies—x-ray, CT, myelogram, diskogram

D. Nursing management

1. To relieve pain and muscular spasm

   a. Administer appropriate medications (analgesics, NSAIDs, muscle relaxants, e.g., cyclobenzaprine)

   b. Apply moist heat/cool 20–30 minutes four times a day

   c. Bedrest; client in Fowler position with moderate hip and knee flexion

   d. Use firm mattress, bedboard, or floor for back support

2. To regain normal elasticity of affected muscle

   a. Isometric exercises for abdominal muscles

   b. Daily exercise program

3. To return joint to normal function

   a. Assist with exercises for abdominal muscles

   b. ROM exercises

4. Good body mechanics

   a. Do not lean forward without bending knees

   b. Exercise under direction of health care provider

   c. Do not stand in one position for prolonged time

   d. Sleep in side-lying position with knees and hips bent

E. Client teaching

1. Exercise daily but avoid strenuous exercises

2. Correct posture at all times

3. Avoid prolonged sitting, standing, walking, and driving

4. Rest at intervals

5. Use hardboard for bed, or firm mattress

6. Avoid prone position

7. Avoid straining or lifting heavy objects

F. Management specific to herniated lumbar disk

1. Conservative therapy—combination of medication, heat/ice therapy, ultrasound, transcutaneous electrical nerve stimulation (TENS)

2. Surgical therapy

   a. Percutaneous laser diskectomy; herniated portion of disk is lasered

   b. Diskectomy—partial removal of lamina

   c. Laminectomy—excision of a portion of the lamina to expose the affected disk for removal

   d. Laminectomy with fusion—involves several disk herniations; operation includes use of bone graft to strengthen the weakened vertebral column

   e. Postlaminectomy care

      1) Maintain body alignment

      2) Log roll every 2 hours

      3) Calf exercises

      4) Assess for sensations and circulatory status, especially of lower extremities

      5) Monitor elimination

      6) Assist with ambulation

   f. Interbody cage fusion with bone graft

SELECTED MUSCULOSKELETAL TRAUMA/INJURIES AND DISORDERS

A. Assessment

  1. Contusions—injuries to soft tissue

    a. Ecchymosis

    b. Hematoma

  2. Strains/sprains—pulled muscle/torn ligament

    a. Pain

    b. Swelling

  3. Joint dislocations—displacement of joint bones; articulating surfaces lose all contact

    a. Pain

    b. Deformity

  4. Fractures—break in continuity of bone (see Figure 10-2)

    a. Swelling

    b. Pallor, ecchymosis

    c. Loss of sensation to body parts

    d. Deformity

    e. Pain and/or acute tenderness

    f. Muscle spasms

    g. Loss of function

    h. Abnormal mobility

    i. Crepitus (grating sound on movement of ends of broken bone)

    j. Shortening of affected limb

    k. Decreased or absent pulses distal to injury

    l. Affected extremity colder than contralateral part

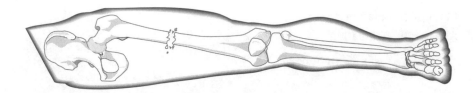

A. Complete: break across entire cross-section of bone

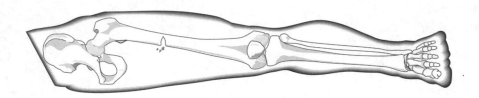

B. Incomplete: break through portion of bone

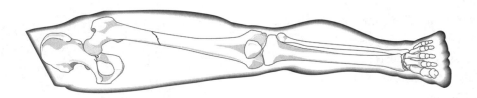

C. Closed: no external communication

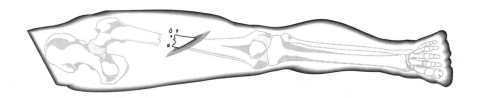

D. Open: extends through skin

Figure   10-2.   TYPES OF FRACTURES

B. Types
   1. Avulsion—tearing away of a fragment of bone by a ligament or tendon pulling the fragment away
   2. Comminuted—a fracture in which the bone is crushed or broken into a number of pieces
   3. Greenstick—an incomplete fracture in which the bone is bent, but fractured only on the outer arc of the bend
   4. Longitudinal—a fracture along the long axis of the bone
   5. Oblique—a slanted fracture of the shaft on the long axis of a bone
   6. Impacted—a bone break in which the adjacent fragmented ends of the fractured bone are wedged together
   7. Interarticular—a fracture within a movable joint
   8. Pathologic—a fracture resulting from a weakness in the bone tissue

9. Spiral—a bone break in which the disruption of bone tissue is spiral, oblique, or transverse to the long axis of the bone

10. Stress—a fracture in the bones of the leg, ankle, or foot caused by repeated, prolonged, or abnormal weight-bearing stress (jogging, running, etc.)

11. Displaced—a traumatic bone break in which two ends of a fractured bone are separated (can cause an open or compound fracture)

C. Complications of fractures
   1. Types
      a. Fat emboli—caused after fracture of long bones when fat globules move into bloodstream; may occlude major vessels; symptoms include shortness of breath, chest pain, anxiety, decreased oxygen saturation, chest petechiae
      b. Hemorrhage
      c. Delayed union—healing of fracture is slowed; caused by infection or distraction of fractured fragments; will see increase in bone pain
      d. Nonunion—healing has not occurred 4–6 months after fracture; insufficient blood supply, repetitive stress on fracture site, infection, inadequate internal fixation; treated by bone grafting, internal fixation, electric bone stimulation
      e. Sepsis
      f. Compartment syndrome—high pressure within a muscle compartment of an extremity compromises circulation; pressure may be internal (bleeding) or external (casts); if left untreated neuromuscular damage occurs within 4–6 hours; limb can become useless within 24–48 hours; will see unrelenting pain out of proportion to injury and unrelieved by pain medication, decreased pulse strength and pale cool extremity
      g. Peripheral nerve damage

D. Nursing management
   1. Contusions—treated with cold application for 24 hours, followed by moist heat; apply elastic bandage
   2. Strains/sprains—treated with rest and elevation of affected part; intermittent ice compresses for 24 hours, followed by heat application; apply elastic pressure bandage; minimize use
   3. Dislocations—considered an orthopedic emergency; treated with immobilization and reduction (e.g., the dislocated bone is brought back to its normal position, usually under anesthesia); bandages and splints are used to keep affected part immobile until healing occurs
   4. Fractures
      a. Provide emergency care
         1) Immobilization before client is moved by use of splints; immobilize joint below and above fracture
         2) In an open fracture, cover the wound with sterile dressings or cleanest material available
         3) Emergency department—give narcotic adequate to relieve pain, except in presence of head injury
      b. Treatment
         1) Splinting/immobilization of the affected part to prevent soft tissue from being damaged by bony fragments
         2) Internal fixation—use of metal screws, plates, nails, and pins to stabilize reduced fractures
         3) Open reduction/surgical dissection and exposure of the fracture for reduction and alignment

5. Traction (see Figures 10-3 through 10-7)

  a. Purposes

    1) Immobilize fracture

    2) Alleviate pain and muscle spasm

    3) Prevent or correct deformities

    4) Promote healing

  b. Types of traction

    1) Skin (Buck's extension, balanced suspension, Russell's, pelvic traction)—noninvasive (does not penetrate the skin)

    2) Skeletal (halo fixation device, Crutchfield tongs)—invasive (penetrates the skin)

  c. Nursing management

    1) Maintain straight alignment of ropes and pulleys

    2) Assure that weights hang free

    3) Frequently inspect skin for breakdown

    4) Maintain position for countertraction

    5) Encourage movement of unaffected areas

    6) Investigate every complaint immediately and thoroughly

    7) Maintain continuous pull

    8) Clean pins with half-strength peroxide and sterile swabs 1–2 times/d

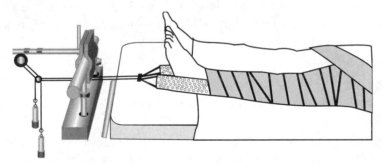

Figure 10-3. BUCK'S TRACTION

Relieves muscular spasm of legs and back; if no fracture, may turn to either side; with fracture, turn to unaffected side. 8–20 lb used; 40 lb for scoliosis. Elevate foot of bed for countertraction. Use trapeze for moving. Place pillow beneath lower legs, not heel. Don't elevate knee gatch.

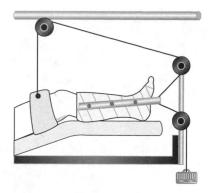

Figure   10–4.   RUSSELL'S TRACTION

"Pulls" contracted muscles; elevate foot of bed with shock blocks to provide counter-traction; sling can be loosened for skin care; check popliteal pulse. Place pillows under lower leg. Make sure heel is off the bed. Must not turn from waist down. Lift client, not leg, to provide assistance.

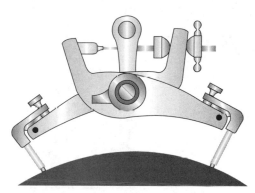

Figure   10–5.   CERVICAL (SKULL TONGS)

Realigns fracture of cervical vertebrae and relieves pressure on cervical nerve; never lift weights—traction must be continuous. No pillow under the head during feeding; hard to swallow, may need suctioning.

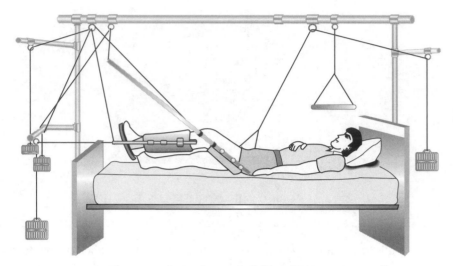

Figure   10–6.   BALANCED SUSPENSION

Realigns fractures of the femur; uses pulley to create balanced suspension by counter-traction to the top of the thigh splint. Thomas splint (positioned under anterior thigh) with Pearson attachment (supports leg from knee down) frequently used.

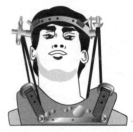

Figure   10–7.   HALO FIXATION DEVICE (VEST)

Provides immobilization of cervical spine; pins are used to maintain traction; care of insertional site includes cleansing area around pins using sterile technique. If prescribed by health care provider, clean with half-strength peroxide or saline and sterile swabs 1–2 times/d.

6. Casting—provides rigid immobilization of affected body part for support and stability; may be plaster or fiberglass
   a. Immediate care
      1) Avoid covering cast until dry (48 hours or longer), handle with palms, not fingertips (plaster cast)
      2) Avoid resting cast on hard surfaces or sharp edges
      3) Keep affected limb elevated above heart on soft surface until dry; no heat lamp
      4) Watch for danger signs (e.g., blueness or paleness, pain, numbness or tingling sensations on affected area); if present, elevate casted area; if it persists, contact health care provider
      5) Elevate arm cast above level of heart
   b. Intermediate care
      1) When cast is dry, client should be mobilized
      2) Encourage prescribed exercises (isometrics)
      3) Report to health care provider any break in cast or foul odor from cast
      4) Tell client not to scratch skin underneath cast; skin may break and infection can set in
      5) If fiberglass cast gets wet, dry with hair dryer on cool setting
   c. After-cast care
      1) Wash skin gently
      2) Apply baby powder, cornstarch, or baby oil
      3) Have client gradually adjust to movement without support of cast
      4) Inform client that swelling is common after cast is removed; elevate limb and apply elastic bandage

FRACTURED HIP

A. Assessment
   1. Leg shortened, adducted, externally rotated
   2. Pain
   3. Hematoma, ecchymosis
   4. Confirmed by x-rays

B. Gerontologic considerations—increased risk of vision and hearing deficits, orthostatic hypotension, medications; decreased fat and muscle mass; gait and balance problems

C. Diagnosis
   1. Commonly seen with elderly women with osteoporosis, postural hypotension, gait and balance problems, vision and hearing problems, medications, decreased fat and muscle mass
   2. Potential nursing diagnoses
      a. Impaired physical mobility
      b. Risk for peripheral neurovascular dysfunction
      c. Risk for impaired gas exchange
      d. Acute pain

D. Plan/Implementation

1. Total hip replacement—acetabulum, cartilage, and head of femur replaced with artificial joint (see Figure 10-8)

2. Abduction of affected extremity (use splints, wedge pillow, or 2 or 3 pillows between legs)

3. Turn client as ordered; keep heels off bed

4. Ice to operative site

5. Overbed trapeze to lift self onto fracture bedpan

6. Prevention of thromboembolism–low-molecular-weight heparin (LMWH) and warfarin; do not sit for prolonged periods

7. Initial ambulation with walker

8. Crutch walking—three-point gait

9. Chair with arms, wheelchair, semireclining toilet seat

10. Medications—anticoagulants to prevent pulmonary embolism, antibiotics to prevent infection

11. Don't sleep on operated side

12. Don't flex hip more than 90°

13. Use adaptive devices for dressing–extended handles, shoe horns

14. Report increased hip pain to health care provider immediately

15. Cleanse incision daily with mild soap and water; dry thoroughly

16. Inspect hip daily for redness, heat, drainage; if present, call health care provider immediately

17. Complications

   a. Dislocation of prosthesis

   b. Excessive wound drainage

   c. Thromboembolism

   d. Infection

18. Postoperative discharge teaching

   a. Maintain abduction

   b. Avoid stooping

   c. Do not sleep on operated side until directed to do so

   d. Flex hip only to 90°

   e. Never cross legs

   f. Avoid position of flexion during sexual activity

   g. Walking is excellent exercise; avoid overexertion

   h. In 3 mo, will be able to resume ADLs, except strenuous sports

19. Prevention

   a. Vitamin D and calcium supplementation

   b. Estrogen replacement therapy

   c. Bisphosphonates

   d. Aerobic and weight-bearing exercise

   e. Safety issues

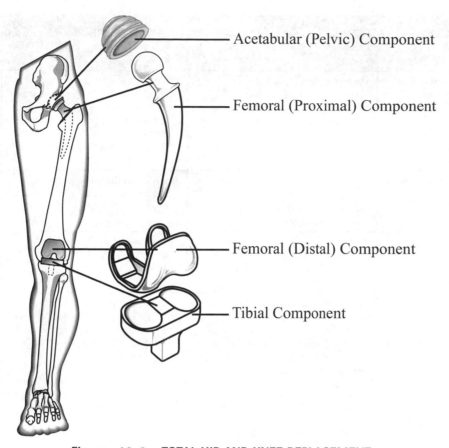

Figure   10-8.   TOTAL HIP AND KNEE REPLACEMENT

AMPUTATION

A. Causes

1. Trauma

2. Peripheral vascular disease

3. Osteogenic sarcoma

4. Gerontologic considerations—decreased peripheral circulation, diabetic neuropathy, decreased immune response

B. Types

1. Disarticulation—resection of an extremity through a joint

2. Above-the-knee amputation

3. Below-the-knee amputation

4. Guillotine or open surface

    a. Amputation in which a straight, guillotine cut is made without skin flaps

    b. Open amputation performed if infection is probable, developing, or recurrent (to allow drainage until the infection clears)

5. Closed or flap

    a. Amputation in which one or two broad flaps of muscular and cutaneous tissue is/are retained to form a cover over the end of the bone

    b. Performed when no infection is present

	Table 10-1 POSTOPERATIVE CARE OF AMPUTATION	
TYPE OF CARE	**DELAYED PROSTHETIC FITTING**	**IMMEDIATE PROSTHETIC FITTING**
Residual limb care	Observe dressings for signs of excessive bleeding; keep large tourniquet on hand to apply around residual limb in event of hemorrhage	Observe rigid dressing for signs of oozing; if blood stain appears, mark area and observe every 10 min for increase; report excessive oozing immediately to health care provider; provide cast care; guard against cast slipping off
Positioning	Elevate foot of the bed for the first few hours to hasten venous return and prevent edema; do not elevate on pillows—hip contracture may result	Lay residual limb flat on the bed; rigid cast acts to control swelling
Turning	Turn client to prone position for short time first postop day, then 30 min 2–3 times daily to prevent hip contracture; have client roll from side to side	Same; however, rigid cast acts to prevent both hip and joint contractures
Exercises	Have client start exercises to prevent contractures as soon as possible (1st or 2nd day postop) including active range of motion, especially of affected leg; strengthening exercises for upper extremities; hyperextension of residual limb	Exercises not as essential because rigid dressing prevents contractures; also early ambulation prevents all immobilization disabilities
Ambulation	Dangle and transfer client to wheelchair and back within 1st or 2nd day postop; crutch-walking started as soon as client feels sufficiently strong	Dangle and ambulate client with walker for short period 1st day; increase length of ambulation each day; in physical therapy, client uses parallel bars, then crutches, then cane
Psychological support	Observe for signs of depression, despondency; remind depressed client that the prosthesis will be fitted when his wound heals	Observe for signs of depression; clients usually less depressed if they awaken with prosthesis attached
Discharge	Teach residual limb care—inspect daily for abrasions, wash, expose to air, do not apply lotions, use only cotton or wool socks	Same
Comfort	Administer medication for pain; phantom limb pain possible; reality that limb is missing; client indicating he/she wants the limb disposed of will help	Same

C. Postoperative management (see Table 10-1)
   1. Delayed prosthesis fitting—residual limb covered with figure-eight wrapping dressing and ACE bandage or residual limb socks; note if Penrose drain is inserted; reapply bandages every 4–6 hours
   2. Immediate prosthesis fitting—residual limb covered with dressing and rigid plastic dressing; Penrose drains usually not inserted; rigid dressing helps prevent bleeding by compressing residual limb

D. Nursing management
   1. Prevent bleeding
   2. Promote circulation

3. Prevent complications of immobility—ROM exercises, trapeze with overhead frame, prone position every 3–4 hours

4. Provide comfort and relieve pain—propranolol, antiseizure medications, and antispasmodics used for phantom limb pain

5. Provide psychological and emotional support

6. Client teaching, regarding residual limb care

DISEASES OF THE MUSCULOSKELETAL SYSTEM

A. Rheumatoid arthritis (RA)

1. Description—systemic crippling condition characterized by inflammation of synovial membrane of the joints with periods of remission and exacerbation

2. History
   a. Autoimmunity
   b. Environmental factors
   c. Viral or streptococcal infection
   d. Genetic

3. Assessment
   a. Joint pain and swelling
   b. Limited joint movement
   c. Contractures; deformities
   d. Weakness, fatigue
   e. High fever and rheumatoid rash, particularly seen in juvenile RA
   f. Nodules over bony prominences
   g. Ulnar deviation
   h. Periods of remissions and exacerbations

4. Diagnostic tests
   a. Blood studies
      1) ASO titer (JRA)
      2) Latex fixation—rheumatoid factor
      3) C-reactive protein
      4) Sedimentation rate
      5) ESR, ANA
   b. Aspiration of synovial fluid
   c. X-rays

5. Nursing management
   a. Relieve pain and discomfort
      1) Application of heat (e.g., warm tub baths, warm, moist compresses, paraffin dips)
      2) If inflammatory process is acute, application of cold packs or ice bag is sometimes effective
      3) Support joints with splints; cervical collar in late stages
      4) Administer analgesics and anti-inflammatory medications
      5) Administer disease modifying antirheumatic medications (e.g., gold, hydroxychloroquine)
      6) Administer immunosuppressive medications (e.g., methotrexate, azathioprine)
      7) Administer antitumor necrosis medications (e.g., etanercept)

      b. Promote rest and mobility

         1) Proper positioning—avoid position flexion

         2) Use firm mattress or bedboard

         3) ROM exercises as tolerated

         4) Encourage independence and acceptance of limitations

      c. Reduce inflammation—administer antiinflammatory medications

      d. Provide adequate dietary intake; appropriate diet for obesity

      e. Provide operative care for clients undergoing musculoskeletal surgery (e.g., arthroplasty—total hip replacement)

      f. Preoperative teaching

         1) Teach partial weight-bearing use of crutches, isometric exercises, and transfer techniques

         2) Familiarize client with overbed traction frame, trapeze, and abduction splint

      g. Postoperative care

         1) Position client flat in bed with affected extremity in abduction

         2) Apply ice to operative area to reduce edema

         3) Assess circulation of affected extremity

         4) Administer medications to prevent postoperative complications

            a) Pulmonary embolism—anticoagulants

            b) Infection—antibiotics

         5) Encourage active foot and ankle motion the day following surgery to prevent circulatory stasis

         6) Help client ambulate gradually with walker, then crutches, using three-point gait

      h. Postoperative discharge teaching

         1) Maintain abduction

         2) Avoid stooping

         3) Do not sleep on operated side until directed to do so

         4) Flex hip only to 1/4 circle

         5) Never cross legs

         6) Avoid position of flexion during sexual activity

         7) Walking is excellent exercise; avoid overexertion

         8) In 3 mo, will be able to resume ADLs, except strenuous sports

B. Juvenile rheumatoid arthritis—(JRA)

  1. Pathophysiology—much the same as adult RA

  2. Characteristic clinical manifestations—same as RA, in addition:

      a. Intermittent fever and chills

      b. Rheumatoid rash (salmon pink, macular rash on chest, thighs, and upper arms)

      c. Iridocyclitis (inflammation of the iris and ciliary body)

      d. Growth restriction

  3. Diagnosis—latex fixation test for RA in adult is seldom positive for JRA

  4. Problems—same as RA plus impaired social and personality development

  5. Treatment and nursing management—same as RA; assist child in adjusting to chronic illness and encourage regular ophthalmologic examination for iridocyclitis

C. Ankylosing spondylitis (Marie-Strümpell disease)
1. Description—chronic progressive disorder that primarily affects the spine
2. Pathophysiology—synovitis, fibrosis, ankylosis of the vertebral joints
3. Clinical manifestations
   a. Pain and stiffness
   b. Kyphosis
   c. Iritis
   d. Decreased respiratory function
4. Diagnostic tests—x-rays (bony growths, called syndesmophytes, that bridge the adjacent vertebrae are visible)
5. Problems
   a. Alteration in comfort (pain)
   b. Decreased mobility
   c. Potential for respiratory difficulty
   d. Potential for poor body image and low self-esteem
6. Treatment and nursing management
   a. Analgesics; promote comfort
   b. Antiinflammatory medications, salicylates
   c. Administer disease modifying antirheumatic medications (e.g., methotrexate)
   d. Administer antitumor necrosis medications (e.g., infliximab)
   e. Physical therapy, heat application
   f. Promote body alignment, especially of the spine
      1) Postural exercises
      2) Splinting; bracing
   g. Improve mobility
      1) ROM exercises
      2) Assist with ADLs
   h. Prevent respiratory complications

D. Degenerative joint disease (osteoarthritis)
1. Description—nonsystemic, progressive degenerative condition that affects the joints; no remissions
2. Pathophysiology—articular cartilage degenerates, new bone forms (spur), joint spaces close
3. History
   a. Poor posture
   b. Trauma
   c. Stress on joints
   d. Obesity
   e. Smoking
4. Assessment
   a. Muscular spasm, pain, limitation of motion, stiffness; impaired ADL performance
   b. Contractures, deformities
   c. Heberden's nodes on fingers and Bouchard's nodes of hand
   d. Obesity/debilitation

5. Diagnostic test—x-rays and MRI of joints show narrowing of joint spaces, ESR, high-sensitivity C-reactive protein

6. Risk factors

   a. Increased age—bone and joint changes

   b. Obesity and sedentary lifestyle

   c. Trauma to joints due to repetitive use

      1) Carpet installer

      2) Construction worker

      3) Farmer

      4) Sports injuries

7. Nursing management

   a. Reduce pain and discomfort

      1) Balance rest with activity

      2) Administer analgesics and antiinflammatory drugs (e.g., NSAIDs or acetaminophen), topical medication (e.g., Lidocaine)

      3) Gerontologic considerations—increased risk of adverse effects with NSAIDs

   b. Heat application or cold application

   c. Maintain mobility

      1) ROM

      2) Encourage usual ADLs that involve using all joints

   d. Provide adequate nutrition; obese clients should be put on appropriate diet

   e. Complementary and alternative therapies—acupuncture, topical capsaicin, glucosamine, chondroitin

E. Gout

   1. Description—nonsystemic inflammation of the joints characterized by remissions and exacerbations

   2. Pathophysiology—disturbed purine metabolism leads to elevated uric acid in the blood, causing tophi (deposits in the joints)

   3. Predisposition—genetic defect of purine metabolism

      a. Swollen, reddened, painful joints, often in the great toe

      b. Limitation of motion

      c. Deformity—tophi

   4. Diagnostic tests

      a. X-rays

      b. Blood tests—WBC, sedimentation rate, uric acid level

      c. Synovial aspiration

   5. Nursing management

      a. Relieve pain and discomfort

         1) Rest affected joint

         2) Administer analgesics

      b. Reduce urate level in the blood

         1) Eliminate purine food from diet, e.g., liver, sardines

         2) Administer medication (cholchicine, probenecid) (see Table 10-2)

F. Bursitis

1. Description—inflammation of connective tissue sac between muscles, tendons, and bones, particularly affecting shoulder, elbow, and knee

2. History

   a. Stress on joints

   b. Toxins

   c. Infections

3. Assessment

   a. Pain

   b. Decreased mobility, especially on abduction

Table 10-2 ANTIGOUT MEDICATIONS		
MEDICATION	ADVERSE EFFECTS	NURSING CONSIDERATIONS
Colchicine	GI upset Agranulocytosis Peripheral neuritis	Antiinflammatory Give with meals Check CBC, I and 0
Probenecid	Nausea, constipation Skin rash	Reduces uric acid Check BUN, renal function tests Encourage fluids Give with milk, food, antacids Alkaline urine helps prevent renal uric acid stones
Sulfinpyrazone	Renal colic, peptic ulcer Blood dyscrasias	Reduces uric acid in the blood Check BUN, CBC, renal function tests Encourage fluids Give with food, milk, antacids
Allopurinol	GI upset Headache, dizziness, drowsiness	Blocks formation of uric acid Encourage fluids Check I and 0 Check CBC and renal function tests Give with meals Alkaline urine helps prevent renal uric acid stones

4. Interventions

   a. Rest

   b. Immobilize affected joint by use of pillows, splints, slings

   c. Administer pain medication, muscle relaxants (diazepam), steroids, NSAIDs

   d. Apply heat/cold packs to decrease swelling

   e. Promote exercise (ROM)

   f. Assist in performance of ADLs by modifying activities relative to limitations

   g. Assist with cortisone injection, draining of bursae

G. Paget's disease

1. Description—disease of unknown cause characterized by enlargement of bones, bone deformities, and increasing vascularity of bones; typical client is male and older than 50 years

2. Pathophysiology—bone resorption, disordered bone formation, vascularity of bone tissue

3. Assessment
   a. Pain and tenderness; long bone, spine and rib pain
   b. Enlarged skull
   c. Kyphosis
   d. Bowed legs
   e. Waddling gait
   f. Decrease in height
   g. Pathologic fractures

4. Nursing management
   a. Administer analgesics
   b. Encourage rest
   c. Prevent pathological fractures by using safety precautions
   d. Administer specific medications to prevent bone destruction

H. Osteoporosis
   1. Description—degenerative disease characterized by generalized loss of bone density and tensile strength
   2. Pathophysiology—reduction in the amount of bone mass without change in mineral composition
   3. History
      a. Age greater than 60
      b. Small-framed and lean body build
      c. Caucasian or Asian race
      d. Decreased estrogen (menopause)
      e. Low calcium intake
      f. Vitamin D deficiency
      g. Malabsorptive disease of the GI tract
      h. Immobility
      i. Hyperthyroidism
      j. Hyperparathyroidism
      k. Prolonged use of steroids
      l. Older women—decreased bone mass, increased bone resorption after menopause, less calcium intake over lifetime

   4. Assessment
      a. Lower back pain
      b. Kyphosis
      c. Decrease in height

   5. Diagnostic tests—x-rays

   6. Nursing management
      a. Provide optimal nutrition diet—high in calcium, protein, and vitamin D
      b. Teach about medications (see Table 10-3)
      c. Promote mobility and strength
         1) Encourage weight-bearing on the long bones

2) ROM exercises

3) Physiotherapy

d. Prevent pathological fractures—safety precautions

e. Promote comfort and relieve pain
   1) Bedrest
   2) Use of back brace or splint for support
   3) Use of bedboards or hard mattress

f. Prevent bone resorption—administer calcitonin, a thyroid hormone that slows bone loss

Table 10-3 CALCIUM AND VITAMIN D MEDICATIONS		
	ADVERSE EFFECTS	NURSING CONSIDERATIONS
Oral calcium medication		
Calcium carbonate Calcium citrate	Chalky taste Mild constipation Alkalosis Milk-alkali syndrome (with calcium carbonate)	Contraindicated in clients with a history of calcium renal calculi, hypercalcemia, or hypercalciuria Assess BP and ECG; serum magnesium, potassium, and phosphorus; BUN; and serum creatinine as therapy begins Monitor BP, ECG, electrolytes, and renal function Monitor for signs and symptoms of hypercalcemia Chewable tablets should be chewed well and taken with a full glass of water 30 minutes to 1 hour after meals
Other medications		
Alendronate Risedronate Calcitonin-salmon	Used in the prevention and treatment of osteoporosis and Paget's disease	Prevents and treats osteoporosis Longer-lasting treatment for Paget's disease Take in AM at least 30 min before other medication, food, water, or other liquids Should sit up for 30 min after taking medication Use sunscreen and wear protective clothing

I. Osteomyelitis

   1. Description—infection of the bone, usually caused by *Staphylococcus aureus*, carried by the blood from a primary site of infection

   2. Pathophysiology—inflammation; abscess formation; necrosis of the bone

   3. History

      a. Chronic skin problems, e.g., pressure injury, gangrene

      b. Compound fractures

      c. Malnutrition

      d. Immunosuppression

   4. Assessment

      a. Pain

      b. Swelling, redness, warmth on affected area (localized infection)

      c. Fever (systemic infection)

   5. Diagnostic tests

      a. Leukocytosis

      b. Elevated sedimentation rate

      c. Culture and sensitivity

      d. X-ray of affected part

   6. Nursing management

      a. Promote comfort, relieve pain

         1) Bedrest

         2) Administer analgesics

         3) Support affected extremity with pillows, splints to maintain proper body alignment

         4) Provide cool environment and lightweight clothing

      b. Reduce inflammatory process

         1) Administer antibiotics and antipyretics

         2) Avoid exercise and heat application to the affected area

         3) Encourage fluid intake

         4) Monitor I and O

      c. Promote skin integrity

         1) Asepsis

         2) General skin care

         3) Aseptic wound care

      d. Provide emotional support

         1) Allow for expression of fear and anxiety

         2) Provide diversionary activities

      e. Improve nutritional status

         1) High-protein diet with sufficient carbohydrates, vitamins, and minerals

         2) Small, frequent feedings

J. Osteomalacia

1. Description—decalcification of bones due to inadequate intake of vitamin D, absence of exposure to sunlight, intestinal malabsorption, chronic renal disease

2. Pathophysiology—calcium deficit leads to porosity and softening of the bones

3. Assessment

   a. Bone pain and tenderness

   b. Muscle weakness

   c. Bowed legs

   d. Kyphosis

4. Diagnostic tests—x-rays (porous bones)

5. Nursing interventions

   a. Relief of pain

      1) Administration of analgesics

      2) Bedrest as needed

      3) Maintain good body alignment

   b. Promote mineralization of bone—administer vitamin D, calcium, and exposure to sunlight and/or ultraviolet irradiation

   c. Promote safety

      1) Assist with performance of ADLs to prevent pathological fractures

      2) Regular medical follow-up

   d. Instruct about high vitamin D foods (milk, eggs, vitamin D enriched cereals and bread products)

Table 10-4 HERBAL SUPPLEMENTS FOR MUSCULOSKELETAL SYSTEM		
MEDICATION	**ADVERSE EFFECTS**	**NURSING CONSIDERATIONS**
Glucosamine	Nausea, heartburn, diarrhea	Antirheumatic Contraindicated if shellfish allergy, client is pregnant or lactating May worsen glycemic control Must be taken on regular basis to be effective
Chondroitin	Headache Restlessness Nausea Vomiting Anorexia	Given alone or with glucosamine Interactions with anticoagulants, NSAIDs, salicylates

Chapter 11

SENSORY AND NEUROLOGICAL FUNCTION

Sections	Concepts Covered
1. Sensation and Perception Functions	Sensory Perception
2. Alterations in Vision	Sensory Perception, Client Education: Providing
3. Alterations in Hearing	Sensory Perception, Client Education: Providing

SENSATION AND PERCEPTION FUNCTIONS

ANATOMY AND PHYSIOLOGY

A. Neuron (see Figure 11-1)

1. Basic component of the nervous system

2. Composed of cell body, axon, and dendrites
   a. Cell body is the center of metabolism
   b. Axons are long fibers that conduct impulses away from the cell body; there is usually one axon for each cell body
   c. Dendrites are short, unsheathed fibers that receive nerve impulses from other axons and transmit impulses to cell body

3. Myelin sheath—covering that protects nerve fiber and facilitates the speed of impulse conduction
   a. Both axons and dendrites may or may not have myelin sheath
   b. Most axons leaving the central nervous system are heavily myelinated with Schwann cells
   c. Gaps in myelin sheath are termed nodes of Ranvier
   d. Gerontologic considerations—myelin sheath degeneration; decreased nerve conduction

4. Primary function is transmission of nerve impulses
   a. Afferent (sensory) neurons: transmit impulses from peripheral receptors to the central nervous system
   b. Efferent (motor) neurons: transmit impulses from the central nervous system to muscles and organs
   c. Action potentials travel along axon; at end of nerve fiber, impulse is transmitted across junction between nerve cells (synapse) by chemical interaction
   d. Gerontologic considerations—less coordination of nerve impulse transmission; decreased ability to maintain blood pressure and body temperature; decreased sense of pain, touch, and temperature

5. Neuroglia—glial cells
   a. Provide support, nourishment, and protection for neurons

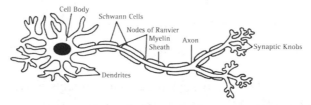

Figure 11–1. ANATOMY AND PHYSIOLOGY OF THE NEURON

B. Peripheral nervous system (PNS)—contains cranial nerves, spinal nerves, autonomic nervous system (unconscious reflexes), ANS sympathetic division (accelerates activity), and parasympathetic division (slows body processes)

C. Central nervous system (CNS)—contains brain and spinal cord (see Figure 11-2)

1. Cerebrum—divided into left and right hemispheres by a longitudinal fissure; each cerebral hemisphere contains frontal, parietal, occipital, and temporal lobes; loss of neurons with aging; increased risk of Alzheimer's disease (see Figure 11-3)

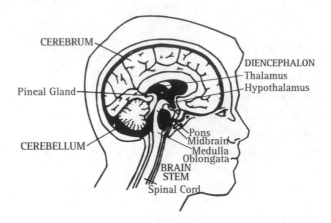

Figure 11-2. CENTRAL NERVOUS SYSTEM (CNS)

a. Frontal lobes
   1) Precentral gyrus—motor function, contralateral movement: face, arm, leg, trunk
   2) Broca's area—in the dominant hemisphere is responsible for the formation of words or speech
   3) Supplementary motor area—contralateral head and eye turning
   4) Prefrontal areas—personality, initiative
   5) Paracentral lobule—cortical inhibition of bladder and bowel

b. Parietal lobes
   1) Important in concept of body image and awareness of external environment (ability to construct shapes)
   2) Postcentral gyrus—registers bodily sensations (temperature, touch, pressure, pain) from opposite side of body

c. Occipital lobes—visual center; comprehension of written word

d. Temporal lobes
   1) Dominant hearing of language; taste, smell
   2) Memory
   3) Wernicke's speech area—recognition of language

2. Basal ganglia—regulate and integrate skeletal voluntary and autonomic motor activity originating in cerebral cortex

3. Diencephalon—connects the cerebrum and brain stem; contains several small structures, the most important of which are the thalamus and hypothalamus
   a. Thalamus—relay station for discrimination of sensation (pain, temperature, touch) received from the periphery; several nuclei in the thalamus, each with specific functions, such as integration of sensory stimuli necessary for abstract thinking and reasoning, vision, hearing; relay station for fibers going to the limbic system
   b. Hypothalamus is responsible for maintaining homeostasis through the secretion of hormones and central control of the autonomic nervous system

      1) Controls vital functions such as water balance, blood pressure, sleep, appetite, body temperature

      2) Affects some emotional responses (pleasure, fear)

      3) Control center for pituitary function

      4) Affects both divisions of the autonomic nervous system

  c. Limbic system influences affective (emotional) behaviors and basic drives such as sexual behavior, aggression

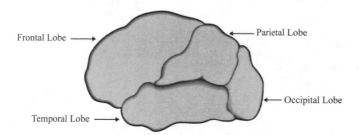

Figure 11-3. DIVISIONS OF THE BRAIN

4. Brain stem—contains midbrain, pons and medulla oblongata, extending from the cerebral hemispheres to the foramen magnum at the base of the skull

  a. Contains nuclei of the fifth, sixth, seventh, and eighth cranial nerves and ascending sensory and descending motor tracts

  b. Contains vital centers of respiratory, vasomotor, and cardiac functions

  c. Reticular formation—relays sensory information; controls vasomotor and respiratory activity

  d. Decreased number of neurons with aging

5. Ventricular system and cerebral spinal fluid (CSF)—supports and cushions the central nervous system

  a. Removes metabolic wastes

  b. Compensatory mechanisms for intracranial volume/pressure

  c. Produces 55 mL/d of CSF; 130–150 mL average amount in system; CSF production decreases with age

  d. Ventricles enlarge and widen with aging

6. Cranial meninges

  a. Dura mater—dense, fibrous, outermost layer serves as periosteum for cranial bones

  b. Arachnoid mater

    1) Delicate, avascular membrane lying under dura

    2) Surrounds brain loosely

    3) Subarachnoid spaces contain CSF, arteries, veins

    4) Contains arachnoid granulations that enable CSF to pass from subarachnoid space into the venous system

  c. Pia mater

    1) Most delicate and inner meningeal layer

    2) Barrier system

  d. Gerontologic considerations—increased subdural space due to cerebral atrophy

7. Cerebellum—control of muscle movement, balance, coordination; trunk mobility and equilibrium; decreased number of neurons with aging, increased problems with balance and coordination

8. Spinal cord—communications link between CNS and PNS; ascending pathways transmit sensory information and descending pathways relay motor instructions

ALTERATIONS IN NEUROLOGICAL FUNCTION

A. Assessment—signs and symptoms

1. Headache

2. Dizziness

3. Changes in level of consciousness

4. Increased intracranial pressure

5. Pupillary reactions—reaction to light, size

6. Seizures—focal or generalized

7. Changes in vital signs—increasing systolic BP, decreasing diastolic BP, bradycardia

8. Hyperpyrexia

9. Ocular movements—six cardinal fields of gaze

10. Skeletal motor function; muscle strength

11. Neurogenic bladder

12. Cranial nerve function (see Table 11-1)

13. Coma—Glasgow coma scale (see Table 11-2): score of 3–8 indicates severe head injury; score of 15 indicates client is alert and oriented

14. Verbal response

B. Specific conditions

1. Loss of consciousness

   a. Assessment—unable to rouse client; use Glasgow coma scale to assess response to stimuli

   b. Management—caring for the unconscious client

      1) Protective measures

         a) Ensure adequate oxygenation and circulation

         b) Keep side rails in elevated position—or mattress on floor

         c) Place in lateral recumbent position

         d) Maintain proper body alignment and range of motion (ROM)

         e) Prevent skin breakdown

         f) Maintain excretory function—catheter, stool softeners, laxatives, enemas

         g) Maintain fluid, electrolyte balance nutrition—IV, nasogastric feeding

         h) Explain all procedures—speak often to client

Table 11-1 CRANIAL NERVE ASSESSMENT

(#)/NERVE	FUNCTION	NORMAL FINDINGS	NURSING CONSIDERATIONS
(I) Olfactory	Sense of smell	Able to detect various odors in each nostril	Have client smell a nonirritating substance such as coffee or tobacco with eyes closed Test each nostril separately
(II) Optic	Sense of vision	Clear (acute) vision near and distant	Snellen eye chart for far vision Read newspaper for near vision Ophthalmoscopic exam
(III) Oculomotor	Pupil constriction, raising of eyelids	Pupils equal in size and equally reactive to light	Instruct client to look up, down, inward Observe for symmetry and eye opening Shine penlight into eye as client stares straight ahead Ask client to watch your finger as you move it toward his/her face
(IV) Trochlear	Downward and inward movement of eyes	Able to move eyes down and inward	(See Oculomotor)
(V) Trigeminal	Motor—jaw movement Sensory—sensation on the face and neck	Able to clench and relax jaw Able to differentiate between various stimuli to the face and neck	Test with pin and wisp of cotton over each division on both sides of face Ask client to open jaw, bite down, move jaw laterally against pressure Stroke cornea with wisp of cotton
(VI) Abducens	Lateral movement of the eyes	Able to move eyes in all directions	(See Oculomotor)
(VII) Facial	Motor—facial muscle movement Sensory—taste on the anterior two-thirds of the tongue (sweet and salty)	Able to smile, whistle, wrinkle forehead Able to differentiate tastes among various agents	Observe for facial symmetry after asking client to frown, smile, raise eyebrows, close eyelids against resistance, whistle, blow Place sweet, sour, bitter, and salty substances on tongue
(VIII) Acoustic	Sense of hearing and balance	Hearing intact Balance maintained while walking	Test with watch ticking into ear, rubbing fingers together, Rinne test, Weber test Test posture, standing with eyes closed Otoscopic exam
(IX) Glossopharyngeal	Motor—pharyngeal movement and swallowing Sensory—taste on posterior one-third of tongue (sour and bitter)	Gag reflex intact, able to swallow Able to taste	Place sweet, sour, bitter, and salty substances on tongue Note ability to swallow and handle secretions Stimulate pharyngeal wall to elicit gag reflex
(X) Vagus	Swallowing and speaking	Able to swallow and speak with a smooth voice	Inspect soft palate—instruct to say "ah" Observe uvula for midline position Rate quality of voice

Table 11-1 CRANIAL NERVE ASSESSMENT *(CONTINUED)*			
(#)/NERVE	FUNCTION	NORMAL FINDINGS	NURSING CONSIDERATIONS
(XI) Spinal accessory	Motor—flexion and rotation of head; shrugging of shoulders	Able to flex and rotate head; able to shrug shoulders	Inspect and palpate sternocleidomastoid and trapezius muscles for size, contour, tone Ask client to move head side to side against resistance and shrug shoulders against resistance
(XII) Hypoglossal	Motor—tongue movements	Can move tongue side to side and stick it out symmetrically and in midline	Inspect tongue in mouth Ask client to stick out tongue and move it quickly from side to side Observe midline, symmetry, and rhythmic movement

Table 11-2 GLASGOW COMA SCALE																				
Eyes Open	Spontaneously	4																		
	To speech	3																		
	To pain	2																		
	None	1																		
Best Verbal Response	Oriented	5																		
	Confused	4																		
	Inappropriate words	3																		
	Incomprehensible sounds	2																		
	None	1																		
Best Motor Response	Obeys commands	6																		
	Localizes pain	5																		
	Flexes to pain	4																		
	Flexor posture	3																		
	Extensor posture	2																		
	No response	1																		

2. Increased intracranial pressure (ICP)
  a. Characteristics
    1) Causes
       a) Cerebral edema
       b) Hemorrhage
       c) Space-occupying lesions

    2) Complications
       a) Cerebral hypoxia
       b) Decreased cerebral perfusion
       c) Herniation—pupil dilation

    3) Early signs of developing increased intracranial pressure: first stimulates, then depresses vital signs

  b. Caring for the client with increased intracranial pressure
    1) Assess for altered level of consciousness (LOC)—often earliest sign of elevated ICP
       a) Confusion
       b) Restlessness
       c) Pupillary changes—blurred vision, diploplia, papilledema

    2) Maintain respiratory function and patent airway
    3) Observe seizure precautions
    4) Elevate head 15–30° to promote venous drainage from brain; monitor response to position change
    5) Avoid neck flexion and head rotation—support in cervical collar or neck rolls
    6) Reduce environmental stimuli
    7) Prevent the Valsalva maneuver; avoid coughing, sneezing, bending forward
    8) Administer stool softeners
    9) Teach client to exhale while turning or moving in bed

Table 11-3 ANTICONVULSANT MEDICATIONS		
MEDICATION	ADVERSE EFFECTS	NURSING CONSIDERATIONS
Clonazepam	Drowsiness Dizziness Confusion Respiratory depression	Benzodiazepine Do not discontinue suddenly Avoid activities that require alertness
Diazepam	Drowsiness, ataxia Hypotension Tachycardia Respiratory depression	IV push doses shouldn't exceed 2 mg/minute Monitor vital signs—resuscitation equipment available if given IV Alcohol increases CNS depression After long-term use, withdrawal leads to symptoms such as vomiting, sweating, cramps, tremors, and possiblyconvulsions
Fosphenytoin	Drowsiness Dizziness Confusion Leukopenia Anemia	Used for tonic–clonic seizures, status epilepticus Highly protein-bound Contact healthcare provider if rash develops

MEDICATION	ADVERSE EFFECTS	NURSING CONSIDERATIONS
Levetiracetam	Dizziness Suicidal ideation	Avoid alcohol Avoid driving and activities that require alertness
Phenytoin sodium	Drowsiness, ataxia Nystagmus Blurred vision Hirsutism Lethargy GI upset Gingival hypertrophy	Give oral medication with at least 1/2 glass of water, or with meals to minimize GI irritation Inform client that red-brown or pink discoloration of sweat and urine may occur IV administration may lead to cardiac arrest—have resuscitation equipment at hand Never mix with any other drug or dextrose IV Instruct in oral hygiene Increase vitamin D intake and exposure to sunlight may be necessary with long-term use Alcohol increases serum levels Increased risk toxicity in older adults
Phenobarbital	Drowsiness, rash GI upset Initially constricts pupils Respiratory depression Ataxia	Monitor vital signs—resuscitation equipment should be available if given IV Drowsiness diminishes after initial weeks of therapy Don't take alcohol or perform hazardous activities Nystagmus may indicate early toxicity Sudden discontinuation may lead to withdrawal Tolerance and dependence result from long-term use Folic acid supplements are indicated for long-term use Decreased cognitive function in older adults
Primidone	Drowsiness Ataxia, diplopia Nausea and vomiting	Don't discontinue use abruptly Full therapeutic response may take 2 weeks Shake liquid suspension well Take with food if experiencing GI distress Decreased cognitive function in older adults
Magnesium sulfate	Flushing Sweating Extreme thirst Hypotension Sedation, confusion	Monitor intake and output Before each dose, deep tendon reflexes should be tested Vital signs should be monitored often during parenteral administration Used for pregnancy-induced hypertension Monitor magnesium levels
Valproic acid	Sedation Tremor, ataxia Nausea, vomiting Prolonged bleeding time	Agent of choice in many seizure disorders of young children Do not take with carbonated beverage Take with food Monitor platelets, bleeding time, and liver function tests
Carbamazepine	Myelosuppression Dizziness, drowsiness Ataxia Diplopia, rash	Monitor intake and output Supervise ambulation Monitor CBC Take with meals Wear protective clothing due to photosensitivity Multiple drug interactions

Table 11-3 ANTICONVULSANT MEDICATIONS (CONTINUED)

Table 11-3 ANTICONVULSANT MEDICATIONS *(CONTINUED)*		
MEDICATION	**ADVERSE EFFECTS**	**NURSING CONSIDERATIONS**
Gabapentin	Increased appetite Ataxia Irritability Dizziness Fatigue	Monitor weight and behavioral changes. Can also be used to treat postherpetic neuralgia other neuropathic pain, fibromyalgia, prophylaxis of migraine.
Lamotrigine	Diplopia Headaches Dizziness Drowsiness Ataxia Nausea, vomiting Life-threatening rash when given with valproic acid	Take divided doses with meals or just afterward to decrease adverse effects
Topiramate	Ataxia Confusion Dizziness Fatigue Vision problems	Adjunct therapy for intractable partial seizures Increased risk for renal calculi Stop drug immediately if eye problems—could lead to permanent damage
Action	Decreases flow of calcium and sodium across neuronal membranes	
Indications	Partial seizures: Luminal, Mysoline, Tegretol, Neurontin, Lamictal Generalized tonic-clonic seizures: Luminal, Mysoline, Tegretol Absence seizures: Zarontin Status epilepticus: diazepam, lorazepam, phenytoin	
Adverse effects	Cardiovascular depression Respiratory depression Agranulocytosis Aplastic anemia	
Nursing considerations	Tolerance develops with long-term use Don't discontinue abruptly Caution with use of medications that lower seizure threshold (MAO inhibitors) Barbiturates and benzodiazepines also used as anticonvulsants Increased risk reactions in older adults	

10) Monitor vital signs hourly—be alert for widening pulse pressure

11) Restrict fluids to 1,200–1,500 mL/d

12) Administer medications (see Table 11-3)

    a) Osmotic diuretics (mannitol and furosemide) to reduce fluid volume

    b) Corticosteroid therapy (dexamethasone) to reduce cerebral edema

    c) Antiseizure medications—diazepam, phenytoin, phenobarbital

    d) Antipyretics

    e) Monitor during barbiturate coma

3. Caring for the client demonstrating seizure activity (see 11-4)
   a. Protect from injury
   b. Raise siderails or ease client to floor
   c. Keep bed in low position
   d. Use side rails according to agency policy
   e. Loosen restrictive clothing
      1. Do not restrain, provide environment that will prevent injury

Table 11-4 SEIZURE CLASSIFICATIONS		
FOCAL ONSET	GENERALIZED ONSET	UNKNOWN ONSET
Aware/Impaired Awareness	Impaired Awareness	Aware/Impaired Awareness
Motor Onset	*Motor Onset*	*Motor Onset*

automatisms
  atonic
  clonic
  epileptic
spasms
  hyperkinetic
  myoclonic
  tonic
	tonic-clonic
	  myoclonic
	  atonic
		tonic-clonic
		  epileptic spasms

Nonmotor Onset	*Nonmotor Onset (Absence)*	*Nonmotor (Absence)*
autonomic behavior arrest cognitive emotional sensory	typical atypical myoclonic eyelid-myoclonia	behavior arrest

Table 11-4 SEIZURE DEFINITION		
FOCAL ONSET	TYPES	CHARACTERISTICS

Motor Seizure:	Tonic-Clonic	begins with tonic phase
		  immediate loss of consciousness
		  clonic phase:rhythmic jerking of all extremities

	Myoclonic	brief jerking of extremities
	Atonic	sudden loss of muscle tone client falls
	Complex focal	client blacks out for a few seconds automatism may occur
	Simple focal	remains conscious often reports aura
Non Motor Seizure:	Absence, Typical Simple	brief periods of consciousness like day-dreaming, more common in children
	Absence, Typical Complex	brief periods of loss of consciousness with some type of movement like blinking, chewing gestures
	Absence, Atypical	unaware, blank stare with movements like eye blinking, lip smacking, continue as adult, autonomic

    f. Do not try to insert a bite block, padded tongue blade, or oral airway

    g. Protect yourself—client may flail arms

    h. Maintain adequate ventilation

       1) If possible, place client on one side with the head flexed forward to facilitate drainage of secretions

       2) Provide oxygen and suction equipment

       3) If prescribed, administer oxygen by nasal cannula

    i. Monitor status

       1) Onset, duration, and pattern

       2) Level of consciousness (LOC)

       3) Vital signs

       4) Skin color

       5) Responses to interventions

       6) Postseizure—check tongue, provide mouth care, raise head of bed to 30° angle, place in side-lying position

       7) Administer medications: phenobarbital, diazepam, lorazepam, fosphenytoin

       8) Check for adverse effects of phenytoin: gum hypertrophy, dark urine

       9) Provide description of seizures in record

    j. Prevent sensory overload

       1) Explain all tests and treatments to client

       2) Promote rest and comfort

       3) Be aware of cultural factors when providing nursing care

       4) Provide privacy

       5) Position noise-producing mechanical devices in a way that minimizes audibility

    k. Complementary/Alternative therapy

       1) Ketogenic diet to prevent seizures

          a) Diet high in fat and low in carbohydrates mimics effects of fasting and places the body in a constant state of ketosis

          b) Suppresses many types of seizures ; may be effective when other methods of seizure control have failed

C. Prevent sensory deprivation

    1. Involve client in planning own care

    2. Encourage a variety of diversional activities

    3. Provide a continuous means of orientation, e.g., calendar, clock, television

ALTERATIONS IN NEUROLOGICAL FUNCTION

A. Intracranial tumors

    1. Assessment—signs and symptoms vary, depending on location

      a. Motor deficits

      b. Language disturbances

      c. Hearing difficulties

      d. Visual disturbances

      e. Dizziness, coordination problems

f. Paresthesias

g. Seizures—frequently first presenting sign

h. Personality disturbances

Table 11-5 NEUROLOGICAL TESTS

TEST	PURPOSE	PREPARATION/TESTING	POST-TEST NURSING CARE
Cerebral angiography	Identifies aneurysms, vascular malformations, narrowed vessels	Informed consent Explain procedure: Lie flat; dye injection into femoral artery by needle/catheter; fluoroscopy and radiologic films taken after injection Well hydrated Pre-procedure sedation Skin prep, chosen site shaved Mark peripheral pulses May experience feeling of warmth and metallic taste when dye injected	Neurologic assessment every 15–30 min until vital signs are stable Keep flat in bed 12–14 hours Check puncture site every hour Immobilize site for 6–8 hours Assess distal pulses, color, and temperature Observe symptoms of complications, allergic response to dye, puncture site hematoma Force fluids, accurate intake and output
Lumbar puncture (LP)	Insertion of needle into subarachnoid space to obtain specimen, relieve pressure, inject dye or medications	Explain procedure Informed consent Procedure done at bedside or in treatment room Positioned in lateral recumbent fetal position at edge of bed	Neurological assessment every 15–30 min until stable Position flat for several hours Encourage PO fluid to 3,000 mL Oral analgesics for headache Observe sterile dressing at insertion site for bleeding or drainage
Electroencephalogram (EEG)	Records electrical activity of brain	Explain procedure Procedure done by technician in a quiet room Painless Tranquilizer and stimulant medications withheld for 24-48 hours pre-EEG Stimulants such as caffeine, cola, and tea, cigarettes withheld for 24 hours pre-EEG May be asked to hyperventilate 3-4 min and watch bright, flashing light Meals not withheld May be kept awake night before test	Help client remove paste from hair Administer prescribed medication withheld before EEG Observe for seizure activity in seizure-prone clients
Magnetic resonance imaging (MRI)	Body parts visualized by magnetic energy	Screen client for pacemaker or metalparts in body; lie very still for 1 hour	None
CT scan (computed tomography)	Detects hemorrhage, infarction, abscesses, tumors	Written consent Explain procedure Painless Immobile during exam If contrast dye used, may experience flushed, warm face and metallic taste during injection	No specific intervention Assess for allergic responses to contrast dye, e.g., rash, pruritus, urticaria Encourage PO fluids

Table 11-5 NEUROLOGICAL TESTS *(CONTINUED)*			
TEST	**PURPOSE**	**PREPARATION/TESTING**	**POST-TEST NURSING CARE**
Myelogram	Visualizes spinal column and subarachnoid space	Informed consent Explain procedure NPO for 4-6 hours before test Obtain allergy history Phenothiazines, CNS depressants, and stimulants withheld for 48 hours prior to test Table will be moved to various positions during test	Neurologic assessment every 2–4 hours; Bedrest with head of bed elevated 30-45 ° for 3 hours after procedure; assess for allergic responses to contrast dye, e.g., rash, pruritus, urticaria Oral analgesics for headache Encourage PO fluids Assess for distended bladder Inspect injection site
PET (Positron emission tomography)	Used to assess metabolic and physiologic function of brain; diagnose stroke, brain tumor, epilepsy, Parkinson's disease, head injury	Client inhales or is injected with radioactive substance, then is scanned Tell client he/she may experience dizziness, headache Teach relaxation exercises	No specific interventions

    i. Papilledema

    j. Headache

    k. Nausea and vomiting

    l. Drowsiness

    m. Changes in level of consciousness

2. Diagnostics (see Table 11-5)

3. Characteristics

    a. Types—classified according to location

        1) Supratentorial

        2) Infratentorial

    b. Causes—unknown

    c. Medical/surgical management—intracranial surgery (burr holes, craniotomy, cranioplasty), radiation

4. Nursing management—client undergoing neurosurgery

    a. Preoperative care

        1) Detailed neurological assessment for baseline data

        2) Head shave—prep of site

        3) Psychological support

        4) Prepare client for postoperative course

    b. Postoperative care

        1) Maintain patent airway

        2) Elevate head of bed to a 30–45° angle—after supratentorial surgery

        3) Position client flat on either side—after infratentorial surgery

        4) Monitor vital and neurological signs

      5) Observe for complications—respiratory difficulties, increased intracranial pressure, hyperthermia, meningitis, wound infection

      6) Administer medications—corticosteroids, osmotic diuretics, mild analgesics, anticonvulsants, antibiotics, antipyretics, antiemetics, hormone replacement as needed; no narcotics postop

B. Stroke

1. Assessment
   a. Confusion/disorientation
   b. Changes in vital signs
   c. Changes in neurological signs
   d. Change in level of consciousness
   e. Seizures
   f. Aphasia—expressive, receptive, global
   g. Hemiplegia (paralysis on one side of body), hemiparesis (weakness on one side of body)
   h. Bladder and/or bowel incontinence
   i. Headache
   j. Vomiting
   k. Dysphagia—difficulty swallowing
   l. Hemianopsia—loss of half of visual field
   m. Decreased sensation/Neglect syndrome
   n. Emotional liability

2. Preventive measures—identify risk factors
   a. Advanced age
   b. Hypertension
   c. Transient ischemic attacks (TIA)
   d. Diabetes mellitus
   e. Smoking
   f. Obesity
   g. Elevated blood lipids
   h. Oral contraceptives

3. Characteristics
   a. Abrupt onset of neurological deficits resulting from interference with blood supply to the brain
   b. Causes
      1) Thrombosis
      2) Embolism
      3) Hemorrhage—intracerebral, subarachnoid

4. Nursing management
   a. Immediate care
      1) Maintain patent airway
      2) Minimize activity
      3) Keep head in a midline, neutral position
      4) Maintain proper body alignment
      5) Keep side rails in upright position
      6) Administer thrombolytic therapy if appropriate
   b. Intermediate care and rehabilitative needs
      1) Position for good body alignment and comfort
      2) Monitor elimination patterns
      3) Provide skin care

        4) Perform passive and/or active ROM exercises

        5) Orient to person, time, and place

        6) Move affected extremities slowly and gently

        7) Teach use of supportive devices—commode, trapeze, cane, etc.

        8) Address communication needs—e.g., supply pad and pencil, magic slate

    c. Gerontologic considerations—ability to perform ADLs, loss of independence, altered relationship with significant other

C. Organic brain syndrome

  1. Assessment

    a. Acute organic brain syndrome

      1) Memory loss

      2) Confusion

      3) Delirium

      4) Hallucinations

      5) Delusions

    b. Chronic organic brain syndrome

      1) Memory deficit

      2) Deterioration of intellectual functioning

      3) Incoherent communication

      4) Irritability

      5) Mood swings

      6) Incontinence

      7) Unkempt appearance

  2. Characteristics

    a. Acute organic brain syndrome—reversible condition

      1) Fluid and electrolyte imbalance

      2) Malnutrition

      3) Metabolic imbalance

      4) Trauma

      5) Infection

      6) Stress

    b. Chronic organic brain syndrome—irreversible condition

      1) Cerebral arteriosclerosis

      2) Tumor

      3) Korsakoff's psychosis

      4) Alzheimer's disease

    c. Nursing management

      1) Decrease disorientation by frequent reorientation

      2) Decrease confusion

      3) Reduce anxiety—provide calm environment

      4) Maximize independent functioning

      5) Refer to occupational therapy, as indicated

D. Intellectual delay (see Table 11-6)

  1. Definition: sub-average intellectual function (IQ less than 70) with concurrent impairment in adaptive functioning; onset under the age of 18

  2. Delay—general

a. Assessment
   1) Sensory deficits
   2) Physical anomalies
   3) Delayed growth and development

b. Characteristics
   1) Lack of, or destruction of, brain cells
   2) Causes—heredity, infection, fetal anoxia, cranial or chromosomal abnormalities, intracranial hemorrhage

c. Nursing management
   1) Assist parents with adjustment
   2) Provide sensory stimulation
   3) Encourage socially acceptable behavior
   4) Provide emotional support
   5) Encourage school training, education, vocational development as appropriate

Table 11-6 INTELLECTUAL DELAY				
CLASSIFICATION	IQ RANGE	PRESCHOOL GROWTH AND DEVELOPMENT	SCHOOL TRAINING AND EDUCATION	ADULT SOCIAL/ VOCATIONAL LEVEL
I. Mild	55–70	Slow to walk, feed self, and talk compared with other children	With special education, can learn reading and math skills for third- to sixth-grade level	Can achieve social/ vocational self-maintenance May need occasional psychosocial support
II. Moderate	40–55	Delays in motor development Can do some self-help activities	Responds to training Does not progress with reading or math skills Poor communication skills	Sheltered, usually incapable of self-maintenance
III. Severe	25–40	Marked delay in development May be able to help self minimally	Can profit from habit training Has some understanding of speech	Dependent on others for care Can conform to routine
IV. Profound	Under 25	Significant delay, minimal-capacity functioning	May respond to skill training Shows basic emotional responses	Incapable of self-maintenance, needs nursing care

3. Down syndrome
   a. Assessment
      1) Mental capacity—IQ range from 20 to 70
      2) Marked hypotonia; short stature
      3) Altered physical development—epicathal folds, low set ears, protruding tongue, low nasal bridge

   b. Characteristics
      1) Trisomy 21—chromosomal abnormality involving an extra chromosome number 21
      2) Causes—unknown; associated with maternal age greater than 35

   c. Nursing management
      1) Provide stimulation—OT, PT, special education

      2) Observe for signs of common physical problems: 30–40% have heart disease; 80% have hearing loss; respiratory infections are common

      3) Establish and maintain adequate nutrition, parental education and support

E. Learning delay

  1. Assessment

    a. Hyperkinesis (sometimes absent)

    b. Decreased attention span, i.e., attention deficit disorder (ADD) (see Table 11-7)

    c. Perceptual deficits

    d. Aggression/depression

  2. Characteristics—learning and behavioral disorders that occur because of CNS malfunctioning

    a. Neuropsychological testing—reveals individual differences

    b. Average to high IQ

  3. Nursing management

    a. Reduce frustration

    b. Special educational intervention; small class size

    c. Provide safety and security

    d. Administer medications, e.g., methylphenidate hydrochloride, dextroamphetamine sulfate

    e. Refer to appropriate resources—special education, parent support groups

F. Cranial nerve disorders

  1. Trigeminal neuralgia (tic douloureux)

    a. Assessment

      1) Stabbing or burning facial pain—excruciating, unpredictable, and paroxysmal

      2) Twitching, grimacing of facial muscles

      3) Social isolation

    b. Characteristics

      1) Type of neuralgia involving one or more branches of the fifth cranial nerve (trigeminal)

      2) Causes—unknown; infections of sinuses, teeth, and mouth, irritation of nerve due to pressure are aggravating factors

    c. Nursing management

      1) Identify and avoid stimuli that exacerbate the attacks (light touch)

      2) Administer medications—carbamazepine and pain relievers when prescribed

      3) Administer appropriate diet

      4) Treatment—carbamazepine, alcohol injection to nerve, resection of the nerve, microvascular decompression

  2. Bell's palsy (facial paralysis)

    a. Assessment

      1) Inability of eye to close

      2) Increased lacrimation

      3) Speech difficulty

      4) Loss of taste

      5) Distortion of one side of face

    b. Characteristics

1) Peripheral involvement of the seventh cranial nerve

2) Causes—unknown; predisposing factors are vascular ischemia, viral disease, edema, inflammatory reactions

Table 11-7 ATTENTION DEFICIT DISORDER MEDICATIONS		
MEDICATION	**ADVERSE EFFECTS**	**NURSING CONSIDERATIONS**
Methylphenidate	Nervousness, palpitations Insomnia Tachycardia Weight loss, growth suppression	May precipitate Tourette's syndrome Monitor CBC, platelet count Has paradoxical calming effect in ADD Monitor height/weight in children Monitor BP Avoid drinks with caffeine Give at least 6 hours before bedtime Give pc
Dextroamphetamine sulfate	Insomnia Tachycardia, palpitations	Controlled substance May alter insulin needs Give in AM to prevent insomnia Don't use with MAO inhibitor (possible hypertensive crisis)
Dexmethylphenidate	Abdominal discomfort Anorexia Fever Nausea Insomnia Weight loss	Obtain baseline height and weight and monitor for growth restriction in children Children are more likely to develop the adverse effects of abdominal pain, anorexia, insomnia, and weight loss May lower the seizure threshold in those with a history of seizures Do not administer in the afternoon or evening because it can cause insomnia Monitor CBC, WBC count with differential, and platelet count
Action	Increase level of catecholamines in cerebral cortex and reticular activating system	
Indications	Attention deficit disorder (ADD) Narcolepsy	
Adverse effects	Restlessness Insomnia Tremors Tachycardia Seizures	
Nursing considerations	Monitor growth rate in children	

c. Nursing management

1) Comfort measures—protect head from cold or drafts, administer analgesics and appropriate diet

        2) Improve facial muscle tone—assist with electric stimulation, teach isometric exercises of face

        3) Provide emotional support for altered body image

        4) Prevent corneal abrasions

        5) Treatment—electrical stimulation, analgesics, steroid therapy

3. Acoustic neuroma
   a. Assessment
      1) Deafness—partial, initially
      2) Tinnitus
      3) Dizziness

   b. Characteristics
      1) Benign tumor of the vestibulocochlear nerve (cranial nerve VIII)
      2) Treatment—surgical excision of tumor

   c. Nursing management
      1) Pre- and postoperative care for posterior fossa craniotomy (see Table 11-8)
      2) Comfort measures—assist with turning of head and neck

G. Head injury
1. Assessment
   a. Battle's sign (ecchymosis over mastoid bone may indicate a lower skull fracture); racoon eyes (bruising around the eyes); rhinnorrhea, otorrhea
   b. Concussion—transient mental confusion or loss of consciousness, headache, no residual neurological deficit, possible loss of memory surrounding event, long-term effects (lack of concentration, personality changes)
   c. Contusion—varies from slight depression of consciousness to coma, with decorticate posturing (flexion and internal rotation of forearms and hands) or decerebrate posturing (extension of arms and legs, pronation of arms, plantar flexion, opisthotonos), indicates deeper dysfunction, generalized cerebral edema
   d. Hemorrhage/hematoma
      1) Epidural—short period of unconsciousness, followed by lucid interval with ipsilateral pupillary dilation, weakness of contralateral extremities, rapid neurologic deterioration
      2) Subdural—decreased level of consciousness, ipsilateral pupillary dilation, contralateral weakness, personality changes; increased risk with aging and chronic alcohol conumption

2. Characteristics
   a. Theory—skull is a closed vault with a volume ratio of three components: brain tissue, blood, and CSF; sudden increase in any of these can cause brain dysfunction
   b. Ingestion of drugs and alcohol may delay manifestations of symptoms of damage
   c. Generalized brain swelling in response to injury

3. Treatment
   a. Minor injury—repair CSF leak, scalp lacerations
   b. Penetrating wounds—surgical repair, antibiotics, and anticonvulsants
   c. Moderate to severe head injury—supportive care of the unconscious client, prophylactic anticonvulsants, prevent and control intracranial hypertension, prevent secondary brain damage from hypotension, prevent anemia, increased arterial carbon dioxide levels

4. Nursing management
   a. Management of increased intracranial pressure (IICP) and cerebral edema

b. Neurological assessment

c. Administer glucocorticoids—dexamethasone, mannitol, furosemide

d. Hypothermia—to decrease metabolic demands

e. Barbiturate therapy—to decrease cerebral metabolic rate

f. Minimal procedures, e.g., suctioning, turning, positioning (HOB elevated at 30° or more) in acute phase

g. Prevention of complications of immobility

Table 11-8 CRANIAL NERVE DISORDERS			
	TRIGEMINAL NEURALGIA (TIC DOULOUREUX)	BELL'S PALSY (FACIAL PARALYSIS)	ACOUSTIC NEUROMA
Assessment	Stabbing or burning facial pain—excruciating, unpredictable, paroxysmal Twitching, grimacing of facial muscles	Inability to close eye Decreased corneal reflex Increased lacrimation Speech difficulty Loss of taste Distortion of one side of face	Deafness—partial, initially Twitching, grimacing of facial muscles Dizziness
Analysis	Type of neuralgia involving one or more branches of the fifth cranial nerve Causes—infections of sinuses, teeth, mouth, or irritation of nerve from pressure	Peripheral involvement of the seventh cranial nerve Predisposing factors—vascular ischemia, viral disease, edema, inflammatory reactions	Benign tumor of the eighth cranial nerve
Nursing considerations	Identify and avoid stimuli that exacerbate the attacks Administer medications—carbamazepine and analgesics Treatment—carbamazepine, alcohol injection to nerve, resection of the nerve, microvascular decompression Avoid rubbing eye Chew on opposite side of mouth	Protect head from cold or drafts Administer analgesics Assist with electrical stimulation Teach isometric exercises for facial muscles (blow and suck from a straw) Massage, warm packs Provide emotional support for altered body image Prevent corneal abrasions (artificial tears) Treatment—electrical stimulation, analgesics, steroid therapy, antiviral medications Recovery takes 3–5 wk	Pre- and postoperative care for posterior fossa craniotomy Comfort measures—assist with turning of head and neck Treatment—surgical excision of tumor

H. Spinal cord injury (see Table 11-9)

1. Assessment

   a. Loss of sensory function below injury

   b. Loss of motor function below injury

   c. Spinal shock symptoms

      1) Flaccid paralysis of skeletal muscles

      2) Complete loss of all sensation

      3) Suppression of somatic (pain, touch, temperature) and visceral reflexes

   d. Postural hypotension, bradycardia

    e. Circulatory problems—edema

    f. Alterations in normal thermoregulation

2. Extent of neurological deficit (see Table 11-9)

3. Characteristics

    a. Types of spinal cord injuries

        1) Concussion without direct trauma

        2) Penetrating wound or fracture dislocation

        3) Hemorrhage

        4) Compression of blood supply

    b. Categories of neurological deficit

        1) Complete—no voluntary motor activity or sensation below level of injury

        2) Incomplete—some voluntary motor activity or sensation below level of injury

        3) Paraplegia—thoracic vertebral injury or lower; lower extremities affected

        4) Tetraplegia (quadriplegia)—cervical vertebral injury; all four extremities involved

Table 11-9 SPINAL CORD INJURY		
LEVEL OF INJURY	**FUNCTIONAL ABILITY**	**SELF–CARE CAPABILITY**
C3 and above	Inability to control muscles of breathing	Unable to care for self, life-sustaining ventilatory support essential
C4	Movement of trapezius and sternocleidomastoid muscles, no upper extremity muscle function, minimal ventilatory capacity	Unable to care for self, may self-feed with powered devices (depending on respiratory function)
C5	Neck movement, possible partial strength of shoulder and biceps	Can drive electric wheelchair, may be able to feed self with powered devices
C6	Muscle function in C5 level; partial strength in pectoralis major	May self-propel a lightweight wheelchair, may feed self with devices, can write and care for self, can transfer from chair to bed
C7	Muscle function in C6 level; no finger muscle power	Can dress lower extremities, minimal assistance needed, independence in wheelchair, can drive car with hand controls
C8	Muscle function in C7 level; finger muscle power	Same as C7; in general, activities easier
T1–T4	Good upper extremity muscle strength	Some independence from wheelchair, long-leg braces for standing exercises
T5–L2	Balance difficulties	Still requires wheelchair, limited ambulation with long-leg braces and crutches
L3-L5	Trunk-pelvis muscle function intact	May use crutches or canes for ambulation
L5-S3	Waddling gait	Ambulation

    c. Causes

       1) Trauma due to accidents—more common in young men

       2) Neoplasms

    d. Complication—autonomic dysreflexia

    e. Treatment

       1) Skeletal traction—Gardner-Wells, Crutchfield, Vinke tongs, halo traction

       2) Surgical stabilization—reduction and stabilization by fusion, wires, and plates

       3) Steroid therapy

       4) Hyperbaric oxygen therapy

       5) Antispasmodics (e.g., baclofen, diazepam)

4. Nursing management

    a. Ensure patent airway

    b. Maintenance of cardiovascular functioning

    c. Move client by log-rolling technique; use turning frames

    d. Provide good skin care

    e. Emotional support

    f. Ensure adequate nutrition

    g. Reduce aggravating factors that cause spasticity

    h. Bladder and bowel training

    i. Client and family education to cope with detailed care at home

5. Gerontologic concerns—fall prevention strategies; greater risk of complications after SCI

I. Guillain-Barré syndrome

1. Assessment

    a. Diffuse inflammatory response occurring in peripheral nervous system, resulting in compression of nerve roots and peripheral nerves; demyelination occurs and slows or alters nerve conduction

    b. Possible etiologies

       1) Infective/viral

       2) Autoimmune response

       3) May follow immunizations

    c. Course

       1) Acute, rapid, ascending sensory and motor deficit that may stop at any level of CNS

       2) Protracted, develops slowly, regresses slowly

       3) Prolonged course with phases of deterioration and partial remission

2. Characteristics

    a. Abrupt onset of presenting signs

       1) Paresthesias/pain often occurring in stocking-and-glove distribution

       2) Motor losses symmetrical, usually beginning in lower extremities, then extend upward to include trunk, upper extremities, cranial nerves, and vasomotor function; deep tendon reflexes disappear; respiratory muscle compromise

       3) Excessive or inadequate autonomic function

          a) Hypotension/tachycardia

          b) Vasomotor flushing

        c) Paralytic ileus

        d) Profuse sweating

    4) Plateau period—progress to peak severity between 2–4 weeks

    5) Recovery period—2 wk to 24 mo

3. Nursing management
   a. Intervention is symptomatic
   b. Steroids in acute phase
   c. Plasmapheresis, IV immunoglobulins, adrenocorticotropic hormone, corticosteroids
   d. Aggressive respiratory care
   e. Utilize principles of immobility
   f. Maintain adequate nutrition
   g. Physical therapy
   h. Pain-reducing measures
   i. Eye care
   j. Prevention of complications—UTI, aspiration, constipation, urinary retention
   k. Psychosocial
      1) Fear/anxiety
      2) Altered body image

J. Herpes zoster (shingles)
1. Assessment
   a. Herpesvirus; causative agent is identical to varicella (chickenpox)
   b. Results from reactivation of the varicella virus, which has remained dormant
   c. Most commonly affects (in descending order):
      1) Ophthalmic branch of the trigeminal nerve
      2) Thoracic branch
      3) Cervical branch
      4) Sacral branch

2. Characteristics
   a. Severe pain in specific dermatome for 1–2 days before skin changes
   b. Vesicular blisters on affected areas
   c. Muscle weakness in the affected area and distal to blisters
   d. Headache

3. Nursing management
   a. No specific treatment
      1) Analgesics
      2) Topical medication (e.g., permethrin, crotamiton)
      3) Antiviral medication (e.g., famciclovir, valacyclovir)

K. Ménière's disease
1. Assessment
   a. Rare neurological syndrome manifested by recurrent attacks of vertigo with sensorineural hearing loss
   b. Possible etiology—degeneration of the cochlear hair cells of the labyrinth

2. Characteristics
   a. Signs and symptoms
      1) Nausea and vomiting
      2) Incapacitating vertigo
      3) Tinnitus
      4) Feeling of pressure/fullness in the ear
      5) Fluctuating hearing loss (deafness after repeated episodes)
      6) Nystagmus
      7) Diagnostic tests—Weber and Rinne test, CT

   b. Course—attacks are recurrent several times a week with periods of remission lasting several years

3. Nursing management
   a. Antihistamines in acute phase (epinephrine, diphenhydramine)
   b. Antiemetics
   c. Bedrest during acute phase
   d. Provide protection when ambulatory
   e. Maintain adequate nutrition

L. Amyotrophic lateral sclerosis (Lou Gehrig's disease)
   1. Assessment
      a. Progressive, degenerative disease involving the lower motor neurons of the spinal cord and cerebral cortex; the voluntary motor system is particularly involved, with progressive degeneration of the corticospinal tract, leads to a mixture of spastic and atrophic changes in cranial and spinal musculature
      b. No specific pattern exists—involvement may vary in different parts of the same area
      c. Possible etiologies
         1) Genetic/familial
         2) Chronic (slow) viral infection
         3) Autoimmune disease
         4) Environmental factors

   2. Characteristics
      a. Signs and symptoms
         1) Tongue fatigue/atrophy with fasciculations
         2) Nasal quality to speech/dysarthria
         3) Dysphagia/aspiration
         4) Muscular wasting/atrophy/spasticity
            a) Usually begins in upper extremities
            b) Distal portion affected first
            c) Fasciculations
         5) Emotional lability, cognitive dysfunction
         6) Respiratory insufficiency (usual cause of death)
         7) No alteration in autonomic, sensory, or mental function

3. Nursing management
   a. No known treatment proven effective
   b. Current approach remains supportive/symptomatic
   c. Apply principles of care of client with progressive, terminal disease
   d. Treat self-care deficits symptomatically
   e. Maintain adequate nutrition
   f. Physical therapy/speech therapy
   g. Adaptive home equipment
   h. Psychosocial support
   i. Administer riluzole—extends survival time; risk of liver toxicity

M. Encephalitis
   1. Assessment
      a. Virus most common cause
      b. May be sequelae of:
         1) Viral disease, e.g., measles
         2) Prophylactic inoculations
         3) Obscure illness of viral origin
      c. Pathogens
         1) Arboviruses
            a) Eastern equine, Western equine, St. Louis, Powassan
            b) Reservoir in ticks, mosquitoes
         2) Enteroviruses—polio, ECHO, Coxsackie
         3) Other viruses (latent)
            a) Herpes simplex Type 1
            b) Herpes zoster
            c) Mumps
            d) Cytomegalovirus, Epstein-Barr virus
            e) Rabies
         4) Other
            a) Bacteria/spirochetes
            b) Fungal—cryptococcus
            c) Protozoal, metazoal—malaria, toxoplasmosis

2. Characteristics
   a. Signs and symptoms
      1) Prodromal illness—headache, fever, myalgia, malaise, sore throat preceding onset of neurological signs
      2) Behavioral disturbances
      3) Alterations in consciousness from lethargy to coma
      4) Confusion/disorientation
      5) Bilateral motor/sensory deficits
      6) Seizures
      7) Meningeal signs
      8) Increased ICP
   b. CSF abnormalities

3. Management
   a. Medical management
      1) Symptomatic/supportive
      2) Antiserum—rabies
      3) Antiviral agents—adenine arabinoside (ARA-A), cytosine arabinoside (ARA-C), acyclovir
   b. Surgical management—decompression and necrotic tissue excision
   c. Nursing management
      1) Symptomatic care
      2) Prevent complications

N. Meningitis
   1. Assessment—access routes
      a. Blood—most common
         1) Septicemia/bacteremia
         2) Septic emboli—bacterial endocarditis, URI
      b. Direct pathogen invasion
         1) Traumatic—penetrating wounds, skull fracture, operative procedures
         2) Nontraumatic—secondary to otitis media, sinusitis, teeth infections
      c. Cerebrospinal fluid
         1) CSF leak—otorrhea, rhinorrhea
         2) Lumbar puncture
      d. Pathogens
         1) Bacteria—Gram-positive/negative organisms
         2) Virus—enteroviruses, mumps, measles
         3) Mycobacteria—*Mycobacterium tuberculosis*
         4) Fungal—*Cryptococcus neoformans*
         5) Spirochetes/parasites

    e. Host factors

       1) Immunoglobulin deficiency

       2) Long-term radiation therapy

       3) Immunosuppressive therapy

    f. Types

       1) Septic—organisms isolated by routine culture

       2) Aseptic—nonbacterial inflammatory disorder

2. Characteristics

    a. Signs and symptoms

       1) Headache/fever/photophobia

       2) Meningeal signs

          a) Nuchal rigidity

          b) Kernig's sign—when hip flexed to 90°, complete extension of the knee is restricted and painful

          c) Brudzinski's sign—attempts to flex the neck will produce flexion at knee and thigh

          d) Opisthotonic position—extensor rigidity, with legs hyperextended, forming an arc with the trunk

       3) Alterations in mental status—confusion to coma

       4) Seizures

       5) Infants

          a) Refusal of feedings

          b) Vomiting/diarrhea

          c) Bulging fontanelles

          d) Vacant stare

          e) High-pitched cry

3. Management

    a. Medical management

       1) Antibiotic therapy

       2) Antifungal therapy—amphotericin

       3) *Mycobacterium*—INH, streptomycin

       4) Viral—supportive therapy

    b. Surgical placement of ventricular catheter to drain CSF from ventricles

    c. Nursing management

       1) Decrease temperature

       2) Analgesia for headache

       3) Provide nonstimulating, dark environment

       4) Seizure precautions

       5) Monitor for shock and embolic complications

       6) Droplet precautions for *Haemophilus influenzae*, type b, and *Neisseria meningitidis*

O. Brain abscess
   1. Assessment
      a. Similar to meningitis assessment
      b. Asymptomatic until reaching considerable size if located in frontal or temporal lobe, mimics space-occupying lesion (e.g., a tumor)

   2. Characteristics
      a. Chills, fever
      b. Anorexia, malaise, lethargy
      c. Leukocytosis
      d. Meningeal signs
      e. Focal neurological signs—depending on area of lesion
         1) Seizures
         2) Motor/sensory deficits
         3) Visual disturbances
         4) Speech disturbances
         5) Personality changes
         6) Cranial nerve palsies
      f. Signs of increased intracranial pressure
      g. Increased white cell count, ESR
      h. CT, MRI

   3. Management
      a. Nonsurgical—appropriate antibiotic therapy
      b. Surgical—extensive drainage and/or repeated aspiration
      c. Nursing care/goals—similar to meningitis/encephalitis
      d. Evaluation—minimal neurological deficit remains

P. Migraine headache
   1. Assessment
      a. Prodromal—depression, irritability, feeling cold, food cravings, anorexia, change in activity level, increased urination
      b. Aura—light flashes and bright spots, numbness and tingling (lips, face, hands), mild confusion, drowsiness, dizziness, diploplia
      c. Headache—throbbing (often unilateral), photophobia, nausea, vomiting, 4 to 72 hours
      d. Recovery—pain gradually subsides, muscle aches in neck and scalp, sleep for extended period

   2. Diagnosis
      a. Episodic events or acute attacks
      b. Seen more often in women before menses
      c. Familial disorders due to inherited vascular response to different chemicals
      d. Precipitating factors stress, menstrual cycles, bright lights, depression, sleep deprivation, fatigue, foods containing tyramine, monosodium glutamate, nitrites, or milk products (aged cheese, processed foods)

3. Plan/Implementation
   a. Prevention and treatment
      1) Medications
         a) Beta blockers
         b) Triptan preparations—activate serotonin receptors
         c) Acetaminophen, NSAIDS
         d) Topiramate
         e) Ergotamines—dihydroergotamine (DHE); take at start of headache

4. Implementation
   a. Avoid triggers
   b. Comfort measures
   c. Quiet dark environment
   d. Elevate head of bed 30°

5. Complementary/Alternate therapy
   a. Riboflavin (vitamin B_2) supplement
      1) 400 mg daily may reduce the number and duration but not the severity of the headaches
      2) Take as an individual supplement
   b. Massage, meditation, relaxation techniques

Q. Huntington's disease
   1. Assessment—a rare, familial, progressive, degenerative disease passed from generation to generation (dominant inheritance)
   2. Characteristics
      a. Depression and temper outbursts
      b. Choreiform movements
         1) Slight to severe restlessness
         2) Facial grimacing
         3) Arm movements
         4) Irregular leg movements
         5) Twisting, turning, struggling nature
         6) Tongue movements
         7) Person is in constant motion by end of disease progression
      c. Personality changes
         1) Irritability; demanding behavior
         2) Paranoia
         3) Memory loss
         4) Decreased intellectual function
         5) Dementia
         6) Psychosis seen at end stage
   3. Management
      a. Therapeutic intervention
         1) Disease progresses until client is completely helpless and speechless
         2) Treatment is symptomatic

       b. Drug therapy—intended to reduce movement and subdue behavior changes

          1) Chlordiazepoxide

          2) Haloperidol

          3) Chlorpromazine

       c. Nursing management

          1) Supportive, symptomatic

          2) Genetic counseling for all family members

R. Parkinson's disease

  1. Description—chronic progressive disease; degeneration of dopamine-producing neurons in the substantia nigra of the midbrain, resulting in disturbed transmission of nerve impulses

  2. Assessment

       a. Tremors (pill-rolling motion)

       b. Bradykinesia (loss of automatic movements)

       c. Restlessness

       d. Rigidity and propulsive gait

       e. Weakness

       f. Monotonous speech

       g. Increased salivation, dysphagia

       h. Depression, insomnia, dementia

       i. Mask-like facial expression

       j. Constipation

       k. Urinary incontinence

  3. Nursing management

       a. Promote rest, comfort, and sleep

       b. Keep client as functional and productive as possible

          1) Encourage finger exercises, e.g., typing, piano-playing

          2) Range of motion (ROM) as appropriate

          3) Teach client ambulation modification, refer to physical therapy

             a) Goose-stepping walk

             b) Walk with wider base

             c) Concentrate on swinging arms while walking

             d) Turn around slowly, using small steps

             e) Look ahead, not down

       c. Promote family understanding of the disease

          1) Client's intellect is not impaired

          2) Sight and hearing are intact

          3) Disease is progressive but slow

       d. Refer for speech therapy, potential stereotactic surgery

       e. Administer medications for symptomatic relief (see Table 11-10)

       f. Other medications include ropinirole and pramipexole

       g. Antihistamines may also be used to manage tremors

4. Complementary/Alternative therapy

    a. Coenzyme Q10 supplements

        1) Made naturally in the body; used by cells to produce energy and as an antioxidant

        2) 1,200 mg/d causes decreased deterioration in feedings, bathing, walking

S. Myasthenia gravis

  1. Description—autoimmune process; deficiency of acetylcholine at myoneural junction

  2. Assessment

    a. Extreme skeletal muscle weakness, quickly produced by repeated movement but disappears following rest

    b. Tiredness on slight exertion

    c. Diplopia, ptosis

    d. Impaired speech

    e. Choking and aspiration of food

    f. Respiratory distress

Table 11-10 PARKINSON'S DISEASE MEDICATIONS		
MEDICATION	**ADVERSE EFFECTS**	**NURSING CONSIDERATIONS**
Apomorphine Pramipexole Ropinirole	Nausea Dizziness Constipation Rhinitis Sleepiness Postural hypotension	A centrally acting dopamine agonist, which reduces tremors and rigidity and improves movement, posture, and equilibrium Overdose may require supportive measures to maintain BP Monitor BP and heart rate and rhythm Use cautiously in clients with a history of cardiac dysrhythmias, confusion, or hallucinations Daily administration usually given in 3 divided doses
Benztropine mesylate Trihexyphenidyl	Drowsiness, nausea, vomiting Atropine-like effects—blurred vision, mydriasis Antihistaminic effects—sedation, dizziness	Acts by lessening cholinergic effect of dopamine deficiency Suppresses tremor of parkinsonism Most adverse effects are reversed by changes in dosage Additional drowsiness can occur with other CNS depressants
Levodopa	Nausea and vomiting, anorexia Postural hypotension Mental changes: confusion, agitation, mood alterations Cardiac dysrhythmias Twitching	Precursor of dopamine Thought to restore dopamine levels in extrapyramidal centers Administered in large prolonged doses Contraindicated in glaucoma, hemolytic anemia Give with food Monitor for postural hypotension Avoid OTC meds that contain vitamin B_6 (pyridoxine); reverses effects
Bromocriptine mesylate	Dizziness, headache, hypotension Tinnitus Nausea, abdominal cramps Pleural effusion Orthostatic hypotension	Give with meals May lead to early postpartum conception Monitor cardiac, hepatic, renal, hematopoietic function

Table 11-10 PARKINSON'S DISEASE MEDICATIONS *(CONTINUED)*		
MEDICATION	ADVERSE EFFECTS	NURSING CONSIDERATIONS
Carbidopa–levodopa	Hemolytic anemia Dystonic movements, ataxia Orthostatic hypotension Dysrhythmias GI upset, dry mouth	Levodopa agent Don't use with MAO inhibitors Advise to change positions slowly Take with food
Amantadine	CNS disturbances, hyperexcitability Insomnia, vertigo, ataxia Slurred speech, convulsions	Antiviral drug Enhances effect of l-dopa Contraindicated in epilepsy, arteriosclerosis Antiviral
Selegiline Rasagiline	Nausea, dyskinesia, agitation, rigidity	Inhibits MAO and increases dopamine levels
Entacapone Tolcapone	Nausea, dyskinesia, agitation, rigidity	Used only with Carbidopa-levodopa

3. Diagnosis—Tensilon test

4. Management

    a. Medications

        1) Anticholinergics

        2) Corticosteroids, immunosuppressants

        3) Surgical therapy—thymectomy

        4) Plasmapheresis

    b. Nursing

        1) Promote comfort, rest, and sleep; balanced diet

        2) Relieve symptoms by administering medications (anticholinesterase, corticosteroids, immunosuppressants)

        3) Teach client

            a) Use of Medic-Alert band

            b) Be aware of factors that may precipitate myasthenia crisis, e.g., infections, emotional stress, use of streptomycin or neomycin (they produce muscular weakness), surgery

            c) Be alert for myasthenia crisis—sudden inability to swallow, speak, or maintain a patent airway

T. Multiple sclerosis

    1. Description—chronic progressive disease characterized by demyelinization and scarring throughout the brain and spinal cord

    2. History—onset between 15–50 years of age

        a. Viral

        b. Autoimmunity

        c. Genetic factors

    3. Assessment

        a. Ataxia

        b. Weakness

        c. Spasticity

    d. Vertigo, tinnitus

    e. Nystagmus, patchy blindness

    f. Chewing and swallowing difficulties

    g. Scanning speech

    h. Paresthesias

    i. Incontinence/retention of urine, constipation

    j. Emotional lability

    k. Sexual impairment

4. Nursing management

    a. Promote comfort, rest, and sleep

    b. Promote maximum function, avoid stress

       1) Relaxation and coordination exercises

       2) Progressive resistance exercises, ROM

    c. Encourage fluid intake 2000 mL/day

    d. Administration of medications

       1) Corticosteriods (e.g., methylprednisolone)

       2) Immunosuppressive medications (e.g., cyclophosamide)

       3) Immune modulators (e.g., Interferon beta—Avonex, Betaseron, Rebif)

       4) Monoclonal antibody (e.g., natalizumab, glatiramer acetate)

    e. Wide-based walk, use of cane or walker

    f. Use of weighted bracelets and cuffs to stabilize upper extremities

    g. Bladder and bowel training (care of Foley catheter if appropriate)

    h. Self-help devices

    i. Eye patch for diplopia

    j. Occupational therapy

    k. Nutritional therapy

    l. Provide emotional support

    m. Referrals—National Multiple Sclerosis Society

U. Alzheimer's disease—chronic, progressive, degenerative disease characterized by a loss of memory, judgment, visuospatial perception, and personality

  1. Etiology—changes in structure and chemistry of the brain; exact cause unknown

    a. Structure—enlargement of the ventricles, widening of the cerebral sulci, narrowing of the gyri

    b. Reduction in neurotransmitters

    c. Vascular degeneration

  2. Assessment

    a. Stages—client may or may not progress through them in sequence

       1) Early, Stage 1: Forgets names, misplaces household items, short attention span, problems with judgment, decreased performance when stressed, decreased knowledge of current events, unable to travel alone to new destinations, inability to make decisions, increased confusion at night ("sundowning"), hoarding, wandering

2) Moderate, Stage 2: Gross intellectual impairments, complete disorientation to time, place, and events; agitated, possible depression, loss of ability to care for self, speech and language deficits, visuospatial deficits

3) Severe, Stage 3: Completely incapacitated, motor and verbal skills lost, general and focal neurological deficits, totally dependent in ADL

3. Nursing management
   a. Structure the environment—prevent overstimulation, provide consistency, prepare client for changes in routine, reality and validation therapy, present change gradually
   b. Promote independence in ADL—use occupational therapy as resource
   c. Promote bowel and bladder continence—take client to bathroom frequently throughout the day, less frequently at night
   d. Assist with facial recognition—encourage presence of family pictures and reminiscing
   e. Medication therapy—use of donepezil and galantamine to improve cognitive function; also, antidepressants and other psychotropic medications may be appropriate to relieve hallucinations and delusions, promote sleep, NMDA receptor antagonists (e.g. memantine)

4. Complementary/Alternative therapy
   a. Ingesting fish (a source of omega-3 fatty acids) one or more times per week may decrease the incidence of Alzheimer's
   b. Vitamin E 1,000 International Units BID to delay loss of activities of daily living; progression to a rating score of 3 or death
   c. Ginko biloba

ANATOMY OF THE EYE

(See Figure 11-4)

A. Three layers
   1. Sclera—fibrous outer coat
   2. Choroid—middle vascular coat
   3. Retina—inner nerve coat

B. Cornea
   1. Dome-like structure that forms most of the anterior portion of the eye
   2. Main refracting surface of the eye

C. Lens
   1. Lies behind pupil and iris
   2. Held in position by suspensory ligament attached to the ciliary body
   3. Elastic qualities allow accommodation to focus image on retina

D. Iris
   1. Colored portion of eye
   2. Attached around circumference by ciliary body
   3. Opening at center—pupil
   4. Controls the amount of light entering eye

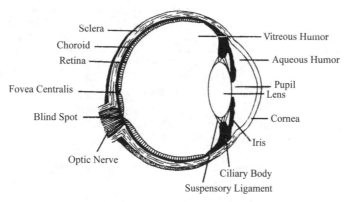

Figure 11-4. ANATOMY OF THE EYE

E. Retina
   1. Innermost lining of the eye
   2. Contains rods and cones
      a. Rods function with colorless, twilight vision
      b. Cones function with perception of color and bright, daylight vision
      c. Optic disk
         1) Point of entrance of nerve and blood vessels

2) Blind spot

3) Most prominent structure visible on the fundus (retina lining at the back of eye)

    a) Excessive pallor signals optic atrophy, a partial or complete destruction of the optic nerve

    b) Excessive redness—may signal beginning papilledema inflammation

    c) Papilledema (choked disks: severe form)

       i.   May be caused by inflammation

       ii. May signal passive congestion from ICP

F. Gerontologic considerations

1. Cornea thickens and flattens; increased incidence of astigmatism

2. Lens thickens; decreased anterior chamber size; intraocular pressure increases; increased risk glaucoma

3. Lens opacity increases; increased risk of cataracts

4. Retina degeneration—decreased visual acuity and color perception

5. Lacrimal apparatus—decreased tear production

6. Iris rigidity—smaller pupils; decreased response to light stimulation

VISUAL FUNCTION

A. Assessment (see Table 11-11)

Table 11-11 VISUAL FUNCTION TESTS		
TEST	**PROCEDURE**	**CLIENT PREPARATION**
Tonometry— measures intraocular pressure	Cornea is anesthetized Tonometer registers degree of indentation on cornea when pressure is applied Pressure increased in glaucoma	Client will be recumbent or sitting Remove contact lenses Advise not to squint, cough, or hold breath during the procedure
Visual fields—measurement of range of vision (perimetry)	Client is seated a measured distance from chart of concentric circles Client asked to fix eyes on a point on a chart at center of circle Client instructed to indicate when he/she first sees pointer; this point is recorded as a point in field of vision This procedure is repeated around 360° of a circle Normal visual fields for each eye are approximately a 50° angle superiorly, 90° laterally, 70° inferiorly, and 60° medially	None
Snellen test— test of visual acuity	Client stands 20 ft from chart of letters One eye is covered at a time Client reads chart to smallest letter visible Test results indicate comparison of distance at which this client reads to what normal eye sees at 20 ft	None

B. Signs and symptoms of eye problems
1. Redness, pain and burning
2. Edema
3. Increased lacrimation and exudate
4. Headache
5. Nausea and vomiting
6. Squinting
7. Visual disturbances
8. Disorders of accommodation (see Table 11-12)

Table 11-12 DISORDERS OF ACCOMMODATION	
TYPES	NURSING CONSIDER- ATIONS
Myopia (nearsightedness)—light rays refract at a point in front of the retina	Corrective lenses
Hyperopia (farsightedness)—light rays refract behind the retina	Corrective lenses
Presbyopia with aging	Commonly occurs after age 35 Corrective lenses
Astigmatism—uneven curvature of cornea causing blurring of vision	Corrective lenses

C. Treatments
1. Eye irrigation—method
   a. Tilt head back and toward the side of affected area
   b. Allow irrigating fluid to flow from the inner to the outer canthus
   c. Use a small bulb syringe or eye dropper to dispense fluid
   d. Place small basin close to head to collect excess fluid and drainage

2. Eyedrop instillation
   a. Equipment must be sterile
      1) Wash hands before instillation
      2) Do not allow dropper to touch eye
      3) Do not allow drops from eye to flow across nose into opposite eye
   b. Tilt head back and look up; pull lid down
   c. Place drops into center of lower conjunctival sac
      1) Instruct client not to squeeze eye
      2) Teach client to blink between drops
   d. To prevent systemic absorption, press the inner canthus near the bridge of the nose for 1–2 minutes

	Table 11-13 INSTILLATION OF EYE DROPS
A.	Equipment must be sterile. 1. Teach hand washing before instillation. 2. Do not allow dropper to touch eye. 3. Do not allow drops from one eye to flow across nose or into opposite eye.
B.	Tilt head back. Allow overflow to go out temporal side of eye.
C.	Place drops into lower conjunctival sac. 1. Instruct client not to squeeze eye. 2. Teach client to blink between drops.
D.	To prevent systemic absorption, press the inner angle of eye after instillation.

D. Nursing management of eye emergencies
1. Prevent eye injuries
   a. Provide safe toys
   b. Use of eye protectors when working with chemicals, tools
   c. Use of eye protectors during sports
   d. Protect eyes from ultraviolet light
   e. Instructions for first aid

2. Emergency treatment
   a. Burns (see Table 11-14)
   b. Trauma (see Table 11-15)

Table 11-14 BURNS OF THE EYE	
TYPES	**NURSING CONSIDERATIONS**
Chemical Acids, cleansers, insecticides	Eye irrigation with copious amounts of water for 15–20 min
Radiation Sun, lightning, eclipses	Prevention—use of eye shields
Thermal Hot metals, liquids, other occupational hazards	Use of goggles to protect the cornea; patching; analgesics

Table 11-15 EYE TRAUMA	
TYPES	**NURSING CONSIDERATIONS**
Nonpenetrating—abrasions	Eye patch for 24 hours
Nonpenetrating—contusions	Cold compresses, analgesics
Penetrating—pointed or sharp objects	Cover with patch; refer to surgeon

LOSS OF VISUAL FUNCTION

A. Assessment

1. Adjustment to vision loss depends upon:
   a. Age of onset
   b. Degree of suddenness

2. Principles of working with blind persons
   a. Facilitate normal lifestyle patterns
      1) Adapted household equipment
      2) Books and newspapers with large print for partially sighted
      3) Provide information concerning aids for the blind
      4) Braille
      5) Canes
      6) Guide dogs
      7) Facilitate developmental patterns
      8) Encourage social development
      9) Provide for education and employment

3. Nursing management of the blind client
   a. Enhance communication
      1) Address client by name
      2) Always introduce self
      3) State reason for being there
      4) Inform client when leaving the room

   b. Provide sense of safety and security
      1) Explain all procedures in detail
      2) Keep furniture arrangement consistent
      3) Provide hand rail
      4) Doors should never be half open
      5) Have client follow attendant when walking by lightly touching attendant's elbow (1/2 step ahead)
      6) Instruct client in use of lightweight walking stick when walking alone

   c. Foster sense of independence
      1) Provide assistance only when needed
      2) Identify food and location on plate or tray
      3) Encourage recreational and leisure time activities

CARE FOR THE CLIENT UNDERGOING EYE SURGERY

A. Preoperative care

1. Assessment of visual acuity
2. Preparation of periorbital area
3. Orientation to surroundings

4. Preoperative teaching—prepare for postoperative course

5. Teach postop necessity to avoid straining with stool, stooping

B. Postoperative care

1. Observe for complications—hemorrhage, sharp pain, infection

2. Avoid sneezing, coughing, straining with stool, bending down

3. Protect from injury; restrict activity

4. Keep signal bell within reach

5. Administer medications as ordered; medication for nausea, vomiting, restlessness

6. Shield worn for protective purposes

7. Discharge teaching—avoid stooping or straining at stool; use proper body mechanics

SELECTED DISORDERS OF THE EYE

A. Detached retina

1. History

   a. Flashes of light

   b. Blurred or "sooty" vision, "floaters"

   c. Sensation of particles moving in line of vision

   d. Delineated areas of vision blank

   e. A feeling of a coating coming up or down

   f. Loss of vision

   g. Confusion, apprehension

2. Characteristics

   a. Separation of the retina from the choroid

   b. Cause

      1) Trauma

      2) Aging process

      3) Diabetes

      4) Tumors

   c. Medical management

      1) Sedatives and tranquilizers

      2) Surgery—retina to adhere to choroid

3. Nursing management

   a. Bedrest, do not bend forward, avoid excessive movements

   b. Affected eye or both eyes may be patched to decrease movement of eye(s)

   c. Specific positioning—area of detachment should be in the dependent position

   d. Take precautions to avoid bumping head, moving eyes rapidly, or rapidly jerking the head

   e. Hairwashing delayed for 1 wk

   f. Avoid strenuous activity for 3 mo

B. Cataracts

1. History

   a. Objects appear distorted and blurred

   b. Annoying glare

   c. Pupil changes from black to gray to milky white

2. Assessment

   a. Partial or total opacity of the normally transparent crystalline lens

   b. Cause

     1) Congenital

     2) Trauma

     3) Aging process

     4) Associated with diabetes mellitus, intraocular surgery

     5) Medications—steroid therapy

   c. Surgical management—laser surgery

     1) Extracapsular extraction—cut through the anterior capsule to express the opaque lens material

     2) Intracapsular extraction (method of choice)—removal of entire lens and capsule

     3) Lens implantation

3. Nursing management

   a. Observe for postoperative complications

     1) Hemorrhage

     2) Increased intraocular pressure

     3) Slipped suture(s)

     4) If lens implant, pupil should remain constricted; if aphakic, pupil remains dilated

   b. Avoid straining and no heavy lifting

   c. Bend from the knees only to pick things up

   d. Instruct about instillation of eye drops, use of night shields

   e. Protect eye from bright lights

   f. Adjustments needed in perception if aphakic

   g. Diversional activities

C. Glaucoma

1. Assessment

   a. Cloudy, blurry, or loss of vision

   b. Artificial lights appear to have rainbows or halos around them

   c. Loss of vision

   d. Decreased peripheral vision

   e. Pain, headache

   f. Nausea, vomiting

   g. Tonometer readings exceed normal intraocular pressure (10–21 mm Hg)

2. Characteristics
   a. Abnormal increase in intraocular pressure leading to visual disability and blindness—obstruction of outflow of aqueous humor
   b. Types
      1) Angle-closure (closed angle); sudden onset, emergency
      2) Open-angle (primary); most common; blockage of aqueous humor flow
   c. Causes
      1) Closed-angle glaucoma—associated with ocular diseases, trauma
      2) Open-angle glaucoma—associated with aging, heredity, retinal vein occlusion
   d. Treatment of closed-angle glaucoma (see Table 11-16)
      1) Medications—miotics, carbonic anhydrase inhibitors, oral glycerin (Osmoglyn) and mannitol
      2) Surgery
   e. Treatment of open-angle glaucoma
      1) Medications—miotics, carbonic anhydrase inhibitors, anticholinesterase beta-blocking agents, adrenergic agonists, prostaglandin agonists
      2) Surgery—laser trabeculoplasty, standard glaucoma surgery
   f. Common nursing diagnosis—sensory/perceptual/visual alteration

3. Nursing management
   a. Compliance with medical therapy
   b. Avoid tight clothing (e.g., collars)
   c. Reduce external stimuli
   d. Avoid heavy lifting, straining at stool
   e. Avoid use of mydriatics
   f. Educate public to five danger signs of glaucoma:
      1) Brow arching
      2) Halos around lights
      3) Blurry vision
      4) Diminished peripheral vision
      5) Headache or eye pain

Table 11-16 EYE MEDICATIONS		
MEDICATION	**ADVERSE EFFECTS**	**NURSING CONSIDERATIONS**
Methylcellulose	Eye irritation if excess is allowed to dry on eyelids	Lubricant Use eyewash to rinse eyelids of "sandy" sensation felt after administration
Polyvinyl alcohol	Blurred vision Burning	Artificial tears Applied to contact lenses before insertion
Tetrahydrozoline	Cardiac irregularities Pupillary dilation, increased intraocular pressure Transient stinging	Used for ocular congestion, irritation, allergic conditions Rebound congestion may occur with frequent or prolonged use Apply light pressure on lacrimal sac for 1 min following instillation
Timolol maleate	Eye irritation Hypotension	Beta-blocking agent Reduces intraocular pressure in management of glaucoma Apply light pressure on lacrimal sac for 1 min following instillation Monitor BP and pulse
Action	Causes vasoconstriction by local adrenergic action	
Indications	Ocular irritation	
Adverse effects	Headache Dizziness Transient stinging in eye Pupillary dilation Photophobia	
Nursing considerations	Apply light pressure on lacrimal sac for 1 min after instilling drops Rebound congestion may occur with prolonged use	

ALTERATIONS IN HEARING

ANATOMY AND PHYSIOLOGY OF EAR

(See Figure 11-5)

A. External ear
1. Pinna or auricle
2. External acoustic meatus
3. External auditory canal

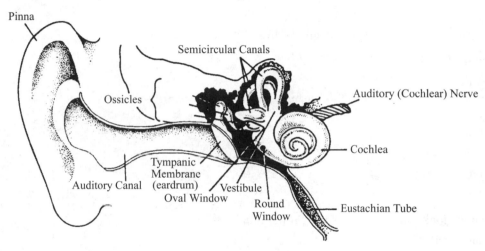

Figure 11-5. ANATOMY AND PHYSIOLOGY OF THE EAR

B. Middle ear
1. Located in temporal bone
2. Contains ossicles
   a. Malleus
   b. Incus
   c. Stapes
3. Eustachian tube—connects middle ear to the throat and assists in equalizing pressure in middle ear
4. Physiology of sound
   a. Sound waves enter external auditory canal to tympanic membrane
   b. Tympanic membrane vibrates, triggering ossicles (malleus, incus, stapes)
   c. Vibration transmitted to oval window to acoustic nerve and brain

C. Inner ear
1. Contains vestibule, semicircular canals, and cochlea (labyrinth)
2. Movement of the sensory hairs signals changes in position; aids in maintaining stable posture

D. Gerontologic considerations
1. Ear canal narrows

2. Cerumen glands atrophy; dried cerumen

3. Tympanic membrane flexibility decreases; decreased sound transmission in middle ear

4. Decreased ability to hear high frequency sounds

ALTERATIONS IN FUNCTION

A. Assessment

1. Signs and symptoms
   a. Pain, fever
   b. Headache
   c. Discharge
   d. Altered growth and development
   e. Personality changes, e.g., irritability, depression, suspiciousness, withdrawal

2. Diagnostics
   a. Audiogram—quantitative, i.e., degree of loss
   b. Tuning fork—qualitative, i.e., type of loss

B. Types of hearing loss

1. Conductive loss—disorder in auditory canal, eardrum, or ossicles
   a. Causes
      1) Infection
      2) Inflammation
      3) Foreign body
      4) Trauma

   b. Complications—meningitis resulting from initial infection
   c. Management
      1) Heat
      2) Antibiotics
      3) Ear drops, ointments, irrigation
      4) Surgery
      5) Hearing aid

2. Perceptive (sensorineural loss)—due to disorder of the organ of Corti or the auditory nerve
   a. Causes
      1) Congenital—maternal exposure to communicable disease
      2) Infection, drug toxicity
      3) Trauma
      4) Labyrinth dysfunction—Ménière's disease

   b. Complications
      1) Vertigo
      2) Tinnitus
      3) Vomiting

    c. Management
      1) Medication
      2) Surgery
      3) Combined loss—conductive and sensorineural
      4) Psychogenic loss—functional

C. Nursing management of ear infections

  1. Ear irrigation—method

    a. Tilt head toward side of affected ear; gently direct stream of fluid against sides of canal

    b. After procedure, instruct client to lie on affected side to facilitate drainage

    c. Contraindicated if there is evidence of swelling or tenderness

  2. Ear drop instillation—method

    a. Position the affected ear uppermost

    b. Pull outer ear upward and backward for preschoolers through adults (3 years of age and older)

    c. Pull outer ear downward and backward for infants and toddlers (under 3 years of age)

    d. Place drops so they run down the wall of ear canal

    e. Have client lie on unaffected ear to encourage absorption

D. Nursing management for clients undergoing ear surgery

  1. Preoperative care

    a. Assessment of preoperative symptoms

    b. Prep depends on nature of incision

    c. Encourage client to wash hair prior to surgery

    d. Teaching—expect postoperative hearing loss and discuss need for special position of operative ear as ordered

  2. Postoperative care

    a. Reinforce dressing only. Avoid nose blowing, sneezing, and coughing

    b. Observe for possible complications

      1) Facial nerve damage—may be transient

      2) Infection

      3) Vertigo, tinnitus

      4) Do not apply pressure if bleeding is noted on internal ear surgery—notify health care provider immediately

      5) Administer medications

      6) Provide for client safety

    c. Discharge teaching—avoid getting water in ear, flying, drafts, crowds, exercise caution around people with respiratory infections

SELECTED DISORDERS

A. Acute otitis media

  1. Assessment

    a. Fever, chills

    b. Headache

    c. Ringing in ears

    d. Deafness

        e. Sharp pain

        f. Head rolling, crying, ear tugging (child)

        g. Nausea, vomiting

        h. Red bulging tympanic membrane

   2. Characteristics

        a. Infection of middle ear

        b. Cause—pathogenic organisms, i.e., bacteria and viruses

        c. Complications

           1) Chronic otitis media—children more susceptible due to short eustachian tube

           2) Residual deafness

           3) Perforation of tympanic membrane

           4) Cholesteatoma growth

           5) Mastoiditis or meningitis

        d. Medical and surgical management

           1) Antibiotics—organism-specific

           2) Antihistamines for allergies

           3) Nasal decongestants

           4) Ventilatory tubes—inserted in eustachian tube for continuous ventilation

           5) Myringotomy—typanic membrane incision to relieve pressure and release purulent fluid

        e. Nursing management

           1) Administer medication as ordered

           2) Report persistent symptoms to health care provider

           3) Following a myringotomy—no water can be allowed to enter the ear

           4) Bedrest if temperature is elevated

           5) Position on side of involved ear to promote drainage

B. Mastoiditis

   1. Assessment

        a. Fever, chills

        b. Headache, dizziness

        c. Deafness

        d. Auricle discharge

        e. Pain, tenderness

        f. Stiff neck

        g. Facial paralysis

        h. Vomiting

        i. Can cause meningitis

   2. Characteristics

        a. Inflammation of mastoid

        b. Cause—middle ear infection

   3. Medical/surgical treatment

        a. Antibiotic therapy

        b. Mastoidectomy—removal of mastoid cells

4. Nursing management
   a. Observe for postoperative complications
      1) Facial nerve injury—facial paralysis
      2) Infection
      3) Vertigo
   b. Administer medications as ordered

C. Ménière's disease
1. Assessment
   a. Decreased hearing on involved side
   b. Tinnitus
   c. Headache, nystagmus, rapid eye movements
   d. Vertigo
   e. Anxiety
   f. Nausea, vomiting

2. Characteristics
   a. Dilation of the membrane of the labyrinth
   b. Complication—hearing loss
   c. Medical and nursing management
      1) Salt-free and neutral ash diet (Furstenberg diet)—restrict water and salt intake
      2) Symptomatic treatment, i.e., antiemetics, antihistamines, vasodilators, antivertigo medications, diuretics
      3) Decompression of endolymphatic sac with Teflon shunt (method of choice)
      4) Total labyrinthectomy—last resort with the possible complication of Bell's palsy
      5) Cochlear implant
      6) Client education
         a) Need to slow down body movements—jerking or sudden movements may precipitate attack
         b) Need for self-protection and to lie down when an attack takes place
         c) If driving, pull over and stop car
         d) Occupational counseling—if occupation involves operating machinery

Chapter 12

ONCOLOGY

Sections	Concepts Covered
1. Cancer	Cellular Regulation, Comfort
2. Leukemia	Cellular Regulation, Coagulation
3. Skin Cancer	Cellular Regulation, Skin Integrity
4. Intracranial Tumors	Intracranial Regulation, Cellular Reguation
5. Pancreatic Tumors	Metabolism, Cellular Regulation
6. Carcinoma of the Larynx	Gas Exchange, Cellular Regulation

CANCER

A group of many diseases of multiple causes that can arise in any cell that is able to evade regulatory controls over cell proliferation and differentiation

A. Assessment
1. American Cancer Society warning signs
    a. Change in bowel, bladder habits
    b. A sore that does not heal
    c. Unusual bleeding or discharge from any body orifice
    d. Thickening or a lump in the breast or elsewhere
    e. Indigestion or difficulty in swallowing
    f. Obvious change in a wart or mole
    g. Nagging cough or hoarseness

B. Etiology
1. Defect in cellular proliferation
    a. Proliferation is indiscriminate and continuous
    b. Continuous growth of tumor mass: pyramid effect

2. Defect in cellular differentiation
    a. Oncogenes interfere with normal cell expression, causing cells to be malignant
    b. Cells regain fetal appearance and function
    c. Some cells produce hormones; others produce proteins

3. Development of cancer (multifactorial)
    a. Physical
        1) Radiation—excessive exposure to sunlight, ultraviolet radiation, and ionizing radiation
        2) Chronic irritation
        3) Foreign bodies

    b. Malignancies correlated with physical factors
        1) Leukemias
        2) Lymphoma
        3) Thyroid cancer
        4) Bone cancer
        5) Lung cancer (asbestos-related)

    c. Chemical
        1) Food additives, e.g., nitrates
        2) Dietary factors
        3) Pharmaceutical, e.g., stilbestrol
        4) Smoking
        5) Alcohol

    d. Malignancies correlated with chemical factors
       1) Vaginal cancer
       2) Acute myelogenous leukemia
       3) Non-Hodgkin's lymphoma
       4) Multiple myeloma
       5) Lung cancer

    e. Genetic
       1) Strong predisposition
       2) Inherited chromosomal abnormalities

    f. Cancers with a genetic component
       1) Lung cancer
       2) Breast cancer
       3) Leukemia
       4) Uterine cancer
       5) Colon cancer
       6) Neuroblastoma

    g. Viral—incorporated into cell genesis
       1) DNA and RNA viruses induce malignancies
       2) Epstein-Barr virus, Burkitt's lymphoma

    h. Stress—inhibits immune surveillance system

  4. Classifications
    a. Carcinoma/adenocarcinoma—epithelial tissue
    b. Sarcoma—connective tissue
    c. Lymphoma—lymphoid tissue
    d. Leukemia—blood-forming tissue (WBCs and platelets)
    e. Multiple myeloma—plasma
    f. Neuroblastoma—nerve cells
    g. Meningeal sarcoma—meninges

C. Nursing management
  1. Chemotherapy (see Tables 12-1 through 12-8)
  2. Radiotherapy—gamma, beta, and alpha rays
    a. External radiation (e.g., cobalt); external beam (teletherapy)
       1) Leave radiology markings intact on skin
       2) Avoid creams or lotions, deodorants, perfumes (only vitamin A and D ointment permitted)
       3) Use lukewarm water to cleanse area
       4) Assess skin for redness, cracking
       5) Administer antiemetics for nausea, analgesics for pain
       6) Observe skin, mucous membranes, and hair follicles for adverse effects
       7) No hot water bottle, tape; don't expose area to cold or sunlight
       8) Wear cotton clothing

    b. Internal radiation (e.g., cesium, radium, gold); brachytherapy

       1) Sealed source—mechanically positioned source of radioactive material placed in body cavity or tumor

          a) Lead container and long-handled forceps in room in event of dislodged source

          b) Save all dressings, bed linens until source is removed; then discard dressings and linens as usual

          c) Urine, feces, and linens not radioactive

          d) Do not stand close or in line with radioactive source

          e) Client on bedrest while implant in place

          f) Position of source verified by radiography

       2) Unsealed source of radiation—unsealed liquid given orally, or instilled in body cavity (e.g., iodine [^{131}I])

          a) All body fluids contaminated

          b) Greatest danger from body fluids during first 24–96 hours

       3) Nursing management for client with internal radiation

          a) Assign client to private room

          b) Place "Caution: Radioactive Material" sign on door

          c) Wear dosimeter film badge at all times when interacting with client (offers no protection but measures amount of exposure; each nurse has individual badge)

          d) Do not assign pregnant nurse to client

          e) Rotate staff caring for client

          f) Organize tasks so limited time is spent in client's room

          g) Limit visitors

          h) Encourage client to do own care

          i) Provide shield in room

          j) Use antiemetics for nausea

          k) Consider body image (e.g., alopecia)

          l) Provide comfort measures, analgesic for pain

          m) Provide good nutrition

3. Skin care

    a. Avoid use of soaps, powders, lotions

    b. Wear cotton, loose-fitting clothing

4. Mouth care

    a. Stomatitis—develops 5–14 days after chemotherapy begins

    b. Symptoms—erythema, ulcers, bleeding

    c. Oral rinses with saline or soft-bristled toothbrush

    d. Avoid hot (temperature) or spicy foods

    e. Topical antifungals and anesthetics

5. Hair care

    a. Alopecia commonly seen, alters body image; alopecia temporary

    b. Assist with wig or hairpiece

    c. Scarves, hats

6. Nutritional changes
    a. Anorexia, nausea, and vomiting commonly seen with chemotherapy
    b. Malabsorption and cachexia (wasting) common
    c. Make meals appealing to senses
    d. Conform diet to client preferences and nutritional needs
    e. Small, frequent meals with additional supplements between meals (high-calorie, high-protein diet)
    f. Encourage fluids but limit at mealtimes
    g. Perform oral hygiene and provide relief of pain before mealtime
    h. TPN as needed

7. Neutropenic precautions—prevent infection among clients with immunosuppression
    a. Assess skin integrity every 8 hours; auscultate breath sounds, presence of cough, sore throat; check temperature every 4 hours; report if greater than 101°F (38°C); monitor CBC and differential daily
    b. Private when possible
    c. Thorough hand hygiene before entering client's room
    d. Allow no staff with cold or sore throat to care for client
    e. No fresh flowers or standing water
    f. Clean room daily
    g. Low microbial diet; no fresh salads, unpeeled fresh fruits and vegetables
    h. Deep breathe every 4 hours
    i. Meticulous body hygiene
    j. Inspect IV site, meticulous IV site care

8. Pain relief—three-step ladder approach
    a. For mild pain—nonnarcotic meds (acetaminophen) along with antiemetics, antidepressants, glucocorticoids
    b. For moderate pain—weak narcotics (codeine) and nonnarcotics
    c. For severe pain—strong narcotics (morphine)
    d. Give pain meds on regularly scheduled basis (preventative approach), additional analgesics given for breakthrough pain

9. Activity level
    a. Alternate rest and activity
    b. Maintain normal lifestyle

10. Psychosocial issues
    a. Encourage participation in self-care and decision-making
    b. Provide referral to support groups, organizations
    c. Hospice care

11. Complementary/Alternative therapy
    a. Vitamin E administered with cisplatin decreases the incidence and severity of treatment-associated neurotoxicity

Table 12–1 ANTINEOPLASTIC MEDICATIONS: ALKYLATING AGENTS	
Examples	Cyclophosphamide
Actions	Interferes with rapidly reproducing cell DNA
Indications	Leukemia
	Multiple myeloma
Adverse effects	Bone marrow suppression
	Nausea, vomiting
	Stomatitis
	Alopecia
	Gonadal suppression
	Renal toxicity (cisplatin)
	Ototoxicity (Cisplatin)
Nursing considerations	Used with other chemotherapeutic agents
	Check hematopoietic function weekly
	Encourage fluids (10-12 glasses/day)

Table 12–2 ANTINEOPLASTIC MEDICATIONS: ANTIMETABOLITES	
Examples	Fluorouracil
	Mercaptopurine
	Methotrexate
Actions	Closely resembles normal metabolites, "counterfeits" fool cells; cell division halted
Indications	Acute lymphatic leukemia
	Rheumatoid arthritis
	Psoriasis
	Cancer of colon, breast, stomach, pancreas
	Sickle cell anemia
Adverse effects	Nausea, vomiting
	Diarrhea
	Oral ulceration
	Hepatic dysfunction
	Bone marrow suppression
	Renal dysfunction
	Alopecia
Nursing considerations	Monitor hematopoietic function
	Good mouth care
	Small frequent feedings
	Counsel about body image changes (alopecia); provide wig
	Good skin care
	Photosensitivity precautions
	Infection control precautions

Table 12-3 ANTINEOPLASTIC MEDICATIONS: ANTITUMOR ANTIBIOTICS	
Examples	Dactinomycin Doxorubicin
Actions	Interferes with DNA and RNA synthesis
Indications	Hodgkin's disease Non-Hodgkin's lymphoma Leukemia Many cancers
Adverse effects	Bone marrow depression Nausea, vomiting Alopecia Stomatitis Heart damage Septic shock
Nursing considerations	Monitor closely for septicemic reactions Monitor for manifestations of extravasation at injection site (severe pain or burning that lasts minutes to hours, redness after injection is completed, ulceration after 48 hours)instruct client urine and tears may be red in color Monitor for signs of heart failure

Table 12-4 ANTINEOPLASTIC MEDICATIONS: HORMONAL	
Examples	**Antiestrogens:** Tamoxifen **Aromatase Inhibitors:** Anastrozole, Letrozole, Exemestane **Gonadotropin-Releasing Hormone Agonist:** Leuprolide **Gonadotropin-Releasing Hormone Antagonists:** Degarelix
Actions	Tamoxifen–antiestrogen (competes with estrogen to bind at estrogen receptor sites on malignant cells) Leuprolide–progestin (causes tumor cell regression by unknown mechanism) Testolactone–androgen (used for palliation in advanced breast cancer)
Indications	Breast cancer
Adverse effects	Hypercalcemia Jaundice Increased appetite Masculinization or feminization Sodium and fluid retention Nausea, vomiting Hot flashes Vaginal dryness
Nursing considerations	Baseline and periodic gyn exams Not given IV Discuss pregnancy prevention

Table 12-5	ANTINEOPLASTIC MEDICATIONS: VINCA ALKALOIDS
Examples	Vinblastine sulfate Vincristine sulfate
Actions	Interferes with cell division
Indications	Hodgkin's disease Lymphoma Cancers
Adverse effects	Bone marrow suppression (mild with vincristine) Neuropathies (vincristine) Stomatitis
Nursing considerations	Same as antitumor antibiotics

Table 12-6	ANTINEOPLASTIC MEDICATIONS: DNA TOPOISOMERASE
Examples	Irinotecan Topotecan
Actions	Binds to enzyme that breaks the DNA strands
Indications	Ovary, lung, colon, and rectal cancers
Adverse efects	Bone marrow suppression Diarrhea Nausea, vomiting Hepatotoxicity

Table 12-7 ANTINEOPLASTIC MEDICATIONS: OVERVIEW

MEDICATION	ADVERSE EFFECTS	NURSING CONSIDERATIONS
Alkylating Agents		
Busulfan	Bone marrow depression	Check CBC (applies to all medications in this table) Most chemotherapy causes stomatitis and requires extra fluids to flush system
Chlorambucil	Nausea, vomiting, bone marrow depression, sterility	Monitor for infection Avoid IM injections when platelet count is low to minimize bleeding
Cyclophosphamide	Alopecia, bone marrow depression, hemorrhagic cystitis, dermatitis, hyperkalemia, hypoglycemia, amenorrhea	Report hematuria, force fluids Monitor for infection Give antiemetics
Platinum Compound		
Cisplatin	Anaphylactic-type reaction, seizures, hearing loss, renal toxicity, leukopenia, thrombocytopenia	Monitor dosing Assess frequently for ototoxicity assess for reanl toxicity
Antimetabolites		
Fluorouracil	Nausea, stomatitis, GI ulceration, diarrhea, bone marrow depression, liver dysfunction, alopecia	Monitor for infection Avoid extravasation
Methotrexate	Oral and GI ulceration, liver damage, bone marrow depression, stomatitis, alopecia, bloody diarrhea, fatigue	Good mouth care, avoid alcohol Monitor hepatic and renal function tests
Mercaptopurine	Liver damage, bone marrow depression, infection, alopecia, abdominal bleeding	Check liver function tests
Cytarabine	Hematologic abnormalities, nausea, vomiting, rash, weight loss	Force fluids Good oral hygiene
Hydroxyurea	Bone marrow depression, GI symptoms, rash	Teach client to report toxic GI symptoms promptly
Antibiotic Antineoplastics		
Doxorubicin	Red urine, nausea, vomiting, stomatitis, alopecia, cardiotoxicity, blisters, bone marrow depression	Check EKG, avoid IV infiltration Monitor vital signs closely Good mouth care
Bleomycin	Nausea, vomiting, alopecia, edema of hands, pulmonary fibrosis, fever, bone marrow depression	Observe for pulmonary complications Treat fever with acetaminophen Check breath sounds frequently
Dactinomycin	Nausea, bone marrow depression	Give antiemetic before administration
Vinca Alkaloids		
Vinblastine	Nausea, vomiting, stomatitis, alopecia, loss of reflexes, bone marrow depression	Avoid IV infiltration and extravasation Give antiemetic before administration Acute bronchospasm can occur if given IV Zyloprim given to increase excretion and decrease buildup of urates (uric acid)
Vincristine	Peripheral neuritis, loss of reflexes, bone marrow depression, alopecia, GI symptoms	Avoid IV infiltration and extravasation Check reflexes, motor and sensory function Zyloprim given to increase excretion and decrease buildup of urates (uric acid)
Hormonal Agents		
Tamoxifen	Transient fall in WBC or platelets Hypercalcemia, bone pain	Check CBC Monitor serum calcium Nonsteroidal antiestrogen

Table 12-8 ANTINEOPLASTIC MEDICATIONS: NURSING IMPLICATIONS FOR ADVERSE EFFECTS	
Bone marrow suppression	Monitor bleeding: bleeding gums, bruising, petechiae, guaiac stools, urine and emesis
	Avoid IM injections and rectal temperatures
	Apply pressure to venipuncture sites
Nausea, vomiting	Monitor intake and output ratios, appetite and nutritional intake
	Prophylactic antiemetics as ordered
	Smaller, more frequent meals
Altered immunologic response	Prevent infection by handwashing
	Timely reporting of alterations in vital signs or symptoms indicating possible infection
Impaired oral mucous membrane; stomatis	Oral hygiene measures
Fatigue	Encourage rest and discuss measures to conserve energy
	Use relaxation techniques, mental imagery

LEUKEMIA

Fatal neoplastic disease that involves the blood-forming tissues of the bone marrow, spleen, and lymph nodes

A. Outstanding characteristic—abnormal, uncontrolled, and destructive proliferation of one type of white cell and its precursors

B. Classification of the leukemias

1. Acute leukemia—rapid onset and progresses to a fatal termination within days to months; more common among children and young adults

2. Chronic leukemia—gradual onset with a slower, more protracted course; more common between ages 25 and 60

C. Assessment

1. Severe infection (e.g., ulcerations of the mouth and throat, pneumonia, septicemia)—high leukocyte count (15,000–500,000/mm^3 or higher), immature or abnormal, and consequently are unable to fight and destroy microorganisms

2. Anemia accompanied by fatigue, lethargy, hypoxia, and hemorrhage (e.g., gum bleeding, ecchymoses, petechiae, retinal hemorrhages) due to thrombocytopenia—occurs because rapidly proliferating leukocytes "crowd out" the developing erythrocytes and thrombocytes, bone and joint pain

3. Enlarged organs cause pressure on adjacent structures (e.g., splenomegaly, hepatomegaly, lymphadenopathy, bone marrow hypercellularity)—distention of tissues occurs from accumulation of high numbers of white cells

4. Increased metabolic rate accompanied by weakness, pallor, and weight loss

   a. Increased production of leukocytes requires large amounts of amino acids and vitamins

   b. Increased destruction of cells leads to increased release of metabolic wastes, which must be disposed of by the body

5. Uric acid stones, which cause renal pain, obstruction, and infection—uric acid is released as a result of the destruction of large numbers of leukocytes by antileukemic medications

6. Renal insufficiency with uremia as a late development—abnormal leukocytes infiltrate into the kidneys

7. Central nervous system symptoms (e.g., headache, disorientation, convulsions)—abnormal white cells infiltrate into the brain and nervous system

8. Diagnosis

   a. Elevated leukocyte count with a "shift to the left" (presence of large numbers of immature neutrophils)

   b. A differential leukocyte count in which one type of white cell is overwhelmingly predominant

   c. A bone marrow specimen that contains massive numbers of leukocytes

   d. A blood smear that reveals many "blast" cells

   e. The presence of anemia, bleeding, tenderness, sternal tenderness, and organ enlargement

D. Factors associated with development of leukemia

1. Viruses

2. Ionizing radiation

3. Genetic predisposition

4. Absorption of certain chemicals (e.g., benzene, pyridine, and aniline dyes)

E. Nursing management

1. Monitor for signs of bleeding, e.g., petechiae, bruising, bleeding gums; follow bleeding precautions

2. Monitor for signs of infection, e.g., changes in vital signs, chills

3. Provide mouth care

4. Provide high-calorie, high-vitamin diet

5. Provide frequent feedings of soft, easy-to-eat food

6. Provide antiemetics, as ordered, for nausea and vomiting

7. Neutropenic precautions if necessary

8. Strict hand washing

9. Prevent skin breakdown

10. Administer and monitor blood transfusions (whole blood, platelets)

11. Administer medications, as ordered, and observe for adverse effects

    a. Chemotherapy

        1) Nausea, vomiting, diarrhea

        2) Stomatitis, alopecia, skin reactions

        3) Bone marrow depression

    b. Radiation or radioisotope therapy—bone marrow transplants

SKIN CANCER

A. Assessment

1. Basal cell carcinoma—small, waxy nodule on sun-exposed areas of body (e.g., face); may ulcerate and crust

2. Squamous cell carcinoma—rough, thick, scaly tumor seen on arms or face

3. Malignant melanoma—variegated color (brown, black mixed with gray or white) circular lesion with irregular edges seen on trunk or legs

B. Types

1. Basal cell carcinoma—most common type of skin cancer; rarely metastasizes but commonly recurs

2. Squamous cell carcinoma—may metastasize to blood or lymph

3. Malignant melanoma—most lethal of skin cancers; frequently seen in ages 20–45; highest risk persons with fair complexions, blue eyes, red or blond hair, and freckles; metastasizes to bone, liver, spleen, CNS, lungs, lymph

4. Diagnosed by skin lesion biopsy

C. Nursing management

1. Postop care following surgical excision

2. Teach prevention

   a. Avoid exposure to sun 10 AM to 3 PM

   b. Use sunscreen with SPF (solar protection factor) to block harmful rays (especially important for children)

   c. Reapply sunscreen after swimming or prolonged time in sun

   d. Use lip balm with sunscreen protection

   e. Wear hat when outdoors

   f. Do not use tanning lamps or booths

   g. Teach client to examine skin surfaces monthly

3. Teach how to identify danger signs of melanoma—change in size, color, shape of mole or surrounding skin

4. Chemotherapy for metastases

5. Complementary/Alternative therapy

   a. Fish oil, vitamin E from food, normal levels of selenium, green tea, and soy may decrease risk of melanoma

   b. Nonsteroidal anti-inflammatory drugs (NSAIDs) may reduce risk of melanoma

INTRACRANIAL TUMORS

INTRACRANIAL TUMORS

A. Assessment—signs and symptoms vary depending on location
1. Motor deficits
2. Language disturbances
3. Hearing difficulties (temporal lobe), visual disturbances (occipital lobe)
4. Dizziness, paresthesia (cerebellum), coordination problems
5. Seizures (motor cortex)—frequently first presenting sign
6. Personality disturbances (frontal lobe)
7. Papilledema
8. Nausea and vomiting
9. Drowsiness, changes in level of consciousness

B. Types
1. Types—classified according to location
   a. Supratentorial—incision usually behind hairline; surgery within the cerebral hemisphere
   b. Infratentorial—incision made at nape of neck around occipital lobe; surgery within brain stem and cerebellum
2. Causes—unknown
3. Medical/surgical management—intracranial surgery (burr holes, craniotomy, cranioplasty), radiation

C. Nursing management
1. Preoperative care
   a. Detailed neurological assessment for baseline data
   b. Head shave—prep site
   c. Psychological support
   d. Prepare client for postoperative course

2. Postoperative care
   a. Maintain patent airway
   b. Elevate head of bed 30–45° after supratentorial surgery
   c. Position client flat and lateral on either side after infratentorial surgery
   d. Monitor vital and neurological signs
   e. Observe for complications—respiratory difficulties, increased intracranial pressure, hyperthermia, meningitis, wound infection
   f. Administer medications—corticosteroids, osmotic diurectics, mild analgesics, anticonvulsants, antibiotics, antipyretics, antiemetics, hormone replacement as needed; no narcotics postoperatively (masks changes in LOC)

PANCREATIC TUMORS

A. Assessment
1. Weight loss
2. Vague upper or midabdominal discomfort
3. Abnormal glucose tolerance test (hyperglycemia)
4. Jaundice, clay-colored stools, dark urine

B. Types
1. Tumors may arise from any portion of the pancreas (head or tail); each has unique clinical manifestations

C. Diagnostic tests—CT, CT-guided needle biopsy, MRI

D. Nursing/medical management
1. Medical
   a. High-calorie, bland, low-fat diet; small, frequent feedings
   b. Avoid alcohol
   c. Anticholinergics
   d. Chemotherapy, radiation therapy, stent placement

2. Surgery (Whipple procedure)—removal of head of pancreas, distal portion of common bile duct, the duodenum, and part of the stomach

3. Postop care
   a. Monitor for peritonitis and intestinal obstruction
   b. Monitor for hypotension
   c. Monitor for steatorrhea
   d. Administer pancreatic enzymes
   e. Monitor for diabetes mellitus

CARCINOMA OF THE LARYNX

Section 6

CARCINOMA OF THE LARYNX

A. Assessment
1. Pain radiating to the ears
2. Hoarseness, dysphagia, foul breath
3. Dyspnea
4. Enlarged cervical nodes
5. Hemoptysis

B. Diagnostic tests
1. Laryngoscopy, bronchoscopy
2. Biopsy
3. CT, MRI
4. X-rays

C. Causes
1. Industrial chemicals
2. Cigarette smoking and alcohol use
3. Straining of the vocal cords
4. Chronic laryngitis
5. Family predisposition

D. Nursing management
1. Caring for the client with a laryngectomy or laser surgery
   a. Preoperative care
      1) Explain compensatory methods of communication
      2) Referral to speech therapy

   b. Postoperative care
      1) Laryngectomy care—stoma care, suction
      2) Place in semi-Fowler position
      3) Turn, cough, and deep breathe
      4) Nasogastric gastrostomy or jejunostomy enteral nutrition
      5) Provide humidified oxygen
      6) Suction oral secretions
      7) Monitor condition of skin flap

   c. Observe for postoperative complications after laryngectomy
      1) Respiratory difficulties
      2) Fistula formation
      3) Rupture of carotid artery
      4) Stenosis of trachea

    d. Monitor weight, food intake, and fluid I and O

    e. Communication for total laryngectomy clients

        1) Esophageal speech

        2) Artificial larynx—commonly used mechanical device for speech

        3) Radiation therapy—small, localized cancers; sore throat, increased hoarseness, dysphagia

        4) Chemotherapy—alone or with radiation therapy and surgery

Chapter 13

MATERNITY AND GYNECOLOGICAL NURSING

Sections	Concepts Covered
1. The Reproductive System	Reproduction, Sexuality, Client Education: Providing
2. Childbearing—Antepartal Care	Reproduction
3. Labor and Delivery	Fluid/Electrolyte Balance, Comfort, Perfusion, Emotional Process
4. Postpartum	Fluid/Electrolyte Balance
5. The Neonate	Gas Exchange, Fluid/ Electrolyte Balance
6. Childbearing—Maternal Complications	Coagulation, Perfusion, Infection
7. Childbearing—Neonatal Complications	Fluid/Electrolyte Balance, Gas Exchange, Infection

THE REPRODUCTIVE SYSTEM

HUMAN REPRODUCTION

A. Female

1. Anatomy

   a. External structures

      1) Mons veneris—fat pad covered with pubic hair, over symphysis pubis

      2) Labia majora—crescent-shaped fatty tissue containing folds of skin; extends down from mons veneris to perineum

      3) Labia minora—narrow folds of hairless skin between labia majora and vagina

      4) Clitoris—short, sensitive, erectile tissue, anterior junction of the vulva

      5) Perineum—area between vaginal opening and anus composed of muscles and fascia, which supports pelvic structures

      6) Hymen—membranous tissue over vaginal opening

      7) Urethral opening—beneath clitoris

   b. Internal organs and structures

      1) Ovaries—small oval organs located on each side of the uterus in the upper part of the pelvis; function in the development and expulsion of ova

      2) Fallopian tubes (oviduct)—two tubes, each closely adjoining an ovary

         a) Each has two openings—one into the abdominal cavity and one into the uterine cavity

         b) Function to conduct the released ovum from the ovary to the uterus

      3) Uterus—hollow, pear-shaped, thick-walled muscular structure, located between the bladder and the rectum in the pelvic cavity

         a) Composed of three sections: fundus, body, and cervix

         b) Consists of:

            i. The myometrium—involuntary muscle fibers that provide for expansion and support during pregnancy and for expulsion of fetus and control of hemorrhage during labor and delivery

            ii. The endometrium—highly vascular lining that provides for implantation of fertilized ovum, shed during menstruation

         c) During labor, expels the products of conception

      4) Vagina—distensible mucous membrane-lined passage (birth canal) located between the bladder and rectum

      5) Pelvis—the bony ring through which the fetus passes during labor and delivery; consists of four united bones (two hip or innominate bones, the sacrum, and the coccyx) between the trunk and the thighs

         a) Pelvic types

            i. Gynecoid—classic female pelvis inlet, well rounded (oval); ideal for delivery

            ii. Android—resembling a male pelvis, narrow and heart-shaped; usually requires cesarean section or difficult forceps delivery

        iii. Platypelloid—flat, broad pelvis; usually not adequate for vaginal delivery

        iv. Anthropoid—similar to pelvis of anthropoid ape; long, deep, and narrow; usually adequate for vaginal delivery

    b) Measurements—may be obtained by internal and external pelvic examination (using a pelvimeter), x-ray pelvimetry (used rarely in pregnancy and only late in third trimester or in labor), and ultrasound

  6) Breasts—pair of accessory glands of female reproduction responsible for lactation

    a) Externally covered by skin with darker-colored nipple and areola containing Montgomery's glands that lubricate the nipples

    b) Internally contain the alveoli that produce the colostrum (premilk) and breast milk late in pregnancy and after delivery, as well as lactiferous or mammary ducts to eject the milk

2. Physiology

  a. Menstrual cycle—four phases (dates assume a 28-d cycle):

    1) Menstrual phase (day 1 to 5)—degeneration and discharge of most of endometrium if conception does not occur

    2) Proliferative phase (day 6 to 14)—graafian follicle is approaching maximum development in ovary (follicular fluid contains estrogen, which is responsible for the thickening of the endometrium)

    3) Secretory/luteal phase (day 14 to 28)—corpus luteum secretes progesterone, which changes the character of the uterine lining to prepare for implantation of fertilized ovum

    4) Ischemic phase—occurs if fertilization does not occur; corpus luteum degenerates; decrease in estrogen and progesterone levels; menstrual flow begins

  b. Hormonal control of menstrual cycle—pituitary gland

    1) Anterior lobe: follicle-stimulating hormone (FSH) rises slightly in the proliferative phase until just before ovulation, when both FSH and luteinizing hormone (LH) rise rapidly, triggering the rupture of the follicle

    2) Posterior lobe: secretes oxytocin and causes uterine contractions

  c. Menstrual irregularities

    1) Amenorrhea—absence of menstrual flow when normally expected: may result from congenital abnormalities, physical or emotional disorders, hormonal disturbances, and most often, pregnancy

    2) Oligomenorrhea—scanty flow

    3) Menorrhagia—excessive flow

    4) Dysmenorrhea—painful menstruation

  d. Menopause—cessation of menses and fertility, average age 50 years old

    1) Assessment—may be symptoms associated with hormonal changes, e.g., lighter or heavier flow before cessation, hot flashes and night sweats, emotional disturbances, atrophy of genitals, and decreased bladder support

    2) Management—estrogen replacement therapy (ERT), contraindicated if client/family has history of uterine or breast cancer, hypertension, or thromboembolic disease; Kegel exercises for strengthening pelvic muscle support, supplemental calcium (1 g HS) to slow osteoporosis, regular exercises and good nutrition

3) Complementary/Alternative therapy
    a) Black cohosh
        i.   Relieves hot flashes
        ii. May increase hypotensive effect of antihypertensives
        iii. Do not take for more than 6 months

3. Nursing management during female reproductive cycle
   a. Assessment
      1) Client's understanding of anatomy and the importance of periodic pelvic examinations and Pap smears
      2) Assist with pelvic examination, cultures, and Pap smear—advise no douching for at least 12 hours prior to test, have client empty bladder just before exam, place client in lithotomy position

   b. Interventions
      1) Appropriate information and referrals
      2) Less emphasis on monthly breast self-exam (BSE) but more important to develop breast self-awareness. This involves becoming familiar with how breasts look and feel. Many women do this through performing breast self-exams.
      3) Instruct client in breast self-examination
         a) Perform examination one week after the onset of each menstrual period; if nonmenstruating, a routine monthly time, e.g., the first day of the month
         b) Inspect breasts in the mirror first with arms at sides, second with arms above head, and third with hands on hips, always looking for asymmetry, changes in skin color or texture, dimpling, or retractions
         c) While lying on the back and using a circular motion of the fingertips in a circular pattern around breast and into the axilla, palpate all of the tissue to detect unusual growths
         d) Examine nipples for discharge
      4) Contraception—assess understanding, desired form, risk factors (see Table 13-1)

B. Normal male anatomy
  1. External organs and structures
    a. Scrotum—external pouch containing the testes, epididymis, and vas deferens at a temperature slightly lower than normal body temperature
    b. Penis—organ of copulation composed of erectile tissue; allows for passage of urine and semen

  2. Internal organs of reproduction
    a. Testes—site of testosterone and sperm production; sperm produced continuously from puberty
    b. Canal system
      1) Seminiferous tubules—site of sperm production
      2) vas deferens—sperm storage and transport
      3) Interstitial cells—secrete testosterone
      4) Urethra—passage for ejaculate as well as urine
    c. Prostate gland—accessory gland of male reproduction that enhances the transmission of sperm

Table 13-1 METHODS OF CONTRACEPTION

METHOD	NURSING CONSIDERATIONS
Oral contraceptives—"the pill"	1. Action—inhibits the release of FSH, resulting in anovulatory menstrual cycles; close to 100% effective 2. Adverse effects—nausea and vomiting (usually occurring the first 3 months), increased susceptibility to vaginal infections 3. Contraindications—hypertension, thromboembolic disease, and history of circulatory disease, varicosities, or diabetes mellitus 4. Teaching—swallow whole at the same time each day; one missed pill should be taken as soon as remembered that day or two taken the next day; more than one missed pill requires use of another method of birth control for the rest of the cycle; consume adequate amounts of vitamin B; report severe/persistent chest pain, cough and/or shortness of breath, severe abdominal pain, dizziness, weakness and/or numbness, eye or speech problems, severe leg pain
Hormone injections—methoxyprogesterone estradiol	Injectable progestin that prevents ovulation for 12 weeks. Convenient because it is unrelated to coitus (requires no action at the time of intercourse) and is 99.7% effective. Injections must be given every 12 weeks. The site should not be massaged after the injection because this accelerates the absorption and decreases the effectiveness time. Menstrual irregularity, spotting, and breakthrough bleeding are common. Return to fertility is 6 to 12 months A monthly injectable contraceptive. Similar to oral contraceptives in chemical formulation, but has the advantage of monthly rather than daily dosing. Provides effective, immediate contraception within 5 days of the last normal menstrual period (LNMP) Menstrual periods less painful and with less blood loss Return to fertility is 2 to 4 months
Intrauterine device (IUD)	1. Action—presumed either to cause degeneration of the fertilized egg or render the uterine wall impervious to implantation; nearly 100% effective 2. Inserted by health care provider during the client's menstrual period, when the cervix is dilated 3. Adverse effects—cramping or excessive menstrual flow (for 2–3 months), infection 4. Teaching—check for presence of the IUD string routinely, especially after each menstrual period; report unusual cramping, late period, abnormal spotting/bleeding, abdominal pain or pain with intercourse, exposure to STDs, infection, missing/shorter/longer IUD string
Condom—rubber sheath applied over the penis	1. Action—prevents the ejaculate and sperm from entering the vagina; helps prevent sexually transmitted disease; effective if properly used; OTC 2. Teaching—apply to erect penis with room at the tip every time before vaginal penetration; use water-based lubricant, e.g., K-Y jelly, never petroleum-based lubricant; hold rim when withdrawing the penis from the vagina; if condom breaks, partner should use contraceptive foam or cream immediately
Female (vaginal) condom	Allows the woman some protection from disease without relying on the male condom. The device is a polyurethane pouch inserted into the vagina, with flexible rings at both ends. The closed end with its ring functions as a diaphragm. The open end with its ring partially covers the perineum. The female condom should not be used at the same time that the male partner is using a condom. Failure rates are high with the female condom, at about 21%. Increased risk of infections.
Diaphragm—flexible rubber ring with a latex-covered dome inserted into the vagina, tucked behind the pubic bone, and released to cover the cervix	1. Action—prevents the sperm from entering the cervix; highly effective if used correctly 2. Must be fitted by health care provider and method of inserting practiced by the client before use 3. Risk—urinary tract infection (UTI) and toxic shock syndrome (TSS) 4. Teaching—diaphragm should not be inserted more than 6 hours prior to coitus; best used in conjunction with a spermicidal gel applied to rim and inside the dome before inserting; additional spermicide is necessary if coitus is repeated; remove at least once in 24 hours to decrease risk of toxic shock syndrome; report symptoms of UTI and TSS

METHOD	NURSING CONSIDERATIONS
Vaginal spermicides (vaginal cream, foam, jellies)	1. Action—interferes with the viability of sperm and prevents their entry into the cervix; OTC 2. Teaching—must be inserted before each act of intercourse; report symptoms of allergic reaction to the chemical
Natural family planning (rhythm method, basal body temperature, cervical mucus method)	1. Action—periodic abstinence from intercourse during fertile period; based on the regularity of ovulation; variable effectiveness 2. Teaching—fertile period may be determined by a drop in basal body temperature before and a slight rise after ovulation and/or by a change in cervical mucus from thick, cloudy, and sticky during nonfertile period to more abundant, clear, thin, stretchy, and slippery as ovulation occurs
Coitus interruptus	Action—man withdraws his penis before ejaculation to avoid depositing sperm into vagina; variable effectiveness
Sterilization	1. Vasectomy (male)—terminates the passage of sperm through the vas deferens 2. Usually done in health care provider's office under local anesthesia; permanent and 100% effective 3. Teaching—postprocedure discomfort and swelling may be relieved by mild analgesic, ice packs, and scrotal support; sterility not complete until the proximal vas deferens is free of sperm (about 3 months), another method of birth control must be used until two sperm-free semen analyses; success of reversal by vasovasostomy varies from 30 to 85% 4. Tubal ligation (female)—fallopian tubes are tied and/or cauterized through an abdominal incision, laparoscopy, or minilaparotomy 5. Teaching—usual postop care and instructions; intercourse may be resumed after bleeding ceases 6. Success of reversal by reconstruction of the fallopian tubes is 40- 75%

Table **13-1** **METHODS OF CONTRACEPTION** *(CONTINUED)*

3. Nursing management of male reproduction
   a. Assessment—client's knowledge of reproduction
   b. Teach testicular self-examination
      1) Support testes in palm of one hand and roll each testis between the thumb and forefinger
      2) Best palpated in the shower when cremaster muscles are relaxed and testes are pendulous
      3) Report any changes in color and shape, lumps, or swelling

ASSESSMENT AND DIAGNOSTIC TOOLS—FEMALE

Table 13-2 FEMALE REPRODUCTIVE SYSTEM: DIAGNOSTIC TESTS AND PROCEDURES		
STANDARD TESTS	**CLIENT PREPARATION**	**NURSING CONSIDERATIONS**
Culdoscopy–visualization of ovaries, fallopian tubes, uterus via lighted tube inserted into vagina and through cul-de-sac	Local anesthetic and/or light sedation	Knee-chest position during procedure Position on abdomen after procedure Observe for vaginal bleeding Avoid douching and intercourse for 2 wk
Colposcopy–visualization of cervix and vaginal tissues for color, shape, by a lighted scope	Similar to pelvic exam Performed between menstrual periods Takes 20 min	Lithotomy position Cervix is washed with dilute acetic acid
Laparoscopy–visualization of pelvic cavity through an incision beneath the umbilicus to view structures	Carbon dioxide introduced to enhance visualization General anesthesia Foley catheter inserted for bladder decompression	Out of bed after procedure Regular diet
Cultures and smears–samples of tissues are taken to identify infectious processes or abnormal cells	No anesthetic needed	*Chlamydia* smear needs media preparation by laboratory
Papanicolaou (Pap) Test microscopic examination of cervical cells	no vaginal intercourse or douching 24 hours before test lithotomy position	client in mid menstrual cycle manage discomfot
Biopsy–sample tissue taken to identify unusual cells	No anesthesia May have cramping sensation Expect restrictions on intercourse, douching, and swimming for 3 days	Provide written instructions Refrain from douching and intercourse

A. Culdoscopy–lighted tube inserted through vagina to directly examine ovaries, fallopian tubes, uterus, and small intestines; used to rule out ectopic pregnancy, evaluate ovarian disorders and pelvic masses

1. Local anesthetic and/or light sedation

2. Knee-chest position during procedure

3. Air entering the abdominal cavity during the procedure can cause irritation of the phrenic nerve of the diaphragm; client may complain of severe shoulder pain when she sits up; postprocedure the client should be positioned on her abdomen with a pillow underneath to expel the air

4. Postprocedure–assess vital signs; observe for vaginal bleeding; offer analgesic and/or back rub to relieve temporary discomfort; instruct client to avoid douching and intercourse for 2 wk

B. Colposcopy–colposcope (magnifies tissue) inserted into the vagina through the speculum to observe tissues for color, shape, vasculature, and lesions

C. Laparoscopy—lighted laparoscope inserted through an incision beneath the umbilicus to view structures in the pelvic cavity; done under general anesthesia
   1. A straight or indwelling urinary catheter is inserted to maintain bladder decompression
   2. Carbon dioxide may be introduced to distend the abdomen and enhance visualization
   3. At the end of the procedure, the CO_2 is released and the incision is covered with a dressing
   4. After the procedure, routine postoperative care is provided; client may be out of bed and have a regular diet as tolerated

D. Smears—done to identify infectious processes, the presence of abnormal cells, and hormonal changes

E. Cultures—taken from exudate of the vagina, cervix, or breast to diagnose syphilis, gonorrhea, genital herpes, chlamydia (requires laboratory-prepared media), or mastitis

F. Biopsies—samples of tissue are taken to confirm or locate a malignant lesion
   1. Cervical—to detect cancer of the cervix
      a. Punch biopsy may be done as office procedure without anesthesia; cone biopsy requires anesthesia in an operating room
      b. Postprocedural tampon for vaginal packing is left in place for 8–24 hours
   2. Endometrial—usually an office procedure with or without anesthesia; afterward the client is allowed to rest until cramping stops and advised to refrain from douching and intercourse until discharge stops
   3. Dilation and curettage (D and C)—cervix dilated and the uterus scraped for biopsy tissue or aspirated for bleeding tissue
   4. Breast biopsy—obtained by incision or aspiration under general or local anesthesia

G. Radiographic examinations—to detect abnormal tissue, presence and position of structures, patency of ducts
   1. Mammography—used to detect tumors of the breast before clinical symptoms appear; no cream, powder, or deodorant is to be used before the test
   2. Thermography—detects changes in circulation in breast tissue: increased heat in areas of increased blood supply indicates a tumor process

PROBLEMS OF THE FEMALE REPRODUCTIVE TRACT

(See Table 13-3)

A. Infectious processes
   1. Vaginal
      a. Simple vaginitis—characterized by a yellow discharge, itching, burning, and edema; treated with dilute vinegar douche, antibiotics, sitz baths
      b. Nonspecific vaginitis (Gardnerella)—presumed to be bacterial
         1) Gray-white discharge with foul/fishy odor; itching; "clue" cells on saline wet slide
         2) May be treated locally with sulfa vaginal cream; more commonly with oral metronidazole, tetracycline (both of which are contraindicated in pregnancy), or ampicillin
      c. *Candida albicans*—overgrowth of vaginal yeast
         1) Odorless, cheesy white discharge; itching, inflamed vagina and perineum
         2) Treated with topical clotrimazole, nystatin, or oral (fluconazole)

      d. *Trichomonas vaginalis—protozoan infection*

         1) Profuse green/yellow/white, malodorous, frothy discharge; irritated genitalia, itching; "strawberry" cervix

         2) Client and partner(s) are treated with metronidazole and advised to use a condom during intercourse; concurrent alcohol ingestion with metronidazole causes severe GI symptoms (disulfiram-type reaction)

      e. Atrophic vaginitis—occurs after menopause

         1) Pale, thin, dry mucosa, itching, dyspareunia

         2) Treated with topical estrogen cream, water-soluble vaginal lubricants, and sometimes antibiotic vaginal suppositories and ointments

2. Toxic shock syndrome (TSS)

    a. Characterized by sudden onset of high fever, vomiting, diarrhea, drop in systolic blood pressure, diffuse sunburnlike macular red rash, later desquamation of palms and soles; usually *Staphylococcus aureus*

    b. Potential involvement of kidneys, CNS, gastrointestinal system, hematological system, and/or cardiovascular system; therefore, early diagnosis and treatment are important

    c. Managed with antibiotics, fluid and electrolyte replacement, education about tampon use

3. Pelvic inflammatory disease (PID)—local infection, usually gonorrhea and/or chlamydia, spreads to the fallopian tubes, ovaries, and other organs

    a. Characterized by lower abdominal pain and tenderness, malaise, fever, leukocytosis, and purulent vaginal discharge

    b. Potential to cause adhesions that produce sterility and contribute to ectopic pregnancy

    c. Risk factors include 20 years old or younger, multiple sexual partners, IUD, vaginal douching, smoking, history of STDs, history of PID

    d. Management includes noting amount, color, and odor of drainage; systemic antibiotics; warm douches to increase circulation and promote drainage; rest and comfort measures; STD prevention

B. Problems related to the breast

1. Fibrocystic disease

    a. Characterized by multiple soft, tender, freely moving cysts that become enlarged during menstruation and subside during pregnancy, lactation, or after menopause

    b. Management includes aspiration to relieve discomfort and instructing the client to report to the health care provider any changes in shape or size

Table 13-3 PROBLEMS OF THE REPRODUCTIVE TRACT		
DISORDER	**ASSESSMENT**	**NURSING CONSIDERATIONS**
Infertility	Inability to conceive after a year of unprotected intercourse Tests include check of tubal patency, sperm Affects approximately 10-15% of all couples analysis	Support and assist clients through tests Allow expression of feelings and refer to support groups as needed Alternatives include artificial insemination, *in vitro* fertilization, adoption
Simple vaginitis	Yellow discharge, itching, burning	Douche, antibiotics, sitz baths
Atrophic vaginitis	Occurs after menopause Pale, thin, dry mucosa, itching, dyspareunia	Treated with topical estrogen cream, water-soluble vaginal lubricants, antibiotic vaginal suppositories and ointments
Candida albicans	Odorless, cheesy white discharge Itching, inflamed vagina and perineum	Topical clotrimazole, Diflucan, Nystatin
Toxic shock syndrome (TSS)	Sudden-onset fever, vomiting, diarrhea, drop in systolic blood pressure, and erythematous rash on palms and soles	Early diagnosis critical to avoid involvement with other organ systems Managed with antibiotics, fluid and electrolyte replacement Educate about use of tampons
Pelvic inflammatory disease (PID)	Local infection spreads to the fallopian tubes, ovaries, and other organs Malaise, fever, abdominal pain, leukocytosis, and vaginal discharge	Managed with antibiotics, fluid and electrolyte replacement, warm douches to increase circulation, rest Can cause adhesions that produce sterility
Mastitis	Reddened, inflamed breast Exudate from nipple Fever, fatigue, leukocytosis, pain	Systemic antibiotics, warm packs to promote drainage, rest, breast support
Fibrocystic changes	Multiple cyst development Free-moving, tender, enlarged during menstrual period and about 1 wk before	Review importance and technique of breast self-exam Provide frequent monitoring for changes Prepare for possibility of aspiration, biopsy, or surgery Diet changes and vitamin supplements Benign, but associated with increased risk of breast cancer
Cancer of the cervix	Early—asymptomatic Later—abnormal bleeding, especially postcoital	Preparation for tests, biopsy Internal radiation therapy Pap smear
Breast cancer	Small, fixed, painless lump Rash, or in more advanced cases, change in color, puckering or dimpling of skin, pain and/or tenderness, nipple retraction or discharge Axillary adenopathy	Mammography screening Prepare for surgery and/or radiation, chemotherapy
Uterine fibroids (myomas)	Low back pain, fertility problems Menorrhagia	Benign tumors of myometrium Size and symptoms determine action Prepare for possible hysterectomy (removal of uterus) or myomectomy (partial resection of uterus)
Uterine displacement/ prolapse	Weak pelvic support, sometimes after menopause Pain, menstrual interruption, fertility problems Urinary incontinence	Kegel exercises—isometric exercises of the muscle that controls urine flow (pubococcygeus, or PC muscle) can improve pelvic musculature support Pessary—device inserted into vagina that gives support to uterus in cases of retroversion or prolapse; must be inserted and rechecked by health professional Surgical intervention—colporrhaphy (suturing fascia and musculature to support prolapsed structures)

Table 13-3 PROBLEMS OF THE REPRODUCTIVE TRACT *(CONTINUED)*		
DISORDER	**ASSESSMENT**	**NURSING CONSIDERATIONS**
Endometriosis	Found in colon, ovaries, supporting ligaments, causes inflammation and pain Causes dysmenorrhea and infertility, backache Most common in young nulliparous women	Advise client that oral contraceptives suppress endometrial buildup or that surgical removal of tissue is possible Inform client that symptoms abate after childbirth and lactation

Uterine cancer	Watery discharge, irregular menstrual bleeding, menorrhagia
	Diagnosed by endometrial biopsy or curettage
		Internal radiation implants:
		  Must restrict movements; bedrest with air mattress
		  Enema, douche, low-residue diet, ample fluids
		  Indwelling catheter and fracture pan for elimination
		  Visitors and professionals wear protective garments and limit exposure time
		  Dislodged implant must be handled with special tongs and placed in lead-lined container for removal; call hospital radiation therapy specialist first
		Hysterectomy:
		  Subtotal—removal of fundus only
		  Total—removal of the uterus (vagina remains intact)
		  Total abdominal hysterectomy with bilateral salpingo-oophorectomy (TAH-BSO)—removal of uterus, fallopian tubes, and ovaries
		  Radical—removal of lymph nodes as well as TAH-BSO
		  Assess for hemorrhage, infection, thrombophlebitis
		  If ovaries removed, estrogen replacement therapy (ERT) may be needed

Ovarian cyst	Pelvic discomfort Palpable during routine exam	May do biopsy or removal to prevent necrosis Monitor by sonography
Ovarian cancer	Family history of ovarian cancer, client history of breast, bowel, endometrial cancer, nulliparity, infertility, heavy menses, palpation of abdominal mass (late sign), diagnosis by ultrasound, CT, x-ray, IVP	Surgical removal, chemotherapy, staging of tumor after removal Foster verbalization of feelings, ensure continuity of care, encourage support systems
Orchitis (male)	Complication of mumps, virus, STD; may cause sterility, pain, and swelling	Prophylactic gamma-globulin if exposed to mumps virus Administration of medications specific for organism Ice packs to reduce swelling, scrotal support, bedrest
Prostatitis (male)	May be complication of lower UTIs Acute—fever, chills, dysuria, purulent penile discharge; elevated WBC and bacteria in urine Chronic—backache, urinary frequency, enlarged, firm, slightly tender prostate	Antibiotics, sitz baths Increased fluid intake Activities to drain the prostate

Table 13-3 PROBLEMS OF THE REPRODUCTIVE TRACT *(CONTINUED)*		
DISORDER	**ASSESSMENT**	**NURSING CONSIDERATIONS**

Benign prostatic hyperplasia (BPH) (male)	Enlargement of the glandular and cellular tissue of the prostate, resulting in compression on the urethra and urinary retention; most often in men over 50 years old
	Dysuria, frequency, urgency, decreased urinary stream, hesitancy, and nocturia; later symptoms may be cystitis, hydronephrosis, or urinary calculi
	KUB, x-ray, IVP, and cystoscopy demonstrate prostate enlargement and urinary tract changes
		Preoperative:
		  Promote urinary drainage
		  Assure nutrition
		  Correct fluid and electrolyte balance
		  Antibiotics
		  Acid-ash diet to treat infection
		Postoperative:
		  Assure patency of three-way Foley catheter; may have continuous irrigation with normal saline to remove clots
		  If traction on catheter (pulled taut and taped to abdomen or leg to prevent bleeding), keep client's leg straight
		  Monitor drainage (should be reddish-pink that progresses to clear)
		  Discourage attempts to void around catheter; control/treat bladder spasms
		  Teach bladder retraining by contracting and relaxing sphincter; instruct to avoid heavy lifting, straining at bowel movement, prolonged travel; inform about potential for impotence and discuss alternative ways of expressing sexuality

Prostate cancer (male)	Urinary urgency, frequency, retention Back pain or pain radiating down leg	Hormonal and chemotherapy; surgical removal
Phimosis	Stenosis of the distal foreskin of the penis, resulting in an inability to retract the foreskin in the uncircumcised male Associated symptoms include urinary retention and balanitis (inflammation of the glans penis)	Physiologic phimosis is present in infants and young children because the foreskin normally is not retractable until ages 3 to 5 years. In adults, phimosis is frequently associated with adhesions due to recurrent inflammation and infection.
Inguinal hernia	Protrusion of a bowel loop through the inguinal ring; usually soft and painless and decreases or disappears (reduces) with gentle pressure	With the client in the supine position, gentle pressure on the visible hernia causes the bowel loop to return to the abdominal cavity. Direct assessment of an inguinal hernia requires the examiner to insert a finger into the inguinal canal and ask the client to strain or cough, causing the bowel loop to be palpable. Hernias that fail to reduce require immediate medical attention.
Varicocele	Abnormal dilation and tortuosity of the veins along the spermatic cord Client may complain of a pulling sensation, dull ache, or scrotal pain. The veins above the testis may be palpated as a thickened area in the scrotum	Cause is often multifactorial, but is thought to be caused by differences in venous drainage between the right and left sides. Most commonly affects boys and young men, and most often on the left side. Is a cause of male infertility because of increased testicular pressure.
Testicular cancer	Painless testicular mass discovered by the client on self-examination or by the sexual partner. If pain is an initial symptom, usually indicates that the mass has caused bleeding within the testicle or has caused testicular torsion.	Most common malignancy in men 20 to 34 years of age. Those at greatest risk have a history of undescended testicle(s) at birth (cryptorchidism). Teaching and practice of testicular self-examination (TSE) is critically important in early detection.

2. Hypoplasia or hyperplasia of the breast—may affect a woman's self-concept; cosmetic surgery may be done to increase or reduce breast size
    a. Augmentation mammoplasty—inserts are placed under breast tissue
    b. Reduction mammoplasty—excessive tissue removed and the nipple is relocated

3. Mastitis—infection of the breast (occurring most often during lactation) caused by inadequate cleanliness of the breast, infection in the infant, blood-borne infections, or plugged lactiferous ducts

    a. Characterized by reddened, inflamed, and tender breasts; exudate from the nipple; fever, fatigue, leukocytosis; and pain from stagnation of milk

    b. Management includes administering systemic antibiotics, warm packs to promote drainage, and instructing the client to wear a brassiere to support the breasts

4. Cancer of the breast—rapidly growing tumor

    a. Assessment—small, immobile, painless lump; rash, or in more advanced cases, change in color, puckering or dimpling of skin, pain and/or tenderness, nipple retraction or discharge; axillary adenopathy; detection by mammography

    b. Risk factors include family history of mother, sister, or daughter developing premenopausal breast cancer; age greater than 50; menses beginning age less than 12; no children; first pregnancy occurs age greater than 30; menopause age greater than 55

    c. May be managed by surgery, radiation therapy, and/or chemotherapy

    d. Types of mastectomies

      1) Partial (lumpectomy)—removal of involved tissue while preserving contour and muscle function; usually followed by radiation

      2) Subcutaneous (adenomastectomy)—removal of breast tissue but skin and nipple remain intact; used with premalignant lesions

      3) Simple—removal of the entire breast; a skin flap may be left for cosmetic reconstruction

      4) Radical—removal of the breast as well as the major and minor pectoral muscles, all lymph nodes, fat, and fascia; a skin graft may be used to cover the area

      5) Modified radical—removal of all of above, except the major and minor pectoral muscles

      6) Extended radical—the chest wall is resected, as well as all of above

      7) Superradical—the sternum is split and lymph nodes are dissected from the mediastinum

    e. Nursing care in addition to routine postop care:

      1) Inspect dressing and incision for bleeding

      2) To prevent lymphedema (pooling of lymph circulation in involved arm), elevate it on a pillow, turn client to back and unaffected side; avoid constricting clothing and using the arm for blood pressure measurement, IVs, injections, blood draws

      3) To prevent muscle contractures, encourage an exercise program with gradual progression from those that do not stress the incision to adduction and external rotation

      4) Promote acceptance of new body image by providing emotional support

C. Problems of the uterus

  1. Fibroids (myomas)—benign tumors on the myometrium

    a. Assessment—backache, constipation, menorrhagia, and pain

    b. May predispose to uterine cancer

    c. Management includes hysterectomy (surgical removal of the uterus) or myomectomy (partial resection of the uterus)

  2. Uterine displacements—caused by weakening of pelvic muscles; may be retrograde (retroversion and/or retroflexion) or forward displacement (anteversion and/or anteflexion)

    a. Assessment—discomfort, dysmenorrhea

    b. May contribute to infertility

    c. Management includes muscle-strengthening exercises, insertion of a pessary, or surgery to shorten the muscles

3. Uterine prolapse—collapse of the uterus into the vagina due to weakened pelvic musculature

    a. Assessment—urinary incontinence, retention, constipation, backache, and vaginal discharge

    b. Management by insertion of a pessary or by surgical removal of the uterus

4. Cancer of the cervix—malignant tumor cells invade the cervix

    a. Assessment—often asymptomatic; with invasion, the primary sign is painless vaginal bleeding, later a watery, foul-smelling discharge progressively becomes darker; irregular menstrual bleeding, and menorrhagia, confirmed positive Pap smear and positive cervical biopsy

    b. Risk factors include family history of mother, sister, or daughter developing premenopausal breast cancer; age greater than 50 years; menses begin before age 12; no children or first pregnancy occurs after age 30; menopause after age 55; human papilloma virus (HPV) infection, multiple sex partners

    c. Loop electrosurgical excision procedure (LEEP); laser therapy, cryotherapy, conization

    d. Managed by intravaginal radiation implants to deter tumor growth and metastatic invasion or by hysterectomy

    e. Types of hysterectomy

        1) Subtotal—removal of the fundus only

        2) Total—removal of the uterus (vagina remains intact)

        3) Panhysterosalpingo-oophorectomy—removal of the uterus, fallopian tubes, and ovaries

        4) Radical—removal of the lymph nodes in addition to the uterus, fallopian tubes, and ovaries

    f. Nursing care—appropriate for internal radiation therapy or routine preoperative and postoperative care of client with malignancy

5. Uterine (endometrial) cancer—slowly growing malignancy most often occurring postmenopausally

    a. Assessment—usually asymptomatic during early development; primary symptom is postmenopausal vaginal bleeding, followed by low pelvic and lower back pain, palpable uterine mass; diagnosis by endometrial biopsy

    b. Risk factors include age greater than 55, postmenopausal bleeding, obesity, diabetes mellitus, hypertension, unopposed estrogen-replacement therapy

    c. Management includes internal and sometimes external radiation therapy; surgery (see cancer of the cervix); chemotherapy in advanced cases, hormonal therapy

D. Problems related to the ovaries

1. Ovarian cysts—benign tumors (rare after menopause); may or may not be painful; surgical removal may be recommended during fertile years for cysts larger than 8 cm

2. Ovarian cancer—leading cause of death from female reproductive malignancies because of rapid growth and spread and lack of early symptoms; related to excessive exposure to estrogen

    a. Assessment—family history of ovarian cancer, client history of breast, BRCA-1 and BRCA-2 genetic mutation, bowel, endometrial cancer, nulliparity, infertility, heavy menses, palpation of abdominal mass (late sign); diagnosis by ultrasound, CT, x-ray, IVP

    b. Management—Elective salpingo-oophorectomy, hysterectomy, chemotherapy, staging of tumor after removal

    c. Nursing care—foster verbalization of feelings, continuity of care, encourage support systems

E. Other alterations of female reproductive structures

1. Endometriosis—proliferation of aberrant endometrial tissue in the uterus, ovaries, fallopian tubes, and within the abdominal cavity and vagina

   a. Assessment—backache, menstrual irregularities, and increasing dysmenorrhea

   b. May potentially cause adhesions, which can result in sterility

   c. Management includes hormonal contraceptives (ovulation is the stimulus for the proliferation of tissue), NSAIDs, GnRH agonists (e.g., leuprolide)

2. Cancer of the vulva—rarely occurring tumor

3. Cystocele—protrusion of the bladder through the vaginal wall

   a. Assessment—interference with voiding and stress incontinence

   b. Management includes Kegel's exercises; surgery (anterior colporrhaphy) to surgically shorten the muscles that support the bladder

4. Rectocele—protrusion of the rectum through the vaginal wall characterized by rectal pressure, heaviness, and hemorrhoids; kegel exercises; pelvic support with pessaries; surgical repair

ASSESSMENT AND DIAGNOSTIC TOOLS—MALE

A. Cystoscopy—insertion of a lighted cystoscope through the urethra to the bladder; used to visualize the prostate and bladder; to remove tumors, stones, prostate tissue; to implant radium

1. Pretest nursing care—routine preop care; may be general anesthesia requiring client NPO or local anesthesia

2. Post-test nursing care—monitor I and O and vital signs (VS); check for more than pink-tinged hematuria and large clots; provide warm sitz baths and mild analgesics for discomfort; report signs and symptoms of infection

B. Prostatic smear—detects microorganisms or tumor cells in the prostate: health care provider massages the prostate through the rectum and the client voids into a sterile specimen container

C. Testicular biopsy—to detect abnormal cells and presence of sperm, obtained by incision or aspiration

D. Prostatic acid phosphatase—blood test used to detect prostatic cancer

E. Prostate-specific antigen (PSA)—another blood test used to detect prostatic cancer

PROBLEMS OF THE MALE REPRODUCTIVE TRACT

A. Infection

1. Testicular (orchitis)—complication of mumps, virus, STD; may cause sterility

   a. Assessment—pain and swelling

   b. Management—administration of prophylactic gamma globulin, if exposed to mump virus; administration of medications specific for organism; ice packs to reduce swelling; bedrest; scrotal support

2. Prostatitis—may be complication of lower UTIs

   a. Assessment

      1) Acute fever, chills, dysuria, purulent penile discharge; elevated WBC and bacteria in urine

      2) Chronic—backache, urinary frequency; enlarged, firm, slightly tender prostate

   b. Management—antibiotics, sitz baths, increased fluid intake, activities to drain the prostate

B. Problems of the prostate

1. Benign prostatic hyperplasia (BPH)—enlargement of the glandular and cellular tissue of the prostate, resulting in compression on the urethra and urinary retention; most often in men over 50 years old

   a. Assessment—dysuria, frequency, urgency, decreased urinary stream, hesitancy, and nocturia; later symptoms may be cystitis, hydronephrosis, or urinary calculi; KUB x-ray, IVP, and cystoscopy demonstrate prostate enlargement and urinary tract changes

   b. Management—prostatic massage to reduce prostatic congestion and surgical intervention (suprapubic prostatectomy, retropubic prostatectomy, perineal approach, transurethral resection [TURP], radical prostatectomy)

   c. Medications—5-alpha reductase inhibitor (e.g., finasteride); alpha-blocking agents (e.g., tamsulosin)

   d. Complementary and alternative therapies—saw palmetto extract, lycopene

   e. Nursing care

      1) Preoperative—promote urinary drainage, assure nutrition, and correct fluid and electrolyte balance; antibiotics and acid-ash diet to treat infection

      2) Postoperative

         a) Assure patency of three-way Foley catheter, may be continuous irrigation to remove clots; if traction on catheter (pulled taut and taped to abdomen or leg to prevent bleeding), keep leg straight, monitor drainage (should be reddish-pink initially, progresses to clear)

         b) Discourage attempts to void around catheter; control/treat bladder spasms

         c) Teach bladder retraining by contracting and relaxing sphincter; instruct to avoid heavy lifting, straining at bowel movement, prolonged travel; inform about potential for impotence complications and discuss alternative ways of expressing sexuality

2. Cancer—proliferation of cells originating in the posterior lobe of the prostate

   a. Assessment—urinary urgency, frequency, and retention; back pain or pain radiating down the leg; stony hard prostate with irregularities or indurations by palpation; confirmation by biopsy

   b. Diagnosis—prostatic-specific antigen serum biomarker, ultrasound biopsy

   c. Management—hormonal and chemotherapy (palliative measures to relieve pain and retard metastasis) and/or surgical intervention (removal of the prostate gland and, if there is metastasis, the seminal vesicles and part of the urethra)

   d. Nursing care as appropriate to the management plan

PROBLEMS OF INFERTILITY

Inability to conceive after at least one year of regular unprotected sexual intercourse; may be related to female, male, or most often, to multiple factors or conditions in both

A. Factors in the male
   1. Conditions
      a. Anatomical abnormalities of the penis, urethra, prostate, or seminal vesicle difficulties
      b. Testicular infection (orchitis); varicosities, abnormalities, e.g., cryptorchidism (undescended testicles); retrograde ejaculation; hypospadias (placement of urethral meatus on underside of penis) and/or chordee (painful downward curvature of penis with erection), torsion (twisting of spermatic cord causing ischemia and, eventually, necrosis of testis; surgical emergency)
      c. Illnesses, surgeries, and/or medications
      d. Social factors, e.g., stress, smoking, alcohol, and/or drugs, nutritional inadequacies
      e. Spermatozoal abnormalities
   2. Specific tests
      a. Semen analysis/sperm adequacy—evaluates the quantity, number, motility, and morphology of sperm
      b. Postcoital test evaluates for sperm placement, receptivity of cervical mucus, and ability of sperm to migrate

B. Factors in the female
   1. Anatomical defects of the vagina, cervix, uterus, tubes, ovaries
   2. Endocrine abnormalities, e.g., pituitary dysfunction, deficient estrogen or progesterone
   3. Endometriosis/endometritis
   4. Social factors, e.g., coital problems
   5. Chronic disease states
   6. Immunologic reactions to sperm

C. Specific tests
   1. Basal body temperature and cervical mucus for estimate of ovulation and hormonal assessment of ovulatory function
   2. Hysterosalpingogram/hystogram—x-ray with radiopaque substance to evaluate tubal patency; may be therapeutic by removing tubal obstruction
   3. Pelvic ultrasound
   4. Laparoscopy

D. Nursing management
   1. Assessment
      a. Obtain detailed health, sexual, reproductive, psychosocial, and family history
      b. Assist with complete physical examination
      c. Provide information, rationale, and instructions for the tests; reinforce necessity to comply with scheduled tests
   2. Encourage couple to relate feelings; support groups may be helpful
   3. Discuss appropriate alternatives
      a. Artificial insemination by partner and/or donor
      b. *In vitro* fertilization

c. Adoption

d. Accepting childlessness

SEXUALLY TRANSMITTED INFECTION (STI)

(See Table 13-4)

A. Definition—contagious disease spread by contact during sexual intercourse

B. Overall picture

1. Prevention involves education and contact investigation

2. Measures to control spread include prophylactic vaccine development

C. Signs of sexually transmitted infections

Table 13-4 SEXUALLY TRANSMITTED INFECTIONS				
TYPE	SYMPTOMS	DIAGNOSTIC TESTS	TRANSMISSION AND INCUBATION	NURSING CONSIDERATIONS
Syphilis	Stage 1: painless chancre disappears within 4 weeks	VDRL, RPR, FTA-ABS, MHA-TP (to confirm syphilis when VDRL and RPR are positive) Darkfield microscopy	Mucous membrane or skin; congenital; kissing, sexual contact 10-90 days	Prevention—condoms Treat with penicillin G IM
	Stage 2: copper-colored rash on palms and soles; low-grade fever			For PCN allergy—erythromycin for 10-15 days Ceftriaxone and tetracyclines (nonpregnant females)
	Stage 3: cardiac and CNS dysfunction			Retest for cure Abstinence from sexual activity until treatment complete Reportable disease
Gonorrhea	Thick discharge from vagina or urethra Frequently asymptomatic in females If female has symptoms, usually has purulent discharge, dysuria, and dyspareunia (painful intercourse) Symptoms in male include painful urination and a yellow-green discharge	Culture of discharge from cervix or urethra Positive results for other STD diagnostic tests	Mucous membrane or skin; congenital; vaginal, orogenital, anogenital sexual activity 2–7 days	IM ceftriaxone 1 time and PO doxycycline BID for 1 week; azithromycin IM aqueous penicillin with PO probenecid (to delay penicillin urinary excretion) PO azithromycin or doxycycline is used to treat chlamydia, which coexists in 45% of cases Spectinomycin if allergy to ceftriaxone Monitor for complications, pelvic inflammatory disease

Table 13-4 SEXUALLY TRANSMITTED INFECTIONS *(CONTINUED)*				
TYPE	SYMPTOMS	DIAGNOSTIC TESTS	TRANSMISSION AND INCUBATION	NURSING CONSIDERATIONS
Genital Herpes (HSV-2)	Painful vesicular genital lesions Difficulty voiding Recurrence in times of stress, infection, menses	Direct examination of cells HSV antibodies	Mucous membrane or skin; congenital Virus can survive on objects such as towels 3–14 days	Acyclovir (not cure) Emotional support Sitz baths Local medication Notification of contacts Monitor Pap smears on regular basis—increased incidence of cancer of cervix Precautions about vaginal delivery
Chlamydia	Men—dysuria, frequent urination, watery discharge Women—may be asymptomatic, thick discharge with acrid odor, pelvic pain, yellow-colored discharge; painful menses	Direct examination of cells Enzyme-linked ELISA	Mucous membrane; sexual contact 1–3 weeks	Notification of contacts May cause sterility Treat with azithromycin, doxycycline, erythromycin
Condylomata acuminata (genital warts)	Initially single, small papillary lesion spreads into large cauliflowerlike cluster on perineum and/or vagina or penis; may be itching/burning	Direct exam Biopsy HPV	Majority due to human papilloma virus (HPV) Mucous membrane; sexual contact; congenital 1–3 months	Curettage, cryotherapy with liquid nitrogen or podophyllin resin Kerotolytic agents Avoid intimate sexual contact until lesions are healed Strong association with incidence of genital dysplasia and cervical carcinoma Atypical, pigmented, or persistent warts should be biopsied Notify contacts

CHILDBEARING—ANTEPARTAL CARE

FERTILIZATION–union of ovum and spermatozoon

A. Cells of the human body develop from chromosomes

1. Normal human cell tissue contains 46 chromosomes—22 pairs of homologous autosomes (any chromosome other than a sex chromosome) and one pair of sex chromosomes; one chromosome of each pair of chromosomes is received from the mother and the other one from the father

2. Sex determination occurs at the moment of conception as a result of the sex chromosome contributed by the male; an X-carrying sperm fertilizing the ovum produces a female (XX), a Y-carrying sperm produces a male (XY)

3. Aberrations in the number of chromosomes result in abnormal offspring or spontaneous abortion

B. Process of fertilization (conception)—only one sperm penetrates ovum

1. Usually occurs in the outer third of the fallopian tube

2. Implantation usually occurs in the upper part of the uterus about 7–10 days after fertilization when the developing zygote burrows into the endometrium, which has undergone changes to provide for its nourishment and is now called the decidua

3. There are 3 groups of cells in the developing embryo:

   a. Outer layer (ectoderm)—develops into the following structures: hair, nails, sebaceous glands, sweat glands, epithelium of nasal and oral passages

   b. Middle layer (mesoderm)—develops into the following structures: muscles, bones, sexual structures, heart, kidneys, teeth dentin

   c. Inner layer (endoderm)—develops into the following: epithelium of digestive tract, respiratory tract, bladder

STRUCTURES OF PREGNANCY

A. Fetal membranes—2 layers

1. Amnion—the smooth, slippery membrane enclosing the fluid-filled space that develops around the embryo (the "bag of waters") wherein the fetus floats and moves

   a. Fluid functions to maintain fetal temperature and cushion the fetus from injury

   b. At full term, contains about 500 to 1,000 mL of clear, slightly yellowish liquid with a characteristic but not foul odor; later in the pregnancy, fetus contributes to the fluid through urine excretion and absorbs from it by swallowing; hydramnios or polyhydramnios (greater than 2,000 mL) or oligohydramnios (less than 500 mL) indicate an abnormal process

2. Chorion—the outer membrane that gives rise to the placenta, which is formed by the union of chorionic villi and decidua basalis

B. The umbilical cord—connects the placenta and the fetus; is about 20 inches in length and about 3/4 of an inch in diameter; contains two arteries and one large vein

C. Placenta—organ of pregnancy that permits an exchange across two closed vascular systems by diffusion, active transport, pinocytosis, and leakage (which allows for a slight mixing of blood)

1. Functions

   a. Transfers nutrients from maternal bloodstream by a number of mechanisms

      b. Transfer of oxygen from mother to fetus by diffusion

      c. Removes waste products of fetal metabolism into mother's bloodstream, from which these will be excreted

      d. Produces hormones of pregnancy

         1) Early in pregnancy, the human chorionic gonadotropin supports the corpus luteum in the continued production of progesterone and estrogen necessary for the maintenance of the secretory phase of the endometrium

         2) After the second month of pregnancy, the placenta takes over the production of estrogen and progesterone from the ovaries

         3) High levels of estrogen and progesterone during gestation also function to suppress the secretion of prolactin from the anterior pituitary gland, thereby delaying the onset of lactation until after delivery of the placenta, when the estrogen and progesterone levels drop significantly

      e. Passes antibodies to fetus from mother

      f. Provides a barrier to some but not all harmful substances; microorganisms, especially viruses, and medications may cross

  2. Perfusion (blood flow) is influenced by:

      a. Maternal BP

      b. Condition of maternal blood vessels

      c. Uterine contractions have inhibiting effect

      d. Maternal position, i.e., in supine position the gravid uterus compresses the inferior vena cava and descending aorta, causing reduced venous return and cardiac output, which may cause hypotension and decreased blood flow to the brain (dizziness, pallor, clamminess), the kidneys, and placenta (decreased fetal heart rate); corrected by left side-lying

FETAL DEVELOPMENT

(See Table 13-5)

A. Stages

  1. Ovum (10–14 d)—implantation

      a. HCG is secreted by cells of chorionic villi to ensure continued estrogen and progesterone secretion; progesterone is absolutely necessary for implantation and maintenance of decidua

      b. Possible abnormal events

         1) Spontaneous abortion/ectopic pregnancy

         2) Maternal infection (e.g., rubella), resulting in multiple anomalies

         3) Genetic defects before 3 wk may result in spontaneous abortion

Table 13-5 FETAL DEVELOPMENT		
AGE	SIZE	DEVELOPMENTAL FACTORS
4 wk	0.25 in	Recognizable traces of all organs; heart formed and beating; backbone bent with head touching tip of tail
8 wk	1 in	Head very large in proportion to rest of body; some discernible facial features Tail less prominent Some movement
12 wk	3 in 1–1.6 oz	All organ systems are formed Well-differentiated genitals; rudimentary kidneys that secrete urine Able to suck and swallow
16 wk	6 in 4 oz	External genitalia obvious; able to distinguish sex; meconium in bowel
20 wk	10 in 10 oz	Fetal heartbeat can be heard; fetal movement should be felt by mother Fine hairs over body (lanugo)
24 wk	12 in 1.5 lb	Skin red, wrinkled, little fat Body well proportioned and covered with vernix caseosa
28 wk	14–15 in 2.5 lb	Skin is wrinkled If born at this time, may survive with respiratory support and intensive care
32 wk	16.5 in	Most infants would survive if born; may need support for respiratory system
36 wk	16–19 in 5.5–6 lb	Lanugo disappearing Deposits of subcutaneous fat Chances of survival good; may require some special care
40 wk	20 in 6.5–7.5 lb	Full term; full development Most lanugo has disappeared; vernix caseosa only in skin creases and folds

2. Embryo (13 days through 8 wk)—organ development
   a. Cell growth and tissue differentiation, resulting in formation of all body systems
   b. Possible abnormal events
      1) Time of highest mortality
      2) Malformations related to genetic defects, poor maternal health, teratogens (nongenetic factors that can cause fetal malformations)

3. Fetus (9 wk to term)—refinement of organ systems
   a. Growth in body size and organ maturity
   b. Possible abnormal events
      1) Preterm delivery (before 38 wk)—prognosis dependent on CNS maturity to maintain body temperature and respirations, lung development, and availability of clinical technology
      2) Intrauterine growth restriction (IUGR) or small for gestational age (SGA)
      3) Poor organ system development

MATERNAL ADAPTATIONS IN PREGNANCY

A. Anatomical

1. Uterus—changes in size, structure, and position to become a thin-walled, muscular abdominal organ capable of containing the fetus, placenta, and amniotic fluid

   a. In the early months of pregnancy, growth is partly due to formation of new muscle fibers and enlargement of preexisting muscle fibers

   b. After the first trimester, the increase in size is partly mechanical due to the pressure of the developing fetus

   c. The full-term pregnant uterus and its contents weigh about 12 lb

2. Cervix—undergoes increased blood supply, edema, and hyperplasia of the cervical glands contributing to:

   a. Softening (Goodell's sign) about 6 wk

   b. A blue-violet color (Chadwick's sign) about 6–8 wk

   c. Increased friability (bleeds easily after Pap smear and intercourse)

   d. Distention of cervical mucosa glands with mucus, creating a tenacious "mucous plug" that seals the endocervical canal and inhibiting the ascent of bacteria and other substances into the uterus

3. Vagina and external genital organs—enlarge, soften, thicken, and develop blue-violet hue as a result of increased vasculature

   a. Vaginal secretions become alkaline, causing an increased risk of vaginitis

   b. Connective tissue loosens in preparation for labor and delivery

4. Breasts—enlarge early in pregnancy, causing progressive feelings of heaviness, fullness, and tenderness; the nipple and areola become larger, darker in color; blood vessels enlarge and become prominent beneath the skin

5. Body mass—changes with weight gain; total desirable weight gain in pregnancy (for average woman) is about 23–28 lb; 3–4 lb (1.36–1.81 kg) during the first trimester, followed by an average of slightly less than one pound per week for the rest of the pregnancy

6. Skin

   a. Pink or reddish streaks (striae gravidarum) may occur on breasts, abdomen, buttocks, and/or thighs as a result of fat deposits, which cause stretching of the skin

   b. Increased pigmentation can occur on the face as blotchy brown areas on the forehead and cheeks (chloasma or "mask of pregnancy") and on the abdomen as dark line from the symphysis pubis to the umbilicus (linea nigra)

   c. Minute vascular spiders may occur

   d. The umbilicus is pushed outward, and by about the seventh month its depression disappears and becomes a darkened area on the abdominal wall

   e. Sweat and sebaceous glands are more active

7. Musculoskeletal

   a. Change in the center of gravity, decreased muscle tone, and increased weight-bearing cause an accelerated lumbosacral curve, which may lead to lower back pain and difficulty with locomotion

   b. Progesterone-produced relaxation and increased mobility of the pelvic joints may cause discomfort and difficulty in walking

   c. The vertical abdominal muscles may separate (diastasis recti)

B. Physiological

  1. Hormonal

    a. Placental

      1) Estrogen—enlargement of uterus, breasts, genitals; growth of glandular tissue, ducts, alveoli, and nipples of breasts; fat deposition; increased elasticity of connective tissue; altered thyroid function; altered nutrient metabolism; sodium and water retention by kidneys; hypercoagulability of blood; vascular changes

      2) Progesterone—development of decidua; decreased contractility of the uterus; decreased gastric motility (sphincters relaxed); increased sensitivity to CO_2 in respiratory center; decreased tone of smooth muscle; development of secretory portions of lobular-alveolar system in breasts; sodium excretion

      3) Human chorionic somatomammotropin and human placental lactogen; anabolic effect; insulin antagonist

    b. Pituitary gland

      1) Anterior lobe secretes prolactin hormone after delivery of the placenta

      2) Posterior lobe secretes oxytocin during labor and lactation

  2. Blood—total blood volume in body increases during pregnancy by about 30%; normal blood pressure is maintained by peripheral vasodilation

    a. RBC production increases; WBC count increases; clotting factors increase while fibrolytic activity decreases

    b. Hemoglobin and hematocrit levels decrease slightly in response to hemodilution (increased plasma content); hemoglobin less than 10 g/dL or hematocrit less than 35% may indicate anemia

    c. The increased blood volume creates the need for the heart to pump more blood through the aorta (about 50% more blood per minute) resulting in increased heart rate; occasional palpitations (possibly due to sympathetic nervous imbalance in the early months of pregnancy or to intra-abdominal pressure of the enlarged uterus toward the end of the pregnancy)

  3. Respiration—in the later months of pregnancy, the enlarged uterus causes the diaphragm to be displaced upward, putting pressure on the lungs and causing shortness of breath

  4. Digestion

    a. Nausea and vomiting may occur in the first trimester; vomiting that is excessive or persists beyond this time (hyperemesis gravidarum) may require medical management; appetite usually improves as pregnancy advances

    b. Progesterone-induced relaxation of smooth muscle tone, reduction in total acidity of gastric juices, and pressure from the growing uterus may cause heartburn, flatulence, and constipation

    c. Aversions or cravings for certain foods or unusual substances (e.g., pica) may occur

    d. Carbohydrate metabolism is profoundly affected to meet growth and development needs of fetus and the metabolic needs of mother to support tissue expansion

    1) The first half of pregnancy
- a) Maternal glucose is moved across the placenta by active transport; causing maternal glucose levels to fall slightly; her pancreas responds by decreasing production of insulin
- b) Maternal insulin does not cross the placenta
- c) By 8 wk the fetus's own insulin production is consistent with the amount of glucose received from the mother

    2) The second half of pregnancy—the placental hormones impede the mother's ability to utilize insulin; the resulting demand for added insulin can be met by a normally functioning pancreas

5. Urinary system
   a. Urinary output is increased and has a low specific gravity; possible tendency to excrete glucose; reabsorption of sodium and decreased water output (latter half of pregnancy) is a compensatory mechanism to maintain increased blood volume
   b. Ureters become dilated (especially the right ureter) due to the pressure of the enlarged uterus; the dilated ureters are unable to propel urine as efficiently, resulting in stasis of urine and possible urinary tract infection
   c. Bladder—urinary frequency may occur early in pregnancy and later again when "lightening" occurs, result of increased pressure on the bladder from the enlarged uterus

C. Psychological
1. First trimester—maternal ambivalence, even in planned pregnancy, is usual; there may be some anticipation and concern related to fears and fantasies about the pregnancy
2. Second trimester—usually increased maternal feelings of physical and emotional well-being; mother is often described as self-absorbed and introverted
3. Third trimester—possible new fears related to labor and delivery and fantasies about the appearance of the baby; feelings of awkwardness, clumsiness, and decreased femininity related to changes in body image
4. Paternal reactions—may parallel those of mother; some may experience physical symptoms of pregnancy (couvade syndrome)
5. Adaptation of siblings—age and experience related

PRENATAL ASSESSMENT

A. Verifying pregnancy
1. Signs and symptoms
   a. Presumptive—suspicion not proof; predominantly subjective; amenorrhea, nausea/vomiting ("morning sickness"), breast sensitivity, fatigue/lassitude, quickening (maternal perception of fetal movement occurring between 16 and 20 wk of gestation)
   b. Probable—increased suspicion but still no proof; no subjective data; uterine enlargement, souffle and contractions, positive urine pregnancy tests
   c. Positive—definite signs of pregnancy; no subjective data; fetal heartbeat (about 8 wk by Doptone and by 20 wk auscultation), palpation of fetal movement, outline of fetal skeleton by sonogram or x-ray (done only if absolutely necessary late in pregnancy)
2. Pregnancy test—HCG (human chorionic gonadotropin)
   a. Immunologic tests can detect HCG in woman's urine by 2 wk after missed period; cannot measure the amount of HCG; false readings may occur with inappropriate timing, handling error, or some medications

B. Estimated date of birth (EDB) or estimated date of delivery (term pregnancy is 38 to 42 wk)

1. Naegle's rule: add 7 days to the first day of the last menstrual period (LMP), subtract 3 months, and add 1 year, except if LMP is in the first 3 months of the year (EDC = LMP + 7 days – 3 months + 1 year); assumes a 28-d cycle and no recent use of oral contraceptive

2. Measurement of fundal height from the top of symphysis pubis to the top of the fundus with a flexible, nonstretchable tape measure to be used as a gross estimate of dates

   a. Level of symphysis between 12 and 14 wk

   b. At the umbilicus about 20 wk (measures 20 cm)

   c. Rises about 1 cm/wk until 36 wk, after which it varies

C. History

1. Initial visit

   a. Obstetrical

      1) Gravida—the total number of pregnancies regardless of duration (includes present pregnancy)

      2) Para—number of past pregnancies that have gone beyond the period of viability (capability of the fetus to survive outside of the uterus; currently considered any time after 20-wk gestation), regardless of the number of fetuses or whether the infant was born alive or dead

      3) Abortion—pregnancy that terminates before the period of viability

   b. Health factors that may influence course of pregnancy

      1) Past/concurrent illnesses, surgeries, medications (possible teratogens)

      2) Reproductive factors, e.g., menstrual pattern or problems, contraception, infections

      3) Personal, social, cultural, marital, sexual, environmental, educational, occupational, drugs (including alcohol), cigarette smoking, caffeine (coffee, tea, colas), exercise factors

      4) Nutritional—prepregnancy weight (may indicate long-term malnutrition and depleted nutrient stores), recent weight gain or loss (may denote at-risk situation), adequacy of diet, vitamin supplements

2. Interim history

   a. Frequency, intensity, and management of discomforts of pregnancy

   b. Abnormal signs and symptoms or risk factors

   c. Changes in emotional, financial, marital status

   d. Nutritional status

      1) Weight gain should be within expected parameters; based on pre-pregnancy weight

    2) Increased nutrient requirements

      a) Calories—300 kcal/d; may need adjustment for prepregnant under/overweight

      b) There should be no attempt at weight reduction during pregnancy

      c) Carbohydrates—needed to prevent unsuitable use of fats/proteins for added energy needs; important to avoid "empty" calorie sources

      d) Proteins to 60 g/d; additional increase for adolescent/multiple pregnancies; efficient use requires complete protein (contains all essential amino acids; animal sources) or protein source complemented with other protein sources, e.g., legumes, grains, nuts

      e) Iron—to a total of 30 mg/d of elemental iron; usually requires supplement

      f) Calcium to 1,200/d; best obtained from dairy products; if milk is disliked or poorly tolerated, calcium supplement may be necessary

      g) Sodium—should not be restricted without serious indication; excess should be discouraged

    3) 24-h recall/diet diary may be used to evaluate high-risk woman

D. Physical assessment

    1. Initial visit—complete physical exam

      a. Breast exam—nipple formation using "pinch test" in which the areola is pinched gently and pushed in with the examiner's thumb and forefinger; an everted or normal nipple will protrude, an inverted nipple will look flat or turned inward, indicating potential difficulty with breastfeeding

      b. Pelvic exam—Pap smear; culture for gonorrhea and herpes if appropriate; smear for chlamydia; bimanual (palpation of reproductive organs between abdominal and vaginal hands) to establish uterine size, consistency, and contour; pelvic measurements

    2. Routine visits—every 4 wk until 32 wk, then every 2 wk until 36 wk, then weekly until delivery to monitor vital signs, weight, fetal heart tones, fundal height and outline

E. Laboratory screening

    1. Initially and at routine visits, urine dipstick for glucose, protein (pregnancy-induced hypertension and UTI)

    2. Repeat GC culture late third trimester (more often if indicated; based on pre-pregnancy BMI)

    3. Maternal serum alpha-fetoprotein (AFP) at 16–18 wk to identify risk of neural tube defect in fetus

    4. Glucose screening between 24–28 wk to detect gestational diabetes

    5. Rh antibody titers for Rh-negative woman at 24, 28, 32, 36, and 40 wk

F. Discomforts associated with pregnancy (see Table 13-6)

1. First trimester

   a. Nausea and vomiting ("morning sickness") related to altered hormone levels and metabolic changes; advise small snacks of dry crackers before arising, small feedings of bland food, milk; avoid strong odors and greasy foods

   b. Urinary frequency and urgency without dysuria; fluid intake should not be restricted

   c. Increased vaginal discharge; manage with good hygiene (but no douching) and loose-fitting cotton underwear; report signs or symptoms of vaginitis

   d. Breast soreness due to hormonal changes; suggest wearing a well-fitting, supportive brassiere

   e. Headache due to tension from emotional and physical stresses at any time during pregnancy; provide reassurance, suggest relaxation techniques; inform client to report persistent and/or severe episodes

2. Second and third trimesters

   a. Heartburn may be related to tension and vomiting in early pregnancy, progesterone-induced decreased motility and relaxation of the cardiac sphincter, displacement of the stomach by the growing uterus; encourage small, frequent meals and discourage overeating, ingesting fried/fatty foods, lying down soon after eating, use of sodium bicarbonate (would interfere with sodium balance)

   b. Constipation related to progesterone-induced hypoperistalsis, compression/displacement of the bowel by the enlarging uterus, poor food choices, lack of fluids, and/or iron supplementation; advise bulk foods, fruits and vegetables, exercise, and generous fluid intake; avoid laxatives

   c. Hemorrhoids due to pelvic congestion related to pressure from enlarged uterus; suggest regulation of bowel habits, gentle reinsertion into rectum with use of lubricant, relief measures, e.g., ice packs, topical ointments, sitz baths, lying down with legs elevated

   d. Uterine contractions (Braxton-Hicks) due to tension on the round ligaments as a result of displacement of the uterus; instruct client to rest, change position or activity

   e. Backache due to increased spinal curvature; educate the client on the importance of good posture; pelvic tilt exercises

   f. Faintness related to vasomotor lability or postural hypotension; instruct the client to use slow, deliberate movements when rising, avoid prolonged standing and warm, stuffy environments; elastic hose may be needed

   g. Leg cramps related to pressure on the nerves supplying the lower extremities, aggravated by poor peripheral circulation or fatigue; instruct the client to increase calcium and decrease phosphorus intake; encourage dorsiflexion of feet

   h. Ankle edema related to decreased venous return from lower extremities, instruct the client to avoid wearing anything that constricts blood flow, elevate legs when sitting or resting, and dorsiflex feet when sitting or standing for any length of time; medical management if edema persists in AM, is pitting, involves the face, or associated with elevated BP, proteinuria, persistent headaches

   i. Varicosities of extremities or vulva related to uterine compression of venous return, increased vein wall distensibility from progesterone-initiated relaxation, or inherited tendency; suggest elevating legs frequently, avoid sitting with legs crossed, standing/sitting for long periods of time, or wearing constrictive clothing; support/elastic stockings may be helpful

Table 13-6 DISCOMFORTS OF PREGNANCY	
ASSESSMENT	NURSING CONSIDERATIONS
Nausea and vomiting (morning sickness)	May occur any time of day Eat dry crackers on arising Eat small, frequent meals
Constipation, hemorrhoids	Bulk foods, fiber Generous fluid intake Encourage regularity, routine
Leg cramps	Increase calcium intake Flex feet, local heat
Breast soreness	Well-fitting bra Bra may be worn at night
Backache	Emphasize posture Careful lifting Good shoes
Heartburn	Small, frequent meals Antacids—avoid those containing phosphorus Decrease amount of fatty and fried foods
Dizziness	Slow, deliberate movements Support stockings Monitor intake
Vertigo, light-headedness	Vena cava or supine hypotensive syndrome Turn on left side
Urinary frequency	Kegel exercises Decrease fluids before bed Report signs of infection

FETAL ASSESSMENT

A. Fetal heart rate (FHR)—a significant predictor of fetal well-being; should be monitored at all routine prenatal and any acute care visits

B. Fetal movements (FM)—a regular pattern of 10 movements in one hour is a good indicator of fetal well-being; less than 10 movements in a 3-h period should be reported

LABOR AND DELIVERY

A. Critical factors affecting the process of labor

1. Passage (maternal)—size and type of pelvis, ability of the cervix to efface and dilate, and distensibility of vagina and introitus

2. Passenger (fetal)

   a. Size—primarily related to fetal skull

   b. Fetopelvic relationships

      1) Lie—relationship of spine of fetus to spine of mother; longitudinal (parallel), transverse (right angles), oblique (slight angle off a true transverse lie)

      2) Presentation—part of fetus that presents to (enters) maternal pelvic inlet

         a) Cephalic/vertex—head presentation (greater than 95% of labors)

         b) Breech presentation (3–4%)

            i. Frank (most common)—flexion of hips and extension of knees

            ii. Complete—flexion of hips and knees

            iii. Footling/incomplete—extension of hips and knees

         c) Shoulder (transverse lie)—rare

      3) Attitude—relationship of fetal parts to each other; usually flexion of head and extremities on chest and abdomen to accommodate to shape of uterine cavity

      4) Position—relationship of fetal reference point to mother's pelvis (see Figure 13-1)

         a) Fetal reference point

            i. Vertex presentation—dependent upon degree of flexion of fetal head on chest; full flexion—occiput (O); full extension—chin (M); moderate extension—brow (B)

            ii. Breech presentation—sacrum (S)

            iii. Shoulder presentation—scapula (SC)

         b) Maternal pelvis is designated per her right/left and anterior/posterior

         c) Expressed as standard three letter abbreviation; e.g., LOA = left occiput anterior, indicating vertex presentation with fetal occiput on mother's left side toward the front of her pelvis

      5) Station—level of presenting part of fetus in relation to imaginary line between ischial spines (zero station) in midpelvis of mother (see Figure 13-2)

         a) -5 to -1 indicates a presenting part above zero station (floating); +1 to +5, a presenting part below zero station

         b) Engagement—when the presenting part is at station zero

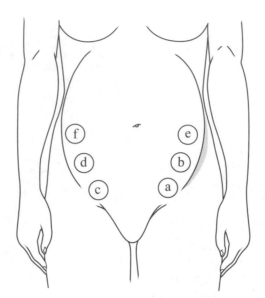

Figure 13-1. DETERMINING POSITION

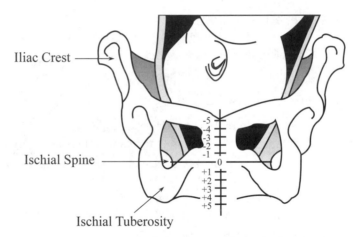

Figure 13-2. STATION OF PRESENTING PART

3. Powers—force expelling the fetus and placenta
   a. Primary—involuntary uterine contractions
      1) Three phases
         a) Increment—steep crescent slope from beginning of a contraction until its peak
         b) Acme/peak—strongest intensity
         c) Decrement—diminishing intensity

      2) Characteristics of contractions
         a) Frequency—time frame in minutes from the beginning of one contraction to the beginning of the next one; frequency of less than every 2 min should be reported
         b) Duration—time frame in seconds from the beginning of a contraction to its completion; greater than 90 seconds should be reported because of potential risk of uterine rupture or fetal distress

      c) Intensity—the strength of a contraction at acme; may be assessed by subjective description from the woman, palpation (mild contraction would feel like the tip of the nose, moderate like the chin, strong like the forehead), or electronic intrauterine pressure catheter (IUPC)

   b. Secondary—voluntary bearing-down efforts

4. Psychological state of the woman—fear and anxiety may lead to increased perception of pain and impede progress of labor; preparation and support for childbirth may enhance coping efforts
   a. Preparation for childbirth education about the birthing process and methods to decrease discomfort and tension
      1) Relaxation of voluntary muscles
      2) Distraction, focal point, imagery
      3) Breathing techniques with each contraction
         a) Always begin and end with "cleansing" or "relaxing" breath (inhale deeply through nose and exhale passively through relaxed, pursed lips)
         b) Hyperventilation—may cause maternal respiratory alkalosis and compromise fetal oxygenation; characterized by light-headedness, dizziness, tingling of fingers and/or circumoral numbness; managed by having woman breathe into her cupped hands or a paper bag

   b. Support person/"coach" should be involved in the formal preparation

5. Position (maternal)
   a. Side-lying enhances blood flow to the utero-feto-placental unit and maternal kidneys
   b. Upright (standing, walking, squatting) enlists gravity to aid in fetal descent through the birth canal
   c. Frequent changes relieve fatigue and improve circulation

B. Cardinal mechanisms/movements of labor in vertex presentation—usually flow smoothly and often overlap; failure to accomplish one or more usually requires obstetrical intervention
1. Descent—progress through the maternal pelvis; continuous throughout labor
2. Flexion—as a result of resistance from maternal pelvis and musculature, the head flexes so that a smaller diameter enters pelvis
3. Internal rotation—head rotates from occiput transverse or oblique position (usual position as it enters the pelvis) to anterior/posterior at pelvic outlet; head is under symphysis pubis and neck is twisted
4. Extension—the head is moved backward as it proceeds under the symphysis pubis and baby is born by extension over the perineum
5. Restitution and external rotation—movement of head to align itself with face and shoulders (restitution) and then rotation bringing shoulders into anteroposterior diameter appears as one movement
6. Expulsion—first the anterior shoulder under the symphysis pubis, then the posterior shoulder over the perineum, followed rapidly by the rest of the body; time of birth is recorded at this time

C. Signs and symptoms of labor
1. Impending—may begin several weeks prior to labor
   a. Lightening—settling of uterus and fetal presenting part into pelvis; sensation of decreased abdominal distention
   b. Increased Braxton-Hicks contractions (mild, intermittent, irregular, abdominal contractions); decrease/disappear with activity

    c. May be heightened anxiety, and anticipation, fatigue

    d. Weight loss of about 2–3 lb 3–4 days before onset of labor; related to changes in estrogen and progesterone levels

    e. Increased vaginal mucus discharge

    f. Fetal movements may appear less active

    g. May be episodes of false labor (see Table 13-7)

2. Onset

    a. Expulsion of mucous plug; pink/brown-tinged discharge (bloody show)

    b. Regular contractions increasing in frequency, duration, and intensity

    c. Spontaneous rupture of membranes (SROM) may occur before or during labor

       1) Check FHR by auscultation for 1 min and with next contraction

       2) May be a gush or trickle; report strong/foul odor (infection), meconium-stained (in vertex presentation, may indicate fetal anoxia) or wine-colored (indicative of premature separation of placenta)

       3) Questionable leakage of amniotic fluids should be tested for alkalinity to differentiate from urine:

          a) Nitrazine tape turns blue/gray/green (alkaline); urine (acidic) does not change the yellow color

          b) A mixture of cervical mucus and amniotic fluid dried on a slide looks like crystallized ferns by microscopic examination

    d. Cervical changes

       1) Effacement—thinning and shortening of the cervix during late pregnancy and/or labor; measured in percentages (100% is fully effaced)

       2) Dilation—opening and enlargement of the cervical canal; measured in centimeters 0–10 cm (10 cm is fully dilated)

Table 13-7 TRUE VERSUS FALSE LABOR	
TRUE	**FALSE**
Cervix progressively effaced and dilated	Cervical changes do not occur
Contractions—regular with increasing frequency (shortened intervals), duration, and intensity	Contractions—irregular with usually no change in frequency, duration, or intensity
Discomfort radiates from back around the abdomen	Discomfort is usually abdominal
Contractions do not decrease with rest	Contractions may lessen with activity or rest

D. Stages of labor

1. First stage (dilating stage)—from onset of regular contractions to full dilation; averages 13–18 hours for nulliparas and 8–9 hours for multiparas

    a. Latent phase (0–3 cm)—the cervix begins effacing and dilating and contractions become increasingly stronger and more frequent; nulliparas 7–10 hours and multiparas 5–6 hours

    b. Active phase (4–7 cm)—more rapid dilation of cervix and descent of presenting part; approximately 3–4 hours for both

    c. Transition (8–10 cm)—contractions may be every 2 to 3 min and last 60–90 s; should not be more than 3 hours for nulliparas or 1 hour for multiparas

        1) May be accompanied by irritability and restlessness, hyperventilation, and dark heavy show, as well as leg cramps, nausea/vomiting, hiccups, belching

        2) Possible rectal pressure creating a desire to push; should discourage before full dilatation because it may cause maternal exhaustion and cervical and fetal trauma

2. Second stage (complete cervical dilation to delivery of fetus)—from complete dilation of cervix to delivery of the baby; averages 2 hours for nulliparas and 20 min for multiparas

    a. Contractions are now severe, lasting 60–90 s at 2 to 3 min intervals

    b. Bearing down/pushing increases intra-abdominal pressure from voluntary contraction of maternal abdominal muscles and pushes the presenting part against the pelvic floor, causing a stretching, burning sensation and bulging of the perineum; "crowning" occurs when the presenting part appears at the vaginal orifice, distending the vulva

    c. Timing of transfer to delivery room

        1) Nulliparas—during second stage when the presenting part begins to distend the perineum

        2) Multiparas—at the end of first stage when the cervix is dilated 8–9 cm

    d. Delivery

        1) Normal spontaneous vaginal delivery

           a) The mother is encouraged not to push as the head is delivered; the neonate cries (or is encouraged to do so to expand the lungs); if the cord is encircling the neck (nuchal cord), it is gently slipped over the head

           b) Episiotomy (a surgical incision of the perineum) may be done at the end of the second stage of labor to facilitate delivery and to avoid laceration of the perineum

        2) Assisted deliveries

           a) Forceps—two double-curved, spoonlike articulated blades used to extract the fetal head; indicated if mother cannot push fetus out or compromised maternal/fecal status in late second stage; contraindicated in cephalopelvic disproportion (CPD)

           b) Vacuum extractor—delivery with use of a suction device that is applied to the fetal scalp for traction; used in prolonged second stage; contraindicated in CPD and face/breech presentation

    e. A difficult stage for the fetus because of possible trauma or asphyxia as it passes through the birth canal

3. Third stage (birth and delivery of placenta)—from delivery of the baby to delivery of the placenta; if more than 30 min, placenta is considered retained

    a. Separation of placenta from the uterine wall evidenced by a change in the fundus from discoid to globular shape as it becomes firm and rises in the abdomen, a sudden gush/trickle of blood and lengthening of the umbilical cord

    b. Expulsion of the placenta through the vagina by uterine contractions and pushing by mother or by gentle traction on the umbilical cord

    c. Contraction of the uterus following delivery controls uterine hemorrhage and produces placental separation: if necessary, oxytocin (Pitocin) or methylergonovine maleate (Methergine) may be administered to help contract the uterus

4. Fourth stage—immediate recovery period from delivery of placenta to stabilization of maternal systemic responses and contraction of the uterus; from 1 to 4 hours

      a. Mother begins to readjust to nonpregnant state

      b. Areas of concern include discomfort due to contraction of uterus (afterpain) and/or episiotomy, fatigue or exhaustion, hunger, thirst, excessive bleeding, bladder distention, parent-newborn interaction

E. Pharmacological control of discomfort (see Table 13-8)

   1. Principles of use—minimize pain without increasing risk to mother or fetus; type of pain relief is influenced by length of gestation, maternal choice, mother's emotional status, response to pain, previous history with analgesics or anesthesia, and general character of labor process

      a. Timing of administration

         1) Before 5 cm (latent phase)—may retard or stop labor

         2) From 5 to 7 cm (early active phase)—may aid relaxation

         3) After 8 cm (transition phase)—may result in respiratory depression requiring resuscitative measures in sedated neonate

      b. Because most medications cross the placental barrier, FHR is taken frequently before and after administration of medication

   2. Systemic analgesia—functions through alleviation of sensation of pain or enhancement of threshold for pain

      a. Narcotics

         1) Morphine—Rapidly crosses the placenta causing decrease in FHR variability

         2) Fentanyl—less nausea, vomiting, and respiratory depression than meperidine

         3) Mixed narcotic agonist-antagonist compounds (butorphanol [IM/IV], nalbuphine [IV/IM/ SC])—analgesia while decreasing adverse effects but can still produce respiratory depression, nausea and vomiting, light-headedness

         4) Narcotic antagonist (Opioid antagonist—counteracts respiratory depressant effects; may be administered to mother IM/IV 5–15 min prior to delivery or to neonate IV via umbilical vein immediately after birth.
Note: Narcotic antagonist given to a woman who is addicted to narcotics may cause immediate withdrawal symptoms.

      b. Antiemetics—used to decrease nausea, vomiting, and anxiety

         1) Hydroxyzine—can increase effectiveness of opioid; decreases anxiety and N/V; cannot be given IV

         2) Promethazine—reduces N/V; can cause sedation; may contribute to maternal hypotension

   3. Local anesthetics—used to provide nerve blockage in specific areas

      a. Subarachnoid block/"saddle block" (nerves from S1 to S4)—anesthetizes perineum, lower pelvis, and upper thighs; diminishes pushing efforts; high incidence of maternal hypotension and potential for fetal hypoxia

      b. Pudental nerve block—local anesthetic is injected into pudental nerves; provides pain relief in lower vagina, vulva, and perineum

      c. Neuraxial analgesia/anesthesia—produces a loss of sensation or, with opioid use, pain control. Does not interfere with the process of labor. Provided by epidural, intrathecal, and/or spinal injection.

         1) Epidural block—affects the entire pelvis by blocking impulses at level of T12 through S5; may be administered continuously through tubing left in place; incidence of maternal hypotension may be minimized if 500–1000 mL of IV fluid is infused at a rapid rate prior to administration and mother is maintained in side-lying position

a) There must be vigilant monitoring of maternal BP and FHR every 1–2 min × 15 min and every 10–15 min thereafter

b) Treatment of maternal hypotension includes

    i. Mild/moderate—place mother in left lateral position, increase the rate of IV fluid; administer oxygen by mask

    ii. Severe/prolonged—place mother in Trendelenburg position for 2–3 min

2) Combined spinal-epidural—provides rapid onset of pain relief; maternal motor function unimpaired

3) Patient controlled epidural analgesia (PCEA)—placement of an indwelling epidural catheter is completed and the mother can control the amount of analgesia provided

d. General anesthesia—used for emergency cesarean births. All agents cross the placental barrier so fetal depression is of concern

Table 13-8 COMMON ANALGESICS AND ANESTHETICS OF LABOR AND DELIVERY

MEDICATION	ADVERSE EFFECTS	NURSING CONSIDERATIONS
Morphine	Hypotension Bradycardia Respiratory depression	Sedates Anxiety relief Pain control Do not administer within 2 hours expected delivery Have naloxone available for newborn
Nalbuphine	Respiratory depression	Causes less N/V for the mother
Lidocaine	Confusion Tremors Restlessness Hypotension Dysrhythmias Tinnitus Blurred vision	Regional nerve block Relieves uterine or perineal pain If subarachnoid space used, keep client flat for 6–8 hours
Opioid Antagonists		
Naloxone hydrochloride	Tachycardia Hypertension Tremors	IV into umbilical vein for neonates ET is neonate in entubated (0.01 mg/kg) Reverses narcotic depression

F. Fetal monitoring during labor and delivery

  1. Fetal heart rate

    a. Methods

      1) Periodic auscultation of the fetal heart by fetoscope (stethoscope adapted to amplify sound) or Doptone (ultrasound stethoscope) during contractions and for 30 s beyond; best heard over fetal back

      2) Electronic fetal monitoring (EFM)—continuous monitoring providing audio and visual recordings as well as tracing strips

        a) External—indirect, noninvasive method using a lubricated (water-soluble gel) ultrasound transducer attached to the abdomen

        b) Internal—small electrode attached to the fetal scalp; indicated for high-risk maternity client, problematic labor, or with oxytocin use; requires ROM, cervical dilation of at least 2 cm, and presenting part can be reached

b. Alterations in fetal heart rate

   1) Rate

        a) Normal—120–160 BPM during a 10 minute period, excluding fetal heart rate measured during a contraction

        b) Tachycardia (greater than 160 BPM)—associated with prematurity, maternal fever, fetal activity, or fetal hypoxia/infection, medications; if continued for greater than 10 minutes or accompanied by late deceleration, indicates fetal distress

        c) Bradycardia (less than 110 BPM)—associated with fetal hypoxia, maternal drugs/hypotension, prolonged cord compression, congenital heart lesions; persistent bradycardia or persistent drop of 20 beats per min below baseline may indicate cord compression or separation of the placenta

   2) Variability—beat-to-beat fluctuations; measured by internal EFM only

        a) Absent (fluctuation range undetectable)—may be associated with fetal sleep state, fetal prematurity, reaction to medications, congenital anomalies, hypoxia, acidosis

        b) Minimal (fluctuation range less than 5 BPM)—loss of the baseline (beat-to-beat variation) or "smoothing out" of the baseline is often a prelude to neonatet death

        c) Moderate (fluctuation range of 6–25 BPM)—normal; indicates fetus is well-developed and oxygenated

        d) Marked (fluctuation range greater than 25 BPM)—causes may be cord prolapse or compression, maternal hypotension, uterine hyperstimulation, abruptio placentae

   3) Periodic changes

        a) Accelerations—elevation of fetal heart rate more than 15 BPM above the baseline lasting more than 15 seconds and less than 2 minutes; reassuring and commonly seen with fetal movement

        b) Decelerations—transient fall in fetal heart rate; classified as early, late, or variable

           i. Early—characterized by gradual decrease in fetal heart rate; nadir (lowest point) coincides with the peak of the contraction; most often uniform mirror image of contraction on tracing; associated with head compression, commonly in second stage with pushing

          ii. Late—transitory decrease in fetal heart rate; smooth and symmetrical decrease; characterized by nadir occurring after the peak of the contraction; return to baseline does not occur until contraction is over; indicative of fetal hypoxia because of deficient placental perfusion

         iii. Variable deceleration—transient U/V/M-shaped reduction occurring at any time before, during, or after contraction; indicative of cord compression, which may be relieved by change in mother's position; ominous if repetitive, prolonged, severe, or has slow return to baseline

      c) Nursing interventions

          i. For early decelerations—evaluate fetal station and maternal dilation and effacement; usually no intervention is required

          ii. For late decelerations (at the first sign of abnormal tracing)—position mother lying on left side (if no change, move to other side, Trendelenburg or knee/chest position); administer oxygen by mask, start IV or increase flow rate, stop oxytocin if appropriate; if the pattern persists, fetal scalp blood sampling for acidosis (pH greater than 7.25 is normal, 7.20–7.24 is considered preacidotic—repeat in 10–15 min; 7.2 or less indicates serious acidosis; prepare for cesarean section)

          iii. For variable decelerations—reposition the mother to relieve pressure on the cord

G. Intrapartal nursing management

  1. Stage 1

    a. Maternal

      1) Monitor vital signs, fluid and electrolyte balance, frequency, duration, and intensity of uterine contractions and degree of discomfort (hourly, at minimum); urine protein and glucose with every voiding; laboratory results; preparedness; ROM

      2) Provide comfort measures—e.g., positioning, back massage/effleurage (light abdominal stroking in rhythm with breathing during a contraction to ease mild/moderate discomfort), warm/cold compresses, ice chips

      3) Support coping measures—reassure, explain procedures, reinforce/teach breathing techniques, relaxation, focal point

      4) Assist support person

    b. Fetal—monitor status

  2. Stage 2

    a. Maternal

      1) Monitor physical status; assess progress of labor, perineal and rectal bulging, increased vaginal show

      2) Assist in techniques to foster expulsion—encourage bearing down with focus on vaginal orifice (discourage breath holding for more than 5 s), position squatting, side-lying, Fowler as appropriate

      3) Provide comfort measures; support coping measures; assist support person

    b. Fetus/neonate

      1) Monitor fetal heart rate and regularity

      2) Provide immediate neonatal care

          a) Mucus is removed by bulb syringe immediately after the head is delivered (mouth before nose to avoid aspiration)

          b) After delivery of the full body, the cord is clamped twice and cut between the clamps

          c) Record time of birth

          d) Inspect cord for two arteries and one vein

          e) Dry and wrap neonate to prevent heat loss

3. Stage 3
   a. Maternal—observe for signs and symptoms of placental separation; assess amount of blood loss; monitor blood pressure, pulse, and fundus frequently
   b. Neonate
      1) Apgar scores at 1 and 5 min to evaluate condition at birth (see Table 13-9)
         a) Based on five signs: heartbeat, respiratory effort, muscle tone, reflex irritability, color
         b) Each sign rated 0–2 (2 is top score); all the scores are added for total score
         c) 7–10 (good condition) should do well in normal neonatal nursery; 4–6 (fair condition) may require close observation; 0–3 (extremely poor condition) resuscitation and intensive care are required
      2) Maintain temperature—minimize exposure to environmental heat loss (evaporation, radiation, conduction, convection); skin-to-skin with mother or at 97.5–99°F (36.4–37.2°C) skin temperature
      3) Weigh and measure neonate
      4) Place identification band on neonate; footprint neonate and fingerprint mother
      5) Record time of first void and stool (meconium) after delivery; monitor physical status
      6) Initiate parent-child interaction
      7) Instill prophylactic eye ointment—legally required to prevent conjunctival gonococcal infection that could lead to blindness in the neonate; 0.5% erythromycin
      8) Administer intramuscular Aquamephyton—for first 3–4 days of life the neonate is unable to synthesize vitamin K, which is necessary for blood clotting and coagulation

4. Stage 4 (see Table 13-10)
   a. Monitor maternal blood pressure and pulse; uterine contractility tone and location; amount and color of lochia, presence of clots; condition of episiotomy every 15 min × 4
   b. Monitor bladder function
   c. Provide comfort
   d. Evaluate parental interaction

Table 13-9 APGAR SCORE			
	0	1	2
Heart rate	Absent	Slow (less than 100 BPM)	Normal (greater than 100 BPM)
Respiratory effort	Absent	Slow, irregular, weak cry	Good cry
Muscle tone	Flaccid	Some flexion of extremities	Well flexed
Reflexes	No response	Grimace	Vigorous cry
Color	Blue, pale	Body pink, extremities blue	Completely pink
TOTAL _____			

Table 13-10 FOURTH STAGE OF LABOR		
FIRST 1–2 HOURS		**NURSING CONSIDERATIONS**
Vital signs (BP, pulse)	q 15 min	Follow protocol until stable
Fundus	q 15 min	Position—at the level of the umbilicus for the first 12 hours, then descends by one finger breadth each succeeding day, pelvic organ usually by day 10
Lochia (color, volume)	q 15 min	Lochia (endometrial sloughing)—day 1-3 rubra (bloody with fleshy odor; may be clots); day 4–9 serosa (pink/brown with fleshy odor); day 10+ alba (yellow–white); at no time should there be a foul odor (indaicates infection)
Urinary	Measure first void	May have urethral edema, urine retention
Bonding	Encourage interaction	Emphasize touch, eye contact

FROM STAGE 4 UNTIL 6 WEEKS AFTER DELIVERY

A. Involution—(uterus reduced to prepregnant size)
1. Fundus—midline, firm, height
   a. Position—at the level of the umbilicus for the first 12 hours, then descends by one finger breadth each succeeding day, pelvic organ usually by day 10
   b. If deviations, check bladder and have client void; if deviations continue, massage fundus
2. Lochia (endometrial sloughing)—day 1–3 rubra (bloody with fleshy odor; may be clots); day 4–9 serosa (pink/brown with fleshy odor); day 10+ alba (yellow-white); at no time should there be a foul odor (indicates infection)
   a. Blood loss greater than 500 mL after a vaginal birth or 1000 mL after a cesarean birth.
   b. Moderate amount of blood flow is greater than 4 inches but less than 6 inches of flow on the peripad within 1 hour (approximately 25-50 mL)
   c. Large amount of blood flow is greater than 6 inches to saturated peripad within 1 hour (approximately 50-80 mL)
   d. Accurate measurement of blood loss is accomplished by weighing peripad

B. Perineum—possible discomfort, swelling, and/or ecchymosis
1. Managed with analgesics and/or topical anesthetics, ice packs for first 12–24 hours and then 20 min sitz baths 3–4 times/d, tightening buttocks before sitting
2. Monitor episiotomy/laceration (see postoperative care)—teach techniques to prevent infection, e.g., change pads on regular basis, peri care (cleaning from front to back using peri-bottle or surgigator after each voiding and bowel movement), sitz baths

C. Breasts—progress from soft to filling with potential for engorgement (vascular congestion related to increased blood and lymph supply; breasts are larger, firmer, and painful)
1. Nonnursing woman—suppress lactation
   a. Mechanical methods—tight-fitting brassiere, ice packs, minimize breast stimulation
2. Nursing woman—successful lactation is dependent on infant sucking and maternal production and delivery of milk (letdown/milk ejection reflex); monitor and teach preventive measures for potential problems (see Table 13-11)
   a. Nipple irritation/cracking
      1) Nipple care—clean with warm water, no soap, and dry thoroughly; absorbent breast pads if leaking occurs; apply breast milk to nipples and areola after each feeding and air dry; apply warm compresses after each feeding and air dry
      2) Position nipple so that infant's mouth covers a large portion of the areola and release infant's mouth from nipple by inserting finger to break suction
      3) Rotate breastfeeding positions
   b. Engorgement—nurse frequently (every 1/2–3 hours) and long enough to empty breasts completely (evidenced by sucking without swallowing); warm shower or compresses to stimulate letdown; alternate starting breast at each feeding; mild analgesic 20 min before feeding and ice packs between feedings for pronounced discomfort

c. Plugged ducts—area of tenderness and lumpiness often associated with engorgement; may be relieved by heat and massage prior to feeding

d. Expression of breast milk—to collect milk for supplemental feedings, to relieve breast fullness or to build milk supply; may be manually expressed or pumped by a device and refrigerated up to 4 days or frozen in plastic bottles (to maintain stability of all elements) in refrigerator freezer for 6 months ideally but up to 12 months is acceptable; thawed breast milk should never be refrozen

e. Medications—most medications/drugs cross into breast milk; check with health care provider before taking any medication

Table 13-11 LACTATION PRINCIPLES	
BREAST CARE—ANTEPARTUM AND POSTPARTUM	INITIATING BREAST FEEDING
Soap on nipples should be avoided during bathing to prevent dryness	Relaxed position of mother is essential—support dependent arm with pillow
Redness or swelling can indicate infection and should always be investigated	Alternate which breast is offered first at each feeding
	Five minutes on each breast is sufficient at first—teach proper way to break suction
	Most of the areola should be in infant's mouth to ensure proper sucking

D. Elimination

1. Urinary—increased output (postpartum diuresis), urethral trauma, decreased bladder sensation, and inability to void in the recumbent position may cause bladder distention, incomplete emptying and/or urinary stasis increasing the risk of uterine relaxation and hemorrhage and/or UTI; monitor I and O and encourage voiding every 24 hours (early ambulation and pouring warm water over perineum); catheterization may be necessary if no voiding after 8 hours

2. GI—bowel sluggishness, decreased abdominal muscle tone, perineal discomfort may lead to constipation; managed by early ambulation, increased dietary fiber and hydration, stool softeners

E. Afterpains—cramps due to uterine contractions; lasts 2–3 days; more common in multipara and with nursing; may be relieved by lying on abdomen with small pillow, heat, ambulation, mild analgesic (if breast feeding, 1 hour before nursing)

F. Rubella vaccine—for susceptible woman; Rho(D) Immune globulin (IGIM) as appropriate

G. Psychosocial adjustment

1. Attachment/bonding—influenced by maternal psychosocial-cultural factors, infant health status, temperament, and behaviors, circumstances of the prenatal, intrapartal, postpartal, and neonatal course; evidenced initially by touching and cuddling, naming, "en face" positioning for direct eye contact, later by reciprocity and rhythmicity in maternal-infant interaction

2. Phases of adjustment

a. "Taking in"/dependency (day 1–2 after delivery)—preoccupied with self and own needs (food and sleep); talkative and passive; follows directions and is hesitant about making decisions; retells perceptions of birth experience

b. "Taking hold"/dependency-independency (by day 3)—performing self-care; expresses concern for self and baby; open to instructions

c. "Letting go"/independence (evident by weeks 5–6)—assuming new role responsibilities; may be grief for relinquished roles; adjustment to accommodate for infant in family

3. "Postpartum blues" (day 3–7)—normal occurrence of "roller coaster" emotions, weeping, "let-down feeling"; usually relieved with emotional support and rest/sleep; report if prolonged or later onset

4. Sexual activities—abstain from intercourse until episiotomy is healed and lochia has ceased (usually 3–4 wk); may be affected by fatigue, fear of discomfort, leakage of breast milk, concern about another pregnancy; assess and discuss couple's desire for and understanding about contraceptive methods; breastfeeding does not give adequate protection, and oral contraceptives should not be used during breastfeeding

ASSESSMENT—PHYSICAL EXAMINATION

A. Measurements at term

1. Weight—6–9 lb (2,750–4,082 g); normal 5–10% weight loss in first few days should be regained in 1–2 wk

2. Length—19–21 in (48–53 cm)

3. Head circumference—13–14 in (33–35 cm); 1/4 body length

4. Chest—12–13 in (30.5-33 cm) 1 in (2.54 cm) less than head circumference

B. Vital signs

1. Temperature

    a. Rectal not recommended as routine because of potential for rectal mucosa irritation and increased risk of perforation

    b. Axillary—97.7–98.6°F (36.5–37°C); thermometer should remain in place at least 3 min unless an electronic thermometer is used

2. Apical rate—100 BPM (sleep); 120–140 BPM (awake); up to 180 BPM (crying); assessed by auscultation for one full minute when infant not crying

3. Respirations—30–60/min; primarily diaphragmatic and abdominal synchronous with chest movements; may be short (less than 15 s) periods of apnea; since neonate is an obligatory nose breather, it is important to keep nose and mouth clear

4. Blood pressure—averages 65/41 mm Hg (arm and calf) in full-term resting neonate, thigh blood pressure may be 4–8 mm Hg higher than arm or calf blood pressure

C. Posture

1. Maintains fetal position for several days

2. Resistance to extension of extremities

D. Skin—sensitive to drying

1. Erythematous (beefy red) color for a few hours after birth; then pink or as expected for racial background; acrocyanosis (bluish discoloration of hands and feet) is normal for 24 hours

2. Vernix caseosa—protective gray-white fatty substance of cheesy consistency covering the fetal/newborn skin; do not attempt vigorous removal

3. Lanugo—light distribution of downy, fine hair may be over the shoulder, forehead, and cheeks; extensive amount is indicative of prematurity

4. Milia—distended sebaceous glands appearing as tiny, white, pinpoint papules on forehead, nose, cheeks, and chin of neonate that disappear spontaneously in a few days or weeks

5. Pigmentation

    a. Slate gray nevus (congenital dermal melanocytosis)—bluish gray or dark nonelevated pigmentation area over the lower back and buttocks present at birth in some infants, (African American, Hispanic, Asian)

    b. Birthmarks

       1) Telangiectatic nevi ("stork bites")—cluster of small, flat, red localized areas of capillary dilatation usually on eyelids, nose, nape of neck; can be blanched by the pressure of the finger; usually fade during infancy

      2) Nevus vasculosus (strawberry mark)—raised, demarcated, dark red, rough-surfaced capillary hemangioma in dermal and subdural layers; grows rapidly for several months and then begins to fade; usually disappears by 7 years old

      3) Nevus flammeus (port wine stain)—reddish, usually flat discoloration commonly on the face or neck; does not grow and does not fade

E. Head—may appear asymmetrical because of overriding of cranial bones during labor and delivery (molding); head lag less than 45°
1. Fontanelles—"soft spots" at junction of cranial bones
   a. Anterior fontanelle—diamond-shaped, easily felt, usually open and flat (may be moderate bulging with crying/stooling); sustained bulging occurs with increased intracranial pressure, depression with dehydration; may be slight pulsation; closes by 18 months of age
   b. Posterior—triangular, not easily palpated; closes between 8 and 12 wk of life
2. Cephalhematoma—collection of blood under the periosteum of a cranial bone appearing 1–2 days; does not cross suture line; disappears in weeks to months
3. Caput succedaneum—localized soft swelling of the scalp often associated with a long and difficult birth; present at birth; overrides the suture line, fluid is reabsorbed within hours to days after delivery
4. Face—symmetrical distribution and movement of all features; asymmetry may signify paralysis of facial cranial nerve (Bell's palsy)
5. Eyes—may be edematous; yellow-white drainage associated with silver nitrate drops (chemical conjunctivitis), which should disappear in 1–2 days without treatment; areas of subconjunctival hemorrhage
6. Mouth—sucks well when stimulated; hard and soft palate intact when examined with clean-gloved finger
7. Ears—tops (pinnae) should be parallel with the inner and outer canthi of eyes; low-set ears are associated with chromosomal abnormalities, intellectual delay, and/or internal organ abnormalities; hearing is evaluated by an arousal response to loud or moderately loud noise unaccompanied by vibration

F. Chest—breast engorgement lasting up to 2 wk may occur in both males and females

G. Abdomen
1. Cylindrical and slightly protuberant
2. Umbilical cord—initially white and gelatinous, shriveled and black by 2–3 d, falls off within 1–2 wk; foul-smelling discharge is indicative of infection and requires immediate treatment to prevent septicemia
3. First stool is dark green or black, and tarry (meconium), passed within 12–24 hours; followed by thin brown-green transitional stools for first 2–3 days; then 1–2 formed pale yellow stools/day with formula feeding or loose golden yellow stools with every feeding for breastfeeding

H. Genitourinary—urine is present in bladder at birth but neonate may not void for 12–24 hours (may be brick-red spots on diaper from passage of uric acid crystals); thereafter usually voids pale yellow urine 6–10 times/d
1. Female—labia relatively large and approximated; may be normal thick white discharge; a white cheeselike substance (smegma and/or blood tinge [pseudomenstruation])
2. Male—testes can be palpated in scrotum

I. Trunk and extremities

1. Arms and legs symmetric in shape and function

2. Hips abduct to greater than 60°; symmetric inguinal and buttock creases indicating no hip dislocation

3. Foot in straight line

J. Reflexes

1. Rooting and sucking—turns toward any object touching/stroking cheek/mouth, opens mouth, and sucks rhythmically when finger/nipple is inserted into mouth (usually disappears by 4–7 mo)

2. Pupillary—constriction on exposure to light

3. Palmar grasp—pressure on palm elicits grasp (fades by 3–4 mo)

4. Plantar grasp—pressure on sole behind toes elicits flexion (lessens by 8 mo)

5. Tonic neck—fencing position; lying on back with head turned on one side, arm and leg on that side of body will be in extension while extremities on opposite side will be flexed (disappears by 3–4 mo)

6. Moro—elicited by sudden disturbance in the infant's immediate environment, body will stiffen, arms in tense extension followed by embrace gesture with thumb and index finger in a "c" formation (disappears after 3–4 mo)

7. Positive—supporting; infant will stiffen legs and appear to stand when held upright

8. Stepping reflex—when held upright with one foot touching a flat surface, will step alternatingly (generally fades by 4 weeks)

9. Babinski's sign—stroking the sole of the foot from heel upward across ball of foot will cause all toes to fan (reverts to usual adult response by 24 mo)

ROUTINE CARE

A. Monitor vital signs at least once per shift

B. Begin and monitor feeding schedule

    1. Before initiating first formula feeding, check for readiness (active bowel sounds, absence of abdominal distention, and lusty cry) and for absence of gagging, choking, regurgitating associated with tracheoesophageal fistula or esophageal atresia by giving a small amount of sterile water (glucose is irritating to lungs)

    2. Because colostrum is readily absorbed by the gastrointestinal system, breastfeeding may be started immediately after birth

C. Umbilical cord care—clean cord daily, following health care provider prescription; no tub baths until cord falls off; fold diapers below to maintain dry area; report redness, drainage, foul odor

D. Care of penis

    1. Uncircumcised—do not force retraction of foreskin (complete separation of foreskin and glans penis takes 3–5 years); parents should be told to *gently* test for retraction occasionally during the bath, and when it has occurred, *gently* clean glans with soap and water

    2. Circumcised (surgical removal of prepuce/foreskin)

        a. Ensure signed permission before procedure; provide pain control during and after procedure

        b. Postprocedure monitor for bleeding and voiding, apply A and D ointment or petroleum jelly (except when Plastibell is used)

        c. Teach parents to clean area with warm water squeezed over penis and dry gently; a whitish yellow exudate is normal and should not be removed; if Plastibell is used, report to health care provider if it has not fallen off in about 8 days

E. Administer prophylactic medications

    1. Eye prophylaxis—0.5% erythromycin or 1% tetracycline immediately after birth

    2. IM Aquamephyton—neonate unable to synthesize vitamin K immediately after birth

CHILDBEARING—MATERNAL COMPLICATIONS

MONITORING FETAL STATUS

A. Ultrasonography—(visualizes the fetus, placenta, amniotic fluid) can diagnose a pregnancy in the first 6 wk and monitor fetal growth and intrauterine environment throughout the course of pregnancy; adjunct to amniocentesis; no known harmful effects to mother and fetus; woman must drink fluid and not void prior to test

B. Amniocentesis—amniotic fluid is aspirated by a needle inserted through the abdominal and uterine walls; indicated early in pregnancy (14–17 wk) to detect inborn errors of metabolism, chromosomal abnormalities, open NTD (neural tube defect); determine sex of fetus and sex-linked disorders after 28 wk; determine lung maturity after 30 weeks

1. Indicated for pregnant women 35 years and older; couples who already have had a child with a genetic disorder; one or both parents affected with a genetic disorder; mothers who are carriers for X-linked disorders

2. Prior to the procedure, the client's bladder should be emptied; ultrasonography (x-ray only if necessary) is used to avoid trauma from the needle

3. Postprocedure, monitor for signs and symptoms of hemorrhage, labor, premature separation of placenta, fetal distress, amniotic fluid embolism, infection, inadvertent injury to maternal intestines/bladder or fetus; Rho(D) Immune globulin (IGIM) is indicated for Rh (–) mothers

C. Chorionic villus sampling (CVS)—transcervical aspiration of chorionic villi that allows for first trimester (8–12 wk) diagnosing of genetic disorders (Down syndrome, sickle cell anemia, PKU, Duchenne muscular dystrophy) comparable to amniocentesis (except for NTD); preprocedure: there should be full bladder; ultrasound is used as in amniocentesis; postprocedure: precautions as for amniocentesis

D. Estriol levels—serial 24-h maternal urine samples or serum specimens to determine fetoplacental status; falling levels usually indicate deterioration

E. Nonstress test (NST)—evaluates FHR by electronic fetal monitor (EFM) in response to fetal movement (FM); as early as 27 wk; woman should eat 2 hours before and may be given snacks during to enhance FM; monitor for maternal hypotension

1. Indicated 1–2 times/wk for high-risk pregnancy

2. Interpretation

   a. Reactive—FHR accelerations of 15 or more BPM lasting 15 or more seconds with at least 2 FM in a 20-min period; monitor NST 1–2 times/wk

   b. Nonreactive—any one of the above criteria is not met; continue EFM and additional testing; immediate delivery may be necessary; report decelerations

   c. Unsatisfactory—inadequate FM despite snacks/gentle pushing baby/vibroacoustic stimulation or unable to interpret data; repeat NST within 24 hours

F. Biophysical profile—assessment of fetal breathing movements, body movements, muscle tone, amniotic fluid volume by ultrasound, and FHR reactivity by NST; with a score of 0–2 for each, 8–10 is considered normal

G. Contraction/stress test (CCT/OCT)—evaluates FHR in response to contractions initiated by endogenous (nipple stimulation) or exogenous oxytocin (IV); after 28 wk; woman in semi-Fowler or side-lying position

1. Indications—intrauterine growth restriction (IUGR), diabetes, postdates (greater than 42 wk), nonreactive NST, abnormal biophysical profile

2. Contraindications—third-trimester bleeding, previous cesarean delivery (C/S) with classic incision, potential for preterm labor

3. Interpretation

   a. Negative—no late decelerations with at least three contractions lasting 40–60 s in a 10-min period; repeat as necessary or in 1 wk

   b. Positive—late decelerations with at least 50% of contractions; potential fetal risk and cesarean may be necessary

   c. Suspicious—late decelerations in less than half of contractions; other testing and/or repeat stress test in 24 hours

   d. Unsatisfactory—inadequate contraction pattern or tracing; continue test or repeat after mother rests

H. Percutaneous umbilical blood sampling (PUBS)—second- and third-trimester method to aspirate cord blood (location identified by ultrasound) to test for genetic conditions, chromosomal abnormalities, fetal infections, hemolytic or hematological disorders

PRENATAL

A. Factors associated with increased risk—lack of prenatal care, age less than 18 or older than 35, conception within two months of previous delivery, fifth or subsequent delivery, prepregnant weight 20% more or less than normal and/or minimal or no weight gain, fetal anomaly

B. Adolescence—may be interference with normal physical growth and maturation, lack of family acceptance or support, isolation from peers, delayed/no prenatal care, and increased medical and obstetrical risks; requires support for feelings, assistance with decision-making, regular monitoring of health status, instruction in nutrition

C. Substance use/abuse

1. Drugs (including alcohol)—may be increased risk of maternal nutritional deficits, sexually transmitted infections (STIs), AIDS, delayed/no prenatal care, withdrawal symptoms, and fetal intrauterine growth restriction (IUGR), anomalies, spontaneous abortions, death, signs and symptoms of withdrawal or addiction in neonate; educate, reinforce, counsel, and/or refer as necessary; emphasize that a safe level of alcohol has not been identified

2. Cigarettes—increased incidence of intrauterine growth restriction (IUGR), preterm births, low Apgar scores, spontaneous abortions, SIDS; as with drugs

D. Infections

1. Urinary tract infections (UTIs)—characterized by urinary frequency and urgency, dysuria, and sometimes hematuria and manifested in upper tract by fever, malaise, anorexia, nausea, abdominal/back pain; confirmed by greater than 100,000/mL bacterial colony count by clean catch urine; sometimes asymptomatic; treated with sulfa-based medications and ampicillin

2. TORCH test series—group of maternal systemic infections that can be transmitted across the placenta or by ascending infection (after ROM) to the fetus; infection early in pregnancy may produce significant and devastating fetal deformities, whereas later infection may result in overwhelming active systemic disease and/or CNS involvement, causing severe neurological impairment or death of newborn

    a. **T**oxoplasmosis (protozoa; transplacental to fetus)—discourage eating undercooked meat and handling cat litter box

    b. **O**ther

        1) Syphilis

        2) Varicella/shingles (transplacental to fetus or droplet to newborn)—caution susceptible woman about contact with the disease and zoster immune globulin for exposure

        3) Group B beta-hemolytic *Streptococcus* (direct or indirect to fetus during labor and delivery)— treated with penicillin

        4) Hepatitis B (transplacental and contact with secretions during delivery)—screen and immunize maternal carriers; treat newborn with HBIg

        5) AIDS (as with hepatitis)—titers in newborn may be passive transfer of maternal antibodies or active antibody formation

    c. **R**ubella (transplacental)—prenatal testing required by law; caution susceptible woman about contact; vaccine is not given during pregnancy

    d. **C**ytomegalovirus (CMV)—transmitted in body fluids; detected by antibody/serological testing

    e. **H**erpes type 2 (transplacental, ascending infection within 4–6 hours after ROM or contact during delivery if active lesions)—cesarean delivery if active lesions

E. Bleeding

  1. Early (before 20 wk)

    a. Spontaneous abortion characterized by painless (may be cramping) dark-bright red vaginal bleeding (see Table 13-12)

    b. Ectopic pregnancy—implantation outside uterus (commonly in fallopian tube), potentially life-threatening to mother

        1) Characterized by unilateral lower quadrant pain after 4–6 wk of normal signs and symptoms of pregnancy; bleeding may be gradual oozing to frank bleeding; may be palpable unilateral mass in adnexa; low HCG levels; rigid and tender abdomen; signs and symptoms of hemorrhage

        2) Necessary to be alert for signs and symptoms—investigate risk factors especially PID, multiple sexual partners, recurrent episodes of gonorrhea, infertility

        3) Management—monitor Hb and Hct, ultrasound for adnexal mass, may be culdocentesis (indicated by nonclotting blood), laparoscopy and/or laparotomy; adequate blood replacement (type and X match, IV with large-bore needle); prepare for surgery; postoperatively, monitor for infection and paralytic ileus, support for emotional distress, Rho(D) Immune globulin (IGIM) for Rh-negative woman

  2. Late in pregnancy

    a. Placenta previa—may be low-lying in lower segment, marginal at border of internal cervical os, or partial or complete obstuction of the os

        1) Characterized by painless vaginal bleeding, which is usually slight at first and increases in subsequent unpredictable episodes; usually soft and nontender abdomen

        2) Management

            a) Hospitalization initially—bed rest side-lying position for at least 72 hours; ultrasound to locate placenta; no vaginal/rectal exam unless delivery would not be a problem (if becomes necessary, must be done in OR under sterile conditions); amniocentesis for lung maturity; monitor for changes in bleeding and fetal status; daily Hb and Hct; 2 units of cross-matched blood available

b) Home if bleeding ceases and pregnancy to be maintained—limit activity; no douching, enemas, coitus; monitor FM; NST at least every 1–2 wk

c) Delivery by cesarean if evidence of fetal maturity, excessive bleeding, active labor, other complications

Table 13-12 CLINICAL CLASSIFICATIONS OF SPONTANEOUS ABORTION		
TYPE	ASSESSMENT	NURSING CONSIDERATIONS
Threatened	Vaginal bleeding and cramping Soft uterus, cervix closed	Ultrasound for intrauterine sac, quantitative HCG Decrease activity for 24–48 hours, avoid stress, no sexual intercourse for 2 wk after bleeding stops Monitor amount and character of bleeding; report clots, tissue, foul odor
Inevitable, if cervical dilation cannot be prevented	Persistent symptoms, hemorrhage, moderate to severe cramping Cervical dilatation and effacement	Monitor for hemorrhage (save and count pads) and infection; if persistent or increased symptoms, D and C Emotional support for grief and loss
Incomplete	Persistent symptoms, expulsion of part of products of conception	Administer IV/blood, oxytocin D and C or suction evacuation
Complete	As above, except no retained tissue	Possible methylergonovine; no other treatment if no evidence of hemorrhage or infection
Missed—fetus dies in utero but is not expelled	May be none/some abating of above symptoms Cervix is closed If retained greater than 6 wk, increased risk of infection, DIC, and emotional distress	D and C evacuation within 4-6 wk After 12 wk, dilate cervix with several applications of prostaglandin gel or suppositories of laminaria (dried sterilized seaweed that expands with cervical secretions)
Habitual—3 or more	May be incompetent cervix, infertility	Cerclage (encircling cervix with suture)

b. Abruptio placentae—premature separation of normally implanted placenta; may be marginal (near edge) with dark red vaginal bleeding or central (at center) with concealed bleeding; life threatening to fetus and mother

1) Characterized by abdominal pain; uterine rigidity and tenderness; rapid signs and symptoms of maternal shock and/or fetal distress

2) Manage signs and symptoms; prepare for immediate delivery usually, cesarean section

3) Postoperatively monitor for complications
   a) Infection
   b) Renal failure
   c) Disseminated intravascular coagulation (DIC)—massive hemorrhage initiates coagulation process causing massive numbers of clots in peripheral vessels (may result in tissue damage from multiple thrombi), which in turn stimulate fibrolytic activity, resulting in decreased platelet and fibrinogen levels and signs and symptoms of local generalized bleeding (increased vaginal blood flow, oozing IV site, ecchymosis, hematuria, etc.); monitor PT, PTT, and Hct, protect from injury; no IM injections; early anticoagulant therapy is controversial

3. Hydatidiform mole—degenerative anomaly of chorionic villi characterized by elevated HCG levels, uterine size greater than expected for dates, no FHR, minimal dark red/brown vaginal bleeding with passage of grapelike clusters and no fetus by ultrasound, possibly increased nausea and vomiting and associated pregnancy-induced hypertension; treated with curettage to completely remove all molar tissue, which can become malignant; pregnancy is discouraged for 1 year, and HCG levels are monitored during that time (if continue to be elevated, may require hysterectomy and chemotherapy)

F. Diabetes mellitus—interaction of diabetes and pregnancy may cause serious problems for mother and fetus/newborn

1. Classification
   a. Type 1
   b. Type 2
   c. Gestational diabetes (GDM)
   d. Impaired glucose tolerance (IGT)

2. Effect of diabetes on pregnancy—long-standing diabetes and/or poor control before conception can increase risk of maternal infections, pregnancy-induced hypertension (PIH), hydramnios (greater than 2,000 mL amniotic fluid) and consequent preterm labor, macrosomia (large for gestational age but may have immature organ systems), and, in more severe cases, congenital anomalies, IUGR, prematurity, and respiratory distress syndrome (RDS) in neonate; untreated ketoacidosis can cause coma and death of mother and fetus

3. Gestational diabetes—usually normal response to glucose load before and after pregnancy; abnormal response is usually noted after 20 wk, when insulin need accelerates, bringing about symptoms; some gravidas will need exogenous insulin but majority are controlled by diet; oral hypoglycemics must not be used because they may be teratogenic and increase the risk of neonatal hypoglycemia

4. Assessment
   a. Risk factors (GDM)—obesity, family history of diabetes; client history of gestational diabetes, hypertension/PIH, recurrent UTIs, monilial vaginitis, polyhydramnios; previously large infant (9 lb/4,000 g or more), previously unexplained death/anomaly or stillbirths; glycosuria, proteinuria on two or more occasions
   b. Diabetes screening—at 24–28 wk for all gravidas
      1) Screen blood glucose level 1 hour after 50 g concentrated glucose solution
      2) Three-hour glucose tolerance test; normal findings: FBS: less than 92 mg/dL (5.1mmol/L) 1 hour: less than 180 mg/dL (9 mmol/L) 2 hours: less than 153 mg/dL (8.5 mmol/L) 3 hours: less than 140 mg/dL (7.8 mmol/L)
      3) If two or more abnormal findings, significant for diabetes
   c. Glycosylated hemoglobin (HbA_{1c})—measures control over the past 3 mo; elevations (greater than 6–8%) in first trimester are associated with increased risk of congenital anomaly and spontaneous abortion; in the last trimester with macrosomia

5. Management—requires close medical and obstetrical supervision throughout the pregnancy, strict insulin regulation to maintain blood glucose levels between 60 and 110 g/dL (3.3–6.1 mmol/L) to prevent hyperglycemia or hypoglycemia, routine home glucose monitoring, regulated physical activity, and diet individualized to diabetic and pregnancy needs

G. Hypertension

1. Preexisting hypertension (HTN)—diagnosed and treated before the 20th week of pregnancy; requires strict medical and obstetrical management

2. Gestational hypertension—characterized by hypertension (systolic pressure greater than 140 mm Hg and/or diastolic pressure greater than 90 mm Hg) without proteinuria after 20 weeks gestation and resolving by 12 weeks post partum; treated with frequent evaluation of BP and protein in urine

3. Preeclampsia and eclampsia

   a. Assessment—increased risk in African Americans, greater than 35-y-old or less than 17-y-old primigravida, multiple fetuses or history of diabetes and renal disease, family history of PIH; prenatal screening at each visit for symptomatology

Table 13-13	CHARACTERISTICS OF PREECLAMPSIA AND ECLAMPSIA				
CONDITION	BP	PROTEINURIA	SEIZURES	HYPERREFLEXIA	OTHER
Mild preeclampsia	Greater than 140/90 mm Hg after 20 weeks gestation	300 mg/L per 24 hours Greater than 1+ random sample	No	No	Mild facial edema Weight gain (greater than 4.5 lb/wk)
Severe preeclampsia	Greater than 160/110 mm Hg	Greater than 500 mg/L per 24 hours Greater than 3+ random sample	No	Yes	Headache Oliguria Blurred vision RUQ pain Thrombocytopenia HELLP (hemolysis, elevated liver enzymes, low platelet count)
Eclampsia	Greater than 160/110 mm Hg	Marked proteinuria	Yes	No	Same as severe preeclampsia Severe headache Renal failure Cerebral hemorrhage

Table 13-14 PREECLAMPSIA AND ECLAMPSIA TREATMENT	
CONDITION	TREATMENT
Mild preeclampsia	Bed rest in left lateral position Monitor BP daily 6–8 8 oz water/day Frequent follow up
Severe preeclampsia	Depends on fetal age and severity Only cure is delivery of fetus (induction of labor) Control BP (hydralyzine), prevent seizures (magnesium sulfate) Prevent long term morbidity and maternal mortality Emotional support if delivery prior to age of viability
Eclampsia (Medical Emergency)	Support through seizures and potential coma Ensure patent airway, O2 support DIC management Delivery of fetus Emotional support if delivery prior to age of viability In cases of severe hypertension, seizures may still occur 24–48 h postpartum; monitor magnesium sulfate or hydralazine if continued postpartum

Table 13-15 HYPERTENSIVE STATES OF PREGNANCY MEDICATIONS		
MEDICATION	ADVERSE EFFECTS	NURSING CONSIDERATIONS
Magnesium sulfate	Flushing, sweating Symptoms of toxicity: sudden drop in BP, respirations less than 12/min, urinary output less than 25–30 mL/hr, decreased/absent DTRs, toxic serum levels	CNS depressant, anticonvulsant Monitor BP, P, R, FHR at least every 15 min; magnesium sulfate levels and DTR prior to administration, mental status frequently; have resuscitation equipment and calcium **gluconate/chloride (antidote) in room**
Hydralazine	Tachycardia, palpitations Headache Nausea and vomiting Orthostatic hypotension	Vasodilator Maintain diastolic BP 90–100 mm Hg for adequate uteroplacental flow; monitor FHT and neonatal status
Diazepam	Risk of neonatal depression if given within 24 hours of delivery	Sedative, anticonvulsant Monitor FHT and neonatal status
Methyldopa	May mask symptoms of preeclampsia; risk of maternal orthostatic hypotension and decreased pulse and BP in neonate for 2–3 days Hemolytic anemia	Used for chronic HTN Monitor maternal, fetal, and neonatal vital signs Monitor maternal mental status
Propranolol	Decreased heart rate, depression, hypoglycemia	Take apical rate before giving Monitor BP, EKG

CARDIAC DISEASE

A. Assessment

1. Chest pain

2. Dyspnea on exertion; dyspnea at rest; edema

3. Monitor vital signs and do EKG as heart lesion (especially those of the mitral valve) may become aggravated by pregnancy

B. Treatment of heart disease in pregnancy is determined by the functional capacity of the heart, and type of delivery will be influenced by the mother's status and the condition of fetus

C. Nursing management

1. Encourage rest and adequate nutrition during pregnancy

2. Encourage moderation in physical activity

3. Explain importance of avoidance and early treatment of upper respiratory infections

4. Be alert for signs of heart failure: increase of dyspnea; tachycardia; weight gain

5. Monitor activity level

PRECIPITOUS DELIVERY OUTSIDE HOSPITAL SETTING

A. Assessment

1. Determine that transport to hospital/birthing center is not possible

2. Evaluate mother's cognitive status and explain actions

B. Nursing management

1. Remain with client; do not attempt to prevent birth

2. Prepare sterile or clean environment

3. Support infant's head; apply slight perineal pressure to control speed of delivery

4. Slip nuchal cord, if present, over head

5. Gently rotate infant externally as head emerges

6. Deliver shoulders, trunk, holding head downward to facilitate drainage

7. Dry baby and place on mother's abdomen

8. Hold placenta as delivered (keep level with newborn heart or tie the umbilical cord)

9. Wrap infant in blanket and put to breast

10. Check for bleeding and fundal tone

11. Comfort mother and family; arrange transport to hospital

CHILDBEARING–NEONATAL COMPLICATIONS

HIGH-RISK CHILDBEARING–NEONATAL

A. Antepartum risk factor

1. Maternal history

   a. Smoking, alcoholism

   b. Infection

   c. Psychosocial problems

2. Risk factors—fetal

   a. Birth asphyxia

   b. Preterm birth (characteristics)

      1) Little subcutaneous fat

      2) Hair—fine and feathery (lanugo)

      3) Poor resistance to infection

      4) Sole of foot smooth and fine

      5) Limbs—relaxed and extended

      6) Weak, underdeveloped muscles

      7) Weak sucking and swallowing

      8) Absorption problems

      9) Ear cartilage poorly developed—ears fold easily

      10) Female—clitoris is prominent; labia majora poorly developed

      11) Male—scrotum underdeveloped; minimal rugae

      12) Immature respiratory system

      13) Potential impairment of renal functioning

      14) Grasp reflex—grasp is weak

   c. Post-term birth—more than 42 wk gestation

   d. Small-for-gestational age (SGA)—birth weight below 10th percentile expected for gestational age

      1) Characteristics

         a) Reduced subcutaneous fat; loose and dry skin; sparse scalp hair

         b) Diminished muscle mass

         c) Sunken abdomen (should be well rounded)

         d) Thin, yellowish, dry, dull umbilical cord

         e) Wide skull sutures (inadequate bone growth)

         f) Chronic intrauterine hypoxia

         g) Large-for-gestational age (LGA)—birth weight 4,000 g or more

         h) Congenital anomalies

         i) Apgar score less than 7

         j) Early or severe jaundice

          i.   Develops in first 24 hours

          ii.   Bilirubin levels above 15 mg/100 mL in a full-term newborn

B. Assessment of problems

   1. Actual and potential problems of high-risk infants

      a. Difficulty initiating and maintaining respirations (preterm, postterm, SGA)

      b. Malnutrition (preterm, postterm, SGA)

      c. Poor thermoregulation (preterm, postterm, SGA)

      d. CNS trauma (preterm, postterm, SGA, and LGA)

      e. Diminished resistance to infection (preterm, SGA)

      f. Musculoskeletal immaturity (preterm, SGA)

      g. Difficulty maintaining renal function (preterm)

      h. Hematologic problems (preterm)

      i. Fetopelvic disproportion (leading to possible birth trauma and asphyxia) (LGA)

      j. Hypoglycemia (LGA, SGA)

C. Selected neonatal disorders

   1. Respiratory distress syndrome—deficiency of surfactant in the immature lung

      a. Assessment

         1) Labored breathing—retractions, tachypnea, expiratory grunting, nasal flaring

         2) Cyanosis

         3) Development of flaccidness, unresponsiveness, apneic episodes

         4) Breathing satisfactory immediately after birth; distress develops 6–8 hours or 2–3 days after birth

         5) Carries highest risk of long-term neurological complications

         6) PO_2 less than 50 mm Hg; pCO_2 greater than 60 mm Hg

      b. Nursing management

         1) Maintain neutral thermal environment to conserve utilization of oxygen

         2) Provide respiratory support

            a) Oxygen therapy

            b) Maintain patent airway with frequent suctioning

            c) Place in side-lying position with roll under neck for hyperextension to facilitate open airway

            d) PEEP or CPAP—keep prongs in place; high frequency ventilation

         3) Provide adequate hydration and caloric intake with gavage feeding and/or parenteral nutrition (if respiratory rate is increased); minimizes risk of aspiration

   2. Perinatal asphyxia—periods of hypoxia during the birthing process

      a. Assessment of problem

         1) Meconium staining

         2) Abnormal respirations with cyanosis and decreased respiratory rate

         3) Possible intracranial hemorrhage manifested by bradycardia, reduced responsiveness, convulsions

         4) Predisposing conditions

        a) SGA infant

        b) Maternal history of heavy cigarette smoking; preeclampsia-eclampsia; multiple gestations

    b. Basic causes of asphyxia

        1) Asphyxia caused by obstructed airway

        2) Nonresponse of respiratory center in the brain

        3) Atelectasis—areas of collapsed alveoli

        4) Respiratory distress syndrome

        5) Pneumothorax or interstitial emphysema—air admitted and trapped between air sacs, preventing full lung expansion

3. Miscellaneous conditions affecting the respiratory system

    a. Agenesis—absence of one part of lung

    b. Diaphragmatic hernia—abdominal organs/intestines push into the thoracic cavity

    c. Congenital malformations of the heart and great vessels

    d. Cysts in the thoracic cavity

    e. Choanal atresia—obstruction of the posterior nares; infant mouth-breathes; may become cyanotic at feedings; surgery may be indicated

    f. Congenital laryngeal stridor—crowing inspiration caused by a flabby epiglottis; severe deformity may necessitate tracheotomy and/or laryngoplasty

4. Cold stress

    a. Assessment of cold stress

        1) Temperature instability to suboptimal levels

        2) Oxygen consumption and energy are diverted from maintaining normal brain cell and cardiac function and growth to thermogenesis

        3) Development of respiratory and metabolic acidosis

    b. Nursing management

        1) Alter environment to increase infant's temperature

        2) Monitor temperature

        3) Observe for signs of cold stress

            a) Mottling of skin or cyanosis

            b) Abnormal blood gases (acidosis), hypoxia

5. Hypoglycemia—blood sugar less than 30–35 mg/dL (1.7–1.9 mmol/L) in term infants (normal 40–80 mg/dL)(2.2-4.4 mmol/L)

    a. Infants at risk

        1) Low birth weight or dysmature infants

        2) Infant of diabetic mother

        3) Infant of preeclamptic-eclamptic mother

        4) Cold-stressed infants

    b. Assessment—jitteriness, irregular respiratory effort, cyanosis, weak-high pitched cry, lethargy, eye-rolling, seizures

    c. Nursing intervention

        1) Perform frequent blood sugar test

    2) Initiate early feeding either orally or with appropriate parenteral fluid

    3) Administer glucose carefully to avoid rebound hypoglycemia

6. Neonatal hypovolemic shock
    a. Assessment
        1) Characteristic symptoms similar to asphyxia except that heart rate and respiratory rate are increased
        2) May be caused by placenta previa, placenta abruptio, or bleeding from umbilical cord
        3) Anemia may be caused by hypovolemia

    b. Nursing management
        1) Monitor vital signs, especially blood pressure
        2) Immediate transfusion

7. Neonatal sepsis
    a. Assessment
        1) Temperature instability
        2) Poor sucking, vomiting, diarrhea
        3) Lethargy, convulsive activity
        4) Lack of weight gain, dehydration
        5) Predisposing factors
            a) Maternal signs and symptoms of infection
            b) Premature rupture of membranes
            c) Prolonged labor or delivery by cesarean section or forceps

    b. Nursing management
        1) Early identification of symptoms
        2) Administration of prophylactic antibiotics as ordered
        3) Maintain clean environment for neonate

8. Hyperbilirubinemia
    a. Physiologic jaundice (icterus)—yellow coloration of skin and eyes
        1) Normal after first 24 hours of life
        2) Caused by infant's inability to clear away waste of RBC destruction previously done via placental circulation, resolving cephalohematoma

9. Pathologic jaundice (Hemolytic anemia)
    a. May appear during first 24 hours of life
    b. Lasts longer than 7 days in full-term or 10 days in preterm infants
    c. Higher than acceptable bilirubin levels
    d. Associated conditions include immature liver; increased rate of hemolysis due to Rh incompatibility; cephalohematoma; cold stress; asphyxia; hypoglycemia; low serum albumin levels
    e. Treated by phototherapy or exchange transfusions

10. Breast-milk jaundice
    a. Presence of an enzyme in milk of some women inhibits the enzyme (glucuronyl transferase) needed for bilirubin conjugation
    b. Occurs in small proportion of infants
    c. Early onset
        1) Onset 2–4 days
        2) Caused by decreased milk intake because milk supply not established
        3) Encourage mother to breast-feed 10–12 times/day; do not give water supplements
    d. Late onset
        1) Onset 5–7 days
        2) Caused by less frequent stooling; possible factors in breast milk preventing bilirubin conjugation
        3) Increase frequency of breast-feeding; no water supplements; monitor bilirubin levels; phototherapy if needed

11. Rh incompatibility
    a. Rh (–) mother produces antibodies against Rh (+) fetal blood cells, causing excessive hemolysis
    b. Mother sensitized during first pregnancy by Rh (+) fetal cells
    c. Mother may receive Rho(D) Immune globulin (IGIM) postdelivery or postabortion to prevent disease in newborn
        1) Rho(D) Immune globulin (IGIM)–Rh immunoglobulin; not useful in women already sensitized and who have Rh antibodies
        2) Given lM, not into fatty tissues or IV
    d. Nursing management
        1) Early determination of onset
        2) Phototherapy with fluorescent lighting–alters the nature of bilirubin to aid excretion (bilirubin excreted in stool); infant's eyes should be covered
        3) Exchange transfusion, if indicated–removes serum bilirubin and maternal hemolytic antibodies
        4) Parental education and reassurance

12. Hemolytic disease of newborn (erythroblastosis fetalis)
    a. Assessment
        1) Jaundice within 24 hours of birth
        2) Serum bilirubin level elevates rapidly
        3) Hematocrit decreased, anemia due to hemolysis of large number of erythrocytes
        4) Coombs' test–detects antibodies attached to circulating erythrocytes, performed on cord blood sample
    b. Causes
        1) Destruction of RBCs from antigen-antibody reaction
        2) Baby's Rh antigens enter mother; mother produces antibodies; antibodies re-enter baby and cause hemolysis and jaundice
        3) Rare during first pregnancy
    c. Nursing management
        1) Assist in early identification

2) Phototherapy with fluorescent lighting—alters nature of bilirubin to aid excretion; infant's eyes and genitals must be covered

3) Exchange transfusion, if indicated—removes bilirubin and maternal hemolytic antibodies

13. Necrotizing enterocolitis
   a. Assessment
      1) Feeding intolerance, bile-colored vomiting, abdominal distension
      2) Blood in stool
      3) Temperature instability
      4) Hypothermia
      5) Lethargy
      6) Onset 4–10 days after feeding started
      7) Diagnostics
         a) Hematest—positive stools
         b) Abdominal radiograph shows air in bowel wall

   b. Nursing management
      1) Stop oral feedings; NPO; insert nasogastric tube; observe for 24–48 hours
      2) Administer antibiotics and intravenous fluids as ordered
      3) Handle infant carefully; avoid tight diapering
      4) Provide caloric needs via TPN or small oral feedings
      5) Careful handwashing

14. Infant of addicted mother/Neonatal Abstinence Syndrome (NAS)
   a. Assessment
      1) High-pitched cry, hyperreflexivity, decreased sleep
      2) Diaphoresis, tachypnea, excessive mucus
      3) Vomiting, uncoordinated sucking, nonnutritive sucking
      4) Drug withdrawal from narcotics, barbiturates, or cocaine; may manifest as early as 12–24 hours after birth, up to 7–10 days after delivery

   b. Nursing management
      1) Assess muscle tone, irritability, vital signs
      2) Administer phenobarbital, as ordered
      3) Report symptoms of respiratory distress
      4) Reduce environmental stimulation
      5) Provide adequate nutrition/fluids; provide pacifier for nonnutritive sucking
      6) Monitor mother/child interactions

15. Disorders of the eye
   a. Retinopathy of prematurity—a cause of blindness in premature infants
      1) Assessment—ensure that all infants born less than 36 wk or less than 2,000 g at birth have eye exam by qualified provider
      2) Characteristics
         a) High concentrations of oxygen cause the premature infant's retinal vessels to constrict, causing blindness

    b) Sometimes occurs when oxygen concentrations are greater than 40% and when used for longer than 48–72 hours in infants

    c) Planning and implementation

      i. Use minimum amount of oxygen

      ii. Monitor PO_2 continuously

      iii. Maintain PO_2 level within normal limits

      iv. Administer vitamin E as ordered; thought to affect tissue response to oxygen

  b. Conjunctivitis of the newborn

    1) Assessment—redness and swelling of the eyelids with exudate from the eyes

    2) Characteristics

      a) Caused by gonococcus organism

      b) Milder form develops from the silver nitrate instilled in the eyes at birth

    3) Nursing management

      a) Observe for inflammation and exudate from eyes 24–48 hours after birth

      b) Observe for purulent discharge

      c) Administer silver nitrate prophylactically as ordered

      d) Administer antibiotic therapy as ordered

  c. Strabismus

    1) Assessment—eyes do not function as a unit because of an imbalance of the extraocular muscles

      a) Visible deviation of eye

      b) Diplopia

      c) Child tilts head or squints to focus

    2) Nursing management

      a) Therapy

        i. Developing visual acuity in both eyes

        ii. Developing coordinate function

      b) Nonsurgical intervention begins no later than age 6

        i. Occlusion of unaffected eye to strengthen weaker eye

        ii. Corrective lenses combined with other therapy to improve acuity

        iii. Orthoptic exercises designed to strengthen eye muscles

      c) Surgery on rectus muscles of eye

16. Congenital malformations of the urinary tract (see Table 13-16)

Table 13-16	CONGENITAL MALFORMATIONS OF THE URINARY TRACT	
ASSESSMENT	ANALYSIS	NURSING CONSIDERATIONS
Epispadias	Urethral opening on dorsal surface of the penis	No circumcision—foreskin used in surgical repair
Hypospadias	Male urethral opening on the ventral surface of penis, or female urethral opening in vagina	No circumcision—foreskin used in surgical repair
Horseshoe kidney	Kidneys are fused at lower poles	Hydronephrosis can develop Surgical correction
Urethral duplication	Two separate ureters from one kidney	Recurrent UTIs Surgical correction
Hydroureter	Ureter dilatation	Urinary diversion is indicated
Bladder exstrophy	Posterior and lateral surfaces of the bladder are exposed; often seen with epispadias	Immediate reconstructive surgery to close bladder and abdominal wall

D. Basic concepts of management (general for high-risk newborn)

1. Resuscitate immediately
2. Provide warmth—use incubator for thermoregulation
3. Support respiratory function
   a. Provide air or oxygen as indicated; use caution with oxygen concentrations above 40% due to risk of retinopathy of prematurity (ROP)
   b. Provide humidity
   c. Suction
   d. Position
4. Maintain fluid and electrolyte balance—administer parenteral fluids, as indicated
5. Meet nutritional needs
6. Monitor infant's condition
   a. Vital signs—temperature, apical pulse, respiratory rate
   b. Intake and output
   c. Skin—color, turgor
   d. CNS symptoms
      1) Fontanelles—bulging, flat
      2) Convulsions
      3) Reflexes
7. Observe for signs of infection
8. Prevent skin breakdown
9. Promote healthy parent-child relationship

E. Absence of complications of oxygen therapy

1. Retinopathy of prematurity
   a. Occurs primarily in premature infants

      b. High concentrations of oxygen cause damage to the retinal blood supply

      c. The best prophylaxis is to reduce the oxygen concentration to the minimum in amount and time of exposure

  2. Chronic lung disease

      a. Pathologic process that develops in the lungs of infants with hyaline membrane disease who have required assisted ventilation

      b. The disease is characterized by changes and/or damage to the lungs

      c. No specific treatment aside from oxygen therapy and other supportive measures; most infants recover by 6 months to 1 year of age

F. Absence of complications associated with nutrition

  1. Neonatal necrotizing enterocolitis (NEC)

      a. Serious condition, usually of preterm infant, speculated to be related to vascular compromise of the gastrointestinal tract (possibly related to hypoxia or sepsis); result of above is damage to the GI tract

      b. Nonspecific clinical signs include lethargy, vomiting, distended (often shiny) abdomen, blood in stools or gastric contents, and absence of bowel sounds

      c. Treatment includes discontinuation of all oral feedings, institution of abdominal decompression via nasogastric suction, and administration of systemic antibiotics

      d. Complications include bowel perforation requiring surgical resection and creation of ileostomy or colostomy

G. Weight gain

H. Active parent-child interaction

Chapter 14

PEDIATRIC NURSING

Sections	Concepts Covered
1. Growth and Development	Growth and Development
2. Pediatric Assessment/Wellness	Health Promotion, Client Education: Providing
3. Alterations in Pediatric Health	Mobility, Intracranial Regulation, Elimination

GROWTH AND DEVELOPMENT

PHASES OF GROWTH AND DEVELOPMENT

(Ages may vary by theorist and source)

A. Process—sequence is orderly and predictable; rate tends to be variable within (more quickly/slowly) and between (earlier/later) individuals

    1. Growth—increase in size (height and weight); tends to be cyclical, more rapid *in utero*, during infancy, and adolescence

    2. Development—maturation of physiological and psychosocial systems to more complex state

        a. Developmental tasks—skills and competencies associated with each developmental stage that have an effect on subsequent stages of development

        b. Developmental milestone—standard of reference by which to compare the child's behavior at specific ages

        c. Developmental delay(s)—variable of development which lags behind the range of a given age

B. Theoretical approaches to development

    1. Erikson (psychosocial approach) (see Table 14-1)

        a. Social development

        b. Role of play in development

    2. Piaget (cognitive approach)—four stages

        a. Sensorimotor—birth to 2 years old

            1) Simple incremental learning—begins with reflex activity progressing to repetitive behavior, then to imitative behavior

            2) Increased level of curiosity

            3) Sense of self as differentiated and separate from environment

            4) Increasing awareness of object permanence (things exist even if not visible)

        b. Preoperational—2 to 7 years old

            1) Thinking and learning are concrete and tangible, based on what is seen, heard, felt, experienced; cannot make generalizations/deductions

            2) Toward the end of this stage, reasoning is more intuitive; beginning understanding of size, mass, time

AGE	STAGE	ERIKSON'S TASK	POSITIVE OUTCOME	NEGATIVE OUTCOME
Birth to 1 year	Infancy	Trust vs. Mistrust	Trusts self and others	Demonstrates an inability to trust; withdrawal, isolation
1 year to 3 years	Toddler	Autonomy vs. Shame and Doubt	Exercises self-control and influences the environment directly	Demonstrates defiance and negativism
3 to 6 years	Preschool	Initiative vs. Guilt	Begins to evaluate own behavior; learns limits on influence in the environment	Demonstrates fearful, pessimistic behaviors; lacks self-confidence
6 to 12 years	School age	Industry vs. Inferiority	Develops a sense of confidence; uses creative energies to influence the environment	Demonstrates feelings of inadequacy, mediocrity, and self-doubt
12 to 20 years	Adolescence	Identity vs. Role Confusion	Develops a coherent sense of self; plans for a future of work/education	Demonstrates inability to develop personal and vocational identity
20 to 45 years	Young adulthood	Intimacy vs. Isolation	Develops connections to work and intimate relationships	Demonstrates an avoidance of intimacy and vocational/career commitments
45 to 65 years	Middle adulthood	Generativity vs. Stagnation	Involved with established family; expands personal creativity and productivity	Demonstrates lack of interests, commitments; preoccupation with self-centered concerns
65 plus	Late adulthood	Integrity vs. Despair	Identification of life as meaningful	Demonstrates fear of death; life lacks meaning

Table 14-1 OVERVIEW OF ERIKSON'S DEVELOPMENTAL TASKS THROUGHOUT THE LIFE SPAN

   c. Concrete operations—7 to 11 years old

     1) Increasingly logical and coherent in thinking; solves problems in concrete manner

     2) Able to sort, classify, collect, order, and organize facts about the environment

     3) Can manage a number of aspects of a situation at one time but not yet able to deal with abstractions

     4) Can consider other points of view

   d. Formal operations—12 to 15 years old

     1) Able to deal with abstractions and abstract symbols

     2) Flexible and adaptable

     3) Can problem solve, develop hypotheses, test them, and arrive at conclusions

     4) Questions and examines moral, ethical, religious, and social issues as beginning definition of self as an adult

3. Freud (psychological approach)—experiences at different stages influence personality traits

   a. Oral (birth to 1 year)—pessimism/optimism, trust/suspiciousness

   b. Anal (1 to 3 years)—retentiveness/overgenerosity, rigidity/laxity, constrictedness/expansiveness, stubbornness/acquiescence, orderliness/messiness

   c. Phallic (3 to 6 years)—brashness/bashfulness, gaiety/sadness, stylishness/plainness, gregariousness/isolation

   d. Latency (6 to 12 years)—elaboration of previously acquired traits

   e. Genital (12+ y)—preparation for forming relationships and marriage

C. Chronological phases

1. Prenatal—conception until birth; rapid growth and development

2. Neonatal—birth until 4 wk of age; adjustment to extrauterine life

3. Infancy—4 wk to 12 or 18 months (upright locomotion); rapid and incremental growth and motor, cognitive, and social development (see Table 14-2)

Table 14-2 INFANT GROWTH AND DEVELOPMENT	
1 month	**7 months**
Head sags Turns head side to side when prone Lifts head momentarily from bed	Sits for short periods using hands for support Transfers toys hand to hand Fear of strangers begins to appear Lability of mood (abrupt mood shifts) Responds to name
2 months	**8 months**
Closing of posterior fontanelle Diminished tonic neck and Moro reflexes Able to turn from side to back Eyes begin to follow a moving object Social smile first appears	Anxiety with strangers Regular patterns of elimination Sits unsupported Beginning pincer grasp Makes consonant sounds Responds to word "no"
3 months	**9 months**
Can hold rattle Head held erect, steady Follows objects to 180° Smiles in mother's presence Laughs audibly	Elevates self to sitting position Creeps on hands and knees Develops preference for dominant hand Rudimentary imitative expression Responds to parental anger
4 months	**10 months**
Rolls back to side Brings objects to mouth Evidence of pleasure in social contact Drooling Moro reflex absent after 3–4 months	Crawls well Pulls self to standing position with support Brings hands together Vocalizes one or two words
5 months	**11 months**
Birth weight usually doubled Takes objects presented to them Teething may begin Smiles at mirror image	Erect standing posture with support Walks holding on to furniture Drops objects and expects it to be picked up Plays peek-a-boo Shakes head for "no"
6 months	**12 months**
Average weight gain of 3-5 oz per week during second 6 months Can hold bottle Can turn from back to stomach Early ability to distinguish and recognize parents and strangers Can chew and bite	Birth weight usually tripled Needs help while walking Sits from standing position without assistance Eats with fingers Usually says 3-5 words in addition to "mama" and "dada" May need "security blanket" or favorite toy

Table 14-2 INFANT GROWTH AND DEVELOPMENT *(CONTINUED)*	
AGE-APPROPRIATE TOYS	
Birth to 2 months	Mobiles
2–4 months	Rattles, cradle gym
4–6 months	Brightly colored toys (small enough to grasp, large enough for safety)
6–9 months	Large toys with bright colors, movable parts, and noisemakers
9–12 months	Books with large pictures, large push-pull toys, teddy bears

4. Toddler—12/18 months to 3 years; slowed growth; marked physical and personality development characterized by profound activity, curiosity, and negativism (see Table 14-3)
   a. Physical—birth weight quadrupled by 2 1/2 years; height grows about 8 in (20.3 cm); pulse 110, respirations 26, BP 85/37–91/49; 20 teeth by 2 1/2; has sphincter control needed for toilet training; appetite lessens because of decreased growth needs
   b. Motor—walks well forward and backward, stoops and recovers, climbs, runs, jumps in place, throws overhand, voluntarily releases hand, uses spoon, drinks from cup, scribbles

Table 14-3 TODDLER GROWTH AND DEVELOPMENT	
15 months	**24 months**
Walks alone	Early efforts at jumping
Crawls up stairs	Builds 6- to 7-block tower
Builds 2-block tower	Turns book pages one at a time
Throws objects	300-word vocabulary
Grasps spoon	Obeys easy commands
Names commonplace objects	Parallel play
18 months	**30 months**
Anterior fontanelle usually closed	Walks on tiptoe
Walks backward	Jumps with both feet
Climbs stairs	Builds 8-block tower
Scribbles	Stands on one foot
Builds 3-block tower	Has sphincter control for toilet training
Oral vocabulary—10 or more words	
Great at mimicry	
AGE-APPROPRIATE TOYS	
Push-pull toys Low rocking horses Dolls Stuffed animals	

c. Psychosocial—indicates wants by behaviors other than crying, may have temper tantrums; increases vocabulary from 10–20 words to about 900 at 3 years; imitates, helps with household chores; points to body parts, recognizes animals; almost dressing/undressing with help at 18 to 24 months (cannot zipper, button, tie shoes); attachment to "security blanket"/stuffed animal

d. Play—parallel play; appropriate toys include push-pull toys, riding toys, work bench, toy hammers, drums, pots and pans, blocks, puzzles with very few large pieces, finger paints, crayons; dolls/stuffed animals

e. Stresses—separation from parents (bedtime may be seen as desertion); alteration in environment/routine/rituals (expect regression/temper tantrums); toilet training; loud noises/animals

f. Safety—accidents (i.e., motor vehicle, burns, poisoning, falls, choking/suffocation [round, cylindrical, and pliable objects, such as balloons, are most dangerous]) are leading cause of death because of continued clumsiness associated with increased mobility, as well as striving for independence and heightened curiosity accompanied by the ability to open things but without cognitive ability to understand potential dangers; requires vigilant child-proofing and supervision while promoting independence; child restraint in motor vehicles is absolute necessity

g. Three phases of separation anxiety

   1) Protest—cries/screams for parents; inconsolable by others

   2) Despair—crying ends; less active; uninterested in food/play; clutches "security" object if available

   3) Denial—appears adjusted; evidences interest in environment; ignores parent when he/she returns; resigned, not contented

5. Preschool—3 to 6 years; steady growth and development distinguished by acquisition of language, social skills, and imagination as well as enhanced self-control and mastery (see Table 14-4)

   a. Physical—weight increases 4–6 lb/y (1.8–2.7 kg); birth length doubled by 4 years; pulse 90–100, respirations 24–25, BP 85–100/60–70; permanent molars appear behind deciduous teeth, maximum potential for amblyopia/"lazy eye" (reduced visual acuity in one eye); handedness is established

   b. Motor—rides tricycle; walks up (3 years) then down (4 years) stairs alternating feet; hops on one foot, tandem walks; draws circle, then cross, then triangle; dresses with assistance, then with supervision, then alone

   c. Psychosocial—knows first name, then age, then last name; uses plurals and three-word sentences, progressing to complex sentences, follows directions, counts; knows simple songs, names of colors, coins, meaning of many words; asks inquisitive questions; evidence of gender-specific behavior by 5 years; becomes more eager to please; may develop imaginary playmates

Table 14-4 PRESCHOOL GROWTH AND DEVELOPMENT	
3 Years	**5 Years**
Copies a circle	Runs well
Builds bridge with 3 cubes	Jumps rope
Less negativistic than toddler, decreased tantrums	Dresses without help
Rides tricycle	2,100-word vocabulary
Jumps off bottom step	Tolerates increasing periods of separation from parents
Undresses without help	Beginnings of cooperative play
900-word vocabulary, uses sentences	Gender-specific behavior
Increased attention span	Skips on alternate feet
4 Years	Ties shoes
Climbs and jumps well	
Laces shoes	
Brushes teeth	
1,500-word vocabulary	
Skips and hops on one foot	
Throws overhead	
May have imaginary friend	
AGE-APPROPRIATE TOYS AND ACTIVITIES	
Child imitative of adult patterns and roles. Offer playground materials, housekeeping toys, coloring books, tricycles with helmet.	

d. Play—associative/interactive/cooperative play; appropriate toys include tricycles and playground equipment; construction sets, illustrated books, puzzles, modeling clay, paints/crayons, simple games; imitative and dramatic play (dress-up, doll house, puppets); supervised TV

e. Stresses—illogical fears (inanimate objects, the dark, ghosts); separation from parents, may be evidenced as anorexia, insomnia, continued quiet crying, and/or aggression; bodily injury, mutilation (fear that puncture will not close and insides will leak out) and pain; intrusive procedures are threatening

f. Safety—similar to toddler; can understand and learn about potential dangers; shoulder harness and lap belt appropriate when child is either 40 lb, 40 in, or 4 years old

6. School age—6 to 11/12 years; constant progress in physical, mental, and social development, skill, competency, and self-concept (see Table 14-5)
   a. Physical—continued slow growth; begins losing temporary teeth early in this phase and has all permanent teeth, except final molars by the end; bone growth exceeds that of muscle and ligament, resulting in susceptibility to injuries/fractures
   b. Motor—skips, skates, tumbles, tandem walks backward, prints progressing to script, ties knots, then bows
   c. Psychosocial—has significant peer relationships, assumes complete responsibility for personal care; school occupies most of time and has social as well as cognitive impact; developing morality, dominated by moral realism with strict sense of right/wrong until 9 years, then development of moral autonomy recognizing different points of view; able to acknowledge own strengths and weaknesses; developing modesty

Table 14-5 SCHOOL-AGE GROWTH AND DEVELOPMENT	
6 Years	**9 Years**
Self-centered Extreme sensitivity to criticism Begins losing temporary teeth Appearance of first permanent teeth Ties knots Develops concepts of numbers Takes bath without supervision	Skillful manual work possible Conflicts between adult authorities and peer group Better behaved Conflict between needs for independence and dependence Likes school
7 Years	
Temporal perception improving Increased self-reliance for basic activities Team games/sports/organizations Develops concept of time Boys prefer playing with boys and girls with girls	**10–12 Years**
	Remainder of teeth (except wisdom) erupt Uses telephone Responds to advertising Increasingly responsible More selective when choosing friends Develops beginning of interest in opposite sex Loves conversation Raises pets
8 Years	
Friends sought out actively Eye development generally complete Movements more graceful Helps with household chores	
AGE-APPROPRIATE TOYS, GAMES, AND ACTIVITIES	
Construction toys, use of tools, household serving tools, table game sports	Participation in repair, building, and mechanical activities, household chores

d. Play—cooperative group play with leader and organized rules/rituals; usual activities include team games/sports/organizations; board games, books, swimming, hiking, bicycling, skating

e. Stresses—possible school phobia; fear of death, disease/injury, punishment

f. Safety—decreasing incidence of accidents except for injuries associated with sports/activities, requires appropriate supervision and education about proper use and maintenance of equipment and hazards of risk taking

7. Adolescence—approximately 11/12 to 18/20 years (depending on gender and individual rate); rapid and dynamic biological, physical, and personality maturation characterized by emotional and family turmoil, leading to redefinition of self-concept and establishment of independence (see Table 14-6)

a. Physical—vital signs approach adult levels; wisdom teeth appear about 17–21 years; puberty is related to hormonal changes and is universal in pattern but not rate (females tend to develop earlier than males)

   1) Growth spurt occurs early

     a) Girls—height increases approximately 3 in/y, slows dramatically at menarche and ceases around age 16; fat is deposited in thighs, hips, and breasts; pelvis broadens

     b) Boys—height increases 4 in/y starting about age 13 and slows in late teens; weight doubles between 12 and 18 years old, related to increased muscle mass; broader chest

Table 14-6 ADOLESCENT GROWTH AND DEVELOPMENT
Physical Development–Puberty
Attainment of sexual maturity
Rapid alterations in height and weight
Girls develop more rapidly than boys
Onset may be related to hypothalmic activity, which influences pituitary gland to secrete hormones affecting testes and ovaries
Testes and ovaries produce hormones (androgens and estrogens) that determine development of secondary sexual characteristics
Pimples or acne related to increased sebaceous gland activity
Increased sweat production
Weight gain proportionally greater than height gain during early stages
Initial problems in coordination–appearance of clumsiness related to rapid unsynchronized growth of many systems
Rapid growth may cause easy fatigue
Preoccupation with physical appearance
Male Changes
Increase in genital size
Breast swelling
Appearance of pubic, facial, axillary, and chest hair
Deepening voice
Production of functional sperm
Nocturnal emissions
Female Changes
Increase in pelvic diameter
Breast development
Altered nature of vaginal secretions
Appearance of axillary and pubic hair
Menarche–first menstrual period
Physical Development—Adolescent
More complete development of secondary sexual characteristics
Improved motor coordination
Wisdom teeth appear (ages 17-21)
Psychosexual Development
Masturbation as expression of sexual tension
Sexual fantasies
Experimental sexual intercourse
Psychosocial Development
Preoccupied with rapid body changes, what is "normal"
Conformity to peer pressure
Moody
Increased daydreaming
Increased independence
Moving toward a mature sexual identity

2) Sweat production and increased body odor result from increased apocrine gland activity; acne may occur related to increased sebaceous gland activity

3) Sexual characteristics and functioning develop
   a) Females
      i. Increase in pelvic diameter
      ii. Breast development—bud stage with protuberant areola; complete about time of menarche
      iii. Nature of vaginal secretions changes
      iv. Axillary and pubic hair appear
      v. Menarche—first menstrual period occurs around 12 1/2 years; for first 1–2 years anovulatory, frequently irregular menses

   b) Males
      i. Increase in genital size beginning about 13 years is first sign of sexual maturation; continues until reproductive maturity (age 17–18)
      ii. Possible temporary breast swelling of short duration
      iii. Pubic, facial, axillary, and chest hair appear
      iv. Voice deepens
      v. Production of functional sperm
      vi. Nocturnal emissions—normal physiologic reflex to ejaculate buildup of semen occurring during sleep; masturbation increases as a way to release semen
      vii. Motor—often clumsiness associated with growth spurt, motor ability is at adult levels

b. Psychosocial
   1) Early—preoccupied with changing body; ambivalent relationship with parents/authority figures; seeking peer affiliations; may begin "dating"; wide and intense mood swings; limited capability for abstract thinking; seeking to identify values
   2) Middle—very self-centered; rich fantasy life; idealistic; major conflicts with parents/authority figures; strong identification with peer group; multiple "love"/sexual relationships (homosexuality is recognized by this time); tends to be more introspective and withdrawn; enhanced ability for abstract reasoning; concerned with philosophical, political, and social issues
   3) Late—established body image; irreversible sexual identity and gender role definition; independent from and less conflict with parents/authority figures; establishing stable individual friendships with both sexes and committed intimacy relationship; more stability in emotions; able to think abstractly; develops life philosophy (values, beliefs); makes occupational decisions

c. Activities—primarily peer group oriented

d. Stresses—threat of loss of control, fear of altered body image; separation primarily from peer group

e. Safety—accidents, especially related to motor vehicles, sports, firearms, homicide, and suicide are leading causes of death; may be significantly related to drug and/or alcohol use; education is paramount

8. Early and middle adulthood—18/20 to 65 years; developmental state and function characterized by self-sufficiency in pursuit of occupation/vocation and defined interpersonal relationships (see Tables 14-7 and 14-8)

a. Physical/cognitive—stabilized growth state (weight is variable) and functioning, refines formal operational abilities, undergoes menopause, begins physical/physiological degeneration

b. Psychosocial—develops self-sufficiency, pursues vocation/occupation, has intense interpersonal relationships (most frequently marriage and children)

Table 14-7 YOUNG ADULTHOOD GROWTH AND DEVELOPMENT		
20 TO 35 YEARS	**35 TO 40 YEARS**	**40 TO 45 YEARS**
Decreased hero worship	Period of discovery, rediscovery of interests and goals	(There is some overlap in years)
Increased reality	Increased sense of urgency	Self-questioning
Independent from parents	Life more serious	Fear of middle age and aging
Possible marriage, partnership	Major goals to accomplish	Reappraises the past
Realization that everything is not black or white, some "gray" areas	Plateaus at work and marriage, partnership	Discards unrealistic goals
Looks toward future, hopes for success	Sense of satisfaction	Potential changes of work, marriage, partnership
Peak intelligence, memory		"Sandwich" generation—concerned with children and aging parents
Maximum problem-solving ability		Increased awareness of mortality
		Potential loss of significant others

Table 14-8 MIDDLE ADULTHOOD GROWTH AND DEVELOPMENT		
45 TO 55 YEARS	**55 TO 60 YEARS**	**60 TO 65 YEARS**
Graying hair, wrinkling skin	(There is some overlap in years)	Increasingly forgetful
Evaluates past	Increasing physical decline	Accepts limitations
Pains and muscle aches	Sets new goals	Modification of lifestyle
Reassessment	Defines value of life, self	Decreased power
Realization—future shorter time span than past	Assesses legacies— professional, personal	Retirement
Menopause	Serenity and fulfillment	Less restricted time, able to choose different activities
Decreased sensory acuity	Balance between old and young	
Powerful, policy makers, leaders	Accepts changes of aging	
Relates to older and younger generations		

9. Late adulthood—65 years until death (see Table 14-9)
   a. Physical/cognitive—has general slowing of physical and cognitive functioning
   b. Psychosocial—needs to establish highest degree of independence (self-sufficiency) physically possible by adapting environment to ability; reflects on life accomplishments, events, and experiences; continues interpersonal relationships despite changes and loss

Table 14-9 LATE ADULTHOOD GROWTH AND DEVELOPMENT	
65 TO 80 YEARS	**GREATER THAN 80 YEARS**
Physical decline	Signs of aging very evident
Loss of significant others	Few significant relationships
Appraisal of life	Withdrawal, risk of isolation
Appearance of chronic diseases	Self-concern
Reconciliation of goals and achievements	Acceptance of death, faces mortality
Changing social roles	Increased losses
	Decreased abilities

D. Factors affecting growth and development
1. Genetic defects
   a. Increased risk in certain groups of people, e.g., African Americans for sickle cell disease, Northern European descendants of Ashkenazic Jews for Tay-Sachs disease, Mediterranean ancestry for thalassemia; couples with a history of a child with a defect; family history of a structural abnormality or systemic disease that may be hereditary; prospective parents who are closely blood-related; women over 40
   b. Chromosomal alteration—may be numeric or structural
      1) Down syndrome (trisomy 21)—increased in women over 35 years; characterized by a small, round head with flattened occiput; low set ears; large fat pads at the nape of a short neck; protruding tongue; small mouth and high palate; epicanthal folds with slanted eyes; hypotonic muscles with hypermobility of joints; short, broad hands with inward curved little finger; transverse simian palmar crease; mental deficiencies
      2) Turner's syndrome (female with only one X)—characterized by stunted growth, fibrous streaks in ovaries, usually infertile, no intellectual impairment; occasionally perceptual problems
      3) Klinefelter's syndrome (male with extra X)—normal intelligence to mild intellectual delay; usually infertile
   c. Autosomal defects—defects occurring in any chromosome pair other than the sex chromosomes
      1) Autosomal dominant—union of normal parent with affected parent; the affected parent has a 50% chance of passing on the abnormal gene in each pregnancy; BRCA-1 and BRCA-2 breast cancer, Type 2 diabetes, Marfan syndrome, polycystic kidney disease
      2) Autosomal recessive—requires transmission of abnormal gene from both parents for expression of condition; cyctic fibrosis, sickle cell disease
      3) Sex-linked transmission traits—trait carried on a sex chromosome (usually the X chromosome); may be dominant or recessive, but recessive is more prevalent; e.g., hemophilia, color blindness
   d. Inborn errors of metabolism—disorders of protein, fat, or carbohydrate metabolism reflecting absent or defective enzymes that generally follow a recessive pattern of inheritance
      1) Phenylketonuria (PKU)—disorder due to autosomal recessive gene, creating a deficiency in the liver enzyme phenylalanine hydroxylase, which metabolizes the amino acid phenylalanine; results in metabolic accumulation in blood; toxic to brain cells

2) Tay-Sachs disease—autosomal recessive trait resulting from a deficiency of hexosaminidase A, resulting in apathy, regression in motor and social development, and decreased vision

3) Cystic fibrosis (mucoviscidosis or fibrocystic disease of the pancreas)—an autosomal recessive trait characterized by generalized involvement of exocrine glands, resulting in altered viscosity of mucus-secreting glands throughout the body

2. Racial and ethnic influences

3. Environment—may influence development more than genetic factors
   a. Family's socioeconomic factors
   b. Adequate nutrition
   c. Climate

4. Intrapersonal factors
   a. State of health
   b. Emotional state

E. Assessment of growth and development
   1. Growth
      a. Repeated measurements must be done and recorded accurately on regular basis to establish pattern and identify deviations; at least five times in first year and then yearly at every well-child visit and sick-child visit as appropriate
      b. Assessing length/height—infant or toddler positioned supine on exam table with legs extended is measured from crown of head to heels using flexible nonstretchable tape, while another person maintains child's position; for the older child, standing measurement is easier and more accurate
      c. Standardized growth chart
         1) Individual's length/height, weight, and head and chest circumference (until 3 years) is assessed in relation to general population, to previous pattern, and to each other
         2) Necessary to reevaluate and report measurements greater than 97th percentile and less than 3rd percentile or deviations from established pattern

   2. Development—evaluates current developmental function, identifies need for follow-up, helps parents to understand the child's behavior and prepare for new experiences, and provides basis for anticipatory guidance
      a. Evaluation should include all the subsystems of development, biophysical (gross and fine motor), cognitive, language, social, affective
      b. Developmental tools
         1) Denver II—evaluates children from birth to 6 years in four skill areas: personal-social, fine motor, language, gross motor
            a) Age adjusted for prematurity by subtracting the number of months preterm
            b) Questionable value in testing children of minority/ethnic groups
         2) Revised Prescreening Developmental Questionnaire (R-PDQ)—paper and pencil questionnaire from the Denver II for parents to answer to prescreen children

   3. Muscular coordination and control—proceeds in head-to-toe (cephalocaudal), trunk-to-periphery (proximodistal), gross to fine developmental pattern

   4. Intellectual—related to genetic potentialities and environment; intelligence tests used to determine IQ; mental age divided by chronological age multiplied by 100

PEDIATRIC ASSESSMENT/WELLNESS

PEDIATRIC ASSESSMENT

A. Subjective—health history

1. Serves not only to gather information but also to build trust/rapport, establish focus of examination/labwork, enhance knowledge base of caregivers, and to offer support

2. Format

    a. Indirect interview—open-ended questioning

        1) Advantages—may provide opportunity for greater exploration of underlying issues/concerns, for more complex description(s) and for therapeutic responses

        2) Disadvantages—may be time consuming, require sorting through unnecessary/irrelevant information and allow parent to avoid area of concern

    b. Direct questioning—promotes specific responses to specific questions, used especially when time factor is important but tends to inhibit exploration

    c. Questionnaire may be done before visit but must be reviewed with client/caregiver

3. Approach

    a. Child and parent together—provides opportunity to observe parent-child interaction, time for child to get used to practitioner, and opportunity for older child to contribute to interview but may inhibit completeness/accuracy of history

    b. Child and parent separately—provides for more complete discussion of sensitive issues, especially with adolescent; confidentiality should be ensured except in potential situations of harm to self (suicide) or another person by the informant

    c. Avoid "talking down" to child/adolescent, making statements/promises that cannot be accomplished, e.g., "I won't hurt you"; sudden/exaggerated movements and/or staring at young child

B. Physical examination

1. Setting—ensure privacy, comfort, and adequate time

2. Approach

    a. Quiet voice with slow and easy approach appropriate to age of child

    b. Introduce self—use full name and title, clarify role/function, and explain rationale of process for eliciting information

    c. Use complete names except with child/adolescent or when adult is well known and/or gives permission for first name use

3. Examination—utilize same basic skills and techniques; however, the order may vary according to age of child to ensure the safety and comfort of child and to provide for ease of examination and accuracy of finding(s) (see Table 14-10)

Table 14-10	AGE-APPROPRIATE PREPARATION FOR HEALTH CARE PROCEDURES	
AGE	SPECIAL NEEDS	TYPICAL FEARS
Newborn	Include parents Mummy restraint	Loud noises Sudden movements
6–12 months	Model desired behavior	Strangers, heights
Toddler	Simple explanations Use distractions Allow choices	Separation from parents Animals, strangers Change in environments
Preschool	Encourage understanding by playing with puppets, dolls Demonstrate equipment Talk at child's eye level	Separation from parents Ghosts Scary people
School age	Allow questions Explain why Allow to handle equipment	Dark, injury Being alone Death
Adolescent	Explain long-term benefit Accept regression Provide privacy	Social incompetence War, accidents Death

a. Wash hands before exam for cleanliness and to warm hands

b. Basic tools and skills
   1) Observation/inspection—appearance, behavior, activity, interaction with parent; careful visual examination of an area
   2) Palpation
      a) Fine tactile details—fingertip pads
      b) Temperature—back/dorsum of hand
      c) Vibration—palm/palmar surface of fingers
   3) Percussion—assess density
      a) Direct—sinus cavity
      b) Indirect/bimanual—resonance (lungs), tympany (gas-filled, e.g., stomach), dull (organ tissue), flat (bone)
   4) Auscultation
      a) Diaphragm—firmly against surface for high-frequency sounds
      b) Bell—lightly against surface for low-frequency sounds

c. Age-related factors—position, undressing, and sequence of exam
   1) Infant and toddler
      a) Take full advantage of opportunities as they arise; when child is quiet, examine lungs, heart, and abdomen
      b) Observe child's activities while he/she is in waiting and exam rooms
      c) Key to success is distraction—test for developmental milestones in the form of a game before performing general exam

    d) May examine neonate and infant on table until approximately 6 mo, thereafter, on parent's lap; do invasive procedures (ears and throat) last

    e) Uncooperative child must be adequately restrained during invasive procedures to prevent injury

2) Young child

    a) Remove clothing as examination progresses

    b) Allow child to choose between possible alternatives but do not request child's permission to do something if child really has no choice

    c) Do the more invasive/uncomfortable procedures last, protecting child as mentioned

    d) May be helpful to play games

3) Preschool age/early school-age child

    a) Encourage child to remove his/her own clothing (children usually like to keep on underwear and socks); note dexterity

    b) Allow child to choose position for exam

    c) May be helpful to involve child, encourage handling appropriate equipment, allow listening to own heart

4) School-age child

    a) Respect modesty—offer gown to any child beyond early childhood

    b) Explain each step and allow child to participate actively

    c) Can proceed in usual head-to-toe sequence; if child is sick, assess healthy areas first

5) Adolescent

    a) Paramount to provide for privacy and modesty; best to examine genitalia last

    b) Reassure about normalcy of findings as appropriate

    c) Provide health teaching as exam progresses

C. Vital signs
  1. Temperature
     a. Rectally provides precise diagnosis of fever but is contraindicated if less than 1 month of age (due to risk of rectal perforation), diarrhea, recent rectal surgery, anorectal lesions, receiving chemotherapy
     b. Rectally if recent/current vomiting, child unable to keep mouth closed
     c. Axillary if rectal irritation/diarrhea in young child; however, axillary readings may be insensitive and inconsistent
     d. Intrauricular probe allows rapid, noninvasive reading when appropriate
  2. Heart rate—apical/radial counted for one full minute; assess rate and rhythm; PMI in infant is just lateral to nipple; with growth, gradually more medial
  3. Respirations—rate and rhythm; note signs and symptoms respiratory distress, grunting, flaring, retracting
  4. Blood pressure—usually after 3 years old
     a. Methods
        1) Auscultation
        2) Palpation
        3) Doppler
     b. Size of cuff important—should be 1/2–2/3 of area of extremity; too narrow—abnormally high reading; too wide—abnormally low reading

D. Routine lab work
  1. Hb/Hct—at 6–9 mo, between 12 and 18 mo, and during adolescence
  2. Urinalysis—after toilet trained and when necessary for signs and symptoms
  3. Lead screening—at 12 months (6 months if high-risk)
  4. Sickle cell screening—after 6 months in high-risk populations (Sickledex)
  5. Tuberculosis (Tine, Mantoux)—after 12 months old

IMMUNIZATIONS

A. Recommended schedule for infants, children, and adolescents (see Table 14-11 or **CDC.gov/vaccines/schedules**)

Table 14-11

Figure 1. Recommended Immunization Schedule for Children and Adolescents Aged 18 Years or Younger—United States, 2018.
(FOR THOSE WHO FALL BEHIND OR START LATE, SEE THE CATCH-UP SCHEDULE [FIGURE 2]).
These recommendations must be read with the footnotes that follow. For those who fall behind or start late, provide catch-up vaccination at the earliest opportunity as indicated by the green bars in Figure 1. To determine minimum intervals between doses, see the catch-up schedule (Figure 2). School entry and adolescent vaccine age groups are shaded in gray.

Vaccine	Birth	1 mo	2 mos	4 mos	6 mos	9 mos	12 mos	15 mos	18 mos	19-23 mos	2-3 yrs	4-6 yrs	7-10 yrs	11-12 yrs	13-15 yrs	16 yrs	17-18 yrs
Hepatitis B[1] (HepB)	1st dose	◄──2nd dose──►			◄───────────────── 3rd dose ─────────────────►												
Rotavirus[2] (RV) RV1 (2-dose series); RV5 (3-dose series)			1st dose	2nd dose	See footnote 2												
Diphtheria, tetanus, & acellular pertussis[3] (DTaP: <7 yrs)			1st dose	2nd dose	3rd dose		◄─────── 4th dose ───────►					5th dose					
Haemophilus influenzae type b[4] (Hib)			1st dose	2nd dose	See footnote 4		◄── 3rd or 4th dose, See footnote 4 ──►										
Pneumococcal conjugate[5] (PCV13)			1st dose	2nd dose	3rd dose		◄───── 4th dose ─────►										
Inactivated poliovirus[6] (IPV: <18 yrs)			1st dose	2nd dose	◄──────────── 3rd dose ────────────►							4th dose					
Influenza[7] (IIV)					◄──────────── Annual vaccination (IIV) 1 or 2 doses ────────────►									Annual vaccination (IIV) 1 dose only			
Measles, mumps, rubella[8] (MMR)						See footnote 8	◄──── 1st dose ────►					2nd dose					
Varicella[9] (VAR)							◄──── 1st dose ────►					2nd dose					
Hepatitis A[10] (HepA)							◄──── 2-dose series, See footnote 10 ────►										
Meningococcal[11] (MenACWY-D ≥9 mos; MenACWY-CRM ≥2 mos)				◄────────────── See footnote 11 ──────────────►										1st dose		2nd dose	
Tetanus, diphtheria, & acellular pertussis[13] (Tdap: ≥7 yrs)														Tdap			
Human papillomavirus[14] (HPV)														See footnote 14			
Meningococcal B[12]														◄── See footnote 12 ──►			
Pneumococcal polysaccharide[5] (PPSV23)												◄────────── See footnote 5 ──────────►					

■ Range of recommended ages for all children	■ Range of recommended ages for catch-up immunization	■ Range of recommended ages for certain high-risk groups	■ Range of recommended ages for non-high-risk groups that may receive vaccine, subject to individual clinical decision making	□ No recommendation

NOTE: The above recommendations must be read along with the footnotes of this schedule.

FIGURE 2. Catch-up immunization schedule for persons aged 4 months–18 years who start late or who are more than 1 month behind—United States, 2018.

The figure below provides catch-up schedules and minimum intervals between doses for children whose vaccinations have been delayed. A vaccine series does not need to be restarted, regardless of the time that has elapsed between doses. Use the section appropriate for the child's age. Always use this table in conjunction with Figure 1 and the footnotes that follow.

Vaccine	Minimum Age for Dose 1	Dose 1 to Dose 2	Dose 2 to Dose 3	Dose 3 to Dose 4	Dose 4 to Dose 5
		Children age 4 months through 6 years	**Minimum Interval Between Doses**		
Hepatitis B[1]	Birth	4 weeks	8 weeks **and** at least 16 weeks after first dose. Minimum age for the final dose is 24 weeks.		
Rotavirus[2]	6 weeks / Maximum age for first dose is 14 weeks, 6 days.	4 weeks	4 weeks[2] / Maximum age for final dose is 8 months, 0 days.		
Diphtheria, tetanus, and acellular pertussis[3]	6 weeks	4 weeks	4 weeks	6 months	6 months[3]
Haemophilus influenzae type b[4]	6 weeks	4 weeks if first dose administered before the 1st birthday. / 8 weeks (as final dose) if first dose was administered at age 12 through 14 months. / No further doses needed if first dose was administered at age 15 months or older.	4 weeks[4] if current age is younger than 12 months **and** first dose was administered at younger than age 7 months, **and** at least 1 previous dose was PRP-T (ActHib, Pentacel, Hiberix) or unknown. / 8 weeks **and** age 12 through 59 months (as final dose)[5] • if current age is younger than 12 months **and** first dose was administered at age 7 through 11 months; OR • if current age is 12 through 59 months **and** first dose was administered before the 1st birthday, **and** second dose administered at younger than 15 months; OR • if both doses were PRP-OMP (PedvaxHIB, Comvax) **and** were administered before age 12 months. / No further doses needed if previous dose was administered at age 15 months or older.	8 weeks (as final dose) / This dose only necessary for children aged 12 through 59 months who received 3 doses before the 1st birthday.	
Pneumococcal conjugate[5]	6 weeks	4 weeks if first dose administered before the 1st birthday. / 8 weeks (as final dose for healthy children) if first dose was administered at the 1st birthday or after. / No further doses needed for healthy children if first dose was administered at age 24 months or older.	4 weeks if current age is younger than 12 months and previous dose given at <7 months old. / 8 weeks (as final dose for healthy children) if previous dose given between 7–11 months (wait until at least 12 months old); OR if current age is 12 months or older and at least 1 dose was given before age 12 months. / No further doses needed for healthy children if previous dose administered at age 24 months or older.	8 weeks (as final dose) / This dose only necessary for children aged 12 through 59 months who received 3 doses before age 12 months or for children at high risk who received 3 doses at any age.	
Inactivated poliovirus[6]	6 weeks	4 weeks	4 weeks[6] If current age is < 4 years. / 6 months (as final dose) if current age is 4 years or older.	6 months[6] (minimum age 4 years for final dose).	
Measles, mumps, rubella[7]	12 months	4 weeks			
Varicella[8]	12 months	3 months			
Hepatitis A[9]	12 months	6 months			
		Children and adolescents age 7 through 18 years			
Meningococcal[11] (MenACWY-D ≥9 mos; MenACWY-CRM ≥2 mos)	Not Applicable (N/A)	8 weeks[11]	See footnote 11	See footnote 11	
Tetanus, diphtheria; tetanus, diphtheria, and acellular pertussis[10]	7 years[10]	4 weeks	4 weeks if first dose of DTaP/DT was administered before the 1st birthday. / 6 months (as final dose) if first dose of DTaP/DT or Tdap/Td was administered at or after the 1st birthday.	6 months if first dose of DTaP/DT was administered before the 1st birthday.	
Human papillomavirus[14]	9 years	Routine dosing intervals are recommended.[14]			
Hepatitis A[9]	N/A	6 months			
Hepatitis B[10]	N/A	4 weeks	8 weeks **and** at least 16 weeks after first dose.		
Inactivated poliovirus[6]	N/A	4 weeks	4 weeks	6 months[6] / A fourth dose is not necessary if the third dose was administered at age 4 years or older and at least 6 months after the previous dose.	A fourth dose of IPV is indicated if all previous doses were administered at <4 years or if the third dose was administered <6 months after the second dose.
Measles, mumps, rubella[7]	N/A	4 weeks			
Varicella[8]	N/A	3 months if younger than age 13 years / 4 weeks if age 13 years or older.			

NOTE: The above recommendations must be read along with the footnotes of this schedule.

Table 14-11 (*continued*)

Footnotes — Recommended Immunization Schedule for Children and Adolescents Aged 18 Years or Younger, UNITED STATES, 2018

For further guidance on the use of the vaccines mentioned below, see: www.cdc.gov/vaccines/hcp/acip-recs/index.html.
For vaccine recommendations for persons 19 years of age and older, see the Adult Immunization Schedule.

Additional information

- For information on contraindications and precautions for the use of a vaccine, consult the *General Best Practice Guidelines for Immunization* and relevant ACIP statements, at www.cdc.gov/vaccines/hcp/acip-recs/index.html.
- For calculating intervals between doses, 4 weeks = 28 days. Intervals of $\geq$4 months are determined by calendar months.
- Within a number range (e.g., 12–18), a dash (–) should be read as "through."
- Vaccine doses administered $\leq$4 days before the minimum age or interval are considered valid. Doses of any vaccine administered $\geq$5 days earlier than the minimum interval or minimum age should not be counted as valid and should be repeated as age-appropriate. The repeat dose should be spaced after the invalid dose by the recommended minimum interval. For further details, see Table 3-1, *Recommended and minimum ages and intervals between vaccine doses*, in *General Best Practice Guidelines for Immunization* at www.cdc.gov/vaccines/hcp/acip-recs/general-recs/timing.html.
- Information on travel vaccine requirements and recommendations is available at wwwnc.cdc.gov/travel/.
- For vaccination of persons with immunodeficiencies, see Table 8-1, *Vaccination of persons with primary and secondary immunodeficiencies*, in *General Best Practice Guidelines for Immunization*, at www.cdc.gov/vaccines/hcp/acip-recs/general-recs/immunocompetence.html; and Immunization in Special Clinical Circumstances. (In: Kimberlin DW, Brady MT, Jackson MA, Long SS, eds. *Red Book: 2015 report of the Committee on Infectious Diseases. 30th ed.* Elk Grove Village, IL: American Academy of Pediatrics, 2015:68-107).
- The National Vaccine Injury Compensation Program (VICP) is a no-fault alternative to the traditional legal system for resolving vaccine injury claims. All routine child and adolescent vaccines are covered by VICP except for pneumococcal polysaccharide vaccine (PPSV23). For more information; see www.hrsa.gov/vaccinecompensation/index.html.

1. **Hepatitis B (HepB) vaccine. (minimum age: birth)**
   Birth Dose (Monovalent HepB vaccine only):
   - **Mother is HBsAg-Negative:** 1 dose within 24 hours of birth for medically stable infants $\geq$2,000 grams. Infants <2,000 grams administer 1 dose at chronological age 1 month or hospital discharge.
   - **Mother is HBsAg-Positive:**
     o Give **HepB vaccine** and **0.5 mL of HBIG** (at separate anatomic sites) within 12 hours of birth, regardless of birth weight.
     o Test for HBsAg and anti-HBs at age 9–12 months. If HepB series is delayed, test 1–2 months after final dose.
   - **Mother's HBsAg status is unknown:**
     o Give **HepB vaccine** within 12 hours of birth, regardless of birth weight.
     o For infants <2,000 grams, give **0.5 mL of HBIG** in addition to HepB vaccine within 12 hours of birth.
     o Determine mother's HBsAg status as soon as possible. If mother is HBsAg-positive, give **0.5 mL of HBIG** to infants $\geq$2,000 grams as soon as possible, but no later than 7 days of age.

   Routine Series:
   - A complete series is 3 doses at 0, 1–2, and 6–18 months. (Monovalent HepB vaccine should be used for doses given before age 6 weeks.)

   - Infants who did not receive a birth dose should begin the series as soon as feasible (see Figure 2).
   - Administration of **4 doses** is permitted when a combination vaccine containing HepB is used after the birth dose.
   - **Minimum age** for the final (3rd or 4th) dose: 24 weeks.
   - **Minimum Intervals:** Dose 1 to Dose 2: 4 weeks / Dose 2 to Dose 3: 8 weeks / Dose 1 to Dose 3: 16 weeks. (When 4 doses are given, substitute "Dose 4" for "Dose 3" in these calculations.)

   Catch-up vaccination:
   - Unvaccinated persons should complete a 3-dose series at 0, 1–2, and 6 months.
   - Adolescents 11–15 years of age may use an alternative 2-dose schedule, with at least 4 months between doses (adult formulation **Recombivax HB** only).
   - For other catch-up guidance, see Figure 2.

2. **Rotavirus vaccines. (minimum age: 6 weeks)**
   Routine vaccination:
   Rotarix: 2-dose series at 2 and 4 months.
   RotaTeq: 3-dose series at 2, 4, and 6 months.
   If any dose in the series is either RotaTeq or unknown, default to 3-dose series.

   Catch-up vaccination:
   - Do not start the series on or after age 15 weeks, 0 days.
   - The maximum age for the final dose is 8 months, 0 days.
   - For other catch-up guidance, see Figure 2.

3. **Diphtheria, tetanus, and acellular pertussis (DTaP) vaccine. (minimum age: 6 weeks [4 years for Kinrix or Quadracel])**
   Routine vaccination:
   - 5-dose series at 2, 4, 6, and 15–18 months, and 4–6 years.
     o **Prospectively:** A 4th dose may be given as early as age 12 months if at least 6 months have elapsed since the 3rd dose.
     o **Retrospectively:** A 4th dose that was inadvertently given as early as 12 months may be counted if at least 4 months have elapsed since the 3rd dose.

   Catch-up vaccination:
   - The 5th dose is not necessary if the 4th dose was administered at 4 years or older.
   - For other catch-up guidance, see Figure 2.

Table 14-11 (*continued*)

For further guidance on the use of the vaccines mentioned below, see: www.cdc.gov/vaccines/hcp/acip-recs/index.html.

4. *Haemophilus influenzae* **type b (Hib) vaccine.**
   (minimum age: 6 weeks)
   Routine vaccination:
   - **ActHIB, Hiberix, or Pentacel:** 4-dose series at 2, 4, 6, and 12–15 months.
   - **PedvaxHIB:** 3-dose series at 2, 4, and 12–15 months.
   Catch-up vaccination:
   - **1st dose at 7–11 months:** Give 2nd dose at least 4 weeks later and 3rd (final) dose at 12–15 months or 8 weeks after 2nd dose (whichever is later).
   - **1st dose at 12–14 months:** Give 2nd (final) dose at least 8 weeks after 1st dose.
   - **1st dose before 12 months and 2nd dose before 15 months:** Give 3rd (final) dose 8 weeks after 2nd dose.
   - **2 doses of PedvaxHIB before 12 months:** Give 3rd (final) dose at 12–59 months and at least 8 weeks after 2nd dose.
   - **Unvaccinated at 15–59 months:** 1 dose.
   - For other catch-up guidance, see Figure 2.
   Special Situations:
   - **Chemotherapy or radiation treatment**
     12–59 months
     o Unvaccinated or only 1 dose before 12 months: Give 2 doses, 8 weeks apart
     o 2 or more doses before 12 months: Give 1 dose, at least 8 weeks after previous dose.
     Doses given within 14 days of starting therapy or during therapy should be repeated at least 3 months after therapy completion.
   - **Hematopoietic stem cell transplant (HSCT)**
     - 3-dose series with doses 4 weeks apart starting 6 to 12 months after successful transplant (regardless of Hib vaccination history).
   - **Anatomic or functional asplenia (including sickle cell disease)**
     12–59 months
     o Unvaccinated or only 1 dose before 12 months: Give 2 doses, 8 weeks apart.
     o 2 or more doses before 12 months: Give 1 dose, at least 8 weeks after previous dose.
     Unimmunized persons 5 years or older
     o Give 1 dose
   - **Elective splenectomy**
     Unimmunized* persons 15 months or older
     o Give 1 dose (preferably at least 14 days before procedure).

- **HIV infection**
  12–59 months
  o Unvaccinated or only 1 dose before 12 months: Give 2 doses 8 weeks apart.
  o 2 or more doses before 12 months: Give 1 dose, at least 8 weeks after previous dose.
  Unimmunized persons 5–18 years
  o Give 1 dose
- **Immunoglobulin deficiency, early component complement deficiency**
  12–59 months
  o Unvaccinated or only 1 dose before 12 months: Give 2 doses, 8 weeks apart.
  o 2 or more doses before 12 months: Give 1 dose, at least 8 weeks after previous dose.
  *Unimmunized = Less than routine series (through 14 months) OR no doses (14 months or older)

5. **Pneumococcal vaccines. (minimum age: 6 weeks [PCV13], 2 years [PPSV23])**
   Routine vaccination with PCV13:
   - 4-dose series at 2, 4, 6, and 12–15 months.
   Catch-up vaccination with PCV13:
   - 1 dose for healthy children aged 24–59 months with any incomplete* PCV13 schedule
   - For other catch-up guidance, see Figure 2.
   Special situations: High-risk conditions:
   Administer PCV13 doses before PPSV23 if possible.
   Chronic heart disease (particularly cyanotic congenital heart disease and cardiac failure); chronic lung disease (including asthma treated with high-dose, oral, corticosteroids); diabetes mellitus:
   Age 2–5 years:
   - Any incomplete* schedules with:
     o 3 PCV13 doses: 1 dose of PCV13 (at least 8 weeks after any prior PCV13 dose).
     o <3 PCV13 doses: 2 doses of PCV13, 8 weeks after the most recent dose and given 8 weeks apart.
   - No history of PPSV23: 1 dose of PPSV23 (at least 8 weeks after any prior PCV13 dose).
   Age 6-18 years:
   - No history of PPSV23: 1 dose of PPSV23 (at least 8 weeks after any prior PCV13 dose).

Cerebrospinal fluid leak; cochlear implant:
Age 2–5 years:
- Any incomplete* schedules with:
  o 3 PCV13 doses: 1 dose of PCV13 (at least 8 weeks after any prior PCV13 dose).
  o <3 PCV13 doses: 2 doses of PCV13, 8 weeks after the most recent dose and given 8 weeks apart.
- No history of PPSV23: 1 dose of PPSV23 (at least 8 weeks after any prior PCV13 dose).
Age 6–18 years:
- No history of either PCV13 or PPSV23: 1 dose of PCV13, 1 dose of PPSV23 at least 8 weeks later.
- Any PCV13 but no PPSV23: 1 dose of PPSV23 at least 8 weeks after the most recent dose of PCV13
- PPSV23 but no PCV13: 1 dose of PCV13 at least 8 weeks after the most recent dose of PPSV23.

Sickle cell disease and other hemoglobinopathies; anatomic or functional asplenia; congenital or acquired immunodeficiency; HIV infection; chronic renal failure; nephrotic syndrome; malignant neoplasms, leukemias, lymphomas, Hodgkin disease, and other diseases associated with treatment with immunosuppressive drugs or radiation therapy; solid organ transplantation; multiple myeloma:
Age 2–5 years:
- Any incomplete* schedules with:
  o 3 PCV13 doses: 1 dose of PCV13 (at least 8 weeks after any prior PCV13 dose).
  o <3 PCV13 doses: 2 doses of PCV13, 8 weeks after the most recent dose and given 8 weeks apart.
- No history of PPSV23: 1 dose of PPSV23 (at least 8 weeks after any prior PCV13 dose) and a 2nd dose of PPSV23 5 years later.
Age 6–18 years:
- No history of either PCV13 or PPSV23: 1 dose of PCV13, 2 doses of PPSV23 (1st dose of PPSV23 administered 8 weeks after PCV13 and 2nd dose of PPSV23 administered at least 5 years after the 1st dose of PPSV23).
- Any PCV13 but no PPSV23: 2 doses of PPSV23 (1st dose of PPSV23 to be given 8 weeks after the most recent dose of PCV13 and 2nd dose of PPSV23 administered at least 5 years after the 1st dose of PPSV23).

Table 14-11 (*continued*)

For further guidance on the use of the vaccines mentioned below, see: www.cdc.gov/vaccines/hcp/acip-recs/index.html.

- PPSV23 but no PCV13: 1 dose of PCV13 at least 8 weeks after the most recent PPSV23 dose and a 2nd dose of PPSV23 to be given 5 years after the 1st dose of PPSV23 and at least 8 weeks after a dose of PCV13.

Chronic liver disease, alcoholism:

Age 6–18 years:
- No history of PPSV23: 1 dose of PPSV23 (at least 8 weeks after any prior PCV13 dose).

*Incomplete schedules are any schedules where PCV13 doses have not been completed according to ACIP recommended catch-up schedules. The total number and timing of doses for complete PCV13 series are dictated by the age at first vaccination. See Tables 8 and 9 in the ACIP pneumococcal vaccine recommendations (www.cdc.gov/mmwr/pdf/rr/rr5911.pdf) for complete schedule details.

6. **Inactivated poliovirus vaccine (IPV). (minimum age: 6 weeks)**

Routine vaccination:
- 4-dose series at ages 2, 4, 6–18 months, and 4–6 years. Administer the final dose on or after the 4th birthday and at least 6 months after the previous dose.

Catch-up vaccination:
- In the first 6 months of life, use minimum ages and intervals only for travel to a polio-endemic region or during an outbreak.
- If 4 or more doses were given before the 4th birthday, give 1 more dose at age 4–6 years and at least 6 months after the previous dose.
- A 4th dose is not necessary if the 3rd dose was given on or after the 4th birthday and at least 6 months after the previous dose.
- IPV is not routinely recommended for U.S. residents 18 years and older.

Series Containing Oral Polio Vaccine (OPV), *either mixed OPV-IPV or OPV-only series:*
- Total number of doses needed to complete the series is the same as that recommended for the U.S. IPV schedule. See www.cdc.gov/mmwr/volumes/66/wr/mm6601a6.htm?s_cid=mm6601a6_w.
- Only trivalent OPV (tOPV) counts toward the U.S. vaccination requirements. For guidance to assess doses documented as "OPV" see www.cdc.gov/mmwr/volumes/66/wr/mm6606a7.htm?s_cid=mm6606a7_w.
- For other catch-up guidance, see Figure 2.

7. **Influenza vaccines. (minimum age: 6 months)**

Routine vaccination:
- Administer an age-appropriate formulation and dose of influenza vaccine annually.
  o **Children 6 months–8 years** who did not receive at least 2 doses of influenza vaccine before July 1, 2017 should receive 2 doses separated by at least 4 weeks.
  o **Persons 9 years and older** 1 dose
- Live attenuated influenza vaccine (LAIV) not recommended for the 2017–18 season.
- For additional guidance, see the 2017–18 ACIP influenza vaccine recommendations (*MMWR* August 25, 2017;66(2):1-20: www.cdc.gov/mmwr/volumes/66/rr/pdfs/rr6602.pdf).
(For the 2018–19 season, see the 2018–19 ACIP influenza vaccine recommendations.)

8. **Measles, mumps, and rubella (MMR) vaccine. (minimum age: 12 months for routine vaccination)**

Routine vaccination:
- 2-dose series at 12–15 months and 4–6 years.
- The 2nd dose may be given as early as 4 weeks after the 1st dose.

Catch-up vaccination:
- Unvaccinated children and adolescents: 2 doses at least 4 weeks apart.

International travel:
- **Infants 6–11 months:** 1 dose before departure. Revaccinate with 2 doses at 12–15 months (12 months for children in high-risk areas) and 2nd dose as early as 4 weeks later.
- **Unvaccinated children 12 months and older:** 2 doses at least 4 weeks apart before departure.

Mumps outbreak:
- Persons ≥12 months who previously received ≤2 doses of mumps-containing vaccine and are identified by public health authorities to be at increased risk during a mumps outbreak should receive a dose of mumps-virus containing vaccine.

9. **Varicella (VAR) vaccine. (minimum age: 12 months)**

Routine vaccination:
- 2-dose series: 12–15 months and 4–6 years.
- The 2nd dose may be given as early as 3 months after the 1st dose (a dose given after a 4-week interval may be counted).

Catch-up vaccination:
- Ensure persons 7–18 years without evidence of immunity (see *MMWR* 2007;56[No. RR-4], at www.cdc.gov/mmwr/pdf/rr/rr5604.pdf) have 2 doses of varicella vaccine:
  o **Ages 7–12:** routine interval 3 months (minimum interval: 4 weeks).
  o **Ages 13 and older:** minimum interval 4 weeks.

10. **Hepatitis A (HepA) vaccine. (minimum age: 12 months)**

Routine vaccination:
- 2 doses, separated by 6-18 months, between the 1st and 2nd birthdays. (A series begun before the 2nd birthday should be completed even if the child turns 2 before the second dose is given.)

Catch-up vaccination:
- Anyone 2 years of age or older may receive HepA vaccine if desired. Minimum interval between doses is 6 months.

Special populations:
Previously unvaccinated persons who should be vaccinated:
- Persons traveling to or working in countries with high or intermediate endemicity
- Men who have sex with men
- Users of injection and non-injection drugs
- Persons who work with hepatitis A virus in a research laboratory or with non-human primates
- Persons with clotting-factor disorders
- Persons with chronic liver disease
- Persons who anticipate close, personal contact (e.g., household or regular babysitting) with an international adoptee during the first 60 days after arrival in the United States from a country with high or intermediate endemicity (administer the 1st dose as soon as the adoption is planned— ideally at least 2 weeks before the adoptee's arrival).

11. **Serogroup A, C, W, Y meningococcal vaccines. (Minimum age: 2 months [Menveo], 9 months [Menactra].**

Routine:
- 2-dose series: 11-12 years and 16 years.

Catch-Up:
- Age 13-15 years: 1 dose now and booster at age 16-18 years. Minimum interval 8 weeks.
- Age 16-18 years: 1 dose.

For further guidance on the use of the vaccines mentioned below, see: www.cdc.gov/vaccines/hcp/acip-recs/index.html.

Special populations and situations:
Anatomic or functional asplenia, sickle cell disease, HIV infection, persistent complement component deficiency (including eculizumab use):
- **Menveo**
  o 1st dose at 8 weeks: 4-dose series at 2, 4, 6, and 12 months.
  o 1st dose at 7–23 months: 2 doses (2nd dose at least 12 weeks after the 1st dose and after the 1st birthday).
  o 1st dose at 24 months or older: 2 doses at least 8 weeks apart.
- **Menactra**
  o Persistent complement component deficiency:
    — 9–23 months: 2 doses at least 12 weeks apart
    — 24 months or older: 2 doses at least 8 weeks apart
  o Anatomic or functional asplenia, sickle cell disease, or HIV infection:
    — 24 months or older: 2 doses at least 8 weeks apart.
    — **Menactra** must be administered at least 4 weeks after completion of PCV13 series.

Children who travel to or live in countries where meningococcal disease is hyperendemic or epidemic, including countries in the African meningitis belt or during the Hajj, or exposure to an outbreak attributable to a vaccine serogroup:
- Children <24 months of age:
  o **Menveo (2-23 months):**
    — 1st dose at 8 weeks: 4-dose series at 2, 4, 6, and 12 months.
    — 1st dose at 7-23 months: 2 doses (2nd dose at least 12 weeks after the 1st dose and after the 1st birthday).
  o **Menactra (9-23 months):**
    — 2 doses (2nd dose at least 12 weeks after the 1st dose. 2nd dose may be administered as early as 8 weeks after the 1st dose in travelers).
- Children 2 years or older: 1 dose of **Menveo** or **Menactra**.

Note: Menactra should be given either before or at the same time as DTaP. For MenACWY booster dose recommendations for groups listed under "Special populations and situations" above, and additional meningococcal vaccination information, see meningococcal *MMWR* publications at: www.cdc.gov/vaccines/hcp/acip-recs/vacc-specific/mening.html.

12. **Serogroup B meningococcal vaccines (minimum age: 10 years [Bexsero, Trumenba].**

Clinical discretion: Adolescents not at increased risk for meningococcal B infection who want MenB vaccine.

MenB vaccines may be given at clinical discretion to adolescents 16–23 years (preferred age 16–18 years) who are not at increased risk.
- **Bexsero:** 2 doses at least 1 month apart.
- **Trumenba:** 2 doses at least 6 months apart. If the 2nd dose is given earlier than 6 months, give a 3rd dose at least 4 months after the 2nd.

Special populations and situations:
Anatomic or functional asplenia, sickle cell disease, persistent complement component deficiency (including eculizumab use), serogroup B meningococcal disease outbreak
- **Bexsero:** 2-dose series at least 1 month apart.
- **Trumenba:** 3-dose series at 0, 1-2, and 6 months.

Note: Bexsero and Trumenba are not interchangeable.
For additional meningococcal vaccination information, see meningococcal *MMWR* publications at: www.cdc.gov/vaccines/hcp/acip-recs/vacc-specific/mening.html.

13. **Tetanus, diphtheria, and acellular pertussis (Tdap) vaccine. (minimum age: 11 years for routine vaccinations, 7 years for catch-up vaccination)**

Routine vaccination:
- Adolescents 11–12 years of age: 1 dose.
- **Pregnant adolescents:** 1 dose during each pregnancy (preferably during the early part of gestational weeks 27–36).
- Tdap may be administered regardless of the interval since the last tetanus- and diphtheria-toxoid-containing vaccine.

Catch-up vaccination:
- Adolescents 13–18 who have not received Tdap: 1 dose, followed by a Td booster every 10 years.
- **Persons aged 7–18 years not fully immunized with DTaP:** 1 dose of Tdap as part of the catch-up series (preferably the first dose). If additional doses are needed, use Td.

- **Children 7–10 years** who receive Tdap inadvertently or as part of the catch-up series may receive the routine Tdap dose at 11–12 years.
- **DTaP inadvertently given after the 7th birthday:**
  o **Child 7–10:** DTaP may count as part of catch-up series. Routine Tdap dose at 11-12 may be given.
  o **Adolescent 11–18:** Count dose of DTaP as the adolescent Tdap booster.
- For other catch-up guidance, see Figure 2.

14. **Human papillomavirus (HPV) vaccine (minimum age: 9 years)**

Routine and catch-up vaccination:
- Routine vaccination for all adolescents at 11–12 years (can start at age 9) and through age 18 if not previously adequately vaccinated. Number of doses dependent on age at initial vaccination:
  o **Age 9–14 years at initiation:** 2-dose series at 0 and 6–12 months. Minimum interval: 5 months (repeat a dose given too soon at least 12 weeks after the invalid dose and at least 5 months after the 1st dose).
  o **Age 15 years or older at initiation:** 3-dose series at 0, 1–2 months, and 6 months. Minimum intervals: 4 weeks between 1st and 2nd dose; 12 weeks between 2nd and 3rd dose; 5 months between 1st and 3rd dose (repeat dose(s) given too soon at or after the minimum interval since the most recent dose).
- Persons who have completed a valid series with any HPV vaccine do not need any additional doses.

Special situations:
- **History of sexual abuse or assault:** Begin series at age 9 years.
- **Immunocompromised* (including HIV)** aged 9–26 years: 3-dose series at 0, 1–2 months, and 6 months.
- **Pregnancy:** Vaccination not recommended, but there is no evidence the vaccine is harmful. No intervention is needed for women who inadvertently received a dose of HPV vaccine while pregnant. Delay remaining doses until after pregnancy. Pregnancy testing not needed before vaccination.

*See MMWR, December 16, 2016;65(49):1405–1408, at www.cdc.gov/mmwr/volumes/65/wr/pdfs/mm6549a5.pdf.

	Table 14-12 NURSING CONSIDERATIONS FOR THE CHILD RECEIVING IMMUNIZATION	
NAME	**ROUTE**	**NURSING CONSIDERATIONS**
DTaP (diphtheria, tetanus, pertussis)	IM anterior or lateral thigh (No IMs in gluteal muscle until after child is walking)	Potential adverse effects include fever within 24–48 hours, swelling, redness, soreness at injection site More serious adverse effects—continuous screaming, convulsions, high fever, loss of consciousness Do not administer if there is past history of serious reaction
MMR (measles, mumps, rubella)	SC anterior or lateral thigh	Potential adverse effects include rash, fever, and arthritis; may occur 10 days to 2 wk after vaccination May give DTaP, MMR, and IPV at same time if family has history of not keeping appointments for vaccinations Contraindicated with allergies to neomycin Is live attenuated vaccine
IPV	IM	Reactions very rare
HB (hepatitis B)	IM vastus lateralis or deltoid	Should not be given into dorsogluteal site Mild local tenderness at injection site
Tuberculosis test	Intradermal	May be given 4–6 years, and 11–16 years if in high-prevalence areas Evaluated in 48–72 hours PPD (purified protein derivative) 0.1 mL Tine test (multiple puncture) less accurate
TD (tetanus/ diphtheria booster)	IM anterior or lateral thigh	Repeat every 10 years Contraindicated in moderate or severe illness
Live attenuated rubella	SC anterior or lateral thigh	Give once only to women who are antibody-negative for rubella, and if pregnancy can be prevented for 3 months postvaccination
Live attenuated mumps	SC	Give once Prevention of orchitis (and therefore sterility) in susceptible males

B. Overall contraindications to immunizations
   1. Severe febrile illness
   2. Live viruses should not be given to anyone with altered immune system, e.g., undergoing chemotherapy, radiation, or with immunologic deficiency
   3. Previous allergic response to a vaccine
   4. Recently acquired passive immunity, e.g., blood transfusion, immunoglobulin

COMMON CHILDHOOD PROBLEMS

A. Common communicable disease (see Table 14-13)

Table 14-13 COMMON COMMUNICABLE DISEASES OF CHILDHOOD

NAME/ INCUBATION	TRANSMISSION/CLINICAL PICTURE	NURSING CONSIDERATIONS
Chickenpox (Varicella) 13–17 days	Prodromal: slight fever, malaise, anorexia Rash is pruritic, begins as macule, then papule, and then vesicle with successive crops of all three stages present at any one time; lymphadenopathy; elevated temperature Transmission: spread by direct contact, airborne, contaminated object	Isolation until all vesicles are crusted; communicable from 1–2 days before rash Avoid use of aspirin due to association with Reye's syndrome; use acetaminophen and/or ibuprofen Topical application of calamine lotion or baking soda baths Airborne and contact precautions in hospital
Diphtheria 2–5 days	Prodromal: resembles common cold Low-grade fever, hoarseness, malaise, pharyngeal lymphadenitis; characteristic white/gray pharyngeal membrane Transmission: direct contact with a carrier, infected client contaminated articles	Contact and droplet precautions until two successive negative nose and throat cultures are obtained Complete bedrest; watch for signs of respiratory distress and obstruction; provide for humidification, suctioning, and tracheostomy as needed; severe cases can lead to sepsis and death Administer antitoxin therapy
Pertussis (Whooping Cough) 5–21 days, usually 10	Prodromal: upper respiratory infection for 1–2 weeks Severe cough with high-pitched "whooping" sound, especially at night, lasts 4–6 weeks; vomiting Transmission: direct contact, droplet, contaminated articles	Hospitalization for infants; bedrest and hydration Complications: pneumonia, weight loss, dehydration, hemorrhage, hernia, airway obstruction Maintain high humidity and restful environment; suction; oxygen Administer erythromycin and pertussis immune globulin
Rubella (German Measles) 14–21 days	Prodromal: none in children, low fever and sore throat in adolescent Maculopapular rash appears first on face and then on rest of the body Symptoms subside first day after rash Transmission: droplet spread and contaminated articles	Contact precautions Isolate child from potentially pregnant women Comfort measures; antipyretics and analgesics Rare complications include arthritis and encephalitis Droplet precautions Risk of fetal deformity
Rubeola 10–20 days	Prodromal: fever and malaise followed by cough and Koplik's spots on buccal mucosa Erythematous maculopapular rash with face first affected; turns brown after 3 days when symptoms subside Transmission: direct contact with droplets	Isolate until 5th day; maintain bedrest during first 3–4 days Institute airborne and seizure precautions Antipyretics, dim lights; humidifier for room Keep skin clean and maintain hydration
Scarlet fever 2–4 days	Prodromal: high fever with vomiting, chills, malaise, followed by enlarged tonsils covered with exudate, strawberry tongue Rash: red tiny lesions that become generalized and then desquamate; rash appears within 24 hours Transmission: droplet spread or contaminated articles Group A beta-hemolytic streptococci	Droplet precautions for 24 hours after start of antibiotics Ensure compliance with oral antibiotic therapy Bedrest during febrile phase Analgesics for sore throat Encourage fluids, soft diet Administer penicillin or erythromycin
Mononucleosis 4–6 weeks	Malaise, fever, enlarged lymph nodes, sore throat, flulike aches, low-grade temperature Highest incidence 15–30 years old Transmission: direct contact with oral secretions, unknown	Advise family members to avoid contact with saliva (cups, silverware) for about 3 months Treatment is rest and good nutrition; strenuous exercise is to be avoided to prevent spleen rupture Complications include encephalitis and spleen rupture

Table 14-13 COMMON COMMUNICABLE DISEASES OF CHILDHOOD *(CONTINUED)*		
NAME/ INCUBATION	**TRANSMISSION/CLINICAL PICTURE**	**NURSING CONSIDERATIONS**
Tonsillitis (streptococcal)	Fever, white exudate on tonsils Positive culture GpA strep	Antibiotics Teach parents serious potential complications: rheumatic fever, glomerulonephritis
Mumps 14–21 days	Malaise, headache, fever, parotid gland swelling Transmission: direct contact with saliva, droplet	Isolation before and after appearance of swelling Soft, bland diet Complications: deafness, meningitis, encephalitis, sterility

B. Poison control/prevention
1. Assessment
   a. Airway, breathing, circulation (ABC)–treat the client first, then the poison
   b. Identify poison–amount ingested, time of ingestion; save vomitus
   c. Diagnostics
      1) Urine and serum analysis
      2) Long-bone x-rays if suspect lead deposits
      3) CAT scan, EEG
2. Nursing management
   a. Prevention–most toxic ingestions are acute (see Table 14-14)
      1) Child-proofing–store all potentially poisonous substances in locked out-of-reach area
      2) Increased awareness of precipitating factors
         a) Growth and development characteristics–under/overestimating the capabilities of the child
         b) Changes in household routine
         c) Conditions that increase emotional tension of family members

Table 14-14 TEACHING PREVENTION OF ACCIDENTAL POISONING IN CHILDREN	
ACTION	**RATIONALE**
Proper storage–locked cabinets	Once child can crawl, can investigate cabinets and ingest contents of bottles
Never take medicine in front of children	Children are interested in anything their parents take and will mimic taking medicine
Never leave medication in purse, on table, or on kitchen counter	Children will investigate area and ingest bottle contents
Never refer to medicine as candy	Increases interest in taking medicine when unsupervised
Leave medicines, cleaning supplies in original containers	Pill boxes, soda bottles increase attractiveness and inhibit identification of substance should poisoning occur
Provide activities and play materials for children	Encourages child's interest without endangering him/her
Teach need for supervision of small children	Small children cannot foresee potential harm and need protection

    b. Instructions for caretaker in case of suspected poison ingestion

        1) Recognize signs and symptoms of accidental poisoning–change in child's appearance/behavior; presence of unusual substances in child's mouth, hands, play area; burns, blisters and/or suspicious odor around child's mouth; open/empty containers in child's possession

        2) Initiate steps to stop exposure

        3) Call Poison Control Center–be prepared to provide information

           a) Substance–name, time, amount, route

           b) Child–condition, age, weight

        4) Save any substance, vomitus, stool, urine

        5) Induce vomiting if indicated by Poison Control Center

    c. Emergency care in a health care facility

        1) Basic life support

           a) Respiratory–intubate if comatose, seizing, or no gag reflex; frequent blood gases

           b) Circulation–IV fluids; maintain fluid and electrolyte balance; cardiac monitor: essential for comatose child and with tricyclic antidepressant or phenothiazine ingestion

        2) Gastric lavage and aspiration–client is intubated and positioned head down and on left side; large oro/nasogastric tube inserted and repeated irrigations of normal saline instilled until clear; not more than 10 mL/kg; must be done within 60 minutes

        3) Activated charcoal–absorbs compounds, forming a nonabsorbable complex; 5–10 g for each gram of toxin

           a) Give within 1 hour of ingestion and after emetic

           b) Mix with water to make a syrup; given PO or via gastric tube

    d. Hasten elimination

        1) Cathartic–to speed substance through lower GI tract; not recommended

        2) Diuretics–for substances eliminated by kidneys

        3) Chelation–heavy metals (e.g., mercury, lead, and arsenic) are not readily eliminated from body; progressive buildup leads to toxicity; a chelating agent binds with the heavy metal, forming a complex that can be eliminated by kidneys, peritoneal hemodialysis (e.g., deferoxamine, dimercaprol, calcium EDTA)

    e. Prevent recurrence–crisis intervention with nonjudgmental approach; acknowledge difficulty in maintaining constant supervision; explore contributory factors; discuss and educate about growth and development influences as well as passive (child restraint closures) and active safety measures

C. Common substances that cause poisoning

  1. Aspirin (salicylate)–products containing aspirin

    a. Assessment

        1) Tinnitus, nausea, sweating, dizziness, headache

        2) Change in mental status

        3) Increased temperature, hyperventilation (respiratory alkalosis)

        4) Later, metabolic acidosis and respiratory acidosis, bleeding, and hypovolemia

    b. Effects

        1) Toxicity begins at doses of 150–200 mg/kg; 4 gm may be fatal to child

           a) Altered acid–base balance (respiratory alkalosis) due to increased respiratory rate

           b) Increased metabolism causes greater O_2 consumption, CO_2 and heat production

          c) Metabolic acidosis results in hyperkalemia, dehydration, and kidney failure

          d) May result in decreased prothrombin formation and decreased platelet aggregation, causing bleeding

    c. Nursing management

       1) Induce vomiting; initiate gastric lavage with activated charcoal

       2) Monitor vital signs and laboratory values

       3) Maintain IV hydration and electrolyte replacement; monitor I and O, skin turgor, fontanelles, urinary specific gravity, serum potassium (hypokalemia may occur with correct of condition)

       4) Reduce temperature—tepid water baths or hypothermia blankets; prone to seizures

       5) Vitamin K, if needed, for bleeding disorder; guaiac of vomitus/stools

       6) IV sodium bicarbonate enhances excretion

2. Acetaminophen overdose

    a. Assessment

       1) First 2 hours, nausea and vomiting, sweating, pallor, hypothermia, slow-weak pulse

       2) Followed by latent period (1–1.5 d) when symptoms abate

       3) If no treatment, hepatic involvement occurs (may last up to 1 wk) with RUQ pain, jaundice, confusion, stupor, coagulation abnormalities

       4) Diagnostic tests—serum acetaminophen levels at least 4 hours after ingestion; liver function test AST, ALT, and kidney function tests (creatinine, BUN)—change in renal and liver function is a late sign

    b. Effects

       1) Toxicity begins at 150 mg/kg

       2) Major risk is hepatic necrosis

    c. Nursing management

       1) Induce vomiting

       2) *N*-acetylcystine—specific antidote; most effective in 8–10 hours; must be given within 24 hours; given po every 4 hours × 72 hours or IV × 3 doses

       3) Maintain hydration; monitor output

       4) Monitor liver and kidney function

3. Lead toxicity (plumbism)

    a. Assessment

       1) Physical symptoms

          a) Irritability

          b) Sleepiness, decreased activity

          c) Nausea, vomiting, abdominal pain

          d) Constipation

          e) Decreased activity

          f) Increased intracranial pressure (e.g., seizures and motor dysfunction)

       2) Environmental sources

          a) Flaking, lead-based paint (primary source)

          b) Crumbling plaster

          c) Odor of lead-based gasoline

    d) Pottery with lead glaze

    e) Lead solder in pipes

  3) Diagnostic tests

    a) Blood lead level—there is no safe level of lead in the blood. Public health action is recommended with blood levels above 5 mcg/dL (0.24 mcmol/L)

    b) Erythrocyte protoporphyrin (EP) level

    c) CBC—anemia

    d) X-rays (long bone/GI)—may show radiopaque material, "lead lines"

    e) Calcium disodium mobilization/provocative test—to evaluate degree of stored lead; lead levels are measured in urine collected over a specific time after injection of calcium disodium

b. Analysis

  1) Child—practice of pica (habitual and compulsive ingestion of nonfood substances); children absorb more lead than adults; paint chips taste sweet

  2) Pathology—lead is slowly excreted by kidneys and GI tract; stored in inert form in long bones; chronic ingestion affects many body systems

    a) Hematological—blocks formation of hemoglobin, leading to microcytic anemia (initial sign) and increased erythrocyte protoporphyrin (EP)

    b) Renal—toxic to kidney tubules, allowing an abnormal excretion of protein, glucose, amino acids, phosphates

    c) CNS—increases membrane permeability, resulting in fluid shifts into brain tissue, cell ischemia and destruction causing neurological and intellectual deficiencies with low-dose exposure; with high-dose exposure, intellectual delay, convulsions, and death (lead encephalopathy)

c. Nursing management

  1) Chelating agent—promotes lead excretion in urine and stool; dimercaprol (BAL in Oil), calcium disodium, EDTA; succimer; deferoxamine

    a) Maintain hydration

    b) Identify sources of lead and institute deleading procedures; involve local housing authorities as needed

    c) Instruct parents about supervision for pica and ways to encourage other activities for the child

ALTERATIONS IN PEDIATRIC HEALTH

INTERVENTIONS FOR THE HOSPITALIZED CHILD

A. Prevent or minimize the effects of separation on the child
   1. Encourage parental involvement in child's care, especially through rooming-in facilities
   2. Assign the same nurse to care for the child
   3. Provide objects which re-create familiar surroundings (e.g., toys from home)

B. Observe for alterations in parenting
   1. Behavior patterns of parents and child
   2. Identify healthy relationships and unhealthy relationships, e.g., failure to thrive; indications of child abuse

C. Educate parents on proper health care for children
   1. Pediatrician visits; immunization schedules; childhood diseases
   2. Review diet and exercise patterns

SELECTED DISORDERS—INFANTS

A. Cleft lip and palate
   1. Definition—congenital malformation
      a. Cleft lip—small or large fissure in facial process of upper lip or up to nasal septum, including anterior maxilla
      b. Cleft palate—midline, bilateral, or unilateral fissures in hard and soft palate
   2. Basic concepts
      a. Lip is usually repaired during first weeks of life
      b. Palate is usually repaired before child develops altered speech patterns (between 12–18 months)
   3. Clinical manifestations
      a. Parents will have strong reaction to birth of defective infant—provide support and information
      b. Assess infant's ability to suck

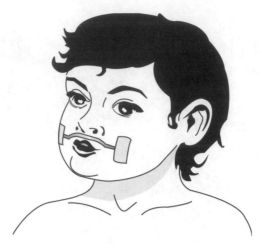

Figure 14-1. LOGAN BOW

4. Nursing management
   a. Preoperative
      1) Maintain adequate nutrition
      2) Feed with soft nipple, special lamb's nipple, Breck feeder, or cup

   b. Postoperative
      1) Maintain airway
         a) Observe for respiratory distress
         b) Provide suction equipment and endotracheal tube at bedside

      2) Guard suture line
         a) Keep suture line clean and dry
         b) Use lip protective devices, i.e., Logan bow device (see Figure 14-1) or tape as ordered
         c) Maintain side-lying position on unaffected side
         d) Minimize crying with comfort measures—rocking, cuddling
         e) Use restraints as needed

      3) Provide nutrition
         a) Use feeding techniques to minimize trauma—usually very slow to feed
         b) Burp baby frequently during feedings

      4) Facilitate parents' positive response to child
      5) Provide referrals to speech therapy and orthodontists as needed

B. Colic (in infants)
   1. Definition—abdominal cramps
   2. Assessment
      a. Abrupt onset of crying with loud screams commonly lasting 3 hours and occurring at least 3 times/week, clenched fists, and legs drawn up to abdomen
      b. Flatus or belching during the vigorous crying spells
      c. Symptoms worse in early evening and night

   3. Analysis
      a. Most frequent in infants of low birth weight
      b. Usually disappears by 3 months of age

      c. Excessive air swallowing

        1) Too rapid feeding

        2) Too vigorous sucking on small nipple holes or an empty bottle

      d. Excessive carbohydrate intake—causes increased fermentation and production of gas

      e. Indigestion from overfeeding

      f. Insufficient emotional satisfaction

  4. Nursing management

      a. Enemas, suppositories, and rectal tubes to relieve distention

      b. Frequent burping of baby during and after feedings

      c. Modification of amount and type of formula

      d. Local application of heat to abdomen

      e. Additional cuddling and closeness

      f. Medications—e.g., antispasmodics for relief

C. Pyloric stenosis

  1. Definition—obstruction of the passageway from the stomach to the duodenum due to enlargement of the sphincter muscle, sometimes twice its normal size

  2. Basic concepts

      a. Inflammation and edema can reduce the size of the opening until there is complete obstruction

      b. Infants usually asymptomatic until the second to fourth week after birth; then, regurgitation develops into projectile vomiting; most frequently seen in Caucasian, male, full-term infants

  3. Clinical manifestations

      a. Upper gastrointestinal x-rays reveal delayed gastric emptying and elongated pyloric channel

      b. Signs of pyloric stenosis include projectile vomiting, weight loss, constipation, dehydration, olive-sized tumor, visible peristaltic waves from left upper quadrant (LUQ) to right upper quadrant (RUQ)

  4. Nursing management

      a. Preoperative

        1) Prevent regurgitation and vomiting

          a) Give small frequent feedings

          b) Position upright after feedings

          c) Keep quiet environment after feeding

        2) Monitor for complications—alkalosis, hypokalemia, dehydration, and shock

        3) Support parents

          a) Allow verbalization of parents' anxieties

          b) Instruct parents on expected progress and behavior

      b. Postoperative

        1) Check incision site; keep incision site clean and dry

        2) Provide parenteral fluids at ordered rate

        3) Monitor warmth

        4) Small, frequent feedings of glucose water or electrolyte solution 4–6 hours post operatively; advance diet gradually

        5) If clear fluids retained start formula 24 hours post op

D. Esophageal atresia and tracheoesophageal fistula

    1. Definition—malformations of the esophagus, often with associated anomalies of the heart or genitourinary systems (see Figure 14-2)

    2. History

        a. During the fifth week of embryological development, the embryonic foregut must lengthen and separate into trachea and esophagus; defects in this development result in blind pouches and/or fistulas

        b. In almost 90% of tracheoesophageal defects, the esophagus ends in a blind pouch and the trachea has a short segment attaching it to the stomach (see panel A in Figure 14-2); the second most common defect is seen in panel B, and the defects seen in panels C and D are very rare

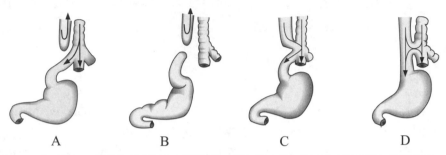

        A   B   C   D

Figure 14-2. ESOPHAGEAL ATRESIA AND TRACHEOESOPHAGEAL FISTULA

    3. Assessment

        a. Excessive saliva

        b. Stomach distention

        c. Choking

        d. Coughing

        e. Cyanosis

    4. Nursing management

        a. Preoperative

            1) Position to prevent saliva aspiration

            2) Facilitate gastrostomy drainage

        b. Postoperative

            1) Care for incision site—observe for inflammation

            2) Prevent pulmonary complications—suction and position

            3) Provide TPN until gastrectomy or oral feedings tolerated

E. Strabismus

    1. Assessment—eyes do not function as a unit because of an imbalance of the extraocular muscles

        a. Visible deviation of eye

        b. Diplopia

        c. Child tilts head or squints to focus

2. Management
   a. Therapy
      1) Developing visual acuity in both eyes
      2) Developing coordinate function

   b. Nonsurgical intervention begins no later than age 6
      1) Occlusion of unaffected eye to strengthen weaker eye
      2) Corrective lenses combined with other therapy to improve acuity
      3) Orthoptic exercises designed to strengthen eye muscles

F. Hydrocephalus
   1. Assessment
      a. Congenital or acquired condition characterized by an increase in the accumulation of CSF within the ventricular system and subsequent increase in ventricular pressure

   2. Etiology
      a. Neoplasm
      b. Aqueductal stenosis—stenosis/obstructions in ventricular system
      c. Spina bifida
      d. Congenital cysts/vascular malformations
      e. Meningitis
      f. Head trauma
      g. Intraventricular hemorrhage in premature infants
      h. Idiopathic

   3. Types
      a. Communicating—due to increased production of CSF or impaired absorption of CSF
      b. Noncommunicating—due to obstruction/blockage of CSF circulation between ventricles and subarachnoid

   4. Characteristics
      a. Signs and symptoms
         1) Fronto-occipital circumference increasing at abnormally fast rate
         2) Splint sutures and widened fontanelles
         3) Prominent forehead
         4) Dilated scalp veins
         5) Distended/tense fontanelles
         6) Sunset eyes, nystagmus
         7) Irritability, vomiting
         8) Unusual somnolence
         9) Convulsions
         10) High-pitched cry

5. Nursing/Medical management
   a. Operative management
      1) Ventriculoperitoneal shunt—ventricles to peritoneal cavity (see Figure 14-3)
      2) Ventricular atrial shunt—ventricles to right atrium
      3) Ventricular drainage—external
      4) Discharge planning/community referral

   b. Nursing care
      1) Observation of shunt functioning/malfunction
      2) Shunt modified as child grows
      3) Observe for increased intracranial pressure and signs of shunt infection (irritability, high pitched cry, lethargy)
      4) Postoperative positioning—on unoperated side in flat position; do not hold infant with head elevated
      5) Continual testing for developmental abnormalities/intellectual delay
      6) Continual testing for developmental abnormalities and cognitive deficiencies
      7) Discharge planning/community referral
      8) Teach parents about increased risk for allergies if myelomeningocele present

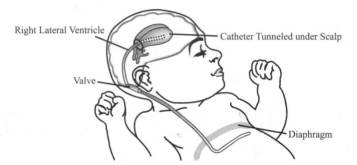

Figure   14–3.   VENTRICULOPERITONEAL SHUNT

G. Congenital heart anomalies (see Table 14-15)
   1. Assessment/symptoms

Table 14–15 CONGENITAL HEART ANOMALIES	
ACYANOTIC TYPE	**CYANOTIC TYPE**
Normal color	Cyanosis usually from birth; clubbing of fingers
Normal CNS function	May have seizures due to hypoxia; fainting; confusion
Possible exercise intolerance	Marked exercise intolerance; may have hypoxic spells following exercise; squats to decrease respiratory distress
Possible weight loss or gain (with fluid retention)	Difficulty eating because of inability to breathe at the same time
Small stature; failure to thrive	Small stature; failure to thrive
Characteristic murmur; increased frequency of respiratory infections	Characteristic murmur; frequent and severe respiratory infections

2. History—predisposing factors
   a. Rubella during pregnancy
   b. Maternal alcoholism
   c. Maternal age over 40 years
   d. Maternal diabetes
   e. Sibling with heart disease
   f. Parent with congenital heart disease
   g. Other congenital anomalies

3. General effects of heart malformation
   a. Increased workload—overloading of chambers resulting in hypertrophy and tachycardia
   b. Pulmonary hypertension (increased vascular resistance) resulting in dyspnea, tachypnea, and recurrent respiratory infections
   c. Inadequate systemic cardiac output, resulting in exercise intolerance and growth failure
   d. Arterial desaturation from shunting of deoxygenated blood directly into the systemic circulation, resulting in polycythemia, cyanosis, cerebral changes, clubbing, squatting, and metabolic acidemia
   e. Murmurs due to abnormal shunting of blood between two heart chambers or between vessels

4. Types of defects
   a. Increased pulmonary blood flow (acyanotic)
      1) Ventricular septal defect (VSD)—abnormal opening between right and left ventricles; may vary in size from pinhole to absence of septum
         a) Characterized by loud, harsh murmur
         b) May close spontaneously by age 3—surgery may be indicated (purse-string closure of defect or pulmonary artery banding)

      2) Atrial septal defect (ASD)—abnormal opening between the two atria; severity depends on the size and location
         a) Small defects high on the septum may result in no apparent clinical symptoms
         b) Murmur audible and distinct for defect
         c) Unless defect is severe, prophylactic closure is done in later childhood

      3) Patent ductus arteriosis (PDA)—failure of that fetal structure to close after birth (in fetus, ductus arteriosis connects the pulmonary artery to the aorta to shunt oxygenated blood from placenta directly into systemic circulation, bypassing the lungs)
         a) PDA allows blood to be shunted from aorta (high pressure) to pulmonary artery (low pressure), causing additional blood to be reoxygenated in the lungs; result is increased pulmonary vascular congestion and right ventricular hypertrophy
         b) Characteristic murmur, widened pulse pressure, bounding pulse, and tachycardia
         c) Treatment is surgical intervention to divide or ligate the patent vessel

   b. Obstruction to blood flow from ventricle (acyanotic)
      1) Coarctation of the aorta—narrowing of the aorta
         a) High blood pressure and bounding pulses in areas receiving blood from vessels proximal to the defect; weak or absent pulses distal to defect, cool extremities, and muscle cramps
         b) Murmur may or may not be present

    c) Surgical treatment involves resection of the coarcted portion and end-to-end anastomosis or replacement of the constricted section using a graft

    d) High incidence of complications if left untreated

2) Pulmonic stenosis—narrowing at the entrance to the pulmonary artery
    a) Resistance to blood flow causes right ventricular hypertrophy

    b) Commonly seen with PDA

    c) Severity depends on degree of defect

    d) Surgery recommended for severe defect (pulmonary valvotomy)

3) Aortic stenosis—narrowing of aortic valve causes decreased cardiac output
    a) Murmur usually heard

    b) Surgery recommended

c. Cyanotic—poorly oxygenated venous blood enters systemic circulation; compensatory mechanisms observed in cyanotic heart disease: tachycardia, polycythemia, and posturing (squatting, knee-chest position)—decreased pulmonary blood flow

1) Tetralogy of Fallot—four defects: ventricular septal defect, pulmonic stenosis, overriding aorta, right ventricular hypertrophy (first three are congenital, fourth is acquired due to increased pressure within the right ventricle)
    a) Cyanosis, clubbing of fingers, delayed physical growth and development

    b) Child often squats or assumes knee-chest position

    c) Treatment is surgical correction

d. Mixed blood flow (cyanotic)
1) Transposition of the great vessels—pulmonary artery leaves the left ventricle, and the aorta leaves from the right ventricle
    a) Unless there is an associated defect to compensate, this condition is incompatible with life

    b) Depending on severity of condition—severely cyanotic to mild heart failure

    c) Treatment is surgical correction

2) Truncus arteriosus—failure of normal septation and embryonic division of pulmonary artery and aorta, resulting in a single vessel which overrides both ventricles, giving rise directly to the pulmonary and systemic circulations
    a) Blood from both ventricles enters the common artery and flows either to the lungs or the aortic arch and body

    b) Cyanosis, left ventricular hypertrophy, dyspnea, marked activity intolerance, and growth restriction

    c) Harsh murmur audible; congestive heart failure usually develops

    d) Palliative treatment—banding both pulmonary arteries to decrease the amount of blood going to lungs

    e) Corrective treatment—closing ventricular septal defect so truncus originates from left ventricle and creating pathway from right ventricle

3) Total anomalous venous return—absence of direct communication between pulmonary veins and left atrium; pulmonary veins attach directly to the right atrium or to various veins draining toward the right atrium
    a) Cyanosis, pulmonary congestion, and heart failure

          b) Murmur audible

          c) Surgical correction involves restoring the normal pulmonary venous circulation

5. Nursing management
   a. Prevent congenital heart disease
      1) Optimal nutrition, prenatal care, and avoidance of drugs and alcohol
      2) Immunization against rubella in females of childbearing age

   b. Recognize early symptoms—cyanosis, poor weight gain, poor feeding habits, exercise intolerance, unusual posturing; carefully evaluate heart murmurs

   c. Help parents adjust to defect
      1) Monitor vital signs and heart rhythm
      2) Prepare client for invasive procedures
      3) Monitor intake and output
      4) Provide calm environment and promote rest

6. Medications
   a. Digoxin
   b. Iron preparations
   c. Diuretics
   d. Potassium

7. Change in feeding pattern for infant
   a. Small amounts every 2 hours
   b. Enlarged nipple hole
   c. Diet—low sodium, high potassium

H. Sudden infant death syndrome (SIDS) (unexplained sudden death during sleep of a child under 1 year old)
   1. Assessment
      a. Occurs during first year of life, peaks at 2 to 4 months
      b. Occurs between midnight and 9 AM
      c. Increased incidence in winter, peaks in January

2. Analysis
   a. Thought to be brainstem abnormality in neurological regulation of cardiorespiratory control
   b. Third leading cause of death in children from 1 wk to 1 year of age
   c. Higher incidence of SIDS
      1) Infants with documented apparent life-threatening events (ALTEs)
      2) Siblings of infant with SIDS
      3) Preterm infants who have pathological apnea
      4) Preterm infants, especially with low birth weight
      5) Infants of African descent
      6) Multiple births
      7) Infants of addicted mothers
      8) Infants who sleep on abdomen
      9) Maternal smoking
      10) Cosleeping with parent(s) or multiple family members
      11) Soft bedding

3. Nursing management
   a. Home apnea monitor
   b. Place all healthy infants in supine position to sleep
   c. Support parents, family
   d. Referral to Sudden Infant Death Foundation

SELECTED NEUROMUSCULAR DISORDERS

A. Spina bifida/neural tube defects
   1. Description—congenital anomaly of the spinal cord characterized by nonunion between the laminae of the vertebrae
   2. Types (see Figure 14-4)
      a. Dimpling at the site (spina bifida occulta)
      b. Bulging, sac-like lesion filled with spinal fluid and covered with thin, atrophic, bluish, ulcerated skin (meningocele)
      c. Bulging, sac-like lesion filled with spinal fluid and spinal cord element (myelomeningocele)

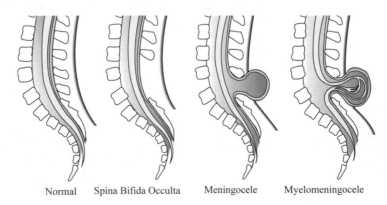

Normal   Spina Bifida Occulta   Meningocele   Myelomeningocele

Figure 14-4. TYPES OF SPINA BIFIDA

3. Risk factors
   a. Maternal folic acid deficiency
   b. Previous pregnancy affected by neural tubal defect

4. Nursing management
   a. Protect lesions from trauma or infection
      1) Observe for irritation, CSF leakage, signs of infection, hydrocephalus
      2) Maintain optimum asepsis; cover lesion with moist sterile dressings
      3) Position client on abdomen or semiprone with sandbags
      4) Provide optimum skin care, especially to perineal area

   b. Identify possible motor and sensory dysfunctions and report immediately
      1) Abnormal movement of extremities
      2) Absent or abnormal reflexes
      3) Incontinence, fecal impaction
      4) Flaccid paralysis of lower extremities

   c. Identify intracranial involvement
      1) Observe for increased intracranial pressure (IICP)
         a) Tense and/or bulging fontanels
         b) Separated cranial sutures
         c) Irritability
         d) High-pitched cry
         e) Distended scalp veins
         f) Changes in feeding habits
         g) Setting-sun sign in the eyes
      2) Observe for alterations in level of consciousness
         a) Similar to IICP
         b) Poor sucking ability
         c) Poor muscle tone
         d) Lack of movement
         e) Weak cry

   d. Provide frequent sources of stimulation appropriate for child's age level
   e. Provide postoperative care—vertebral fusion or surgical repair
      1) Focus observation on detecting signs of meningitis, shock, increased intracranial pressure, and respiratory difficulty
      2) Family teaching on how to care for child at home
      3) Referrals for possible physiotherapy, orthopedic procedures, and bowel and bladder management should be discussed with family

B. Cerebral palsy
1. Description—a neuromuscular disability in which the voluntary muscles are poorly controlled because of brain damage
2. History
   a. Heredity
   b. Maternal diabetes, rubella, toxemia during pregnancy
   c. Rh incompatibility

      d. Birth injuries

      e. Infections

  3. Assessment

      a. Neonate—cannot hold up head, feeble cry, weakness, inability to feed, body noticeably arched

      b. Infants—failure-to-thrive syndrome present

      c. Toddlers and preschoolers—signs of intellectual delay; distorted physical development pattern, especially walking; spasticity of muscles is a dominant characteristic

  4. Nursing managment

      a. Preserve physical and mental capacity of the child

         1) Assist with early diagnosis

         2) Assist with physical and occupational therapy

         3) Give referrals to appropriate agencies

      b. Provide emotional support to parents and client

      c. Encourage measures to allow for normal growth

      d. Provide adequate nutrition

         1) Assist with feeding, e.g., place food at back of mouth or on either side of tongue toward cheek with slight downward pressure of the spoon on the tongue

         2) Never tilt head backward when feeding—leads to choking

         3) Set aside ample time for meals

         4) Administer high-calorie diet

C. Muscular dystrophy

  1. Description—progressive hereditary muscle disorder characterized by muscular weakness

  2. Assessment

      a. Leg weakness, flat feet, stumbling and falling, pelvic muscle weakness

      b. Pseudohypertrophy of muscles

      c. Lordosis, scoliosis

      d. Waddling gait, walking on toes

      e. Contractures of elbows, feet, knees, hips

  3. Diagnostic tests

      a. CPK (creatinine phosphokinase) elevated

      b. Abnormal electromyogram

      c. Abnormal muscle biopsy

  4. Nursing management

      a. Promote safety due to gait and movement disturbances, use of braces or wheelchair

      b. Assist with diagnostic tests

      c. Client/parent education on nature of the disease

      d. Provide emotional support to child and family

      e. Discuss balance between activity and rest for the child

      f. Promote and support growth and development as appropriate

      g. Prevent complications of contractures

      h. Referrals to appropriate agencies

SELECTED MUSCULOSKELETAL DISORDERS

A. Developmental dysplasia of the hip (DDH)

1. Description—inability of the acetabulum to hold the head of the femur

2. Characteristic manifestations

   a. Uneven gluteal folds and thigh creases (more and deeper on involved side)

   b. Limited abduction of hip

   c. Pain on abduction of involved hip

   d. Prominent trochanter

   e. Short limb on affected side

   f. Waddling gait with bilateral dislocation

   g. Limping gait with unilateral dislocation

3. Diagnosis

   a. X-ray evaluations

   b. Clinical signs (see Figure 14-5)

4. Predisposition

   a. Intrauterine position (breech)

   b. Hormonal imbalance

   c. Cultural and environmental influences, e.g., certain groups of people that tightly wrap infants in blankets or strap infant to cradle board

5. Treatment and nursing management—depends on type of dislocation
   a. Splinting for partial dislocation by use of abduction splints (see Figure 14-6)
   b. Hip spica cast after closed reduction for subluxation and complete dislocation (see Figure 14-7)
   c. Open reduction if above measures are unsuccessful, i.e., surgical incision is made to directly visualize and reduce the deformity
   d. Provide for safety, mobility
   e. Prevent deformities

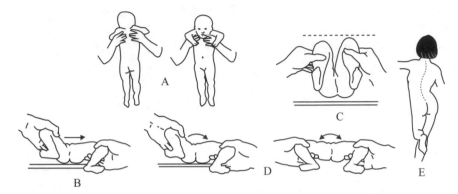

Figure 14-5. DEVELOPMENTAL DYSPLASIA OF THE HIP (DDH)—
Signs of congenital dislocation of hip: (A) asymmetry of gluteal and thigh folds; (B) limited hip abduction as seen in flexion; (C) apparent shortening of femur as indicated by knees in flexion; (D) Ortolani's sign if infant is under 4 wk of age; (E) Trendelenburg on weight bearing. NOTE: Ortolani's sign—palpable click with reduction in abduction and dislocation in adduction; positive sign. Trendelenburg's sign—when standing on dislocated side, unable to elevate pelvis of opposite side.

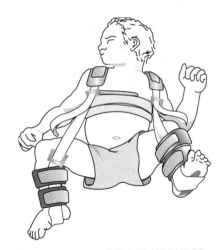

Figure 14-6. PAVLIK HARNESS

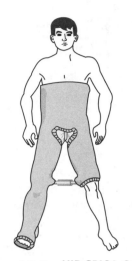

Figure   14-7.   HIP SPICA CAST

B. Fractures

   1. Common fractures in children

      a. Bend

         1) Occurs when the bone is bent but not broken

         2) Associated with the flexibility of the bones in young children

         3) Bones can bend 45° or more before breaking

         4) Occur most often in the ulna and fibula, in association with fractures of the radius and tibia

      b. Buckle fracture

         1) Produced by compression of a porous bone

         2) Appears as a raised or bulging projection at the fracture site

         3) Common in young children

      c. Greenstick fracture

         1) Occurs when a bone bends beyond its limits

         2) Fracture on one side of bone and a bend on the other

   2. Traction

      a. 90-degree-90-degree traction

         1) Common skeletal traction in children

         2) Affected hip and knee are flexed at 90-degree angles

         3) Affected lower leg in boot cast or supported in a sling, Steinmann pin or Kirschner wire placed in distal fragment of femur

      b. Buck extension traction

      c. Russell traction

      d. Balanced suspension traction

   3. Nursing management

      a. Provide care to child with splint

         1) Encourage normal growth and development by allowing child to perform appropriate activities

         2) Teach parents to reapply splints and explain rationale for maintaining abduction

         3) Tell parents to move child from one room to another for environmental change

    4) Discuss with parents modification in bathing, dressing, and diapering

    5) Tell parents to touch and hold child to express affection and reinforce security

  b. Provide care to child in cast

    1) Apply principles of cast care

    2) Teach parents cast care if child is being discharged with cast

C. Club foot (talipes equinovarus)

  1. Description—rigid abnormality of talus bone at birth; does not involve muscles, tendons, nerves, or blood vessels

  2. Assessment

    a. Adduction and inversion of hind and forward part of the foot (see Figure 14-8)

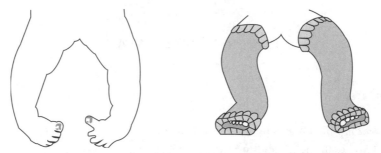

Figure 14-8. CASTING FOR TALIPES EQUINOVARUS

  3. Predisposing factors

    a. Genetics

    b. Environmental

  4. Treatment and management

    a. Foot exercises—manipulation of foot to correct position every 4 hours regularly

    b. Casts and splints correct the deformity in most cases if applied early

    c. Surgery is usually required for older child

  5. Nursing management

    a. Early referral

    b. Care of the child in Denis Browne splint

    c. Care of the child with cast

    d. Support normal growth and development

D. Scoliosis

  1. Description—lateral deviation of one or more vertebrae commonly accompanied by rotary motion

  2. Assessment (see Figure 14-9)

    a. Poor posture

    b. Unevenness of hips or scapulae

  3. Types

    a. Functional—flexible deviation that corrects by bending

    b. Structural—permanent, hereditary deviation

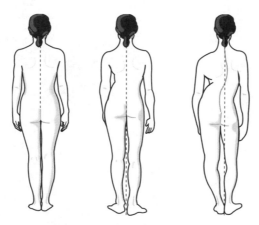

Figure 14-9. SCOLIOSIS

4. Treatment and nursing management
   a. Exercise for functional type
   b. Electrostimulation
   c. Braces
      1) Boston brace and Thoracolumbosacral (TLSO) brace
      2) Milwaukee brace
   d. Risser-turnbuckle cast
   e. Halo traction
   f. Surgery—spinal fusion with Harrington rod insertion; Dwyer instrumentation with anterior spinal fusion; screw and wire (Luque) instrumentation
   g. Assist in prevention of progression of abnormality—teach isometric exercises to strengthen the abdominal muscles
      1) Sit-ups
      2) Pelvic tilt
      3) Push-up with pelvic tilt
   h. Care for client with brace
      1) Skin care on pressure areas
      2) Wear T-shirt under brace to minimize skin irritation
      3) Provide activities consistent with limitations, yet allow positive peer relationships to promote healthy self-concept
   i. Care for client with cast
   j. Care for client in traction
   k. Provide operative care for client undergoing spinal fusion; apply principles of laminectomy care

Chapter 15

PSYCHOSOCIAL INTEGRITY

Sections	Concepts Covered
1. Basic Concepts	Ego Integrity/Self Concept
2. Anxiety	Cognition, Emotional Process
3. Situational Crises	Intracranial Regulation, Emotional Processes
4. Depressive Disorders	Cellular Regulation, Intracranial Regulation, Behavior
5. Bipolar Disorder	Cellular Regulation, Intracranial Regulation, Behavior
6. Altered Thought Processes	Cellular Regulation, Cognition, Intracranial Regulation
7. Social Interactions	Interpersonal Relationships
8. Abuse	Interpersonal Relationship

PSYCHOSOCIAL PROCESSES

A. Psychosocial well-being

1. Appearance, behavior, or mood
   a. Well groomed, relaxed
   b. Self-confident, self-accepting

2. Speech, thought content, and thought processes
   a. Clear, coherent
   b. Reality-based

3. Sensorium
   a. Oriented to person, place, and time
   b. Good memory
   c. Ability to abstract

4. Insight and judgment—accurate self-perception and awareness

5. Family relationships and work habits
   a. Satisfying interpersonal relationships
   b. Ability to trust
   c. Ability to cope effectively with stress
   d. Environmental mastery

B. History

1. Potential support systems or stressors
   a. Religious organization or community support
   b. Family
   c. Socioeconomic resources
   d. Education
   e. Cultural norms

2. Potential risk factors
   a. Family history of mental illness
   b. Medical history—imbalances can cause symptoms resembling emotional illness
   c. Lack of environmental/social support

3. Theorists
   a. Freud—defined parts of the psyche and stages of psychosocial development (see Table 15-1)
      1) Id—unconscious, immediate, pleasure principle
      2) Ego—conscious, compromising, based in reality
      3) Superego—both unconscious and conscious, uncompromising, basis of shame and guilt

Table 15-1 PSYCHOSOCIAL DEVELOPMENT				
AGE	STAGE OF DEVELOPMENT			NORMAL FINDINGS
	Erikson	Freud	Piaget	
Birth– 1 year	Trust vs. mistrust	Oral stage or infancy	Sensorimotor	Recognizes and attaches to primary caretaker, develops simple motor skills, moves from instant gratification to coping with anxiety Learns about self through the environment
1–3 years	Autonomy vs. shame and doubt	Anal stage or toddlerhood	Preoperational	Learns to manipulate environment, learns self-control in toilet training, parallel play Develops expressive language and symbolic play
3–6 years	Initiative vs. guilt	Phallic stage or preschool	Preoperational intuitive	Learns symbols and concepts, assertiveness against environment; learns sex role identity
6–12 years	Industry vs. inferiority	Latency stage or schoolage	Concrete operational	Sees cause and effect and draws conclusions, develops allegiance to friends, uses energy to industriously create and perform tasks, shows competency in school and with friends
12–20 years	Identity vs. role diffusion	Genital stage or adolescence	Formal operational	Thinks abstractly, uses logic and scientific reason, masters independence through rebellion, develops firm sense of self, is strongly influenced by peers, develops sexual maturity, explores sexual relationships
20–45 years	Intimacy vs. isolation			Develops lasting intimate relationships and good work relationships
45–65 years	Generativity vs. stagnation			Establishes a family and oversees next generation, is productive, shows concern for others
65 years to death	Integrity vs. despair			Sees own life as meaningful, is productive, accepts physical changes

b. Erikson—defined stages of psychosocial development throughout life (see Table 15-1)
　　1) Each stage represents developmental milestones
　　2) Completion of one stage is necessary for next stage

c. Sullivan—theory includes the impact of social environment on interpersonal relationships
　　1) Provides basis for many community health models
　　2) Hildegard Peplau (nurse theorist) developed Sullivan's theory into model of nurse-client relationship

C. Requirements for health maintenance
　1. Satisfaction of basic human needs in order of importance (Maslow)
　　a. Physical—oxygen, water, food, sleep, sex
　　b. Safety—physical, security, order
　　c. Love and belonging—affection, companionship, identification
　　d. Esteem and recognition—status, success, prestige
　　e. Self-actualization—self-fulfillment, creativity
　　f. Aesthetic—harmony, spirituality

　2. Potential nursing diagnoses
　　a. Impaired social interactions
　　b. Anxiety

    c. Ineffective coping

    d. Self-esteem disturbance

COMMUNICATION SKILLS OF THE NURSE

A. Therapeutic communication—listening to and understanding client while promoting clarification and insight

  1. Goals

    a. To understand client's message (verbal and nonverbal)

    b. To facilitate verbalization of feelings

    c. To communicate understanding and acceptance

    d. To identify problems, goals, and objectives

  2. Guidelines

    a. Nonverbal communication constitutes 2/3 of all communication and gives the most accurate reflection of attitude

      1) Physical appearance, body movement, posture, gesture, facial expression

      2) Contact—eye contact, physical distance maintained, ability to touch and be touched

    b. The person's feelings and what is verbalized may be incongruent, e.g., client denies feeling sad but appears morose

    c. Implied messages are as important to understand as overt behavior, e.g., continual interruptions may represent loneliness or fear

  3. Phases of a therapeutic relationship

    a. Initiating phase—boundaries of relationship determined

    b. Working phase—client develops insights and learns coping

    c. Terminating phase—work of relationship is summarized

  4. Therapeutic responses—techniques which are the main tools to promote therapeutic exchange between nurse and client (see Table 15-2)

  5. Nontherapeutic responses—responses to avoid (see Table 15-3)

TREATMENT MODALITIES

Techniques that are used to care for the client with psychosocial problems (see Table 15-4)

Table 15-2 THERAPEUTIC RESPONSES		
RESPONSE	**GOAL/PURPOSE**	**EXAMPLES**
Using silence (nonverbal)	Allows client time to think and reflect; conveys acceptance Allows client to take lead in conversation	Use proper nonverbal communication, remain seated, maintain eye contact, sit quietly and wait
Using general leads or broad openings	Encourages client to talk Indicates interest in client Allows client to choose subject Sets tone for depressed client	"What would you like to talk about? Then what? Go on . . ." "What brought you to the hospital?" "What can you tell me about your family?"

Table 15-2 THERAPEUTIC RESPONSES *(CONTINUED)*		
RESPONSE	**GOAL/PURPOSE**	**EXAMPLES**
Clarification	Encourages recall and details of particular experience Encourages description of feelings Seeks clarification, pinpoints specifics Makes sure nurse understands client	"Give me an example." "Tell me more." "And how do you feel when you're angry?" "Who are 'they'?"
Reflecting	Paraphrases what client says Reflects what client says, especially feelings conveyed	"It sounds like you're feeling angry." "In other words, you really felt abandoned." "I hear you saying that it was hard to come to the hospital."

Table 15-3 RESPONSES TO AVOID IN THERAPEUTIC COMMUNICATION	
RESPONSE	**EXAMPLES**
Closed-ended questions that can be answered by a "yes" or "no" or other monosyllabic responses; prevents sharing; puts pressure on client	"How many children do you have?" "With whom do you live?" "Are you feeling better today?"
Advice-giving encourages dependency, may not be right for a particular client	"Why don't you . . . ?" "You really should cut your hair and wear makeup."
Responding to questions that are related to one's qualifications or personal life in an embarrassed or concrete way; keep conversation client-centered	"Yes, I am highly qualified." "You know nurses are not permitted to go out with their clients."
Arguing or responding in a hostile way	"If you do not take your medication, there is really nothing we can do to help you."
Reassuring—client benefits more by exploring own ideas and feelings	"You will start feeling much better any day." "Don't worry, your doctors will do everything necessary for your care."
"Why" questions can imply disapproval and client may become defensive	"Why didn't you take your medication?"
Judgmental responses evaluate client from nurse's values	"You were wrong to do that. " "Don't you think your unfaithfulness has destroyed your marriage?"

Table 15-4	TREATMENT MODALITIES FOR MENTAL ILLNESS	
TYPE	**ASSUMPTIONS**	**FOCUS OF TREATMENT**
Biological	Emotional problem is an illness Cause may be inherited or chemical in origin	Medications, ECT
Psychoanalytical (individual)	Anxiety results when there is conflict between the id, ego, and superego parts of the personality Defense mechanisms form to ward off anxiety	The therapist helps the client to become aware of unconscious thoughts and feelings; understand anxiety and defenses
Milieu therapy	Providing a therapeutic environment will help increase client's awareness of feelings, increase sense of responsibility, and help return to community	Positive physical and social environment Structured groups and activities One-on-one intervention May be token program, open wards, self-medication
Group therapy	Relationship with others will be recreated among group members and can be worked through; members can also directly help one another	Members meet regularly with a leader to form a stable group Members learn new ways to cope with stress and develop insight into their behavior with others
Family therapy	The problem is a family problem, not an individual one Sick families lack a sense of "I" in each member The tendency is to focus on sick member's behavior as the source of trouble The sick member's symptom serves a function in the family	Therapist treats the whole family Helps members to each develop their own sense of identity Points out function of sick member for the rest of the family
Activity therapy	Important group interactions occur when group members work on a task together or share in recreation	Organized group activities created to promote socialization, increase self-esteem
Play therapy	Children express themselves more easily in play than in verbal communication Choice of colors, toys, and interaction with toys is revealing as reflection of child's situation in the family	Provide materials and toys to facilitate interaction with child, observe play, and help child to resolve problems through play
Behavioral therapy and behavior modification	Psychological problems are the result of learning Deficiencies can be corrected through learning	Operant conditioning—use of rewards to reinforce positive behavior; perceived and self-reinforcement becomes more important than the negative behavior

ANXIETY

An uncomfortable feeling of apprehension or dread that occurs in response to internal or external stimuli

A. Assessment (see Table 15-5)
  1. Definition: feeling of dread or fear in the absence of an external threat or disproportionate to the nature of the threat
  2. Levels of anxiety
      a. Mild—high degree of alertness, mild uneasiness, "butterflies in stomach"
      b. Moderate—increased perspiration, light-headedness, muscle tension, urinary frequency, nausea, anorexia, diarrhea, heart-pounding, increased BP, dry mouth, cold, clammy pale skin, selective inattention, poor comprehension
      c. Severe—most symptoms of moderate anxiety intensified, hyperventilation, dizziness, vomiting, tachycardia, panic, inability to hear or speak, further decreased perception, hallucinations, delusions
      d. Panic—symptoms of severe anxiety and inability to function, dread, terror, personality disorganization

  3. Characteristic findings
      a. Cardiovascular
          1) Increased pulse, blood pressure, and respiration
          2) Palpitations
          3) Chest discomfort/pain
          4) Perspiration
          5) Flushing and heat sensations
          6) Cold hands and feet
          7) Headache

      b. Gastrointestinal
          1) Nausea, vomiting, and diarrhea
          2) Belching
          3) Heartburn
          4) Cramps

      c. Musculoskeletal
          1) Increased muscle tension and tendon reflexes
          2) Increased generalized fatigue
          3) Tremors, jerking of limbs
          4) Unsteady voice

      d. Intellectual
          1) Poor comprehension—may be unable to follow directions
          2) Poor concentration

3) Selective inattention

4) Focus on detail

5) Impaired problem solving

6) Unable to communicate

a) Thoughts may become random, distorted, disconnected with impaired logic

b) Rapid, high-pitched speech

e. Social and emotional

1) Feelings of helplessness and hopelessness

2) Feelings of increased threat, dread, horror, anger, and rage

3) Use of defense mechanisms and more primitive coping behaviors

a) Denial

b) Crying, rocking, shouting, curling up, withdrawal

4. Predisposing conditions

a. Prolonged unmet needs of dependency, security, love, and attention

b. Stress threatening security or self-esteem

c. Unacceptable thoughts or feelings surfacing to consciousness, e.g., rage, erotic impulses, flashbacks

d. Older adults—coping mechanisms not as effective when faced with loss of physical or mental function, financial concerns; may have increased physical complaints

B. Ego defense mechanisms (see Table 15-6); used to cope with anxiety and painful feelings

C. Nursing management (see Table 15-7)

1. Institute measures to decrease anxiety

2. Administer medications (see Table 15-8)

3. Goals

a. To understand client's message (verbal and nonverbal)

b. To facilitate verbalization of feelings

c. To communicate understanding and acceptance

d. To identify problems, goals, and objectives

e. Follow guidelines regarding communication skills of the nurse (see Part II of Unit I of this chapter)

Table 15-5 ANXIETY DISORDERS		
TYPE	**ASSESSMENTS**	**NURSING CONSIDERATIONS**
Phobia	Apprehension, anxiety, helplessness when confronted with phobic situation or feared object Examples of specific fears: Acrophobia—heights Claustrophobia—closed areas Agoraphobia—open spaces	Avoid confrontation and humiliation Do not focus on getting client to stop being afraid Systematic desensitization Relaxation techniques General anxiety measures May be managed with antidepressants
Panic disorder	Extreme, overwhelming form of anxiety Experienced when client has a real or perceived threat Palpitations Tachycardia Seating, shaking, nausea Paresthesia Feelings of unreality	Teach, encourage, and support relaxation Teach and support self-evaluation scales Educate and assess medication use and knowledge Support use of distraction and positive self talk Support participation in therapy treatment
Acute stress disorder/ Posttraumatic stress disorder	Develops after a traumatic event Determine timing of event Determine occurrence and timing of symptoms Assess for history of with nine or more symptoms from the 5 categories of; intrusion, negative mood, dissociation, avoidance and arousal	Teach, encourage, and support stress management techniques Educate and assess medication use and knowledge Support participation in therapy treatment Perform passive listening to recount of event
Obsessive-compulsive disorder (OCD)	Obsession—repetitive, uncontrollable thoughts Compulsion—repetitive, uncontrollable acts, e.g., rituals, rigidity, inflexibility	Accept ritualistic behavior Structure environment Provide for physical needs Offer alternative activities, especially ones using hands Guide decisions, minimize choices Encourage socialization Group therapy Managed with clomipramine, SSRIs Stimulus-response prevention
Functional neurologic symptom disorder	Physical symptoms with no organic basis, unconscious behavior—could include blindness, paralysis, convulsions without loss of consciousness, stocking and glove anesthesia; lack of concern about symptoms (la belle indifference)	Diagnostic evaluation Discuss feelings rather than symptoms Promote therapeutic relationship with client Avoid secondary gain

Table 15-6 DEFENSE MECHANISMS		
MECHANISM	DEFINITION	EXAMPLES
Denial	Failure to acknowledge an intolerable thought, feeling, experience, reality	Alcoholic says his drinking is not a problem; terminally ill client makes long-range plans
Displacement	Redirection of feelings to subject that is acceptable or less threatening	Kicking the dog or yelling at one's spouse after a bad day at work
Projection	Attribution to others of one's own unacceptable thoughts, feelings, qualities	Saying someone you are angry with dislikes you; staff nurse complains about the head nurse's poor skills after receiving an unfavorable evaluation
Undoing	An attempt to erase an unacceptable act or thought	Excessively apologizing; buying extravagant gifts for one's spouse while having an affair
Compensation	An attempt to overcome a real or imagined shortcoming	A sickly child becoming an athlete
Substitution	Replacing desired, impractical, or unobtainable object with one that is attainable	Marrying someone who looks like a former fiancée
Introjection	Characteristic of another incorporated into oneself	Wife dies and husband develops symptoms of her illness
Repression	Unacceptable thoughts kept from awareness	Forgetting painful experience
Reaction formation	Expressing attitude directly opposite to unconscious one	Someone with strong dependency needs chooses a "helping" profession
Regression	Returning to an earlier stage of development	Temper tantrums, baby talk, bed-wetting
Dissociation	Detachment of painful emotional experience from consciousness	Amnesia
Rationalization	Attempts to justify, via logical or acceptable explanations, acts or feelings that are not logical or acceptable	A student who is sexually attracted to her teacher tells herself she needs to stay after class for help with a project
Idealization	Glorifying another's characteristics	Only noticing another's positive qualities
Identification	Incorporating certain attributes of another into one's own thoughts or behavior	A person dresses like someone she admires
Acting out	Using action rather than reflection or feelings during emotional conflict	Client gets mad and stays out late

Table 15-7	NURSING INTERVENTIONS IN ANXIETY
GENERAL PRINCIPLES	**EXAMPLES**
Assess level of anxiety	Look at body language, speech patterns, facial expressions, defense mechanisms, and behavior used Distinguish levels of anxiety (symptoms of sympathetic nervous system stimulation)
Keep environmental stresses/stimulation low when anxiety is high	Brief orientation to unit or procedures Written information to read later, when anxiety is lower Pleasant, attractive, uncluttered environment Provide privacy, if presence of other clients is overstimulating Provide physical care if necessary Avoid offering many alternatives or decisions when anxiety is high
Assist client to cope with anxiety more effectively	Acknowledge anxious behavior Always remain with extremely anxious client Assist client in clarifying own thoughts and feelings Encourage measures to reduce anxiety, e.g., exercise, activities, talking with friends, hobbies Assist client in realistically recognizing strengths and capabilities Provide therapy to develop more effective coping and interpersonal skills, e.g., individual, group May need to administer antianxiety medications
Maintain accepting and helpful attitude toward client	Use unhurried speech Acknowledge client's distress and concerns about problem Encourage clarification of feelings and thoughts Evaluate and manage own anxiety while working with client Recognize the value of defense mechanisms and realize that client is attempting to make the anxiety tolerable in the best possible way Do not attempt to remove a defense mechanism at any time

Table 15-8 ANTIANXIETY MEDICATIONS		
MEDICATION	**ADVERSE EFFECTS**	**NURSING CONSIDERATIONS**
Benzodiazepine Derivatives		
Chlordiazepoxide Diazepam	Lethargy, hangover Respiratory depression Hypotension	CNS depressant Use–anxiety, sedation, alcohol withdrawal, seizures May result in toxic build-up in the elderly Potential for physiological addiction/overdose Can develop tolerance and cross-tolerance Cigarette smoking increases clearance of drug Alcohol increases CNS depression Increased sedation, fall risk, and confusion in older adults
Alprazolam Lorazepam Oxazepam	Drowsiness, light-headedness, hypotension, hepatic dysfunction Increased salivation Orthostatic hypotension Memory impairment and confusion	CNS depressant Safer for elderly Don't combine with alcohol or other depressants Check renal and hepatic function Don't discontinue abruptly (true for all antianxiety agents) Teach addictive potential
Midazolam	Retrograde amnesia, euphoria, hypotension, dysrhythmia, cardiac arrest, respiratory depression	CNS depressant, Use–preoperative sedation, conscious sedation for endoscopic procedures and diagnostic tests
Anxiolytics Antianxiety Medications		
Buspirone	Light-headedness Confusion Hypotension, palpitations	Little sedation Requires ≥3 weeks to be effective Cannot be given as a PRN medication Particularly useful for generalized anxiety disorder (GAD) No abuse potential Used for clients with previous addiction Avoid alcohol and grapefruit juice Monitor for worsening depression or suicidal tendencies
Hydroxyzine	Drowsiness, ataxia Leukopenia, hypotension	Produces no dependence, tolerance, or intoxication Can be used for anxiety relief for indefinite periods

Table 15-8 ANTIANXIETY MEDICATIONS *(CONTINUED)*		
MEDICATION	ADVERSE EFFECTS	NURSING CONSIDERATIONS
Herbals		
Kava	Impaired thinking, judgment, motor reflexes, vision, decreased plasma proteins, thrombocytopenia, leukocytopenia, dyspnea, and pulmonary hypertension	Similar activity to benzodiazepines Suppresses emotional excitability and produces mild euphoria Do not take with CNS depressants Should not be taken by women who are pregnant or lactating or by children under the age of 12
Melatonin	Sedation, confusion, headache, and tachycardia	Influences sleep-wake cycles (levels are high during sleep) Used for prevention and treatment of "jet lag" and insomnia Use cautiously if given with benzodiazepines and CNS depressants Contraindicated in hepatic insufficiency, history of cerebrovascular disease, depression, and neurologic disorders
Action	Affects neurotransmitters	
Indications	Anxiety disorders, insomnia, petit mal seizures, panic attacks, acute manic episodes	
Adverse effects	Sedation Depression, confusion Anger, hostility Headache Dry mouth, constipation Bradycardia Elevations in LDH, AST, ALT Urinary retention	
Nursing considerations	Monitor liver function Monitor for therapeutic blood levels Avoid alcohol Caution when performing tasks requiring alertness (e.g., driving car) Benzodiazepines are also used as muscles relaxants, sedatives, hypnotics, anticonvulsants	

CRISIS

Period in which there is a major change in a person's life, either from an event or perceived threat

A. Characteristics

1. Temporary state of disequilibrium precipitated by an event or threat

2. Short duration; self-limiting, usually 4–6 wk

3. May offer opportunity to develop new coping abilities; promote growth and new behaviors

4. Typical precipitating factors—developmental stages, situational factors, threats to self-concept

B. Assessment of crisis (see Table 15-9)

1. Stages of crisis

   a. Denial

   b. Increased tension/anxiety

   c. Disorganization—inability to function

   d. Attempts to escape the problem—pretends problem does not exist; blames others

   e. Attempts to reorganize

   f. General reorganization

2. Precipitating factors

   a. Developmental stages

      1) Birth

      2) Adolescence

      3) Midlife

      4) Retirement

   b. Situational factors

      1) Natural disasters

      2) Financial loss

   c. Threats to self-concept

      1) Loss of job

      2) Failure at school

      3) Onset of serious illness

C. Crisis intervention process

1. Assessment

   a. Explore problem with client

   b. Define the event

   c. Identify client's strengths, previous coping methods used in crisis

   d. Identify client's support system

2. Planning

    a. Evaluate client's abilities realistically

    b. With client, identify potential solutions to the situation

    c. Encourage exploration of all alternatives, using supports and developing new skills

3. Intervention

    a. Focus and clarify problem with client

    b. Assist client in identifying feelings and thoughts

    c. Specific discussion of new strategies and ways to solve problem

    d. Rehearsing and evaluating strategies proposed

4. Evaluation and resolution

    a. Review of the event and changes made to cope with situation

    b. Anticipatory guidance to apply learning to future potential situations

    c. Possible referral for long-term assistance if necessary

D. Nursing management

1. Goal-directed, focus on the here and now

2. Focus on client's immediate problems

3. Explore nurse's and client's understanding of the problem

    a. Define the event (client may truly not know what has precipitated the crisis)

    b. Confirm nurse's perception by reviewing with client

    c. Identify the factors affecting problem solving

    d. Evaluate how realistically client sees the problems or concerns

4. Help client become aware of feelings and validate them

    a. Acknowledge feelings, e.g., "This must be a painful situation for you."

    b. Avoid blaming client for problems and concerns

    c. Avoid blaming others, as this prevents insight

    d. Encourage ventilation with nurse to relieve anxiety

    e. Tell client he will feel better, but it may take 1 or 2 months

5. Develop a plan

    a. Encourage client to make as many arrangements as possible (avoid dependence)

    b. Write out information because comprehension is impaired, e.g., referrals

    c. Maximize client's situational supports

6. Find new coping skills and manage feelings

    a. Focus on strengths and current coping skills

    b. Encourage client to form new coping skills and social outlets—reaching out to others

    c. Facilitate future planning

        1) Ask client "What would you like to do?", "Where would you like to go from here?"

        2) Give referrals when needed—family counseling, vocational counseling, etc.

Table 15-9 SITUATIONAL/TRAUMATIC CRISES		
	GRIEVING CLIENT	DYING CLIENT	RAPE TRAUMA
Assessment	Stages of grief a. Shock and disbelief b. Awareness of the pain of loss c. Restitution Acute grief period 4–8 wk Usual resolution within 1 year Long-term resolution over time	Stages of dying a. Denial b. Anger c. Bargaining d. Depression e. Acceptance	Stages of crisis a. Acute reaction lasts 3–4 wk b. Reorganization is long-term Common responses to rape a. Self-blame, embarrassment b. Phobias, fear of violence, death, injury c. Anxiety, insomnia d. Wish to escape, move, relocate e. Psychosomatic disturbances
Analysis	Potential problems a. Family of deceased or separated – Guilt – Anger – Anxiety b. Client undergoing surgery or loss of body part – Anger – Withdrawal – Guilt – Anxiety – Loss of role	Potential problems a. Avoidance behavior b. Inability to express feelings when in denial c. Feelings of guilt d. Withdrawal e. Lonely, frightened f. Anxiety of client and family	Potential problems a. Fears, panic reactions, generalized anxiety b. Guilt c. Inability to cope Current crisis may reactivate old, unresolved trauma Follow emergency room protocol: may include clothing, hair samples, NPO Be alert for potential internal injuries, e.g., hemorrhage
Intervention	Apply crisis theory Focus on the here and now Provide support to family when loved one dies Provide family privacy Encourage verbalization of feelings Facilitate expressions of anger and rage Emphasize strengths Increase ability to cope Support adjustment to illness, loss of body part	Apply crisis theory Support staff having feelings of loss Keep communication open Allow expression of feelings Focus on the here and now Let client know he/she is not alone Provide comforting environment Be attentive to need for privacy Provide physically comforting care, e.g., back rubs Give sense of control and dignity Respect client wishes (cultural and religious beliefs)	Apply crisis theory Focus on the here and now Write out treatments and appointments for client, as anxiety causes forgetfulness Record all information in chart Give client referrals for legal assistance, supportive psychotherapy, and rape crisis center Follow up regularly until client is improved

E. Grief: self-limiting, normal response to loss (see Table 15-9)
   1. Examples of precipitating events
      a. Separation, divorce, death
      b. Chronic diseases
      c. Trauma, surgery
      d. Newborn with defects or illness
      e. Altered body image

2. Expect a more intense reaction if there is:
    a. Loss of a child
    b. Unresolved conflict with deceased
    c. Few situational, interpersonal supports
    d. Sudden loss
    e. Poor coping in past with losses
    f. Surgery results in loss of visible body part or one that has special significance, e.g., breast and sexuality, or if procedure is palliative rather than curative

3. Management of grief
    a. Encourage expression of memories, feelings
    b. Accept initial dependency of client
    c. Reassure client of normalcy of reaction—pain, crying, anger, guilt
    d. Recognize importance of event for client and need to mourn
    e. Recognize client's potential need for denial and support client when beginning to integrate truth

F. Death and dying—stages of dying are not necessarily an orderly progression; may have various feelings within one period, may skip stage or stay with one or two stages (see Table 15-10 for nursing management)
    1. Denial
    2. Anger
    3. Bargaining
    4. Depression
    5. Acceptance

| Table 15-10 NURSING MANAGEMENT OF DYING CLIENT ||
PROBLEM	INTERVENTION
Caregivers have feelings about dying and dying clients, e.g., need to deny, worries about own mortality, anger, feelings of helplessness	Recognize own thoughts and feelings about death and dying Respect client as having own needs, values, and way of handling situation Clarify situation Focus on positive aspects of care given, e.g., less pain, less anxiety
Need to maintain open communication with client	Explore client's understanding of problem and prognosis Clarify misconceptions, e.g., if client feels he will die tomorrow and there is no indication of terminal phase Use client's questions and statements as guide and focus on feelings Respect denial rather than giving excess information Respect client's wish for more information re: prognosis, treatment
Need for support and hope	Make client aware of what treatment will be provided Explore fears and reassure client that all modalities possible to relieve pain and suffering will be used Emphasize that client will not be abandoned no matter how client's illness progresses Convey idea that day-to-day survival is important and that nurse is interested in client's responses Plan with client to make the most of each day—e.g., visitors, physical comfort, relief of pain, favorite foods brought in by relatives, taking care of personal and business affairs, pleasurable activities

DEPRESSIVE DISORDERS Section 4

DEPRESSIVE DISORDERS

An overwhelming state of sadness, loss of interest or pleasure, feelings of guilt, disturbed sleep and appetite, low energy, and an inability to concentrate

A. Depression—can be manifested as a single episode or recurrent pattern, varies according to age, race, gender; mood disorder
   1. Major depressive disorder (MDD)
      a. Types—melancholia, postpartum, psychotic, agitated, seasonal affective disorder (SAD)
      b. Characterized by symptoms that persist over a minimum 2-week period
      c. MDD involves psychological, biological, and social factors

   2. Dysthymic disorder
   3. Depressive disorder, not otherwise specified (NOS)
   4. Gerontologic considerations
      a. High risk of suicide
      b. Depression underdiagnosed and undertreated
      c. Contributing factors—illness, decreased physical and mental function

B. Assessment
   1. Possible changes in self-esteem/self-confidence
      a. Low self-esteem
      b. Self-deprecation
      c. Feelings of helplessness/hopelessness
      d. Obsessive thoughts and fears
      e. Rumination and worries
      f. Sense of doom, failure
      g. Regressed behavior—immature, demanding

   2. Possible changes in self-care
      a. Unkempt, depressed appearance
      b. Multiple physical complaints
      c. Prone to injury, accidents, and infections
      d. Lack of energy; fatigue
      e. Changes in usual sleep pattern
         1) Insomnia or hypersomnia
         2) Feels unrested after night's sleep
      f. Weight loss, poor appetite, or weight gain
      g. Constipation
      h. Amenorrhea
      i. Lack of sexual desire

3. Possible changes in cognitive/mental functioning
   a. Decreased attention span
   b. Decreased concentration
   c. Slowed speech and thought processes
   d. Slowed motor activity
   e. Impaired reality testing (psychotic depression)
   f. Withdrawn
   g. Ambivalent and indecisive behavior
   h. Agitation and psychomotor restlessness
   i. Suicidal ideation (see Table 15-11)

Table 15-11 BEHAVIORAL CLUES OF IMPENDING SUICIDE
1. Any sudden change in client's behavior
2. Becomes energetic after period of severe depression
3. Improved mood 10–14 days after taking antidepressant may mean suicidal plans made
4. Finalizes business or personal affairs
5. Gives away valuable possessions or pets
6. Withdraws from social activities and plans
7. Appears emotionally upset
8. Presence of weapons, razors, pills (means)
9. Has death plan
10. Leaves a note
11. Makes direct or indirect statements (e.g., "I may not be around then.")

4. Nursing management (see Table 15-12)
   a. Maintain therapeutic environment
      1) Supportive, professional attitude toward client
      2) Continue ongoing assessment
   b. Electroconvulsive therapy (ECT) as ordered (see Table 15-13)
   c. Administer medications as ordered (see Table 15-14)

Table 15-12	NURSING MANAGEMENT OF DEPRESSION
PROBLEM	**INTERVENTION**
Low self-esteem	Calm, accepting attitude; touch when appropriate (not with psychotic clients); sit with client even if silent; encourage client in an unpressured manner; reassure him that depression generally lifts; avoid cheery attitude or pep talks; note improvements and discuss with client; provide tasks client can accomplish to increase sense of mastery
Dependency	Show confidence in client's realistic ability to improve; work with client—avoid doing everything for him or giving advice
Anger	Physical activity to channel psychic energy; encourage expressions of anger when appropriate
Physical needs	Promote eating, offer small frequent feedings, favorite foods; offer companionship during meals

Promote rest, provide quiet sleeping arrangement; stay with client if necessary, offer PRN medication for insomnia; watch client swallow pill |
| Risk for suicide | Monitor for signs of suicidal behavior; remove any potentially dangerous items such as pills, sharp objects, ropelike clothing items, e.g., neckties, pantyhose, belts; close observation—one-to-one; provide concrete assistance, e.g., evaluate resources; give clear explanations and convey sincere desire to help; avoid embarrassment to client by treating him in a dignified, matter-of-fact manner |

Table 15-13 NURSING CONSIDERATIONS FOR ELECTROCONVULSIVE THERAPY (ECT)
1. Prepare client by explaining procedure and telling client about potential temporary memory loss and confusion
2. Informed consent, physical exam, labwork
3. NPO after midnight for an early morning procedure
4. Have client void before ECT
5. Remove dentures, glasses, jewelry
6. Give muscle relaxant to prevent fractures and short-acting barbiturate anesthetic to induce brief general anesthesia
7. Given atropine 30 min before treatment to decrease secretions
8. Have oxygen and suction on hand
9. After procedure, take vital signs, orient client
10. Observe client's reaction and stay with him
11. Observe for sudden improvement and indications of suicidal threats after ECT treatment

Table 15-14 ANTIDEPRESSANT MEDICATIONS OVERVIEW		
MEDICATION	**ADVERSE EFFECTS**	**NURSING CONSIDERATIONS**
Monoamine oxidase inhibitors (MAOIs)		
Isocarboxazid Tranylcypromine sulfate Phenelzine sulfate	Postural hypotension If foods with tyramine ingested, can have hypertensive crisis: headache, sweating, palpitations, stiff neck, intracranial hemorrhage Potentiates alcohol and other medications	Inhibits monoamine oxidase enzyme, preventing destruction of norepinephrine, epinephrine, and serotonin Avoid foods with tyramine—aged cheese, liver, herring, yeast, beer, wine, sour cream, pickled products Avoid caffeine, antihistamines, amphetamines Takes 3-4 weeks to work Avoid tricyclics until 3 weeks after stopping MAO inhibitors Monitor vital signs Sunblock required
Tricyclics		
Amitriptyline hydrochloride Imipramine Desipramine hydrochloride Doxepin Nortriptyline	Sedation/drowsiness, especially with Elavil Blurred vision, dry mouth, diaphoresis Postural hypotension, palpitations Nausea, vomiting Constipation, urinary retention Increased appetite	Increases brain amine levels Suicide risk high after 10–14 days because of increased energy Monitor vital signs Sunblock required Increase fluid intake Take dose at bedtime (sedative effect) Use sugarless candy or gum for dry mouth Delay of 2-6 weeks before noticeable effects
Selective serotonin reuptake inhibitors (SSRI)		
Fluoxetine Paroxetine Sertraline hydrochloride	Palpitations, bradycardia Nausea, vomiting, diarrhea or constipation, increased or decreased appetite Urinary retention Nervousness, insomnia	Decreases neuronal uptake of serotonin Take in AM to avoid insomnia Takes at least 4 weeks to work Can potentiate effect of digoxin, coumadin, and diazepam Used for anorexia
Selective serotonin-norepinephrine reuptake inhibitors (SSNRI)		
Venlafaxine Duloxetine	See above	
Heterocyclics/Atypical		
Bupropion Trazodone	Dry mouth Nausea	May require gradual reduction before stopping Avoid use with alcohol, other CNS depressants for up to 1 week after end of therapy
Herbals		
St. John's wort	Dizziness, hypertension, allergic skin reaction, phototoxicity	Avoid use of St. John's wort and MAOI within 2 weeks of each other Do not use alcohol Contraindicated in pregnancy Avoid exposure to sun and use sunscreen Discontinue 1 to 2 weeks before surgery
Herbal interactions	St. John's wort—interacts with SSRIs; do not take within 2 weeks of MAOI Ginseng may potentiate MAOIs Avoid Ma huang or ephedra with MAOIs Kava kava should not be combined with benzodiazepines or opioids due to increased sedation Increase use of Brewer's yeast with MAOIs can increase blood pressure	

BIPOLAR DISORDER

A. Types
1. Bipolar I and II, cyclothymic disorder
2. Mood disorder in which individuals experience the extremes of mood—depression or euphoria

B. Assessment of mania—lasts from a few days to several months
1. Disoriented, incoherent
2. Euphoria
3. Delusions of grandeur
4. Flight of ideas; impulsive; eccentric
5. Inappropriate dress, excessive makeup and jewelry
6. Lacks inhibition; social blunders
7. Uses sarcastic, profane, and abusive language
8. Quick-tempered, agitated; impaired judgment
9. Talks excessively, jokes, dances, sings; hyperactive
10. Can't stop moving to eat, easily stimulated by environment
11. Happy/festive or angry/hostile
12. Weight loss, decreased appetite
13. Insomnia
14. Regressed behavior
15. Sexually indiscreet, hypersexual

C. Characteristics of depression
1. Weight gain or loss, anorexia
2. Insomnia or hypersomnia
3. Decreased sexual desire
4. Fatigue, decreased activity
5. May feel hopeless, unhappy, helpless, miserable, guilty
6. Regressive thinking—passive, dependent, decreased motivation, concerned with bodily functions, impaired memory, distorted thought content, slow and diminished speech
7. Delusions possible
8. Socially withdrawn
9. Poor self-esteem

D. Etiology

1. Psychodynamics

   a. Bipolar disorder is an affective disorder

   b. Reality contact is less disturbed than in schizophrenia

   c. Elation or grandiosity can be a defense against underlying depression or feelings of low self-esteem

   d. Testing, manipulative behavior results from poor self-esteem

   e. Hypomania (less extreme form)

2. Predisposing factors

   a. Hereditary—genetic

   b. Biochemical

   c. Involvement with alcohol/drugs common (self-medication)

3. Problems

   a. Easily stimulated by surroundings

      1) Hyperactive and anxious

      2) Unable to meet physical needs

   b. Disruptive and intrusive

   c. Denial

   d. Testing, manipulative, demanding behavior

   e. Superficial social relationships

E. Nursing management

1. Institute measures to deal with hyperactivity/agitation

   a. Simplify the environment and decrease environmental stimuli

      1) Assign to a single room away from activity

      2) Keep noise level low

      3) Soft lighting

   b. Limit people

      1) Anticipate situations that will provoke or overstimulate client, e.g., activities, competitive situations

      2) Remove to quiet areas

   c. Distract and redirect energy

      1) Choose activities for brief attention span, e.g., chores, walks

      2) Choose physical activities using large movements until acute mania subsides, e.g., dance

      3) Provide writing materials for busy work when acute mania subsides, e.g., political suggestions, plans

2. Provide external controls

   a. Assign one staff person to provide controls

   b. Do not encourage client when telling jokes or performing, e.g., avoid laughing

   c. Accompany client to room when hyperactivity is escalating

   d. Guard vigilantly against suicide as elation subsides and mood evens out

3. Institute measures to deal with manipulativeness

   a. Set limits, e.g., limit phone calls when excessive

      1) Set firm consistent times for meetings—client often late and unaware of time

2) Refuse unreasonable demands

3) Explain restrictions on behavior and reasons so client does not feel rejected

b. Communicate using a firm, unambivalent, consistent approach
1) Use staff consistency in enforcing rules

2) Remain nonjudgmental, e.g., when client disrobes say, "I will not allow you to undress here."

3) Never threaten or make comparisons with others, as it increases hostility and poor coping

c. Avoid long, complicated discussions
1) Use short sentences with specific straightforward responses

2) Avoid giving advice when solicited, e.g., "I notice you want me to take responsibility for your life."

4. Meet physical needs
a. Meet nutritional needs
1) Encourage fluids; offer water every hour because client will not take the time to drink

2) Give high-calorie finger foods and drinks to be carried while moving, e.g., cupcakes, sandwiches

3) Serve meals on tray in client's room when too stimulated

b. Encourage rest
1) Sedate PRN

2) Encourage short naps

5. Supervise bathing routines when client plays with water or is too distracted to clean self.

6. Administer medications (see Table 15-15)

7. Help decrease denial and increase client's awareness of feelings
a. Encourage expression of real feelings through reflecting

b. Help client acknowledge the need for help when denying it, e.g., "You say you don't need love, but most people need love. It's okay to feel that."

c. Function as a role model for client by communicating feelings openly

d. Help client recognize demanding behavior, e.g., "You seem to want others to notice you."

e. Encourage client to recognize needs of others

f. Have client verbalize needs directly, e.g., wishes for attention

Table 15-15 BIPOLAR DISORDER MEDICATIONS		
MEDICATION	**ADVERSE EFFECTS**	**NURSING CONSIDERATIONS**
Lithium carbonate	Dizziness	Use for control of manic episodes; mood stabilizer
	Headache	Blood levels must be monitored frequently
	Impaired vision	GI symptoms can be reduced if taken with meals
	Fine hand tremors	Therapeutic effects preceded by lag of 1–2 wk
	Reversible leukocytosis	Signs of intoxication—vomiting, diarrhea, drowsiness, muscular weakness, ataxia
		Dosage is usually halved during depressive stages of illness
		Initial blood target level = 1–1.5 mEq/L (1-1.5 mmol/L)
		Maintenance blood target level = 0.8-1.2 mEq/L (0.8-1.2 mmol/L)
		Check serum levels 2–3 times weekly when started and monthly while on maintenance; serum levels should be drawn in AM prior to dose
		Should have fluid intake of 2,500–3,000 mL/day and adequate salt intake
Carbamazepine	Dizziness, vertigo	Mood stabilizer used with bipolar disorder
	Drowsiness	Traditionally used for seizures and trigeminal neuralgia
	Ataxia	Obtain baseline urinalysis, BUN, liver function tests, CBC
	CHF	Shake oral suspension well before measuring dose
	Aplastic anemia, thrombocytopenia	When giving by NG tube, mix with equal volume of water, 0.9% NaCl or D5W, then flush with 100 mL after dose
		Take with food
		Drowsiness usually disappears in 3–4 days
Divalproex sodium	Sedation	Mood stabilizer used with bipolar disorder
	Pancreatitis	Traditionally used for seizures
	Indigestion	Monitor liver function tests, platelet count before starting medication and periodically after medication
	Thrombocytopenia	Teach client symptoms of liver dysfunction (e.g., malaise, fever, lethargy)
	Toxic hepatitis	Monitor blood levels
		Take with food or milk
		Avoid hazardous activities

8. Administer lithium for mania
   a. Physical exam and blood must be done before starting
      1) Contraindications to lithium include:
         a) Cardiovascular disease
         b) Renal disease
         c) Decreased sodium intake (e.g., in hypertensive clients)
   b. Teach client signs of lithium toxicity
      1) Nausea, vomiting, anorexia
      2) Tremors, ataxia
   c. Do not administer drug with diuretics or if toxicity is suspected
   d. Check serum lithium levels, 2–3 times weekly when beginning and monthly on maintenance
      1) Initial level should be between 1–1.5 mEq/L (1-1.5 mmol/L)
      2) Maintenance level should be between 0.8-1.2 mEq/L (0.8-1.2 mmol/L)
      3) Serum levels should be drawn in the AM prior to AM dose

ALTERED THOUGHT PROCESSES

MANIFESTATIONS OF ALTERED THOUGHT PROCESSES

A. Characteristic findings

1. Withdrawal from relationships and from the world
   a. Neologisms, rhyming
   b. Magical thinking
   c. Social ineptitude—aloof and fails to encourage interpersonal relationships

2. Inappropriate or no display of feelings

3. Hypochondriasis, depersonalization

4. Suspiciousness—sees world as a hostile, threatening place

5. Poor reality testing
   a. Hallucinations
   b. Delusions—persistent false beliefs
      1) Grandeur—belief that one is special, e.g., a monarch
      2) Persecutory—belief that one is a victim of a plot
      3) Ideas of reference—belief that environmental events are directed toward the self, e.g., client sees people talking and believes they are discussing the client
   c. Illusions—misperceptions of reality

6. Loose associations

7. Short attention span, decreased ability to comprehend stimuli

8. Psychomotor alteration slow-moving, slow-speaking

9. Hyperactivity
   a. Loud, rapid talking
   b. Inability to sit still (akathisia)

10. Regression

11. Inability to meet basic survival needs
    a. Unable to feed self properly (poor nutritional habits)
    b. Poor personal hygiene
    c. Inappropriate dress for the weather/environment

B. Definitions of characteristic findings

1. Hallucinations—perceptual dysfunction in which false sensory perceptions are experienced in the absence of an external stimulus; visual and auditory hallucinations most common

2. Delusions—persistent false beliefs, rigidly held, which do not stand the test of reality; common types include:
   a. Delusions of grandeur—that one is special in a way that has no basis in reality, e.g., President of the United States
   b. Persecutory—that one is being threatened, e.g., a victim of a plot

     c. Ideas of reference—that situations or events involve them, e.g., thinks people are talking about client; misconstruing trivial remarks

     d. Somatic—that one's body is reacting in a particular way without a basis in reality

  3. Illusion—misperception of reality

  4. Neologisms—privately invented words that people do not understand

  5. Magical thinking—primitive thought process in which one believes thoughts alone can change events

  6. Looseness of associations—incoherent, illogical flow of thoughts and ideas producing confusing language

  7. Autistic thinking—regressive thought process in which subjective, personal interpretations are not validated with objective reality

  8. Word salad—words combined with no logical sequence

C. Types

  1. Conditions predisposing to withdrawal from reality

     a. Senile dementia

     b. Acute drug psychosis

     c. Biochemical interaction

     d. Ineffective family interaction

     e. Schizophrenia—(see Table 15-16)

Table 15-16 SCHIZOPHRENIA	
SUB-TYPES	**PRESENTING SYMPTOMS**
Disorganized	Inappropriate behavior such as silly laughing and regression; transient hallucinations; disorganized behavior and speech
Catatonic	Sudden onset of mutism, bizarre mannerisms; remains in stereotyped position with waxy flexibility; may have dangerous periods of agitation and explosivity
Paranoid	Late onset in life, characterized by suspicion and ideas of persecution and delusions and hallucinations; may be angry or hostile
Undifferentiated	General symptoms of schizophrenia Symptoms of more than one type of schizophrenia
Residual	No longer exhibits overt symptoms

D. Sub-types of schizophrenia

  1. Disorganized —type of schizophrenia characterized by inappropriate or flat affect; social withdrawal extreme; disorganized speech and behavior; silliness, inappropriate laughter, grimacing, and regression common

  2. Catatonic—stuporous condition associated with rigidity, posturing, waxy flexibility (when limb positioned, stays in that position); may alternate with overactivity and agitation; insidious onset

  3. Paranoid—mainly features suspiciousness, distortion, and projection; delusions of grandeur, persecution, or hallucinations may be prominent; if onset occurs later in life, client tends to be less withdrawn from daily activities

4. Undifferentiated—characterized by general symptoms of schizophrenia but does not meet criteria for a particular type (poor overall functioning)

5. Residual—history of at least one psychotic episode, but currently without overt psychotic behavior; may be withdrawn but is able to function

E. Nursing management

1. Maintain client safety

    a. Protect from altered thought processes

        1) Decrease sensory stimuli

        2) Remove from areas of tension

        3) Validate reality

        4) Recognize that client is experiencing hallucination

        5) Do not argue with client

        6) Respond to feeling or tone of hallucination or delusion

        7) Do not reinforce hallucinations

        8) Be alert to hallucinations that command the client to harm self or others or to do destructive acts

    b. Protect from erratic and inappropriate behavior

        1) Communicate in calm, authoritative tone

        2) Address client by name

        3) Observe client for early signs of escalating behavior

    c. Administer antipsychotic medications as indicated (see Table 15-17)

2. Establish a therapeutic relationship—engage in individual therapy

    a. Institute measures to promote trust

        1) Same as general withdrawal from reality (see Table 15-18)

        2) Be consistent and reliable in keeping all scheduled appointments

        3) Avoid direct questions (client may feel threatened)

        4) Accept client's indifference (e.g., failure to smile or greet nurse) and avoidance behavior (e.g., hostility or sarcasm)

        5) Explain staff changes, especially vacations and absences

    b. Encourage client's affect by verbalizing what you observe, e.g., "You seem to think that I don't want to stay."

    c. Tolerate silences—may have to sit through long silences with client who is too withdrawn to speak (catatonic)

    d. Accept regression as a normal part of treatment when new stresses are encountered

        1) With delusional regression, respond to associated feeling, not to the delusion, e.g., client claims he has no heart; nursing response, "You must feel empty."

        2) Help pinpoint source of regression, e.g., anxiety about discharge

3. Meet physical needs of severely regressed clients, e.g., catatonic

    a. Poor basic hygiene—may have to be washed initially

    b. Poor nutritional habits—may have to be fed

        1) Ask client to pick up fork; if unable, then feeding is necessary

        2) When ready, encourage client to eat in dining room with others

4. Engage in family therapy—especially when client is returning to family
    a. Understand the problem involves the family—establish a "family client" in need of support
        1) Family helps maintain pathology
        2) Client is often the scapegoat for family problems
    b. All members must be involved to effect change in client
    c. Decrease fusion—give all members a sense of self and independence

5. Engage in socialization or activity group therapy according to client's ability
    a. Accept nonverbal behavior initially
    b. If client cannot tolerate group, do not force or embarrass
    c. Act as a social role model for client

6. Provide simple activities or tasks to promote positive self-esteem and success
    a. Finger painting and clay are good choices for regressed catatonic client
    b. Encourage attendance at occupational, vocational, and art therapy
    c. Avoid competitive situations with paranoid client; solitary activities are better

Table 15-17 ANTIPSYCHOTIC MEDICATIONS		
MEDICATION	ADVERSE EFFECTS	NURSING CONSIDERATIONS
Conventional high potency		
Haloperidol Haloperidol decanoate Fluphenazine Fluphenazine decanoate	Low sedative effect Low incidence of hypotension High incidence of extrapyramidal adverse effects	Used in large doses for assaultive clients Used with elderly (risk of falling reduced) Decanoate: long-acting form given every 2–4 wk; IM into deep muscle Z-track
Conventional medium potency		
Perphenazine	Orthostatic hypotension Dry mouth Constipation	Can help control severe vomiting Medication is available PO, IM, and IV
Conventional low potency		
Chlorpromazine	High sedative effect High incidence of hypotension Irreversible retinitis pigmentosus at 800 mg/day	Educate client about increased sensitivity to sun (as with other phenothiazines) No tolerance or potential for abuse

Table 15-17 ANTIPSYCHOTIC MEDICATIONS *(CONTINUED)*		
MEDICATION	**ADVERSE EFFECTS**	**NURSING CONSIDERATIONS**
Atypical		
Risperidone Quetiapine Ziprasidone Aripiprazole Clozapine Olanzapine	Moderate orthostatic hypotension Moderate sedation Significant weight gain Doses over 6 mg can cause tardive dyskinesia Moderate orthostatic hypotension Moderate sedation Very low risk of tardive dyskinesia and neuroleptic malignant syndrome ECG changes—QT prolongation	Chosen as first-line antipsychotic due to mild EPS and very low anticholinergic adverse effects Chosen as first-line antipsychotic due to mild EPS and very low anticholinergic adverse effects Effective with depressive symptoms of schizophrenia Low propensity for weight gain
Action	Blocks dopamine receptors in basal ganglia of brain, inhibiting transmission of nerve impulses	
Indications	Acute and chronic psychosis	
Adverse effects	Akathisia (motor restlessness) Dyskinesia (abnormal voluntary movements) Dystonias (abnormal muscle tone producing spasms of tongue, face, neck) Parkinson syndrome (shuffling gait, rigid muscles, excessive salivation, tremors, mask-like face, motor deceleration) Tardive dyskinesia (involuntary movements of mouth, tongue, trunk, extremities; chewing motions, sucking, tongue thrusting) Photosensitivity Orthostatic hypotension Neuroleptic malignant syndrome	
Nursing considerations	Lowers seizure threshold May slow growth rate in children Monitor for urinary retention and decreased GI motility Avoid alcohol May cause hypotension if taken with antihypertensives, nitrates Phenothiazines also used	

F. Managing withdrawn behavior (see Table 15-18)

Table 15-18 NURSING CARE OF CLIENT WHO ACTS WITHDRAWN	
PROBLEM	INTERVENTIONS
Lack of trust and feeling of safety and security	Keep interactions brief, especially orientation
	Structure environment
	Be consistent and reliable; notify client of anticipated schedule changes
	Decrease physical contact
	Eye contact during greeting
	Maintain attentiveness with head slightly leaning toward client and nonintrusive attitude
	Allow physical distance
	Accept client's behavior, e.g., silence; maintain matter-of-fact attitude toward behavior
Hallucinations	Maintain accepting attitude
	Do not argue with client about reality of hallucinations
	Comment on feeling, tone of hallucination, e.g., "That must be frightening to you."
	Encourage diversional activities, e.g., playing cards, especially activities in which client can gain a sense of mastery, e.g., artwork
	Encourage discussions of reality-based interests
Lack of attention to personal needs, e.g., nutrition, hygiene	Assess adequacy of hydration, nutrition
	Structure routine for bathing, mealtime
	Offer encouragement or assistance if necessary, e.g., sit with client or feed client if appropriate
	Decrease environmental stimuli at mealtime, e.g., suggest early dinner before dining room crowds
	Positioning and skin care for catatonic client

G. Managing suspicious behavior (see Table 15-19)

Table 15-19 NURSING CARE OF A CLIENT WHO ACTS SUSPICIOUS	
PROBLEM	**INTERVENTIONS**
Mistrust and feeling of rejection	Keep appointments with clients Clear, consistent communication Allow client physical distance and keep door open when interviewing Genuineness and honesty in interactions Recognize testing behavior and show persistence of interest in client
Delusions	Allow client to verbalize the delusion in a limited manner Do not argue with client or try to convince that delusions are not real Point out feeling tone of delusion Provide activities to divert attention from delusions Solitary activities best at first and then may progress to noncompetitive games or activities Do not reinforce delusions by validating them Focus on potential real concerns of client

H. Managing aggressive/violent behavior (see Table 15-20)

Table 15-20 NURSING CARE OF A CLIENT WHO ACTS VIOLENT	
PROBLEM	**INTERVENTIONS**
Increased agitation/anxiety	Recognize signs of impending violence, e.g., increased motor activity, pacing, or sudden stop—"calm before the storm" Identify yourself, speak calmly but firmly in normal tone of voice Help verbalize feelings Use nonthreatening body language, e.g., arms to side, palm outward, keep distance, avoid blocking exit, avoid body contact Avoid disagreeing with client or threatening client Decrease stimuli—remove threatening objects or people
Violence	Intercede early Continue nonthreatening behavior If client needs to be restrained to protect self or others, get help (at least four people) Move in organized, calm manner, stating that you want to help and that you will not permit client to harm self or others Use restraints correctly, e.g., never tie to bedside rail, check circulation frequently

SOCIAL INTERACTIONS

MANIPULATIVE BEHAVIOR

A. Assessment

1. Characteristic findings
   a. Makes unreasonable requests for time, attention, and favors
   b. Divides staff against each other—attempts to undermine nurse's role
   c. Intimidates others
      1) Uses others' faults to own advantage, e.g., naiveté
      2) Tries to make others feel guilty

   d. Uses seductive and disingenuous approach
      1) Make personal approach to staff, e.g., acts more like friend than client
      2) Takes advantage of others for own gain
      3) Frequently lies and rationalizes

   e. May malinger or behave in helpless manner, e.g., feigns illness to avoid task

2. Predisposing conditions
   a. Substance abuse, alcoholism
   b. Antisocial disorders
   c. Bipolar disorders

3. Goals
   a. Help client set limits on his behavior
   b. Help client learn to see the consequences of his behavior
   c. Help family members understand and deal with client
   d. Promote staff cooperation and consistency in caring for client

B. Nursing management

1. Use consistent undivided staff approach
   a. Clearly define expectations of client
   b. Adhere to hospital regulations
   c. Hold frequent staff conferences to increase staff communication and avoid conflict

2. Set limits
   a. Do not allow behaviors that interfere with the physical and psychological safety of others
   b. Carry out limit-setting, avoid threats and promises
   c. Offer alternatives when possible
   d. Remain nonjudgmental
   e. Avoid arguing or allowing client to rationalize behavior
   f. Be brief in discussion

3. Be constantly alert for potential manipulation
   a. Favors, compliments

b. Attempts to be personal

c. Malingering, helplessness

4. Be alert for signs of destructive behavior
   a. Suicide
   b. Homicide

ALCOHOL ABUSE

A. Intoxication (see Table 15-21)
   1. Mild—blood alcohol 0.05–0.15%
   2. Moderate—blood alcohol 0.15–0.3%
   3. Severe—blood alcohol 0.3–0.5%

Table 15-21 POTENTIAL ALCOHOL INTOXICATION	
ASSESSMENT	**NURSING CONSIDERATIONS**
Drowsiness	Monitor vital signs frequently
Slurred speech	Allow client to "sleep it off"
Tremors	Protect airway from aspiration
Impaired thinking/memory loss	Assess need for IV glucose
	Assess for injuries
Nystagmus	Assess for signs of withdrawal and chronic alcohol dependence
Diminished reflexes	Counsel about alcohol use
Nausea/vomiting	Be alert for potential problems of alcohol poisoning and CNS depression
Possible hypoglycemia	
Increased respiration	
Belligerence/grandiosity	
Loss of inhibitions	
Depression	

B. Nursing management
   1. Counseling the alcoholic
      a. Identify problems related to drinking—in family relationships, work, health, and other areas of life
      b. Help client to see/admit problem
         1) Confront denial with slow persistence
         2) Maintain relationship with client

   2. Establishing control of problem drinking
      a. Identify potential problematic settings that trigger drinking behavior
      b. Alcoholics Anonymous—valuable mutual support group
         1) Peers share experiences
         2) Learn to substitute contact with humans for alcohol
         3) Stress living in the present; stop drinking "one day at a time"
      c. Disulfiram—drug used to maintain sobriety; based on behavioral therapy
         1) Once sufficient blood level reached, disulfiram interacts with alcohol to provide severe reaction

    2) Symptoms of disulfiram–alcohol reaction include flushing, coughing, difficulty breathing, nausea, vomiting, pallor, anxiety

    3) Contraindicated in diabetes mellitus, atherosclerotic heart disease, cirrhosis, kidney disease, psychosis

  d. Assessment of alcohol withdrawal (see Table 15-22)

Table 15–22 ALCOHOL WITHDRAWAL		
WITHDRAWAL	**DELIRIUM TREMENS**	**NURSING CONSIDERATIONS**
Tremors	Tremors	Administer benzodiazepines, chlordiazepoxide, diazepam
Easily startled	Anxiety	
Insomnia	Panic	Monitor vital signs, particularly pulse, BP, temperature
Anxiety	Disorientation, confusion	Seizure precautions
Anorexia	Hallucination	
Alcoholic	Vomiting	Provide quiet, well-lit environment
Hallucinations	Diarrhea	Orient client frequently
	Paranoia	Don't leave hallucinating, confused client alone
	Delusional symptoms	
	Ideas of reference	Administer anticonvulsants as needed
	Suicide attempts	
	Grand mal convulsions (especially first 48 hours after client stops drinking)	Administer thiamine IV or IM as needed
	Potential coma/death	Administer IV glucose as needed 10% mortality rate

3. Counseling the spouse of the alcoholic
  a. Initial goal is to help spouse focus on self
  b. Explore life problems from spouse's point of view
  c. Spouse can attempt to help alcoholic once strong enough

Table 15–23 CHRONIC CNS DISORDERS ASSOCIATED WITH ALCOHOLISM			
	ALCOHOLIC CHRONIC BRAIN SYNDROME (DEMENTIA)	**WERNICKE'S SYNDROME**	**KORSAKOFF'S PSYCHOSIS**
Symptoms	Fatigue, anxiety, personality changes, depression, confusion Loss of memory of recent events Can progress to dependent, bedridden state	Confusion, diplopia, nystagmus, ataxia Disorientation, apathy	Memory disturbance with confabulation, loss of memory of recent events, learning problems Possible problem with taste and smell, loss of reality testing
Nursing considerations	Balanced diet, abstinence from alcohol	IV or IM thiamin, abstinence from alcohol	Balanced diet, thiamin, abstinence from alcohol

      d. Al-Anon: self-help group for spouses and relatives

        1) Learn "loving detachment" from alcoholic

        2) Goal is to try to make one's own life better and not to blame the alcoholic

        3) Provides safe, helpful environment

  4. Counseling children of alcoholic parents

      a. Overcome denial of problem

      b. Establish trusting relationship

      c. Work with parents as well; avoid negative reactions to parents

      d. Referral to Alateen: organization for teenagers of alcoholic parent; self-help, similar to Al-Anon

C. Chronic CNS disorders associated with alcoholism (see Table 15-23)

DRUG ABUSE

A. Definition—a physiological and psychological dependence; increasing doses needed for those drugs that create tolerance

B. Substance abusers—have a low frustration tolerance and need for immediate gratification to escape anxiety

C. Addiction—may result from prolonged use of medication for physical or psychological pain

D. Nursing management

  1. Observe for signs and symptoms of intoxication or drug use

      a. Examine skin for cuts, needle-marks, abscesses, or bruises

      b. Recognize symptoms of individual drug overdose

        1) Hypotension, decreased respirations, constriction(pinpoint) of pupils with narcotics and sedatives

        2) Agitation with amphetamines and hallucinogens

  2. Treat symptoms of overdose

      a. Maintain respiration—airway when needed

      b. IV therapy as necessary

      c. Administer naloxone

        1) Antagonist to narcotics—induces withdrawal, stimulates respirations

        2) Short-acting—symptoms of respiratory depression may return; additional doses may be necessary

      d. Gastric lavage for overdose of sedatives taken orally

      e. Dialysis to eliminate barbiturates from system

  3. Observe for signs of withdrawal, e.g., sweating, agitation, panic, hallucinations

      a. Identify drug type

      b. Seizure precautions

      c. Keep airway on hand

      d. Detoxify gradually

        1) Methadone used for long-term maintenance and acute withdrawal (narcotic)

        2) Decreasing doses of methadone used after initial withdrawal until stabilization is achieved

  4. Treat panic from acute withdrawal and/or marked depression

      a. Hospitalize temporarily for psychotic response

   b. Decrease stimuli, provide calm environment

   c. Protect client from self-destructive behavior

   d. Stay with client to reduce anxiety, panic, and confusion

   e. Assure client that hallucinations are from drugs and will subside

   f. Administer medications as indicated to manage symptoms of withdrawal and panic

   g. Monitor vital signs

5. Promote physical health
   a. Identify physical health needs
      1) Rest
      2) Nutrition
      3) Shelter

   b. Complete physical work-up
      1) Heroin addicts need to be followed for liver and cardiac complications, sexually transmitted infections (STIs), AIDS
      2) Dental care

6. Administer methadone for maintenance when indicated
   a. Synthetic narcotic—blocks euphoric effects of narcotics
   b. Eliminates craving and withdrawal symptoms
   c. Daily urine collected to monitor for other drug abuse while on methadone

7. Implement measures for antisocial personality disorders/manipulative behaviors
   a. Structured, nonpermissive environment
   b. Milieu therapy—peer pressure to conform
   c. Set limits but remain nonjudgmental
   d. Refer to drug-free programs (Synanon, Phoenix House, Odyssey House) for confrontation and support to remain drug-free

8. Treat underlying emotional problems
   a. Individual therapy—give support and acceptance
   b. Group therapy—to learn new ways of interacting
   c. Promote use of self-help groups

9. Assist client with rehabilitation, e.g., work programs, vocational counseling, completion of schooling

Table 15-24 NONALCOHOL SUBSTANCE ABUSE			
MEDICATION/DRUG	SYMPTOMS OF ABUSE	SYMPTOMS OF WITHDRAWAL	NURSING CONSIDERATIONS
Barbiturates			
(downers, barbs, pink ladies, rainbows, yellow jackets) Phenobarbital Nembutal	Respiratory depression Decreased BP and pulse Coma, ataxia, seizures Increasing nystagmus Poor muscle coordination Decreased mental alertness	Anxiety, insomnia Tremors, delirium Convulsions	Maintain airway (intubate, suction) Check LOC and vital signs Start IV with large-gauge needle Give sodium bicarbonate to promote excretion Give activated charcoal, use gastric lavage Hemodialysis
Narcotics			
Morphine Heroin (horse, junk, smack) Codeine Dilaudid Meperidine Methadone — for detoxification and maintenance	Hyperpyrexia Seizures, ventricular dysrhythmias Euphoria, then anxiety, sadness, insomnia, sexual indifference Overdose–severe respiratory depression, pinpoint pupils, coma	Watery eyes, runny nose Loss of appetite Irritability, tremors, panic Cramps, nausea Chills and sweating Elevated BP Hallucinations, delusions	Maintain airway (intubate, suction) Control seizures Check LOC and vital signs Start IV, may be given bolus of glucose Have lidocaine and defibrillator available Treat for hyperthermia Give naloxone to reverse respiratory depression Hemodialysis
Stimulants			
(uppers, pep pills, speed, crystal meth) Cocaine (crack) Amphetamine Benzedrine Dexedrine	Tachycardia, increased BP, tachypnea, anxiety Irritability, insomnia, agitation Seizures, coma, hyperpyrexia, euphoria Nausea, vomiting Hyperactivity, rapid speech Hallucinations Nasal septum perforation (cocaine)	Apathy Long periods of sleep Irritability Depression, disorientation	Maintain airway (intubate, suction) Start IV Use cardiac monitoring Check LOC and vital signs Give activated charcoal, use gastric lavage Monitor for suicidal ideation Keep in calm, quiet environment
Cannabis derivatives			
(pot, weed, grass, reefer, joint, mary jane) Marijuana Hashish	Fatigue Paranoia, psychosis Euphoria, relaxed inhibitions Increased appetite Disoriented behavior	Insomnia, hyperactivity Decreased appetite	Most effects disappear in 5-8 hours as drug wears off May cause psychosis
Hallucinogens			
LSD (acid) PCP (angel dust, rocket fuel) Mescaline (buttons, cactus)	Nystagmus, marked confusion, hyperactivity Incoherence, hallucinations, distorted body image Delirium, mania, self-injury Hypertension, hyperthermia Flashbacks, convulsions, coma	None	Maintain airway (intubate, suction) Control seizures Check LOC and vital signs "Talk down" client Reduce sensory stimuli Small doses of diazepam Check for trauma, protect from self-injury

CHILD ABUSE

A. Definition

1. Intentional physical, emotional, and/or sexual misuse/trauma or intentional omission of basic needs (neglect); usually related to diminished/limited ability of parent(s) to cope with, provide for, and/or relate to child

2. Those at high risk include children born prematurely and/or of low birth weight, children under 3 years and children with physical and/or mental disabilities

B. Assessment

1. Inconsistency between type/location of injury (bruises, burns, fractures, especially chip/spiral) and the history of the incident(s)

2. Unexplained physical or thermal injuries

3. Withdraws or is fearful of parents

4. Sexual abuse—genital lacerations, sexually transmitted diseases

5. Emotional neglect, failure to thrive; disturbed sleep; change in behavior in school

C. Nursing management

1. Provide for physical needs first

2. Mandatory reporting of identified/suspected cases to appropriate agency

3. Nonjudgmental treatment of parents; encourage expression of feelings

4. Provide role modeling to parents

5. Teach growth and development concepts, especially safety, discipline, age-appropriate activities, and human nutrition

6. Provide emotional support for child; play therapy (dolls, drawings, making up stories) may be more appropriate way for child to express feelings

7. Initiate protective placement and/or appropriate referrals for long-term follow-up

8. Documentation should reflect only what nurse saw or was told, not nurse's interpretation or opinion

ELDER ABUSE

A. Assessment

1. Battering, fractures, bruises

2. Over/undermedicated

3. Absence of needed dentures, glasses

4. Poor nutritional status, dehydration

5. Physical evidence of sexual abuse

6. Urine burns, excoriations, pressure injuries

B. Analysis

1. Elderly with chronic illness and depletion of financial resources who are dependent on children and grandchildren are particularly at risk

2. Current population trends indicate a decline in amount of people available to care for elderly

C. Nursing management

1. Provide for safety

2. Provide for physical needs first

3. Report to appropriate agencies (state laws vary)

4. Initiate protective placement and/or appropriate referrals

5. Consider client's rights of self determination

SEXUAL ABUSE

A. Assessment

1. Sexually abused child

   a. Disturbed growth and development

   b. Child becomes protective of others (parents)

   c. Uses defense mechanisms (e.g., denial, dissociation)

   d. Sleep and eating disturbances

   e. Depression and aggression, emotional deadening, amnesia

   f. Poor impulse control

   g. Somatic symptoms (e.g., chronic pain, GI disturbances)

   h. Truancy and running away

   i. Self-destructiveness

2. Adult victims of childhood sexual abuse

   a. Response is similar to delayed posttraumatic stress disorder (PTSD)

   b. Nightmares

   c. Unwanted, intrusive memories

   d. Kinesthetic sensations

   e. Flashbacks

   f. Relationship issues, fear of intimacy, fear of abandonment

3. Sexually abused adult

   a. Uses defense mechanisms (e.g., denial, dissociation)

   b. Relationship issues, abusive relationships, fear of intimacy, fear of abandonment

   c. Somatic complaints

   d. Homicidal thoughts, violence

   e. Hypervigilance, panic attacks, phobias/agoraphobia

   f. Suicidal thoughts/attempts

   g. Self-mutilation

   h. Compulsive eating/dieting, binging/purging

B. Background
1. Victims from every sociocultural, ethnic, and economic group
2. Within the family (incest) and outside the family
3. Usually involves younger, weaker victim
4. Victim is usually urged and coerced, manipulated through fear
5. Difficult to expose abuse; common for child not to be believed

C. Nursing management
1. Establish trusting relationship
2. Use empathy, active support, compassion, warmth
3. Nonjudgmental approach
4. Report to appropriate agencies (state laws vary)
5. Group and individual therapy; appropriate referrals (e.g., legal, shelters)
6. Medications as needed (e.g., antianxiety)

DOMESTIC VIOLENCE

A. Assessment
1. Frequent visits to health care provider's office or emergency room for unexplained trauma
2. Client being cued, silenced, or threatened by an accompanying family member
3. Evidence of multiple old injuries, scars, healed fractures seen on x-ray
4. Fearful, evasive, or inconsistent replies and nonverbal behaviors, such as flinching when approached or touched

B. Background
1. Family violence is usually accompanied by brainwashing (e.g., victims blame themselves, feel unworthy and fear that they won't be believed)
2. Long-term results of family violence are depression, suicidal ideation, low self-esteem, and impaired relationships outside the family
3. Women, children, and female adolescents are the most common victims
4. Cycle of abuse
   a. Tension-building; verbal abuse
   b. Eruption into violent act/behavior
   c. Period of remorse; offering of gifts, thoughtful behaviors, asking forgiveness
   d. Tension builds again

C. Nursing management
1. Provide privacy during initial interview to ensure that the perpetrator of violence does not remain with client; make a statement, e.g., "This part of the exam is always done in private."
2. Carefully document all injuries using body maps or photographs (with consent)
3. Determine the safety of client by specific questions about weapons in the home, substance abuse, extreme jealousy
4. Develop a safety or escape plan with client
5. Refer the client to community resources such as shelters, hotlines, and support groups

Chapter 16

PHARMACOLOGY

Section

1. Listing of Medications

The best way to learn medication information is to use the classification and subclassification systems which group and organize the medications.

Step 1: This section is organized by the most common classifications and subclassifications of medications.

Step 2: Identify the medications included in the classification and subclassification. NCLEX will identify the generic name of the medication.

Step 3: Identify the action or effect of the classification or subclassification.

Step 4: Based on the action of the classification or subclassification, identify the therapeutic use for the medications.

Step 5: Based on the action of the classification or subclassification, identify precautions or contraindications for use of that classification.

Step 6: Adverse effects are more intense effects of the action of the medications included in the classification or subclassification. Knowledge about management of adverse effects is critical when answering questions on NCLEX.

Step 7: Adverse reactions include potentially dangerous consequences related to the action of the medications in the classification or subclassification. The health care provider should be notified when adverse reactions occur.

Step 8: How do you evaluate the effect of the medications in the classification or subclassification? Is it a therapeutic or desired effect? Is it a nontherapeutic or undesired effect?

EMERGENCY MEDICATIONS FOR SHOCK, CARDIAC ARREST, AND ANAPHYLAXIS		
MEDICATION	ADVERSE EFFECTS	NURSING CONSIDERATIONS
Norepinephrine	Headache Palpitations Nervousness Epigastric distress Angina, hypertension **tissue necrosis with extravasation**	Vasoconstrictor to increase blood pressure and cardiac output Reflex bradycardia may occur with rise in BP Client should be attended at all times Monitor urinary output Infuse with dextrose solution, not saline Monitor blood pressure Protect medication from light
Dopamine	Increased ocular pressure Ectopic beats Nausea Tachycardia, chest pain, dysrhythmias	Low-dose–dilates renal and coronary arteries High-dose–vasoconstrictor, increases myocardial oxygen consumption Headache is an early symptom of drug excess Monitor blood pressure, peripheral pulses, urinary output Use infusion pump
Epinephrine	Nervousness Restlessness Dizziness Local necrosis of skin	Stimulates alpha and beta adrenergic receptors Monitor BP Carefully aspirate syringe before IM and subcutaneous doses; inadvertent IV administration can be harmful Always check strength: 1:100 only for inhalation, 1:1,000 for parenteral administration (SC or IM) Ensure adequate hydration
Isoproterenol	Headache Palpitations Tachycardia Changes in BP Angina, bronchial asthma Pulmonary edema	Stimulates beta 1 and beta 2 adrenergic receptors Used for heart block, ventricular arrhythmias, and bradycardia Bronchodilator used for asthma and bronchospasms Don't give at bedtime–interrupts sleep patterns Monitor BP, pulse
Phenylephrine	Palpations Tachycardia Hypertension Dysrhythmia Angina Tissue necrosis with extravasation	Potent alpha 1 agonist Used to treat hypotension
Dobutamine hydrocholoride	Hypertension PVCs Asthmatic episodes Headache	Stimulates beta 1 receptors Incompatible with alkaline solutions (sodium bicarbonate) Administer through central venous catheter or large peripheral vein using an infusion pump Don't infuse through line with other meds (incompatible) Monitor EKG, BP, I and O, serum potassium
Milrinone	Dysrhythmia Thrombocytopenia Jaundice	Positive inotropic agent Smooth muscle relaxant used to treat severe heart failure

EMERGENCY MEDICATIONS FOR SHOCK, CARDIAC ARREST, AND ANAPHYLAXIS *(CONTINUED)*		
MEDICATION	**ADVERSE EFFECTS**	**NURSING CONSIDERATIONS**
Nitroprusside sodium	Hypotension Increased intracranial pressure	Dilates cardiac veins and arteries Decreases preload and afterload Increases myocardial perfusion Keep in dark place after mixing Use an infusion pump
Diphenhydramine HCl	Drowsiness Confusion Insomnia Headache Vertigo Photosensitivity	Blocks effects of histamine on bronchioles, GI tract, and blood vessels
Actions	Varies with med	
Indications	Hypovolemic shock Cardiac arrest Anaphylaxis	
Adverse effects	Serious rebound effect may occur Balance between underdosing and overdosing	
Nursing considerations	Monitor vital signs Measure urine output Assess for extravasation Observe extremities for color and perfusion	

ADRENOCORTICAL MEDICATIONS: GLUCOCORTICOID		
MEDICATION	**ADVERSE EFFECTS**	**NURSING CONSIDERATIONS**
Cortisone acetate Hydrocortisone Dexamethasone Methylprednisolone Prednisone Beclomethasone Betamethasone Budesonide	Increases susceptibility to infection May mask symptoms of infection Edema, changes in appetite Euphoria, insomnia Delayed wound healing Hypokalemia, hypocalcemia Hyperglycemia Osteoporosis, fractures Peptic ulcer, gastric hemorrhage Psychosis	Prevents/suppresses cell-mediated immune reactors Used for adrenal insufficiency Overdosage produces Cushing's syndrome Abrupt withdrawal of drug may cause headache, nausea and vomiting, and papilledema (Addisonian crisis) Give single dose before 9 AM Give multiple doses at evenly spaced intervals Infection may produce few symptoms due to anti-inflammatory action Stress (surgery, illness, psychic) may lead to increased need for steroids Nightmares are often the first indication of the onset of steroid psychosis Check weight, BP, electrolytes, I and O, weight Used cautiously with history of TB (may reactivate disease) May decrease effects of oral hypoglycemics, insulin, diuretics, K$^+$ supplements Assess children for growth restriction Protect from pathological fractures Administer with antacids **Do not stop abruptly** Methylprednisolone also used for arthritis, asthma, allergic reactions, cerebral edema Dexamethosone also used for allergic disorders, cerebral edema, asthma attack, shock
Action	Stimulates formation of glucose (gluconeogenesis) and decreases use of glucose by body cells; increases formation and storage of fat in muscle tissue; alters normal immune response	
Indications	Addison's disease, Crohn's disease, COPD, lupus erythematosus, leukemias, lymphomas, myelomas, head trauma, tumo, to prevent/treat cerebral edema	
Adverse effects	Psychoses, depression, weight gain, hypokalemia, hypocalcemia, stunted growth in children, petechiae, buffalo hump	
Nursing considerations	Monitor fluid and electrolyte balance **Don't discontinue abruptly** Monitor for signs of infection	
Herbal interactions	Senna, celery seed, juniper may decrease serum potassium; when taken with corticosteroids may increase hypoglycemia Ginseng taken with corticosteroids may cause insomnia Echinacea may counteract effects of corticosteroids Licorice potentiates effect of corticosteroids	

ADRENOCORTICAL MEDICATIONS: MINERALOCORTICOID		
MEDICATION	ADVERSE EFFECTS	NURSING CONSIDERATIONS
Fludrocortisone acetate	Hypertension, edema due to sodium retention Muscle weakness and dysrhythmia due to hypokalemia	Give PO dose with food Check BP, electrolytes, I and O, weight Give low-sodium, high-protein, high-potassium diet May decrease effects of oral hypoglycemics, insulin, diuretics, K$^+$ supplements
Action	Increases sodium reabsorption, potassium and hydrogen excretion in the distal convoluted tubules of the nephron	
Indications	Adrenal insufficiency	
Adverse effects	Sodium and water retention Hypokalemia	
Nursing considerations	Monitor BP and serum electrolytes Daily weight, report sudden weight gain to health care provider Used with cortisone or hydrocortisone in adrenal insufficiency	

ANTACID MEDICATIONS		
MEDICATION	**ADVERSE EFFECTS**	**NURSING CONSIDERATIONS**
Aluminum hydroxide gel Calcium carbonate Aluminum hydroxide and magnesium trisilicate	Constipation that may lead to impaction, phosphate depletion	Monitor bowel pattern Compounds contains sodium; check if client is on sodium-restricted diet Aluminum and magnesium antacid compounds interfere with tetracycline absorption Encourage fluids Monitor for signs of phosphate deficiency—malaise, weakness, tremors, bone pain Shake well Careful use advised for kidney dysfunction
Magnesium hydroxide	Excessive dose can produce nausea, vomiting, and diarrhea	Store at room temperature with tight lid to prevent absorption of CO_2 Prolonged and frequent use of cathartic dose can lead to dependence Administer with caution to clients with renal disease
Aluminum hydroxide and magnesium hydroxide	Slight laxative effect	Encourage fluid intake Administer with caution to clients with renal disease
Action	Neutralizes gastric acids; raises gastric pH; inactivates pepsin	
Indications	Peptic ulcer Indigestion Reflux esophagitis Prevent stress ulcers	
Adverse effects	Constipation, diarrhea Acid rebound between doses Acid/base Imbalances	
Nursing considerations	Use medications with sodium content cautiously for clients with cardiac and renal disease Absorption of tetracyclines, quinolones, phenothiazides, iron preparations, isoniazid reduced when given with antacids Effectiveness of oral contraceptives and salicylates may decrease when given with antacids	

ANTI-ANXIETY MEDICATIONS

MEDICATION	ADVERSE EFFECTS	NURSING CONSIDERATIONS
Benzodiazepine Derivatives		
Chlordiazepoxide Diazepam	Lethargy, hangover Respiratory depression Hypotension	CNS depressant Use–anxiety, sedation, alcohol withdrawal, seizures May result in toxic build-up in the elderly Potential for physiological addiction/overdose Can develop tolerance and cross-tolerance Cigarette smoking increases clearance of drug Alcohol increases CNS depression
Alprazolam Lorazepam Oxazepam	Drowsiness, light-headedness, hypotension, hepatic dysfunction Increased salivation Orthostatic hypostension Memory impairment and confusion	CNS depressant Safer for elderly Don't combine with alcohol or other depressants Check renal and hepatic function **Don't discontinue abruptly (true for all antianxiety agents)** Teach addictive potential
Midazolam	Retrograde amnesia Euphoria Hypotension Dysrhythmia Cardiac arrest Respiratory depression	CNS depressant Use–preoperative sedation, conscious sedation for endoscopic procedures and diagnostic tests
Anxiolytics Antianxiety Medications		
Buspirone	Light-headedness Confusion Hypotension, palpitations	Little sedation Requires ≥3 weeks to be effective Cannot be given as a PRN medication Particularly useful for generalized anxiety disorder (GAD) No abuse potential Used for clients with previous addiction Avoid alcohol and grapefruit juice Monitor for worsening depression or suicidal tendencies
Hydroxyzine	Drowsiness, ataxia Leukopenia, hypotension	Produces no dependence, tolerance, or intoxication Can be used for anxiety relief for indefinite periods
Herbals		
Kava	Impaired thinking, judgment, motor reflexes, vision, decreased plasma proteins, thrombocytopenia, leukocytopenia, dyspnea, and pulmonary hypertension	Similar activity to benzodiazepines Suppresses emotional excitability and produces mild euphoria Do not take with CNS depressants Should not be taken by women who are pregnant or lactating or by children under the age of 12
Melatonin	Sedation, confusion, headache, and tachycardia	Influences sleep-wake cycles (levels are high during sleep) Used for prevention and treatment of "jet lag" and insomnia Use cautiously if given with benzodiazepines and CNS depressants Contraindicated in hepatic insufficiency, history of cerebrovascular disease, depression, and neurologic disorders

ANTIANXIETY MEDICATIONS *(CONTINUED)*		
MEDICATION	**ADVERSE EFFECTS**	**NURSING CONSIDERATIONS**
Action	Affects neurotransmitters	
Indications	Anxiety disorders, insomnia, seizures, panic attacks, acute manic episodes	
Adverse effects	Sedation Depression, confusion Anger, hostility Headache Dry mouth, constipation Bradycardia Elevations in LDH, AST, ALT Urinary retention	
Nursing considerations	Monitor liver function Monitor for therapeutic blood levels Avoid alcohol Caution when performing tasks requiring alertness (e.g., driving car) Benzodiazepines are also used as muscles relaxants, sedatives, hypnotics, anticonvulsants	

ANTICHOLINERGIC MEDICATIONS		
MEDICATION	**ADVERSE EFFECTS**	**NURSING CONSIDERATIONS**
Atropine sulfate	Tachycardia Headache, blurred vision Insomnia, dry mouth Dizziness Urinary retention Angina, mydriasis	Used for bradycardia When given PO give 30 minutes before meals Check for history of glaucoma, asthma, hypertension Monitor I and O, orientation When given in nonemergency situations make certain client voids before taking drug Educate client to expect dry mouth, increased respiration and heart rate Client should avoid heat (perspiration is decreased)
Aclidinium Tiotropium Ipratropium plus albuterol	Dry mouth Irritation of pharynx	Used for bronchospasm and long-term treatment of asthma Ipratropium administered as aerosol or in nebulizer Tiotropium administered in powder form by HandiHaler
Benztropine Trihexyphenidyl	Urinary retention Blurred vision Dry mouth Constipation	Used for Parkinson's Disease Increase fluids, bulk foods and exercise Taper before discontinuation Orthostatic hypotension precautions
Scopolamine	Urinary retention Blurred vision Dry mouth Constipation Confusion and sedation	Used for motion sickness Transdermal patch Contraindicated in acute angle glaucoma
Actions	Competes with acetylcholine at receptor sites in autonomic nervous system; causes relaxation of ciliary muscles (cycloplegia) and dilation of pupil (mydriasis); causes bronchodilation and decreases bronchial secretions; decreases mobility and GI secretions	

ANTICHOLINERGIC MEDICATIONS *(CONTINUED)*		
MEDICATION	**ADVERSE EFFECTS**	**NURSING CONSIDERATIONS**
Indications	Atropine—bradycardia, mydriasis for ophthalmic exam, preoperatively to dry secretions Scopolamine—motion sickness, vertigo, mydriasis for ophthalmic exam, preoperative to dry secretions	
Adverse effects	Blurred vision Dry mouth Urinary retention Changes in heart rate	
Nursing considerations	Monitor for urinary retention Contraindicated for clients with glaucoma	

ANTICOAGULANT MEDICATIONS		
MEDICATION	**ADVERSE EFFECTS**	**NURSING CONSIDERATIONS**
Action: Inhibits synthesis of clotting factors		
Heparin	Can produce hemorrhage from any body site (10%) Tissue irritation/pain at injection site Anemia Thrombocytopenia Fever Dose dependant on a PTT	Monitor therapeutic partial thromboplastin time (PTT) at 1.5–2.5 times the control without signs of hemorrhage Lower limit of normal 20–25 sec; upper limit of normal 32–39 sec For IV administration: use infusion pump, peak 5 minutes, duration 2–6 hours For injection: give deep SQ; never IM (danger of hematoma), onset 20–60 minutes, duration 8–12 hours **Antidote: protamine sulfate within 30 minutes** Can be allergenic

Low-molecular-weight heparin
  Enoxaparin
	Bleeding
	  Minimal widespread affect
	  Fixed dose
		Less allergenic than heparin
		Must be given deep SQ, never IV or IM
		Does not require lab test monitoring

Warfarin	Hemorrhage Diarrhea Rash Fever	Monitor therapeutic prothombin time (PT) at 1.5–2.5 times the control, or monitor international normalized ratio (INR) Normal PT 9.5–12 sec; normal INR 2.0–3.5 Onset: 12–24 hours, peak 1.5–3 days, duration: 3–5 days **Antidotes: vitamin K, whole blood, plasma** Teach measures to avoid venous stasis Emphasize importance of regular lab testing Client should avoid foods high in vitamin K: many green vegetables, pork, rice, yogurt, cheeses, fish, milk
Fondaparinux	Hemorrhage Thrombocytopenia	SQ only PT and aPTT aren't suitable monitoring tests
Action: Inhibits activity of clotting		
Dabigatran	Directly inhibits thrombin Used to treat atrial fibrillation Increased risk bleeding age greater than 75, kidney disease, gastrointestinal bleeding, use of NSAIDs	
Action	Heparin blocks conversion of fibrinogen to fibrin Coumadin interferes with liver synthesis of vitamin K–dependent clotting factors	
Indications	For heparin: prophylaxis and treatment of thromboembolic disorders; in very low doses (10–100 units) to maintain patency of IV catheters (heparin flush) For coumadin: management of pulmonary emboli, venous thromboembolism, MI, atrial dysrhythmias, post cardiac valve replacement For Persantine: as an adjunct to coumadin in postop cardiac valve replacement, as an adjunct to aspirin to reduce the risk of repeat stroke or TIAs	

ANTICOAGULANT MEDICATIONS *(CONTINUED)*		
MEDICATION	ADVERSE EFFECTS	NURSING CONSIDERATIONS
Adverse effects	Nausea Alopecia Urticaria Hemorrhage Bleeding/heparin-induced thrombocytopetria (HIT)	
Nursing considerations	Check for signs of hemorrhage: bleeding gums, nosebleed, unusual bleeding, black/tarry stools, hematuria, fall in hematocrit or blood pressure, guaiac-positive stools Client should avoid IM injections, ASA-containing products, and NSAIDs Client should wear medical information tag Instruct client to use soft toothbrush, electric razor, to report bleeding gums, petechiae or bruising, epistaxis, black tarry stools Monitor platelet counts and signs and symptoms of thrombosis during heparin therapy; if HIT suspected, heparin discontinued and non-heparin anticoagulant (lepirudin) given	
Herbal interactions	Garlic, ginger, ginkgo may increase bleeding when taken with warfarin (Coumadin) Large doses of anise may interfere with anticoagulants Ginseng and alfalfa my decrease anticoagulant activity Black haw increases action of anticoagulant Chamomile may interfere with anticoagulants	
Vitamin interaction	Vitamin C may slightly prolong PT Vitamin E will increase warfarin's effect	

ANTICONVULSANT MEDICATIONS		
MEDICATION	ADVERSE EFFECTS	NURSING CONSIDERATIONS
Clonazepam	Drowsiness Dizziness Confusion Respiratory depression	Benzodiazepine **Do not discontinue suddenly** Avoid activities that require alertness
Diazepam	Drowsiness, ataxia Hypotension Tachycardia Respiratory depression	IV push doses shouldn't exceed 2 mg/minute Monitor vital signs–resuscitation equipment available if given IV Alcohol increases CNS depression After long-term use, withdrawal leads to symptoms such as vomiting, sweating, cramps, tremors, and possibly convulsions
Fosphenytoin	Drowsiness Dizziness Confusion Leukopenia Anemia	Used for tonic–clonic seizures, status epilepticus Highly protein-bound Contact healthcare provider if rash develops
Levetiracetam	Dizziness Suicidal ideation	Avoid alcohol Avoid driving and activities that require alertness
Phenytoin sodium	Drowsiness, ataxia Nystagmus Blurred vision Hirsutism Lethargy GI upset Gingival hypertrophy	Give oral medication with at least 1/2 glass of water, or with meals to minimize GI irritation Inform client that red-brown or pink discoloration of sweat and urine may occur IV administration may lead to cardiac arrest–have resuscitation equipment at hand Never mix with any other drug or dextrose IV Instruct in oral hygiene Increase vitamin D intake and exposure to sunlight may be necessary with long-term use Alcohol increases serum levels Increased risk toxicity older adults

ANTICONVULSANT MEDICATIONS *(CONTINUED)*		
MEDICATION	**ADVERSE EFFECTS**	**NURSING CONSIDERATIONS**
Primidone	Drowsiness Ataxia, diplopia Nausea and vomiting	**Don't discontinue use abruptly** Full therapeutic response may take 2 weeks Shake liquid suspension well Take with food if experiencing GI distress Decreased cognitive function older adults
Magnesium sulfate	Flushing Sweating Extreme thirst Hypotension Sedation, confusion	Monitor intake and output Monitor magnesium levels Before each dose, deep tendon reflexes should be tested Vital signs should be monitored often during parenteral administration Used for pregnancy-induced hypertension
Valproic acid	Sedation Tremor, ataxia Nausea, vomiting Prolonged bleeding time	Agent of choice in many seizure disorders of young children Do not take with carbonated beverage Take with food Monitor platelets, bleeding time, and liver function tests
Carbamazepine	Myelosuppression Dizziness, drowsiness Ataxia Diplopia, rash	Monitor intake and output Supervise ambulation Monitor CBC Take with meals Wear protective clothing due to photosensitivity Multiple drug interactions
Ethosuximide	GI symptoms Drowsiness Ataxia, dizziness	Monitor for behavioral changes Monitor weight weekly
Gabapentin	Increased appetite Ataxia Irritability Dizziness Fatigue	Monitor weight and behavioral changes. Can also be used to treat postherpetic neuralgia, other neuropathic pain, fibromyalgia, prophylaxis of migraine
Lamotrigine	Diplopia Headaches Dizziness Drowsiness Ataxia Nausea, vomiting Life-threatening rash when given with valproic acid	Take divided doses with meals or just afterward to decrease adverse effects
Topiramate	Ataxia Confusion Dizziness Fatigue Vision problems	Adjunct therapy for intractable partial seizures Increased risk for renal calculi Stop drug immediately if eye problems—could lead to permanent damage
Action	Decreases flow of calcium and sodium across neuronal membranes	
Indications	Seizures Status epilepticus: diazepam, lorazepam, phenytoin	

ANTICONVULSANT MEDICATIONS *(CONTINUED)*		
MEDICATION	**ADVERSE EFFECTS**	**NURSING CONSIDERATIONS**
Adverse effects	Cardiovascular depression Respiratory depression Agranulocytosis Aplastic anemia	
Nursing considerations	Tolerance develops with long-term use Don't discontinue abruptly Caution with use of medications that lower seizure threshold (MAO inhibitors) Barbiturates and benzodiazepines also used as anticonvulsants Increased risk adverse reactions older adults	

ANTIDEPRESSANT MEDICATIONS: HETEROCYCLICS	
Examples	Bupropion Trazodone
Actions	Does not inhibit MAO; has some anticholinergic and sedative effects; alters effects of serotonin on CNS
Indications	Treatment of depression and smoking cessation
Adverse effects	Dry mouth Nausea Bupropion–insomnia and agitation Trazodone–sedation, orthostatic hypotension
Nursing considerations	May require gradual reduction before stopping Avoid use with alcohol, other CNS depressants for up to 1 week after end of therapy

ANTIDEPRESSANT MEDICATIONS: MONOAMINE OXIDASE (MAO) INHIBITORS

Examples	Phenelzine sulfate, isocarboxazid, tranylcypromine
Actions	Interferes with monoamine oxidase, allowing for increased concentration of neurotransmitters (epinephrine, norepinephrine, serotonin) in synaptic space, causing stabilization of mood
Indications	Depression Chronic pain syndromes
Adverse effects	Hypertensive crisis when taken with foods containing tyramine (aged cheese, bologna, pepperoni, salami, figs, bananas, raisins, beer, Chianti red wine) or OTC medications containing ephedrine, pseudoephedrine Photosensitivity Weight gain Sexual dysfunction Orthostatic hypotension
Nursing considerations	Not first-line medications for depression Should not be taken with SSRIs Administer antihypertensive medications with caution Avoid use of other CNS depressants, including alcohol **Discontinue 10 days before general anesthesia** Medications lower seizure threshold Monitor for urinary retention

ANTIDEPRESSANT MEDICATIONS: SELECTIVE SEROTONIN REUPTAKE INHIBITORS

Examples	SSRIs: Fluoxetine, Citalopram, Escitalopram, Fluvoxamine, Paroxetine, Sertraline SNRIs: Venlafaxine, Duloxetine	
Actions	Inhibits CNS neuronal uptake of serotonin; acts as stimulant counteracting depression and increasing motivation	
Indications	Depression Obsessive-compulsive disorders Obesity Bulimia	
Adverse effects	Headache, dizziness Nervousness Insomnia, drowsiness Anxiety Tremor Dry mouth GI upset	Taste changes Sweating Rash URI Painful menstruation Sexual dysfunction Weight gain
Nursing considerations	Take in AM Takes 4 weeks for full effect Monitor weight Good mouth care Do not administer with MAOIs–risk of serotonin syndrome Monitor for thrombocytopenia, leukopenia, and anemia	

ANTIDEPRESSANT MEDICATIONS: TRICYCLICS	
Examples	Amitriptyline Imipramine
Actions	Inhibits presynaptic reuptake of neurotransmitters norepinephrine and serotonin; anticholinergic action at CNS and peripheral receptors
Indications	Depression Obstructive sleep apnea
Adverse effects	Sedation Anticholinergic effects (dry mouth, blurred vision) Confusion (especially in elderly) Photosensitivity Disturbed concentration Orthostatic hypotension Bone marrow depression Urinary retention
Nursing considerations	Therapeutic effect in 1–3 weeks; maximum response in 6–9 weeks May be administered in daily dose at night to promote sleep and decrease adverse effects during the day Orthostatic hypotension precautions Instruct client that adverse effects will decrease over time Sugarless lozenges for dry mouth Do not abruptly stop taking medication (headache, vertigo, nightmares, malaise, weight change) Avoid alcohol, sleep-inducing medications, OTC medications Avoid exposure to sunlight, wear sunscreen Older adults: strong anticholinergic and sedation effects

ANTIDEPRESSANT MEDICATIONS: OVERVIEW		
MEDICATION	ADVERSE EFFECTS	NURSING CONSIDERATIONS
Monoamine oxidase inhibitors (MAOIs)		
Isocarboxazid Tranylcypromine sulfate Phenelzine sulfate	Postural hypotension If foods with tyramine ingested, can have hypertensive crisis: headache, sweating, palpitations, stiff neck, intracranial hemorrhage Potentiates alcohol and other medications	Inhibits monoamine oxidase enzyme, preventing destruction of norepinephrine, epinephrine, and serotonin Avoid foods with tyramine—aged cheese, liver, herring, yeast, beer, wine, sour cream, pickled products Avoid caffeine, antihistamines, amphetamines Takes 3-4 weeks to work Avoid tricyclics until 3 weeks after stopping MAO inhibitors Monitor vital signs Sunblock required
Tricyclics		
Amitriptyline hydrochloride Imipramine Desipramine hydrochloride Doxepin Nortriptyline	Sedation/drowsiness, especially with amitriptyline Blurred vision, dry mouth, diaphoresis Postural hypotension, palpitations Nausea, vomiting Constipation, urinary retention Increased appetite	Increases brain amine levels Suicide risk high after 10-14 days because of increased energy Monitor vital signs Sunblock required Increase fluid intake Take dose at bedtime (sedative effect) Use sugarless candy or gum for dry mouth Delay of 2-6 weeks before noticeable effects
Selective serotonin reuptake inhibitors (SSRIs)		
Fluoxetine Paroxetine Sertraline hydrochloride Citalopram Venlafaxine	Palpitations, bradycardia Nausea, vomiting, diarrhea or constipation, increased or decreased appetite, urinary retention Nervousness, insomnia	Decreases neuronal uptake of serotonin Take in AM to avoid insomnia Takes at least 4 weeks to work Can potentiate effect of digoxin, warfarin, and diazepam Used for anorexia
Serotonin/norepinephrine reuptake inhibitors (SNRIs)		
Duloxetine	Palpitations, bradycardia Nausea, vomiting, diarrhea or constipation, increased or decreased appetite, urinary retention Nervousness, insomnia	Decreases neuronal uptake of serotonin Take in AM to avoid insomnia Takes at least 4 weeks to work Can potentiate effect of digoxin, warfarin, and diazepam Used for anorexia
Heterocyclics		
Bupropion Trazodone	Dry mouth Nausea	May require gradual reduction before stopping Avoid use with alcohol, other CNS depressants for up to 1 week after end of therapy

ANTIDEPRESSANT MEDICATIONS: OVERVIEW *(CONTINUED)*

MEDICATION	ADVERSE EFFECTS	NURSING CONSIDERATIONS
Herbals		
St. John's wort	Dizziness, hypertension, allergic skin reaction, phototoxicity	Avoid use of St. John's wort and MAOI within 2 weeks of each other Do not use alcohol Contraindicated in pregnancy Avoid exposure to sun and use sunscreen Discontinue 1 to 2 weeks before surgery
Herbal interactions	St. John's wort—interacts with SSRIs; do not take within 2 weeks of MAOI Ginseng may potentiate MAOIs Avoid Ma huang or ephedra with MAOIs Kava kava should not be combined with benzodiazepines or opioids due to increased sedation Increase use of Brewer's yeast with MAOIs can increase blood pressure	

ANTIDIABETIC MEDICATIONS: INSULIN

INSULIN TYPES	ONSET OF ACTION	PEAK ACTION	DURATION OF ACTION	TIME OF ADVERSE REACTION	CHARACTERISTICS
Rapid-acting					
Lispro	15-30 min	0.5–1.5 hours	3–5 hours	Midmorning: trembling, weakness	Client should eat within 5–15 min after injection; also used in insulin pumps
Aspart	15-30 min	1–3 hours	3–5 hours		
Glulisine	10-15 min	1–1.5 hours	3–5 hours		
Short-acting					
Regular insulin	30–60 min	1–5 hours	6–10 hours	Midmorning, midafternoon: weakness, fatigue	Clear solution; given 20–30 min before meal; can be alone or with other insulins
Intermediate-acting					
Isophane (NPH)	1–2 hours	4–12 hours	16 h	Early evening: weakness, fatigue	White and cloudy solution; can be given after meals
Very long-acting					
Glargine	3-4 h	Continuous (no peak)	24 hours	none	Maintains blood glucose levels regardless of meals; cannot be mixed with other insulins; given at bedtime
Determir	unknown	Continuous (no peak)	24 hours (varies)		
Degludec	1 hour	9 hours	24 hours		
Action	Reduces blood glucose levels by increasing glucose transport across cell membranes; enhances conversion of glucose to glycogen				
Indications	Type 1 diabetes; type 2 diabetes not responding to oral hypoglycemic agents; gestational diabetes not responding to diet				
Adverse effects	Hypoglycemia				

ANTIDIABETIC MEDICATIONS: INSULIN *(CONTINUED)*					
INSULIN TYPES	ONSET OF ACTION	PEAK ACTION	DURATION OF ACTION	TIME OF ADVERSE REACTION	CHARACTERISTICS
Nursing considerations	Teach client to rotate sites to prevent lipohypertrophy, fibrofatty masses at injection sites; do not inject into these masses Only regular insulin can be given IV; all can be given SQ				
Herbal interactions	Bee pollen, ginkgo biloba, glucosamine may increase blood glucose Basil, bay leaf, chromium, echinacea, garlic, ginseng may decrease blood glucose				

ANTIDIABETIC MEDICATIONS: ORAL		
MEDICATION	ADVERSE EFFECTS	NURSING CONSIDERATIONS
Sulfonylureas		
Glimepiride Glipizide Glyburide	GI symptoms and dermatologic reactions	Only used if some pancreas beta-cell function Stimulates release of insulin from pancreas Many medications can potentiate or interfere with actions Take with food if GI upset occurs
Biguanides		
Metformin	Nausea Diarrhea Abdominal discomfort	No effect on pancreatic beta cells; decreases glucose production by liver Not given if renal impairment Can cause lactic acidosis Avoid alcohol Do not give with alpha-glucodiase inhibitors
Alpha glucosidase inhibitors		
Acarbose Miglitol	Abdominal discomfort Diarrhea Flatulence	Delays digestion of carbohydrates Must be taken immediately before a meal Can be taken alone or with other agents
Thiazolidinediones		
Rosiglitazone Pioglitazone	Infection Headache Pain Rare cases of liver failure	Decreases insulin resistance and inhibits gluconeogenesis Regularly scheduled liver-function studies Can cause resumption of ovulation in perimenopause
Meglitinides		
Repaglinide	Hypoglycemia GI disturbances URIs Back pain Headache	Increases pancreatic insulin release Medication should not be taken if meal skipped
Gliptins		
Sitagliptin	Upper respiratory infections Hypoglycemia	Enhances action of incretin hormones
Incretin mimetics		
Exanatide	GI upset Hypoglycemia Pancreatitis	Interacts with many medications Administer 1 hour before meals
Indications	Type 2 diabetes	
Adverse effects	Hypoglycemia	

ANTIDIABETIC MEDICATIONS: ORAL *(CONTINUED)*		
MEDICATION	ADVERSE EFFECTS	NURSING CONSIDERATIONS
Nursing considerations	Monitor serum glucose levels Avoid alcohol Teaching for disease: dietary control, symptoms of hypoglycemia and hyperglycemia Good skin care	
Herbal interactions	Bee pollen, ginkgo biloba, glucosamine may increase blood glucose Basil, bay leaf, chromium, echinacea, garlic, ginseng may decrease blood glucose	

HYPOGLYCEMIA MEDICATIONS		
MEDICATION	ADVERSE EFFECTS	NURSING CONSIDERATIONS
Glucagon	Nausea, vomiting	Given SQ or IM, onset is 8–10 min with duration of 12–27 min Should be part of emergency supplies for diabetics May repeat in 15 min if needed
Action	Hormone produced by alpha cells of the pancreas to simulate the liver to change glycogen to glucose	
Indications	Acute management of severe hypoglycemia	
Adverse effects	Hypotension Bronchospasm Dizziness	
Nursing considerations	May repeat in 15 minutes if needed IV glucose must be given if client fails to respond Arouse clients from coma as quickly as possible and give carbohydrates orally to prevent secondary hypoglycemic reactions	

ANTIDIARRHEAL MEDICATIONS

MEDICATION	ADVERSE EFFECTS	NURSING CONSIDERATIONS
Bismuth subsalicylate	Darkening of stools and tongue Constipation	Give 2 hours before or 3 hours after other meds to prevent impaired absorption Encourage fluids Take after each loose stool until diarrhea controlled Notify health care provider if diarrhea not controlled in 48 hours Absorbs irritants and soothes intestinal muscle Do not administer for more than 2 days in presence of fever or in clients less than 3 years of age Monitor for salicylate toxicity Use cautiously if already taking aspirin Avoid use before x-rays (is radiopaque)
Diphenoxylate hydrochloride and atropine sulfate	Sedation Dizziness Tachycardia Dry mouth Paralytic ileus	Onset 45-60 min Monitor fluid and electrolytes Increases intestinal tone and decreases peristalsis May potentiate action of barbiturates, depressants
Loperamide	Drowsiness Constipation	Monitor children closely for CNS effects
Opium alkaloids	Narcotic dependence, nausea	Acts on smooth muscle to increase tone Administer with glass of water Discontinue as soon as stools are controlled
Action	Absorbs water, gas, toxins, irritants, and nutrients in bowel; slows peristalsis; increases tone of smooth muscles and sphincters	
Indications	Diarrhea	
Adverse effects	Constipation, fecal impaction Anticholinergic effects	
Nursing considerations	Not used with abdominal pain of unknown origin Monitor for urinary retention	

ANTIDYSRHYTHMIC MEDICATIONS		
MEDICATION	ADVERSE EFFECTS	NURSING CONSIDERATIONS
CLASS IA TYPE		
Quinidine Procainamide	Hypotension Heart failure	Monitor blood pressure Monitor for widening of the PR, QRS or QT intervals Toxic adverse effects have limited use
CLASS IB		
Lidocaine	CNS: slurred speech, confusion, drowsiness, confusion, seizures Hypotension and bradycardia	Monitor for CNS adverse effects Monitor BP and heart rate and cardiac rhythm
CLASS IC		
Flecainide Propafenone HCL	Bradycardia, Hypotension Dysrhythmias CNS: anxiety, insomnia, confusion, seizures	Monitor for increasing dysrhythmias Monitor heart rate and blood pressure Monitor for CNS effects
CLASS II		
Propanolol Esmolol hydrochloride Acebutolol	Bradycardia and hypotension Bronchospasm Increase in heart failure Fatigue and sleep disturbances	Monitor apical heart rate, cardiac rhythm and blood pressure Assess for shortness of breath and wheezing Assess for fatigue, sleep disturbances Assess apical heart rate for 1 minute before administration
CLASS III		
Amiodarone hydrochloride, Ibutilide fumarate	Hypotension Bradycardia and atrioventricular block Muscle weakness, tremors Photosensitivity and photophobia Liver toxicity	Continuous monitoring of cardiac rhythm during IV administration Monitor QT interval during IV administration Monitor heart rate, blood pressure during initiation of therapy Instruct client to wear sunglasses and sunscreen
CLASS IV		
Verapamil Diltiazem hydrochloride	Bradycardia Hypotension Dizziness and orthostatic hypotension Heart failure	Monitor apical heart rate and blood pressure Instruct clients about orthostatic precautions Instruct clients to report signs of heart failure to health care provider

ANTIEMETIC MEDICATIONS		
MEDICATION	**ADVERSE EFFECTS**	**NURSING CONSIDERATIONS**
Prochlorperazine dimaleate	Drowsiness Orthostatic hypotension Diplopia, photosensitivity	Check CBC and liver function with prolonged use Wear protective clothing when exposed to sunlight
Ondansetron	Headache, sedation Diarrhea, constipation Transient elevations in liver enzymes	New class of antiemetics—serotonin receptor antagonist Administer 30 min prior to chemotherapy
Metoclopramide	Restlessness, anxiety, drowsiness Extrapyramidal symptoms Dystonic reactions	Monitor BP Avoid activities requiring mental alertness Take before meals Used with tube feeding to decrease residual and risk of aspiration Administer 30 min prior to chemotherapy
Meclizine	Drowsiness, dry mouth Blurred vision Excitation, restlessness	Contraindicated with glaucoma Avoid activities requiring mental alertness
Dimenhydrinate	Drowsiness Palpitations, hypotension Blurred vision	Avoid activities requiring mental alertness
Promethazine	Drowsiness Dizziness Constipation Urinary retention Dry mouth	If used for motion sickness, take 1/2 to 1 hour before traveling; avoid activities requiring alertness; avoid alcohol, other CNS depressants Contraindicated in children less than 2 years old
Droperidol	Seizures Arrhythmias Hypotension Tachycardia	Often used either IV or IM in ambulatory care settings; observe for extrapyramidal symptoms (dystonia, extended neck, flexed arms, tremor, restlessness, hyperactivity, anxiety), which can be reversed with anticholinergics
Action	Blocks effect of dopamine in chemoreceptor trigger zone; increases GI motility	
Indications	Nausea and vomiting caused by surgery, chemotherapy, radiation sickness, uremia	
Adverse effects	Drowsiness, sedation Anticholinergic effects	
Nursing considerations	When used for viral infections may cause Reye's syndrome in clients less than 21 years old Phenothiazine medications are also used as antiemetics	
Herbals	Ginger—used to treat minor heartburn, nausea, vomiting; may increase risk of bleeding if taken with anticoagulants, antiplatelets, thrombolytic medication; instruct to stop medication if easily bruised or other signs of bleeding noted, report to health care provider; not approved for morning sickness during pregnancy	

ANTIFUNGAL MEDICATIONS		
MEDICATION	**ADVERSE EFFECTS**	**NURSING CONSIDERATIONS**
Amphotericin B	IV: nicknamed "amphoterrible" GI upset Hypokalemia-induced muscle pain CNS disturbances in vision, hearing Peripheral neuritis Seizures Hematological, renal, cardiac, hepatic abnormalities Skin irritation and thrombosis if IV infiltrates	Refrigerate medication and protect from sunlight Monitor vital signs; report febrile reaction or any change in function, especially nervous system dysfunction Check for hypokalemia Meticulous care and observation of injection site
Nystatin	Mild GI distress Hypersensitivity	Discontinue if redness, swelling, irritation occurs Instruct client in good oral, vaginal, skin hygiene
Fluconazole	Nausea, vomiting Diarrhea Elevated liver enzymes	Drug excreted unchanged by kidneys; dosage reduced if creatine clearance is altered due to renal failure Administer after hemodialysis
Ketoconazole	Headaches, vaginitis, nausea, flu-like symptoms (systemic use)	Reduce dosage hepatic disease Monitor CBC, LFTs, cultures Give tablet with food or milk
Action	Impairs cell membrane of fungus, causing increased permeability	
Indications	Systemic fungal infections (e.g., candidiasis, oral thrush, histoplasmosis)	
Adverse effects	Hepatotoxicity Thrombocytopenia Leukopenia Pruritus	
Nursing considerations	Administer with food to decrease GI upset Small, frequent meals Check hepatic function Teach client to take full course of medication, may be prescribed for prolonged period	

ANTIGOUT MEDICATIONS

MEDICATION	ADVERSE EFFECTS	NURSING CONSIDERATIONS
Colchicine	GI upset Agranulocytosis Peripheral neuritis	Anti-inflammatory Give with meals Check CBC, I and O For acute gout in combination with NSAIDs
Probenecid	Nausea, constipation Skin rash	For chronic gout Reduces uric acid Check BUN, renal function tests Encourage fluids Give with milk, food, antacids Alkaline urine helps prevent renal stones
Allopurinol	GI upset Headache, dizziness, drowsiness	Blocks formation of uric acid Encourage fluids Check I and O Check CBC and renal function tests Give with meals Alkaline urine helps prevent renal stones Avoid ASA because it inactivates drug
Action	Decreases production and reabsorption of uric acid	
Indications	Gout Uric acid stone formation	
Adverse effects	Aplastic anemia Agranulocytosis Renal calculi GI irritation	
Nursing considerations	Monitor for renal calculi	

ANTIHISTAMINE MEDICATIONS

MEDICATION	ADVERSE EFFECTS	NURSING CONSIDERATIONS
Chlorpheniramine maleate	Drowsiness, dry mouth	Most effective if taken before onset of symptoms
Diphenhydramine HCl	Drowsiness Nausea, dry mouth Photosensitivity	Don't combine with alcoholic beverages Give with food Use sunscreen Older adults: greater risk of confusion and sedation
Promethazine HCl	Agranulocytosis Drowsiness, dry mouth Photosensitivity	Give with food Use sunscreen

ANTIHISTAMINE MEDICATIONS *(CONTINUED)*		
MEDICATION	ADVERSE EFFECTS	NURSING CONSIDERATIONS
Loratadine Cetirizine Fexofenadine	Drowsiness	Reduce dose or give every other day for clients with renal or hepatic dysfunction
Action	Blocks the effects of histamine at peripheral H1 receptor sites; anticholinergic, antipruritic effects	
Indications	Allergic rhinitis Allergic reactions Chronic idiopathic urticaria	
Adverse effects	Depression Dry mouth Nightmares GI upset Sedation Bronchospasm Alopecia	
Nursing considerations	Administer with food Good mouth care, sugarless lozenges for dry mouth Good skin care Use caution when performing tasks requiring alertness (e.g., driving car) Avoid alcohol	

ANTI-INFECTIVE MEDICATIONS: AMINOGLYCOSIDES	
Examples	Gentamicin Neomycin Tobramycin Amikacin
Actions	Bacteriocidal Inhibits protein synthesis of many Gram-negative bacteria
Indications	Treatment of severe systemic infections of CNS, respiratory, GI, urinary tract, bone, skin, soft tissues, acute pelvic inflammatory disease (PID), tuberculosis (streptomycin)
Adverse effects	Ototoxicity, Nephrotoxicity Anorexia, nausea, vomiting, diarrhea
Nursing considerations	Check eighth cranial nerve function (hearing) Check renal function (BUN, creatinine) Usually prescribed for 7–10 days Encourage fluids Small, frequent meals

ANTI-INFECTIVE MEDICATIONS: CEPHALOSPORINS	

Examples	Multiple preparations:
	  1st generation example: cephalexin
	  2nd generation example: cefoxitin sodium
	  3rd generation example: ceftriaxone sodium
	  4th generation example: cefepime HCL
	  5th generation example: ceftaroline fosamil

Actions	Bacteriocidal Inhibits synthesis of bacterial cell wall
Indications	Pharyngitis Tonsillitis Otitis media Upper and lower respiratory tract infections Dermatological infections Gonorrhea Septicemia Meningitis Perioperative prophylaxis Urinary tract infections
Adverse effects	Abdominal pain, nausea, vomiting, diarrhea Increased risk bleeding Hypoprothrombinemia Rash Superinfections Thrombophlebitis (IV), abscess formation (IM, IV)
Nursing considerations	Take with food Administer liquid form to children, don't crush tablets Have vitamin K available for hypoprothrombinemia Avoid alcohol while taking medication and for 3 days after finishing course of medication **Cross allergy with penicillins (cephalosporins should not be given to clients with a severe penicillin allergy)** Monitor renal and hepatic function Monitor for Thrombophlebitis

ANTI-INFECTIVE MEDICATIONS: FLUOROQUINOLONES	
Examples	Ciprofloxacin, Levofloxacin
Actions	Broad-spectrum bactericidal; interferes with DNA replication in Gram-negative bacteria
Indications	Treatment of infection caused *by E.coli* and other bacteria, chronic bacterial prostatitis, acute sinusitis, postexposure inhalation anthrax
Adverse effects	Headache Nausea Diarrhea Elevated BUN, AST , ALT, serum creatinine, alkaline phosphatase Decreased WBC and hematocrit Rash Photosensitivity Achilles tendon rupture
Nursing considerations	Culture and sensitivity before starting therapy Take 1 hour before or 2 hours after meals with glass of water Encourage fluids If needed administer antacids 2 hours after medication Take full course of therapy WARNING: Fluoroquinolones can lead to hypoglycemia and possibly hypoglycemic coma, as well as acute psychososis (e.g., agitation, delirium, disorientation, disturbance in attention, memory impairment, and nervousness).

ANTI-INFECTIVE MEDICATIONS: LINCOSAMIDES	
Examples	Clindamycin HCl Phosphate
Action	Both bacteriostatic and bactericidal, it suppresses protein synthesis by preventing peptide bond formation
Indications	Staph, strep, and other infections
Adverse effects	Diarrhea Rash Liver toxicity
Nursing considerations	Administer oral med with a full glass of water to prevent esophageal ulcers Monitor for persistent vomiting, diarrhea, fever, or abdominal pain and cramping, superinfections

ANTI-INFECTIVE MEDICATIONS: MACROLIDES	
Examples	Erythromycin Azithromycin
Actions	Bacteriostatic; bactericidal; binds to cell membrane and causes changes in protein function
Indications	Acute infections Acne and skin infections Upper respiratory tract infections Prophylaxis before dental procedures for clients allergic to PCN with valvular heart disease
Adverse effects	Abdominal cramps, diarrhea Confusion, uncontrollable emotions Hepatotoxicity Superinfections
Nursing considerations	Take oral med 1 hour before or 2–3 hours after meals with full glass of water Take around the clock to maximize effectiveness Monitor liver function Take full course of therapy

ANTI-INFECTIVE MEDICATIONS: PENICILLINS	
Examples	Amoxicillin Ampicillin Methicillin Nafcillin Penicillin G Penicillin V
Actions	Bactericidal; inhibit synthesis of cell wall of sensitive organisms
Indications	Effective against Gram-positive organisms Moderate to severe infections Syphilis Gonococcal infections Lyme disease
Adverse effects	Glossitis, stomatitis Gastritis Diarrhea Superinfections Hypersensitivity reactions
Nursing considerations	Culture and sensitivity before treatment Monitor serum electrolytes and cardiac status if given IV Monitor and rotate injection sites Good mouth care Yogurt or buttermilk if diarrhea develops Instruct client to take missed medications as soon as possible; do not double dose

ANTI-INFECTIVE MEDICATIONS: SULFONAMIDES	
Examples	Sulfasalazine Trimethoprim/Sulfamethoxazole
Actions	Bacteriostatic; competitively antagonize paraminobenzoic acid, essential component of folic acid synthesis, causing cell death
Indications	Ulcerative colitis, Crohn's disease Otitis media Conjunctivitis Meningitis Toxoplasmosis UTIs Rheumatoid arthritis
Adverse effects	Peripheral neuropathy Crystalluria, proteinuria Photosensitivity GI upset Stomatitis Hypersensitivity reactions
Nursing considerations	Culture and sensitivity before therapy Take with a full glass of water Take around the clock Encourage fluid intake (8 glasses of water/day) Protect from exposure to light (sunscreen, protective clothing) Good mouth care

ANTI-INFECTIVE MEDICATIONS: TETRACYCLINES	
Examples	Doxycycline Minocycline Tetracycline HCl
Actions	Bacteriostatic; inhibits protein synthesis of susceptible bacteria
Indications	. Treatment of syphilis, chlamydia, gonorrhea, malaria prophylaxis, chronic periodontitis, acne; treatment of anthrax (doxycycline); as part of combination therapy to eliminate *H. pylori* infections; drug of choice for stage 1 Lyme disease (tetracycline HCl)

ANTI-INFECTIVE MEDICATIONS: TETRACYCLINES *(CONTINUED)*	
Adverse effects	Discoloration and inadequate calcification of primary teeth of fetus if taken during pregnancy Glossitis Dysphagia Diarrhea Phototoxic reactions Rash Superinfections
Nursing considerations	Take 1 hour before or 2–3 hours after meals Do not take with antacids, milk, iron preparations (give 3 hours after medication) Note expiration date (becomes highly nephrotoxic) Protect from sunlight Monitor renal function Topical applications may stain clothing Use contraceptive method in addition to oral contraceptives

ANTI-INFECTIVE MEDICATIONS: VANCOMYCIN	
Examples	Vancomycin
Action	Bacteriocidal Binds to bacterial cell wall, stopping its synthesis
Indications	Treatment of resistant staph infections, pseudomembranous enterocolitis due to *C. difficile* infection
Adverse effects	Thrombophlebitis Abscess formation Nephrotoxicity Ototoxicity
Nursing considerations	Monitor renal function and hearing Poor absorption orally; administer IV: peak 5 minutes, duration 12–24 hours Avoid extravasation during therapy; it may cause necrosis Give antihistamine if "red man syndrome": decreased blood pressure, flushing of face and neck Contact health care provider if signs of superinfection: sore throat, fever, fatigue

ANTI-INFECTIVE MEDICATIONS: OVERVIEW		
MEDICATION	ADVERSE EFFECTS	NURSING CONSIDERATIONS
Penicillins		
Ampicillin Penicillin G potassium Penicillin G sodium	Skin rashes, diarrhea Allergic reactions Renal, hepatic, hematological abnormalities Nausea, vomiting	Obtain C and S before first dose Take careful history of penicillin reaction Observe for 20 minutes post IM injection Give 1–2 hours ac or 2–3 hours pc to reduce gastric acid destruction of drug Monitor for loose, foul-smelling stool and change in tongue Teach to continue medication for entire time prescribed, even if symptoms resolve Check for hypersensitivity to other medications, especially cephalosporins
Sulfonamides		
Sulfasalazine	Nausea, vomiting Skin eruption Agranulocytosis	Advise client to avoid exposure to sunlight Maintain fluid intake at 3,000 mL/day to avoid crystal formation
Trimethoprim/ Sulfamethoxazole	Hypersensitivity reaction Blood dyscrasias Rash	Obtain C and S before first dose IV solution must be given slowly over 60-90 minutes Never administer IM Encourage fluids to 3,000 mL/day
Tetracylines	Photosensitivity GI upset, renal, hepatic, hematological abnormalities Dental discoloration of deciduous ("baby") teeth, enamel hypoplasia	Give between meals If GI symptoms occur, administer with food EXCEPT milk products or other foods high in calcium (interferes with absorption) Assess for change in bowel habits, perineal rash, black "hairy" tongue Good oral hygiene Avoid during tooth and early development periods (fourth month prenatal to 8 years of age) Monitor I and O Caution client to avoid sun exposure Decomposes to toxic substance with age and exposure to light
Doxycycline	Photosensitivity	Check client's tongue for *Monilia* infection
Aminogylcosides	Ototoxicity cranial nerve VIII Nephrotoxicity	Check creatinine and BUN Check peak–2 hours after med given Check trough–at time of dose/prior to med Monitor for symptoms of bacterial overgrowth, photosensitivity Teach to immediately report tinnitus, vertigo, nystagmus, ataxia Monitor I and O Audiograms if given long-term
Neomycin sulfate	Hypersensitivity reactions	Ophthalmic–remove infective exudate around eyes before administration of ointment

ANTI-INFECTIVE MEDICATIONS: OVERVIEW *(CONTINUED)*		
MEDICATION	**ADVERSE EFFECTS**	**NURSING CONSIDERATIONS**
Fluoroquinolones		
Ciprofloxacin	Seizures GI upset Rash	Contraindicated in children less than 18 years of age Give 2 hours pc or 2 hours before an antacid or iron preparation Avoid caffeine Encourage fluids
Macrolides		
Azithromycin Erythromycin	Pain at injection site Nausea, diarrhea	Can be used in clients with compromised renal function because excretion is primarily through the bile
Cephalosporins		

1st generation example:
  Cephalexin
 	
2nd generation example:
  Cefoxitin sodium
 	
3rd generation example:
  Ceftriaxone sodium
 	
4th generation example:
  Cefepime HCL
 	
5th generation example:
  Ceftaroline fosamil
	Diarrhea, nausea
	Dizziness, abdominal pain
	Eosinophilia, superinfections
	Allergic reactions
		Can cause false-positive Coombs' test (which will complicate transfusion cross-matching procedure)
		Cross-sensitivity with penicillins
		Take careful history of penicillin reactions

Glycopeptides		
Vancomycin	Liver damage	Poor absorption orally, but IV peak 5 minutes, duration 12–24 hours Avoid extravasation during therapy—may cause necrosis Give antihistamine if "red man syndrome": decreased blood pressure, flushing of face and neck Contact health care provider if signs of superinfection: sore throat, fever, fatigue
Lincosamides		
Clindamycin HCl phosphate	Nausea Vaginitis Colitis may occur 2–9 days or several weeks after starting meds	Administer oral med with a full glass of water to prevent esophageal ulcers Monitor for persistent vomiting, diarrhea, fever, or abdominal pain and cramping

ANTI-INFECTIVE MEDICATIONS: TOPICAL		
MEDICATION	**ADVERSE EFFECTS**	**NURSING CONSIDERATIONS**
Bacitracin ointment	Nephrotoxicity Ototoxicity	Overgrowth of nonsusceptible organisms can occur
Neosporin cream	Nephrotoxicity Ototoxicity	Allergic dermatitis may occur
Povidone-iodine solution	Irritation	Don't use around eyes May stain skin Don't use full-strength on mucous membranes

ANTI-INFECTIVE MEDICATIONS: TOPICAL *(CONTINUED)*		
MEDICATION	ADVERSE EFFECTS	NURSING CONSIDERATIONS
Silver sulfadiazine cream	Neutropenia Burning	Use cautiously if sensitive to sulfonamides
Tolnaftate cream	Irritation	Use small amount of medication Use medication for duration prescribed
Nystatin cream	Contact dermatitis	Do not use occlusive dressings

ANTIHYPERTENSIVE MEDICATIONS: ANGIOTENSIN II RECEPTOR BLOCKER	
Examples	Candesartan Eprosartan Irbesartan Losartan
Indications	Hypertension Heart failure Diabetic nephropathy Myocardial infarction Stroke prevention
Adverse effects	Angioedema Renal failure Orthostatic hypotension
Nursing considerations	Instruct client about position changes Monitor for edema Instruct client to notify health care provider if edema occurs

ANTIHYPERTENSIVE MEDICATIONS: ANGIOTENSIN-CONVERTING ENZYME (ACE) INHIBITOR	
Examples	Captopril Enalapril Lisinopril Benazepril Fosinopril Quinapril Ramipril
Actions	Blocks ACE in lungs from converting angiotensin I to angiotensin II (powerful vasoconstrictor); causes decreased BP, decreased aldosterone secretion, sodium and fluid loss
Indications	Hypertension CHF

ANTIHYPERTENSIVE MEDICATIONS: ANGIOTENSIN-CONVERTING ENZYME (ACE) INHIBITOR (CONTINUED)

Adverse effects	Gastric irritation, peptic ulcer, orthostatic hypotension
	Tachycardia
	Myocardial infarction
	Proteinuria
	Rash, pruritis
	Persistent dry nonproductive cough
	Peripheral edema
Nursing considerations	Decreased absorption if taken with food—give 1 hour ac or 2 hours pc
	Small, frequent meals
	Frequent mouth care
	Change position slowly
	Can be used with thiazide diuretics

ANTIHYPERTENSIVE MEDICATIONS: ALPHA-1 ADRENERGIC BLOCKER

Examples	Doxazosin
	Prazosin
	Terazosin
Actions	Selective blockade of alpha-1 adrenergic receptors in peripheral blood vessels
Indications	Hypertension
	Benign prostatic hyperplasia
	Pheochromocytoma
	Raynaud's disease
Adverse effects	Orthostatic hypotension
	Reflex tachycardia
	Nasal congestion
	Impotence
Nursing considerations	Administer first dose at bedtime to avoid fainting
	Change positions slowly to prevent orthostatic hypotension
	Monitor BP, weight, BUN/creatinine, edema

ANTIHYPERTENSIVE MEDICATIONS: BETA-ADRENERGIC BLOCKER

Examples	Atenolol
	Nadolol
	Propranolol
	Metoprolol
	Acebutolol
	Carvedilol
	Pindolol
Actions	Blocks beta-adrenergic receptors in heart; decreases excitability of heart; reduces cardiac workload and oxygen consumption; decreases release of renin; lowers blood pressure by reducing CNS stimuli

ANTIHYPERTENSIVE MEDICATIONS: BETA-ADRENERGIC BLOCKER *(CONTINUED)*	
Indications	Hypertension (used with diuretics)
	Angina
	Supraventricular tachycardia
	Prevent recurrent MI
	Migraine headache (propranolol)
	Stage fright (propranolol)
	Heart failure
Adverse effects	Gastric pain
	Bradycardia/tachycardia
	Acute severe heart failure
	Cardiac dysrhythmias
	Impotence
	Decreased exercise tolerance
	Nightmares, depression
	Dizziness
	Bronchospasm (nonselective beta blockers)
Nursing considerations	Do not discontinue abruptly, taper gradually over 2 weeks
	Take with meals
	Provide rest periods
	For diabetic clients, blocks normal signs of hypoglycemia (sweating, tachycardia); monitor blood glucose
	Medications have antianginal and antiarrhythmic actions

ANTIHYPERTENSIVE MEDICATION: CALCIUM CHANNEL BLOCKER	
Examples	Nifedipine
	Verapamil
	Diltiazem
	Amlodipine
	Felodipine
Actions	Inhibits movement of calcium ions across membrane of cardiac and arterial muscle cells; results in slowed impulse conduction, depression of myocardial contractility, dilation of coronary arteries; decreases cardiac workload and energy consumption, increases oxygenation of myocardial cells
Indications	Angina
	Hypertension
	Dysrhythmias
	Interstitial cystitis
	Migraines

ANTIHYPERTENSIVE MEDICATION: CALCIUM CHANNEL BLOCKER *(CONTINUED)*	
Adverse effects	Dizziness
	Headache
	Nervousness
	Peripheral edema
	Angina
	Bradycardia
	AV block
	Flushing, rash
	Impotence
Nursing considerations	Monitor vital signs
	Do not chew or divide sustained-release tablets
	Medications also have antianginal actions
	Contraindicated in heart block
	Contact health care provider if blood pressure less than 90/60
	Instruct client to avoid grapefruit juice
	Monitor for signs of heart failure

HYPERTENSIVE MEDICATIONS: CENTRALLY ACTING ALPHA–ADRENERGIC	
Examples	Clonidine
	Methyldopa
Actions	Stimulates alpha receptors in medulla, causing reduction in sympathetic action in heart; decreases rate and force of contraction, decreasing cardiac output
Indications	Hypertension
Adverse effects	Drowsiness, sedation
	Orthostatic hypotension
	CHF
Nursing considerations	Don't discontinue abruptly
	Monitor for fluid retention
	Older adults: potential for orthostatic hypotension and CNS adverse effects

HYPERTENSIVE MEDICATIONS: DIRECT-ACTING VASODILATOR	
Examples	Hydralazine
	Minoxidil
Actions	Relaxes smooth muscle of blood vessels, lowering peripheral resistance
Indications	Hypertension
Adverse effects	Same as centrally acting alpha adrenergics
Nursing consideratons	Same as centrally acting alpha adrenergics

ANTIHYPERTENSIVE MEDICATIONS: OVERVIEW		
MEDICATION	ADVERSE EFFECTS	NURSING CONSIDERATIONS
Methyldopa	Drowsiness, dizziness, bradycardia, hemolytic anemia, fever, orthostatic hypotension	Monitor CBC Monitor liver function Take at bedtime to minimize daytime drowsiness Change position slowly
Clonidine	Drowsiness, dizziness Dry mouth, headache Dermatitis Severe rebound hypertension	**Don't discontinue abruptly** Apply patch to nonhairy area (upper outer arm, anterior chest)
Atenolol	Bradycardia Hypotension Bronchospasm	Once-a-day dose increases compliance Check apical pulse; if less than 60 bpm hold drug and call health care provider **Don't discontinue abruptly** Masks signs of shock and hypoglycemia
Metoprolol	Bradycardia, hypotension, heart failure, depression	Give with meals Teach client to check pulse before each dose; take apical pulse before administration Withhold if pulse less than 60 bpm
Nadolol	Bradycardia, hypotension, heart failure	Teach client to check pulse before each dose; check apical pulse before administering Withhold if pulse less than 60 bpm **Don't discontinue abruptly**
Hydralazine	Headache, palpitations, edema, tachycardia, lupus erythematosus-like syndrome	Give with meals Observe mental status Check for weight gain, edema
Minoxidil	Tachycardia, angina pectoris, edema, increase in body hair	Teach client to check pulse; check apical pulse before administration Monitor I and O, weight
Captopril Enalapril Lisinopril	Dizziness Orthostatic hypotension	Report swelling of face, lightheadedness ACE-inhibitor medication
Propranolol	Weakness Hypotension Bronchospasm Bradycardia Depression	Beta blocker: blocks sympathetic impulses to heart Client takes pulse at home before each dose **Dosage should be reduced gradually before discontinued**
Nifedipine Verapamil Diltiazem	Hypotension Dizziness GI distress Liver dysfunction Jitteriness	Calcium-channel blocker: reduces workload of left ventricle Coronary vasodilator; monitor blood pressure during dosage adjustments Assist with ambulation at start of therapy Avoid grapefruit juice
Herbal interaction	Ma-huang (ephedra) decreases effect of antihypertensive medications Ephedra increases hypertension when taken with beta blockers Black cohosh increases hypotensive effects of antihypertensives Goldenseal counteracts effects of antihypertensives	

ANTILIPEMIC MEDICATIONS

MEDICATION	ADVERSE EFFECTS	NURSING CONSIDERATIONS
Bile acid sequestrants		
Cholestyramine Colestipol Nicotinic acid	Constipation Rash Fat-soluble vitamin deficiency Abdominal pain and bloating	Increases loss of bile acid in feces; decreases cholesterol Sprinkle powder on noncarbonated beverage or wet food, let stand 2 min, then stir slowly Administer 1 hour before or 4–6 hours after other meds to avoid blocking absorption Instruct client to report constipation immediately
HMG-CoA reductase inhibitors (statins)		
Lovostatin Pravastatin Simvastatin Atorvastatin Fluvastatin Rosuvastatin	Myopathy Increased liver enzyme levels	Decreases LDL cholesterol levels; causes peripheral vasodilation Take with food; absorption is reduced by 30% on an empty stomach; avoid alcohol Contact health care provider if unexplained muscle pain, especially with fever or malaise Take at night Give with caution with ↓ liver function Avoid grapefruit juice
Nicotinic acid		
Niacin	Flushing Hyperglycemia Gout Upper GI distress Liver damage	Decreases total cholesterol, LDL, triglycerides, increases HDL Flushing will occur several hours after med is taken, will decrease over 2 wk Also used for pellagra and peripheral vascular disease Avoid alcohol

Folic acid derivatives
  Fenofibrate
  Gemfibrozil
	Abdominal pain
	Increased risk gallbladder disease
	Myalgia and swollen joints
		Decreases total cholesterol, VLDL, and triglycerides
		Administer before meals
		Instruct clients to notify health care provider if muscle pain occurs

Action	Inhibits cholesterol and triglyceride synthesis; decreases serum cholesterol and LDLs	
Indications	Elevated total and LDL cholesterol Primary hypercholesterolemia Reduce incidence of cardiovascular disease	
Adverse effects	Varies with medication	

ANTILIPEMIC MEDICATIONS (CONTINUED)

MEDICATION	ADVERSE EFFECTS	NURSING CONSIDERATIONS
Nursing considerations	Medication should be used with dietary measures, physical activity, and cessation of tobacco use Lipids should be monitored every 6 wk until normal, then every 4–6 months	
Herbals used to lower cholesterol	Flax or flax seed—decreases the absorption of other medications Garlic—increases the effects of anticoagulants; increases the hypoglycemic effects of insulin Green tea—produces a stimulant effect with the tea contains caffeine Soy	

ANTINEOPLASTIC MEDICATIONS: ANTIMETABOLITES

Examples	Fluorouracil Mercaptopurine Methotrexate
Actions	Closely resembles normal metabolites, "counterfeits" fool cells; cell division halteda
Indications	Acute lymphatic leukemia Rheumatoid arthritis Psoriasis Cancer of colon, breast, stomach, pancreas Sickle cell anemia
Adverse effects	Nausea, vomiting Diarrhea Stomatitis and oral ulceration Hepatic dysfunction Bone marrow suppression Renal dysfunction Alopecia
Nursing considerations	Monitor hematopoietic function Good mouth care Small frequent feedings Counsel about body image changes (alopecia); provide wig Good skin care Photosensitivity precautions Infection control precautions

ANTINEOPLASTIC: ANTIBIOTICS

Examples	Dactinomycin Doxorubicin
Actions	Interferes with DNA and RNA synthesis

ANTINEOPLASTIC: ANTIBIOTICS *(CONTINUED)*	
Indications	Hodgkin's disease Non-Hodgkin's lymphoma Leukemia Many cancers
Adverse effects	Bone marrow depression Nausea, vomiting Alopecia Stomatitis Heart damage Septic shock
Nursing considerations	Monitor closely for septicemic reactions Monitor for manifestations of extravasation at injection site (severe pain or burning that lasts minutes to hours, redness after injection is completed, ulceration after 48 hours) Instruct client urine and tears may be red in color Monitor for signs of heart failure

ANTINEOPLASTIC MEDICATIONS: CYTOXIC AGENTS	
Examples	Busulfan Chlorambucil Cisplatin platinol-AQ Cyclophosphamide
Actions	Interferes with rapidly reproducing cell DNA
Indications	Leukemia Multiple myeloma
Adverse effects	Bone marrow suppression Nausea, vomiting Stomatitis Alopecia Gonadal suppression Renal toxicity (cisplatin) Ototoxicity
Nursing considerations	Used with other chemotherapeutic agents Check hematopoietic function weekly Encourage fluids (10-12 glasses/day)

ANTINEOPLASTICS MEDICATION: HORMONAL

Examples	Antiestrogens: Tamoxifen Aromatase Inhibitors: Anastrozole, Letrozole, Exemestane Gonadotropin-Releasing Hormone Agonist: Leuprolide Gonadotropin-Releasing Hormone Antagonists: Degarelix
Actions	Tamoxifen–antiestrogen (competes with estrogen to bind at estrogen receptor sites on malignant cells) Leuprolide–progestin (causes tumor cell regression by unknown mechanism) Testolactone–androgen (used for palliation in advanced breast cancer)
Indications	Breast cancer
Adverse effects	Hypercalcemia Jaundice Increased appetite Masculinization or feminization Sodium and fluid retention Nausea, vomiting Hot flashes Vaginal dryness
Nursing considerations	Baseline and periodic gyn exams recommended Not given IV Discuss pregnancy prevention

ANTINEOPLASTIC MEDICATIONS: TOPOISOMERASE

Examples	Irinotecan Topotecan
Actions	Binds to enzyme that breaks the DNA strands
Indications	Ovary, lung, colon, and rectal cancers
Adverse effects	Bone marrow suppression Diarrhea Nausea, vomiting Hepatotoxicity

ANTINEOPLASTIC MEDICATIONS: VINCA ALKALOIDS	
Examples	Vinblastine
	Vincristine
Actions	Interferes with cell division
Indications	Hodgkin's disease
	Lymphoma
	Cancers
Adverse effects	Bone marrow suppression (mild with VCR)
	Neuropathies (VCR)
	Stomatitis
Nursing considerations	Same as antitumor antibiotics

ANTINEOPLASTIC MEDICATIONS: OVERVIEW (ALSO SEE EACH INDIVIDUAL TABLE)		
MEDICATION	ADVERSE EFFECTS	NURSING CONSIDERATIONS
Alkylating Medications		
Busulfan	Bone marrow depression	Check CBC (applies to all medications in this table) Most chemotherapy causes stomatitis and requires extra fluids to flush system
Chlorambucil	Nausea, vomiting, bone marrow depression, sterility	Monitor for infection Avoid IM injections when platelet count is low to minimize bleeding
Cyclophosphamide	Alopecia, bone marrow depression, hemorrhagic cystitis, dermatitis, hyperkalemia, hypoglycemia, amenorrhea	Report hematuria, force fluids Monitor for infection Give antiemetics
Antimetabolites		
Fluorouracil	Nausea, stomatitis, GI ulceration, diarrhea, bone marrow depression, liver dysfunction, alopecia	Monitor for infection Avoid extravasation
Methotrexate	Oral and GI ulceration, liver damage, bone marrow depression, stomatitis, alopecia, bloody diarrhea, fatigue	Good mouth care, avoid alcohol Monitor hepatic and renal function tests
Mercaptopurine	Liver damage, bone marrow depression, infection, alopecia, abdominal bleeding	Check liver function tests
Cytarabine	Hematologic abnormalities, nausea, vomiting, rash, weight loss	Force fluids Good oral hygiene
Hydroxyurea	Bone marrow depression, GI symptoms, rash	Teach client to report toxic GI symptoms promptly
Antibiotic Antineoplastics		
Doxorubicin	Red urine, nausea, vomiting, stomatitis, alopecia, cardiotoxicity, blisters, bone marrow depression	Check EKG, avoid IV infiltration Monitor vital signs closely Good mouth care
Bleomycin	Nausea, vomiting, alopecia, edema of hands, pulmonary fibrosis, fever, bone marrow depression	Observe for pulmonary complications, treat fever with acetaminophen Check breath sounds frequently
Dactinomycin	Nausea, bone marrow depression	Give antiemetic before administration
Vinca Alkaloids		
Vinblastine	Nausea, vomiting, stomatitis, alopecia, loss of reflexes, bone marrow depression	Avoid IV infiltration and extravasation Give antiemetic before administration Acute bronchospasm can occur if given IV Allopurinol given to increase excretion and decrease buildup of urates (uric acid)
Vincristine	Peripheral neuritis, loss of reflexes, bone marrow depression, alopecia, GI symptoms	Avoid IV infiltration and extravasation Check reflexes, motor and sensory function Allopurinol given to increase excretion and decrease buildup of urates (uric acid)
Hormonal Medications		
Tamoxifen	Transient fall in WBC or platelets Hypercalcemia, bone pain	Check CBC Monitor serum calcium Nonsteroidal antiestrogen

ANTINEOPLASTIC MEDICATIONS: NURSING IMPLICATIONS FOR ADVERSE EFFECTS	
Bone marrow suppression	Monitor bleeding: bleeding gums, bruising, petechiae, guaiac stools, urine and emesis Avoid IM injections and rectal temperatures Apply pressure to venipuncture sites
Nausea, vomiting	Monitor intake and output ratios, appetite and nutritional intake Prophylactic antiemetics may be used Smaller, more frequent meals
Altered immunologic response	Prevent infection by handwashing Timely reporting of alterations in vital signs or symptoms indicating possible infection
Impaired oral mucous membrane; stomatitis	Oral hygiene measures
Fatigue	Encourage rest and discuss measures to conserve energy Use relaxation techniques, mental imagery

ANTIPARKINSON MEDICATIONS		
MEDICATION	**ADVERSE EFFECTS**	**NURSING CONSIDERATIONS**
Trihexyphenidyl	Dry mouth Blurred vision Constipation, urinary hesitancy Decreased mental acuity, difficulty concentrating, confusion, hallucination	Acts by blocking acetylcholine at cerebral synaptic sites Intraocular pressure should be monitored Supervise ambulation Causes nausea if given before meals Suck on hard candy for dry mouth
Benztropine mesylate	Drowsiness, nausea, vomiting Atropine-like effects—blurred vision, mydriasis Antihistaminic effects—sedation, dizziness	Acts by lessening cholinergic effect of dopamine deficiency Suppresses tremor of Parkinsonism Most adverse effects are reversed by changes in dosage Additional drowsiness can occur with other CNS depressants
Levodopa	Nausea and vomiting, anorexia Postural hypotension Mental changes: confusion, agitation, mood alterations Cardiac arrhythmias Twitching	Precursor of dopamine Thought to restore dopamine levels in extrapyramidal centers Administered in large prolonged doses Contraindicated in glaucoma, hemolytic anemia Give with food Monitor for postural hypotension Avoid OTC meds and foods that contain vitamin B_6 (pyridoxine); reverses effects
Bromocriptine mesylate Pergolide	Dizziness, headache, hypotension Tinnitus Nausea, abdominal cramps Pleural effusion Orthostatic hypotension	Give with meals May lead to early postpartum conception Monitor cardiac, hepatic, renal, hematopoietic function

ANTIPARKINSON MEDICATIONS *(CONTINUED)*		
MEDICATION	**ADVERSE EFFECTS**	**NURSING CONSIDERATIONS**
Carbidopa–Levodopa	Hemolytic anemia Dystonic movements, ataxia Orthostatic hypotension Dysrhythmias GI upset, dry mouth	Stimulates dopamine receptors Don't use with MAO inhibitors Advise to change positions slowly Take with food
Amantadine	CNS disturbances, hyperexcitability Insomnia, vertigo, ataxia Slurred speech, convulsions	Enhances effect of L-Dopa Contraindicated in epilepsy, arteriosclerosis Antiviral
Action	Levodopa–precursor to dopamine that is converted to dopamine in the brain Bromocriptine–stimulates postsynaptic dopamine receptors	
Indications	Parkinson's disease	
Adverse effects	Dizziness Ataxia Confusion Psychosis Hemolytic anemia	
Nursing considerations	Monitor for urinary retention Large doses of pyridoxine (vitamin B_6) decrease or reverse effects of medication Avoid use of other CNS depressants (alcohol, narcotics, sedatives) Anticholinergics, dopamine agonists, MAO inhibitors, catechol-*O*-methyltransferase (COMT) inhibitors, and antidepressants may also be used	

ANTIPLATELET MEDICATIONS		
MEDICATION	**ADVERSE EFFECTS**	**NURSING CONSIDERATIONS**
Adenosine diphosphate (ADP) receptor antagonists Ticlopidine Clopidrogel	Thrombocytopenic purpura GI upset	Prevents platelet aggregation Higher risk of hemorrhage with ticlopidine
Dipyridamole Dipyridamole plus aspirin	Headache Dizziness EKG changes Hypertension, hypotension	Administer 1 hour ac or with meals Monitor BP Check for signs of bleeding
Glycoprotein IIb and IIIa receptor antagonists Eptifibatide Abciximab	GI, retroperitoneal, and urogenital bleeding	Does not increase risk of fatal hemorrhage or hemorrhagic stroke
Salicylates	Short-term use—GI bleeding, heartburn, occasional nausea Prolonged high dosage—salicylism: metabolic acidosis, respiratory alkalosis, dehydration, fluid and electrolyte imbalance, tinnitus	Observe for bleeding gums, bloody or black stools, bruises Give with milk, water, or food, or use enteric-coated tablets to minimize gastric distress Contraindications—GI disorders, severe anemia, vitamin K deficiency Anti-inflammatory, analgesic, antipyretic
Action	Interferes with platelet aggregation	
Indications	Venous thrombosis Pulmonary embolism CVA and acute coronary prevention Postcardiac surgery; postpercutaneous coronary interventions Acute coronary syndrome	
Adverse effects	Hemorrhage, bleeding Thrombocytopenia Hematuria Hemoptysis	
Nursing considerations	Teach client to check for signs of bleeding Inform health care provider or dentist before procedures Older adults at higher risk for ototoxicity Instruct client to contact health care provider before taking any over-the-counter medications Instruct client to avoid gingko, garlic and ginger herbal preparations	
Gerontologic considerations	Dipyridamole causes orthostatic hypotention in older adults Ticlopidine—greater risk of toxicity with older adults	

ANTIPSYCHOTIC MEDICATIONS		
MEDICATION	ADVERSE EFFECTS	NURSING CONSIDERATIONS
Conventional high potency		
Haloperidol Fluphenazine	Low sedative effect Low incidence of hypotension High incidence of extrapyramidal adverse effects	Used in large doses for assaultive clients Used with elderly (risk of falling reduced) Decanoate: long-acting form given every 2–4 wk; IM into deep muscle Z-track
Conventional medium potency		
Perphenazine	Orthostatic hypotension Dry mouth Constipation	Can help control severe vomiting Medication is available PO, IM, and IV
Conventional low potency		
Chlorpromazine	High sedative effect High incidence of hypotension Irreversible retinitis pigmentosus at 800 mg/day	Educate client about increased sensitivity to sun (as with other phenothiazines) No tolerance or potential for abuse
Atypical		
Risperidone	Moderate orthostatic hypotension Moderate sedation Significant weight gain Doses over 6 mg can cause tardive dyskinesia	Chosen as first-line antipsychotic due to mild EPS and very low anticholinergic adverse effects
Quetiapine	Moderate orthostatic hypotension Moderate sedation Very low risk of tardive dyskinesia and neuroleptic malignant syndrome	Chosen as first-line antipsychotic due to mild EPS and very low anticholinergic adverse effects
Ziprasidone Aripiprazole Clozapine Olanzapine	ECG changes—QT prolongation	Effective with depressive symptoms of schizophrenia Low propensity for weight gain
Action	Blocks dopamine receptors in basal ganglia of brain, inhibiting transmission of nerve impulses	
Indications	Acute and chronic psychosis	
Adverse effects	Akathisia (motor restlessness) Dyskinesia (abnormal voluntary movements) Dystonias (abnormal muscle tone producing spasms of tongue, face, neck) Parkinson syndrome (shuffling gait, rigid muscles, excessive salivation, tremors, mask-like face, motor deceleration) Tardive dyskinesia (involuntary movements of mouth, tongue, trunk, extremities; chewing motions, sucking, tongue thrusting) Photosensitivity Orthostatic hypotension Neuroleptic malignant syndrome	
Nursing considerations	Lowers seizure threshold May slow growth rate in children Monitor for urinary retention and decreased GI motility Avoid alcohol May cause hypotension if taken with antihypertensives, nitrates Phenothiazines also used	

ANTIPSYCHOTIC MEDICATIONS: ADVERSE EFFECTS		
MEDICATION	**ADVERSE EFFECTS**	**NURSING CONSIDERATIONS**
Extrapyramidal	Pseudoparkinsonism Dystonia (muscle spasm) Acute dystonic reaction Early signs: tightening of jaw, stiff neck, swollen tongue Late signs: swollen airway, oculogyric crisis Akathisia (inability to sit or stand still, foot tap, pace) Tardive dyskinesia (abnormal, involuntary movements); may be irreversible	Pharmacologic management of Parkinsonian adverse effects: benztropine or trihexyphenidyl Recognize early symptoms of acute dystonic reaction Notify health care provider for IM diphenhydramine protocol
Anticholinergic	Blurred vision Dry mouth Nasal congestion Constipation Acute urinary retention	Educate client that some anticholinergic adverse effects often diminish over time Maintain adequate fluid intake and monitor I and O
Sedative	Sleepiness Possible danger if driving or operating machinery	Monitor sedative effects and maintain client safety
Hypotensive	Orthostatic hypotension is common	Frequent monitoring of BP and advise client to rise slowly
Other	Phototoxicity	Educate client regarding need for sunscreen
Neuroleptic malignant syndrome	Rigidity Fever Sweating Autonomic dysfunction (dysrhythmias, fluctuations in BP) Confusion Seizures, coma	Immediately withdraw antipsychotics Control hyperthermia Hydration Dantroline (muscle relaxant) used for rigidity and severe reactions Bromocriptine (dopamine receptor antogonist) used for CNS toxicity and mild reactions
Atropine psychosis	Skin hot to touch without fever-"red as a beet" (flushed face) Dehydration-"dry as a bone" Altered mental status-"mad as a hatter"	Reduce or discontinue medication Hydration Stay with client while confused, for safety

ANTIPSYCHOTIC MEDICATIONS: DEGREE OF ADVERSE EFFECTS	
ACTION	BLOCKS POSTSYNAPTIC DOPAMINE RECEPTORS IN BRAIN
Indications	Psychotic disorders Severe nausea and vomiting
Adverse effects	Drowsiness Pseudoparkinsonism Dystonia Akathisia Tardive dyskinesia Neuroleptic malignant syndrome Dysrhythmias Photophobia Blurred vision Photosensitivity Lactation Discolors urine pink to red-brown
Nursing considerations	May cause false-positive pregnancy tests Dilute oral concentrate with water, saline, 7-Up, homogenized milk, carbonated orange drink, fruit juices (pineapple, orange, apricot, prune, V-8, tomato) use 60 mL for each 5 mL of medication Do not mix with beverages that contain caffeine (coffee, tea, cola) or apple juice; incompatible Monitor vital signs Takes 4–6 weeks to achieve steady plasma levels Monitor bowel function Monitor elderly for dehydration (sedation and decreased thirst sensation) Avoid activities requiring mental alertness Avoid exposure to sun Maintain fluid intake May have anticholinergic and antihistamine actions

ANTIPSYCHOTIC MEDICATIONS: DEGREE OF ADVERSE EFFECTS FOR SELECTED ANTIPSYCHOTICS				
MEDICATION	EXTRA PYRAMIDAL	ANTI CHOLINERGIC	SEDATIVE	HYPOTENSIVE
Chlorpromazine	↑	↑↑	↑↑↑	↑↑↑
Thioridazine	↑	↑↑↑	↑↑↑	↑↑
Trifluoperazine	↑↑↑	↑	↑	↑
Fluphenazine	↑↑↑	↑	↑	↑
Perphenazine	↑↑↑	↑	↑↑	↑
Haloperidol	↑↑↑	↑	↑	↑
Thiothixene	↑↑	↑	↑	↑↑
KEY: ↑ mild; ↑↑ moderate; ↑↑↑ severe				

ANTIPYRETIC MEDICATIONS		
MEDICATION	ADVERSE EFFECTS	NURSING CONSIDER–ATIONS
Acetaminophen	Overdosage may be fatal GI adverse effects are not common	Do not exceed recommended dose
Salicylates	Short-term use—GI bleeding, heartburn, occasional nausea Prolonged high dosage—salicylism: metabolic acidosis, respiratory alkalosis, dehydration, fluid and electrolyte imbalance, tinnitus	Observe for bleeding gums, bloody or black stools, bruises Give with milk, water, or food, or use enteric-coated tablets to minimize gastric distress Contraindications—GI disorders, severe anemia, vitamin K deficiency Anti-inflammatory, analgesic, antipyretic
Action	Antiprostaglandin activity in hypothalamus reduces fever; causes peripheral vasodilation; anti-inflammatory actions	
Indications	Fever	
Adverse effects	GI irritation Occult bleeding Tinnitus Dizziness Confusion Liver dysfunction (acetaminophen)	
Nursing consid-erations	Aspirin contraindicated for client less than 21 years old due to risk of Reye's syndrome Aspirin contraindicated for clients with bleeding disorders due to anticlotting activity NSAIDS are also used for fever	

ANTITHYROID MEDICATIONS

MEDICATION	ADVERSE EFFECTS	NURSING CONSIDERATIONS
Methimazole Propylthiouracil	Leukopenia, fever Rash, sore throat Jaundice	Inhibits synthesis of thyroid hormone by thyroid gland Check CBC and hepatic function Give with meals Report fever, sore throat to health care provider
Iodine solution Potassium iodide	Nausea, vomiting, metallic taste Rash	Iodine preparation Used 2 weeks prior to surgery; decreases vascularity, decreases hormone release Only effective for a short period Give after meals Dilute in water, milk, or fruit juice Stains teeth Give through straw
Radioactive iodine (^{131}I)	Feeling of fullness in neck Metallic taste Leukemia	Destroys thyroid tissue Contraindicated for women of childbearing age Fast overnight before administration Urine, saliva, vomit radioactive 3 days Use full radiation precautions Encourage fluids
Action		Antithyroid medications—inhibits oxidation of iodine Iodines—reduces vascularity of thyroid gland; increases amount of inactive (bound) hormone; inhibits release of thyroid hormones into circulation
Indications		Hyperthyroidism Thyrotoxic crisis
Adverse effects		Nausea, vomiting Diarrhea Rashes Thrombocytopenia Leukopenia
Nursing considerations		Changes in vital signs or weight and appearance may indicate adverse reactions, which should lead to evaluation of continued medication use

THYROID REPLACEMENT MEDICATIONS

MEDICATION	ADVERSE EFFECTS	NURSING CONSIDERATIONS
Levothyroxine	Nervousness, tremors Insomnia Tachycardia, palpitations Dysrhythmias, angina	Tell client to report chest pain, palpitations, sweating, nervousness, shortness of breath to health care provider
Liothyronine sodium	Excessive dosages produce symptoms of hyperthyroidism	Take at same time each day Take in AM Monitor pulse and BP
Action		Increases metabolic rate of body

THYROID REPLACEMENT MEDICATIONS *(CONTINUED)*

MEDICATION	ADVERSE EFFECTS	NURSING CONSIDERATIONS
Indications	Hypothyroidism	
Adverse effects	Nervousness Tachycardia Weight loss	
Nursing considerations	Obtain history of client's medications Enhances action of oral anticoagulants, antidepressants Decreases action of insulin, digitalis Obtain baseline vital signs Monitor weight Avoid OTC medications	

ANTITUBERCULOTICS MEDICATIONS

MEDICATION	ADVERSE EFFECTS	NURSING CONSIDERATIONS
First-line medications		
Isoniazid	Hepatitis Peripheral neuritis Rash Fever	Pyridoxine (B$_6$): 10–50 mg as prophylaxis for neuritis; 50-100 mg as treatment Teach signs of hepatitis Check liver function tests Alcohol increases risk of hepatic complications Therapeutic effects can be expected after 2–3 weeks of therapy Monitor for resolution of symptoms (fever, night sweats, weight loss); hypotension (orthostatic) may occur initially, then resolve; caution client to change position slowly Give before meals Do not combine with phenytoin, causes phenytoin toxicity
Ethambutol	Optic neuritis	Use cautiously with renal disease Check visual acuity
Rifampin	Hepatitis Fever	Orange urine, tears, saliva Check liver function tests Can take with food
Streptomycin	Nephrotoxicity VIII nerve damage	Check creatinine and BUN Audiograms if given long-term
Second-line medications		
Para-amino-salicyclic acid	GI disturbances Hepatotoxicity	Check for ongoing GI adverse effects
Pyrazinamide	Hyperuricemia Anemia Anorexia	Check liver function tests, uric acid, and hematopoietic studies
Action	Inhibits cell wall and protein synthesis of *Mycobacterium tuberculosis*	

ANTITUBERCULOTICS MEDICATIONS *(CONTINUED)*		
MEDICATION	ADVERSE EFFECTS	NURSING CONSIDERATIONS
Indications	Tuberculosis INH—used to prevent disease in person exposed to organism	
Adverse effects	Hepatitis Optic neuritis Seizures Peripheral neuritis	
Nursing considerations	Used in combination (2 medications or more) Monitor for liver damage and hepatitis With active TB, the client should cover mouth and nose when coughing, confine used tissues to plastic bags, and wear a mask with crowds until three sputum cultures are negative (no longer infectious) In inclient settings, client is placed under airborne precautions and workers wear a N95 or high-efficiency particulate air (HEPA) respirator until the client is no longer infectious	

ANTITUSSIVE/EXPECTORANT MEDICATIONS		
MEDICATION	ADVERSE EFFECTS	NURSING CONSIDERATIONS
Dextromethorphan hydrobromide	Drowsiness Dizziness	Antitussive Onset occurs within 30 min, lasts 3-6 hours Monitor cough type and frequency
Guaifenesin	Dizziness Headache Nausea, vomiting	Expectorant Monitor cough type and frequency Take with glass of water
Action	Antitussives—suppresses cough reflex by inhibiting cough center in medulla Expectorants—decreases viscosity of bronchial secretions	
Indications	Coughs due to URI COPD	
Adverse effects	Respiratory depression Hypotension Bradycardia Anticholinergic effects Photosensitivity	
Nursing considerations	Elderly clients may need reduced dosages Avoid alcohol	

ANTIVIRAL MEDICATIONS		
MEDICATION	**ADVERSE EFFECTS**	**NURSING CONSIDERATIONS**
Acyclovir	Headaches, dizziness Seizures Diarrhea	Used for herpes simplex and herpes zoster Given PO, IV, topically Does not prevent transmission of disease Slows progression of symptoms Encourage fluids Check liver and renal function tests
Ribavarin	Worsening of pulmonary status, bacterial pneumonia Hypotension, cardiac arrest	Used for severe lower respiratory tract infections in infants and children Must use special aerosol-generating device for administration Can precipitate Contraindicated in females who may become pregnant during treatment
Zidovudine	Anemia Headache Anorexia, diarrhea, nausea, GI pain Paresthesias, dizziness Insomnia Agranulocytosis	Used for HIV infection Teach clients to strictly comply with dosage schedule
Zalcitabine	Oral ulcers Peripheral neuropathy, headache Vomiting, diarrhea CHF, cardiomyopathy	Used in combination with zidovudine for advanced HIV
Didanosine	Headache Rhinitis, cough Diarrhea, nausea, vomiting Pancreatitis, granulocytopenia Peripheral neuropathy Seizures Hemorrhage	Used for HIV infection Monitor liver and renal function studies Note baseline vital signs and weight Take on empty stomach Chew or crush tablets
Famciclovir	Fatigue, fever Nausea, vomiting, diarrhea, constipation Headache, sinusitis	Used for acute herpes zoster (shingles) Obtain baseline CBC and renal function studies Remind clients they are contagious when lesions are open and draining
Ganciclovir	Fever Rash Leukemia Seizures GI hemorrhage MI, stroke	Used for retinitis caused by cytomegalovirus Check level of consciousness Monitor CBC, I and O Report any dizziness, confusions, seizures immediately Need regular eye exams

ANTIVIRAL MEDICATIONS *(CONTINUED)*		
MEDICATION	**ADVERSE EFFECTS**	**NURSING CONSIDERATIONS**
Amantadine	Dizziness Nervousness Insomnia Orthostatic hypotension	Used for prophylaxis and treatment of influenza A Orthostatic hypotension precautions Instruct clients to avoid hazardous activities
Oseltamivir Zanamivir	Nausea, vomiting Cough and throat irritation	Used for the treatment of Types A and B influenza Best effect if given within 2 days of infection Instruct clients that medication will reduce flu-symptom duration
Action	Inhibits DNA or RNA replication in virus	
Indications	Recurrent HSV 1 and 2 in immunocompromised clients Encephalitis Herpes zoster HIV infections	
Adverse effects	Vertigo Depression Headache Hematuria	
Nursing considerations	Encourage fluids Small, frequent feedings Good skin care Wear glove when applying topically Not a cure, but relieves symptoms	

ATTENTION–DEFICIT HYPERACTIVITY DISORDER MEDICATIONS		
MEDICATION	**ADVERSE EFFECTS**	**NURSING CONSIDERATIONS**
Methylphenidate	Nervousness, palpitations Insomnia Tachycardia Weight loss, growth suppression	May precipitate Tourette's syndrome Monitor CBC, platelet count Has paradoxical calming effect in ADD Monitor height/weight in children Monitor BP Avoid drinks with caffeine Give at least 6 hours before bedtime Give pc
Dextroamphetamine sulfate	Insomnia Tachycardia, palpitations	Controlled substance May alter insulin needs Give in AM to prevent insomnia Don't use with MAO inhibitor (possible hypertensive crisis)
Action	Increases level of catecholamines in cerebral cortex and reticular activating system	

ATTENTION-DEFICIT HYPERACTIVITY DISORDER MEDICATIONS *(CONTINUED)*		
MEDICATION	**ADVERSE EFFECTS**	**NURSING CONSIDERATIONS**
Indications	Attention-deficit hyperactivity disorder (ADHD) Narcolepsy	
Adverse effects	Restlessness Insomnia Tremors Tachycardia Seizures	
Nursing consider-ations	Monitor growth rate in children	

BIPOLAR DISORDER MEDICATIONS		
MEDICATION	**ADVERSE EFFECTS**	**NURSING CONSIDERATIONS**
Lithium	Dizziness Headache Impaired vision Fine hand tremors Reversible leukocytosis	Use for control of manic episodes in the syndrome of manic-depressive psychosis; mood stabilizer Blood levels must be monitored frequently GI symptoms can be reduced if taken with meals Therapeutic effects preceded by lag of 1–2 weeks Signs of intoxication—vomiting, diarrhea, drowsiness, muscular weakness, ataxia Dosage is usually halved during depressive stages of illness Initial blood target level = 1–1.5 mEq/L(1–1.5 mmol/L) Maintenance blood target level = 0.8–1.2 mEq/L (0.8–1.2 mmol/L) Check serum levels 2–3 times weekly when started and monthly while on maintenance; serum levels should be drawn in AM prior to dose Should have fluid intake of 2,500–3,000 mL/day and adequate salt intake
Carbamazepine	Dizziness, vertigo Drowiness Ataxia CHF Aplastic anemia, thrombocytopenia	Mood stablizer used with bipolar disorder Traditionally used for seizures and trigeminal neuralgia Obtain baseline urinalysis, BUN, liver function tests, CBC Shake oral suspension well before measuring dose When giving by NG tube, mix with equal volume of water, 0.9% NaCl or D_5 W, then flush with 100 mL after dose Take with food Avoid grapefruit juice Drowsiness usually disappears in 3–4 days
Divalproex sodium	Sedation Pancreatitis Indigestion Thrombocytopenia Toxic hepatitis	Mood stablizers used with bipolar disorder Traditionally used for seizures Monitor liver function tests, platelet count before starting med and periodically after med Teach client symptoms of liver dysfunction (e.g., malaise, fever, lethargy) Monitor blood levels Take with food or milk Avoid hazardous activities

BIPOLAR DISORDER MEDICATIONS *(CONTINUED)*		
MEDICATION	**ADVERSE EFFECTS**	**NURSING CONSIDERATIONS**
Action		Reduces amount of catecholamines released into synapse and increases reuptake of norepinephrine and serotonin from synaptic space; competes with Na^+ and K^+ transport in nerve and muscle cells
Indications		Manic episodes
Adverse effects		GI upset Tremors Polydipsia, polyuria
Nursing considerations		Monitor serum levels carefully Severe toxicity: exaggerated reflexes, seizures, coma, death

BONE-RESORPTION INHIBITORS (BISPHOSPHONATES) MEDICATIONS		
MEDICATION	**ADVERSE EFFECTS**	**NURSING CONSIDERATIONS**
Alendronate Risedronate Ibandronate	Esophagitis Arthralgia Nausea, diarrhea	Prevention and treatment of postmenopausal osteoporosis, Paget's disease, glucocorticoid-induced osteoporosis Instruct clients to take medication in the morning with 6–8 ounces of water before eating and to remain in upright position for 30 minutes Bone density tests may be monitored

BRONCHODILATORS/MUCOLYTIC MEDICATIONS		
MEDICATION	**ADVERSE EFFECTS**	**NURSING CONSIDERATIONS**
Terbutaline sulfate	Nervousness, tremor Headache Tachycardia Palpitations Fatigue	Short-acting beta agonist most useful when about to enter environment or begin activity likely to induce asthma attack Pulse and blood pressure should be checked before each dose
Ipratropium bromide Tiotropium	Nervousness Tremor Dry mouth Palpitations	Cholinergic antagonist Don't mix in nebulizer with cromolyn sodium Not for acute treatment Teach use of metered dose inhaler: inhale, hold breath, exhale slowly
Albuterol	Tremors Headache Hyperactivity Tachycardia	Short-acting beta agonist most useful when about to enter environment or begin activity likely to induce asthma attack Monitor for toxicity if using tablets and aerosol Teach how to correctly use inhaler
Epinephrine	Cerebral hemorrhage Hypertension Tachycardia	When administered IV monitor BP, heart rate, EKG If used with steroid inhaler, use bronchodilator first, then wait 5 minutes before using steroid inhaler (opens airway for maximum effectiveness)

BRONCHODILATORS/MUCOLYTIC MEDICATIONS *(CONTINUED)*		
MEDICATION	**ADVERSE EFFECTS**	**NURSING CONSIDERATIONS**
Salmeterol	Headache Pharyngitis Nervousness Tremors	Dry powder preparation Not for acute bronchospasm or exacerbations
Montelukast sodium Zafirlukast Zileuton	Headache GI distress	Used for prophylactic and maintenance therapy of asthma Liver tests may be monitored Interacts with theophylline
Acetylcysteine	Bronchospasm Nausea Vomiting	Mucolytic Administered by nebulization into face mask or mouthpiece Bronchospasm most likely to occur in asthmatics Open vials should be refrigerated and used within 90 hours Clients should clear airway by coughing prior to aerosol

CARBONIC ANHYDRASE INHIBITOR MEDICATIONS		
MEDICATION	**ADVERSE EFFECTS**	**NURSING CONSIDERATIONS**
Acetazolamide	Lethargy, depression Anorexia, weakness Decreased K^+ level, confusion	Used for glaucoma Assess client's mental status before repeating dose
Action	Decreases production of aqueous humor in ciliary body	
Indications	Open-angle glaucoma	
Adverse effects	Blurred vision Lacrimation Pulmonary edema	
Nursing considerations	Monitor client for systemic effects	

CARDIAC GLYCOSIDE (DIGITALIS) MEDICATIONS		
MEDICATION	ADVERSE EFFECTS	NURSING CONSIDERATIONS
Digoxin	Anorexia Nausea Bradycardia Visual disturbances Confusion Abdominal pain	Administer with caution to elderly or clients with renal insufficiency Monitor renal function and electrolytes Instruct clients to eat high-potassium foods Take apical pulse for 1 full minute before administering Notify health care provider if apical pulse less than 60 (adult), less than 90–110 (infants and young children), less than 70 (older children) Digitalizing dose (oral) aimed at administering the drug in divided dosages over a period of 24 hours or days until an "optimum" cardiac effect is reached. Not used frequently. –0.5 to 0.75 mg PO, then 0.25 mg PO every 6–8 hours to a total dose of 1–1.5 mg Digitalizing dose (IV)–0.25 to 0.5 mg IV, then 0.25 mg IV to a total dose of 1 mg Digoxin immune fab–used for treatment of life-threatening toxicity Maintenance dose 0.125–0.5 mg IV or PO (average is 0.25 mg) Teach client to check pulse rate and discuss adverse effects Low K^+ increases risk of digitalis toxicity Serum therapeutic blood levels 0.5–2 ng/mL (0.64–2.56 nmol/L) Toxic blood levels > 2 ng/mL (2.56 nmol/L)
Action	Increases force of myocardial contraction and slows heart rate by stimulating the vagus nerve and blocking the AV node	
Indications	Heart failure, dysrhythmias	
Adverse effects	Tachycardia, bradycardia, heart block Anorexia, nausea, vomiting Halos around dark objects, blurred vision, halo vision Dysrhythmias, heart block	
Nursing considerations	Instruct client to eat high potassium foods Monitor for digitalis toxicity Risk of digitalis toxicity increases if client is hypokalemic	
Herbal interactions	Licorice can potentiate action of digoxin by promoting potassium loss Hawthorn may increase effects of digoxin Ginseng may falsely elevate digoxin levels Ma-huang (ephedra) increases risk of digitalis toxicity	

CYTOPROTECTIVE MEDICATIONS

MEDICATION	ADVERSE EFFECTS	NURSING CONSIDERATIONS
Sucralfate	Constipation Dizziness	Take medication 1 hour ac Should not be taken with antacids or H_2 blockers
Action	Adheres to and protects ulcer's surface by forming a barrier	
Indications	Duodenal ulcer	
Adverse effects	Constipation Vertigo Flatulence	
Nursing considerations	Action lasts up to 6 hours Give 2 hours before or after most medications to prevent decreased absorption	

DISEASE-MODIFYING ANTIRHEUMATIC MEDICATIONS (DMARDS)

MEDICATION	ADVERSE EFFECTS
Nonbiologic DMARDs	
Methotrexate Hydroxychloroquine sulfate Sulfasalazine Cyclosporine	Serious infection Cancer Impaired liver and kidney function
Biologic DMARDs	
Entanercept Infliximab Adalimumab Anakinra Rituximab Abatacept	Bacterial infection Invasive fungal infection Injection site reaction
Action	Non-biologic DMARDs: Interfere with immune system Indirect and nonspecific effect Biologic DMARDs: Interfere with immune system (tumor necrosis factor, interleukins, T- or B-cell lymphocytes)
Indications	Rheumatoid arthritis Psoriasis Inflammatory bowel disease

DISEASE-MODIFYING ANTIRHEUMATIC MEDICATIONS (DMARDS) *(CONTINUED)*	
MEDICATION	**ADVERSE EFFECTS**
Adverse effects	Stomatitis
	Liver toxicity
	Bleeding
	Anemia
	Infections
	Hypersensitivity
	Kidney failure
Nursing consider-ations	Precautions: infections, bleeding disorders
	Monitor liver function tests
	Monitor BUN and creatinine
	Monitor for signs of infection
	Monitor response to medication
	Teach client about risk of live vaccines
	Teach client to avoid alcohol
	Teach client about risk of infection

DIURETIC MEDICATIONS		
MEDICATION	**ADVERSE EFFECTS**	**NURSING CONSIDERATIONS**
Thiazide diuretics		
Hydrochlorothiazide	Hypokalemia	Monitor electrolytes, especially potassium
Chlorothiazide	Hyperglycemia	I and O
	Blurred vision	Monitor BUN and creatinine
	Loss of Na$^+$	Don't give at bedtime
	Dry mouth	Weigh client daily
	Hypotension	Encourage potassium-containing foods
Potassium–sparing		
Spironlactone	Hyperkalemia	Used with other diuretics
	Hyponatremia	Give with meals
	Hepatic and renal damage	Avoid salt substitutes
	Tinnitus	containing potassium
	Rash	Monitor I and O
Loop diuretics		
Furosemide	Hypotension	Monitor BP, pulse rate, I and O
Ethacrynic acid	Hypokalemia	Monitor potassium
	Hyperglycemia	Give IV dose over 1–2 minutes → diuresis in 5–10 min
	GI upset	After PO dose diuresis in about 30 min
	Weakness	Weigh client daily
		Don't give at bedtime
		Encourage potassium-containing foods

DIURETIC MEDICATIONS *(CONTINUED)*		
MEDICATION	**ADVERSE EFFECTS**	**NURSING CONSIDERATIONS**
Ethacrynic acid Bumetanide	Potassium depletion Electrolyte imbalance Hypovolemia Ototoxicity	Supervise ambulation Monitor blood pressure and pulse Observe for signs of electrolyte imbalance
Osmotic diuretic		
Mannitol	Dry mouth Thirst	I and O must be measured Monitor vital signs Monitor for electrolyte imbalance
Other		
Chlorthalidone	Dizziness Aplastic anemia Orthostatic hypotension	Acts like a thiazide diuretic Acts in 2–3 hours, peak 2–6 hours, lasts 2–3 days Administer in AM Monitor output, weight, BP, electrolytes Increase K^+ in diet Monitor glucose levels in diabetic clients Change position slowly
Action	Thiazides—inhibits reabsorption of sodium and chloride in distal renal tubule Loop—inhibits reabsorption of sodium and chloride in loop of Henle and distal renal tubules Potassium-sparing—blocks effect of aldosterone on renal tubules, causing loss of sodium and water and retention of potassium Osmotic—pulls fluid from tissues due to hypertonic effect	
Indications	Heart failure Hypertension Renal diseases Diabetes insipidus Reduction of osteoporosis in postmenopausal women	
Adverse effects	Dizziness, vertigo Dry mouth Orthostatic hypotension Leukopenia Polyuria, nocturia Photosensitivity Impotence Hypokalemia (except for potassium-sparing) Hyponatremia	

DIURETIC MEDICATIONS *(CONTINUED)*		
MEDICATION	**ADVERSE EFFECTS**	**NURSING CONSIDERATIONS**
Nursing considerations	Take with food or milk Take in AM Monitor weight and electrolytes Protect skin from the sun Diet high in potassium for loop and thiazide diuretics Limit potassium intake for potassium-sparing diuretics Used as first-line medications for hypertension	
Herbal interactions	Licorice can promote potassium loss, causing hypokalemia Aloe can decrease serum potassium level, causing hypokalemia Gingko may increase blood pressure when taken with thiazide diuretics	

ELECTROLYTES AND REPLACEMENT SOLUTIONS		
MEDICATION	**ADVERSE EFFECTS**	**NURSING CONSIDERATIONS**
Calcium carbonate Calcium chloride	Dysrhythmias Constipation	Foods containing oxalic acid (rhubarb, spinach), phytic acid (bran, whole cereals), and phosphorus (milk, dairy products) interfere with absorption Monitor EKG Take 1–1.5 hours pc if GI upset occurs
Magnesium chloride	Weak or absent deep tendon reflexes Hypotension Respiratory paralysis	Respirations should be greater than 16/min before medication given IV Test deep tendon reflexes before each dose Monitor I and O
Potassium chloride Potassium gluconate	Dysrhythmias, cardiac arrest Abdominal pain Respiratory paralysis	Monitor EKG and serum electrolytes Take with or after meals with full glass of water or fruit juice
Sodium chloride	Pulmonary edema	Monitor serum electrolytes

ELECTROLYTE MODIFIER MEDICATION

Action	Alkalinizing agents—release bicarbonate ions in stomach and secrete bicarbonate ions in kidneys
	Calcium salts—provide calcium for bones, teeth, nerve transmission, muscle contraction, normal blood coagulation, cell membrane strength
	Hypocalcemic agents—decrease blood levels of calcium
	Hypophosphatemic agents—bind phosphates in GI tract lowering blood levels; neutralize gastric acid, inactivate pepsin
	Magnesium salts—provide magnesium for nerve conduction and muscle activity and activate enzyme reactions in carbohydrate metabolism
	Phosphates—provide body with phosphorus needed for bone, muscle tissue, metabolism of carbohydrates, fats, proteins, and normal CNS function
	Potassium exchange resins—exchange Na^+ for K^+ in intestines, lowering K^+ levels
	Potassium salts—provide potassium needed for cell growth and normal functioning of cardiac, skeletal, and smooth muscle
	Replacement solution—provide water and Na^+ to maintain acid-base and water balance, maintain osmotic pressure
	Urinary acidifiers—secrete H^+ ions in kidneys, making urine acidic
	Urinary alkalinizers—convert to sodium bicarbonate, making the urine alkaline
Indications	Fluid and electrolyte imbalances
	Renal calculi
	Peptic ulcers
	Osteoporosis
	Metabolic acidosis or alkalosis
Adverse effects	See individual medications
Nursing considerations	Monitor clients with HF, hypertension, renal disease

GENITOURINARY MEDICATIONS

MEDICATION	ADVERSE EFFECTS	NURSING CONSIDERATIONS
Nitrofurantoin	Diarrhea Nausea, vomiting Asthma attacks	Anti-infective Check CBC Give with food or milk Avoid acidic foods (cranberry juice, prunes, plums) which increase drug action Check I and O Monitor pulmonary status
Phenazopyridine	Headache Vertigo	Urinary tract analgesic, spasmolytic Inform client that urine will be bright orange Take with meals
Anticholinergics		
Oxybutynin Darifenacin Solifenacin Tolterodine	Drowsiness Blurred vision Dry mouth Constipation Urinary retention	Used to reduce bladder spasms and treat urinary incontinence Increase fluids and fiber in diet Oxybutynin—older adults require higher dose and have greater incidence of adverse effects
Anti-impotence		

GENITOURINARY MEDICATIONS *(CONTINUED)*		
MEDICATION	ADVERSE EFFECTS	NURSING CONSIDERATIONS
Sildenafil Vardenafil Tadalafil	Headache Flushing Hypotension Priapism	Treatment of erectile dysfunction Take 1 hour before sexual activity Never use with nitrates—could have fatal hypotension Do not take with alpha blockers, e.g., doxazosin (Cardura)-risk of hypotension Do not drink grapefruit juice
Testosterone inhibitors		
Finasteride	Decreased libido Impotence Breast tenderness	Treatment of benign prostatic hyperplasia (BPH) by Proscar; male hair loss by Propecia Pregnant women should avoid contact with crushed drug or client's semen—may adversely affect male fetus

GI ULCER DISEASE MEDICATIONS		
MEDICATION	ADVERSE EFFECTS	NURSING CONSIDERATIONS
H$_2$-antagonists		
Cimetidine Ranitidine Famotidine Nizatidine	Diarrhea Confusion and dizziness (esp. in elderly with large doses) Headache	Bedtime dose suppresses nocturnal acid production Compliance may increase with single-dose regimen Avoid antacids within 1 hour of dose Dysrhythmias Cimetidine–greater incidence of confusion and agitation with older adults
Antisecretory agents		
Omeprazole Lansoprazole Rabeprazole Esomeprazole Pantoprazole	Dizziness Diarrhea	Typically administered 30 to 60 minutes before breakfast Do not crush sustained-release capsule; contents may be sprinkled on food or instilled with fluid in NG tube
Prostaglandin analogs		
Misoprostol	Abdominal pain Diarrhea (13%) Miscarriage	Notify health care provider if diarrhea more than 1 week or severe abdominal pain or black, tarry stools
Nursing considerations	Other medications may be prescribed, including antacids (time administration to avoid canceling med effect) and antimicrobials to eradicate *H. pylori* infections Client should avoid smoking, alcohol, ASA, and caffeine, all of which increase stomach acid	

EYE MEDICATIONS: OVERVIEW		
MEDICATION	**ADVERSE EFFECTS**	**NURSING CONSIDERATIONS**
Methylcellulose	Eye irritation if excess is allowed to dry on eyelids	Lubricant Use eyewash to rinse eyelids of "sandy" sensation felt after administration
Polyvinyl alcohol	Blurred vision Burning	Artificial tears Applied to contact lenses before insertion
Tetrahydrozoline	Cardiac irregularities Pupillary dilation, increased intraocular pressure Transient stinging	Used for ocular congestion, irritation, allergic conditions Rebound congestion may occur with frequent or prolonged use Apply light pressure on lacrimal sac for 1 min instillation
Timolol maleate Levobunolol	Eye irritation Hypotension	Beta-blocking agent Reduces intraocular pressure in management of glaucoma Apply light pressure on lacrimal sac for 1 min following instillation Monitor BP and pulse
Proparacaine HCl Tetracaine HCl, cocaine	Corneal abrasion	Topical anesthetic Remind client not to touch or rub eyes while anesthetized Patch the eye to prevent corneal abrasion
Prednisolone acetate	Corneal abrasion	Topical steroid Steroid use predisposes client to local infection
Gentamicin Tobramycin	Eye irritation; itching, redness	Anti-infective agent Clean exudate from eyes before use
Idoxuridine	Eye irritation Itching lids	Topical antiviral agent Educate client about possible adverse effects
Dipivefrin HCl	Increase in heart rate and blood pressure	Adrenergic Monitor vital signs because of systemic absorption
Flurbiprofen	Platelet aggregation disorder	Nonsteroidal anti-inflammatory agents Monitor client for eye hemorrhage Client should not continue wearing contact lens
Nursing considerations	Place pressure on tear ducts for one minute Wash hands before and after installation Do not touch tip of dropper to eye or body	

EYE MEDICATIONS: MIOTIC		
MEDICATION	**ADVERSE EFFECTS**	**NURSING CONSIDERATIONS**
Pilocarpine	Painful eye muscle spasm, blurred or poor vision in dim lights Photophobia, cataracts, or floaters	Teach to apply pressure on lacrimal sac for 1 min following instillation Used for glaucoma Caution client to avoid sunlight and night driving
Carachol	Headache If absorbed systemically, can cause sweating, abdominal cramps, and decreased blood pressure	Cholinergic (ophthalmic) Similar to acetylcholine in action Produces pupillary miosis during ocular surgery
Action	Causes contraction of sphincter muscles of iris, resulting in miosis	

EYE MEDICATIONS: MIOTIC *(CONTINUED)*		
MEDICATION	ADVERSE EFFECTS	NURSING CONSIDERATIONS
Indications	Pupillary miosis in ocular surgery Primary open-angle glaucoma	
Adverse effects	Headache Hypotension Bronchoconstriction	
Nursing considerations	Teach how to instill eye drops correctly Apply light pressure on lacrimal sac for 1 minute after medication instilled Avoid hazardous activities until temporary blurring disappears Transient brow pain and myopia are common initially, disappear within 10-14 days	

EYE MEDICATIONS: MYDRIATIC AND CYCLOPLEGIC		
MEDICATION	ADVERSE EFFECTS	NURSING CONSIDERATIONS
Atropine sulfate	Blurred vision, photophobia Flushing, tachycardia Dry mouth	Contraindicated with narrow-angle glaucoma Suck on hard candy for dry mouth
Cyclopentolate	Photophobia, blurred vision Seizures Tachycardia	Contraindicated in narrow-angle glaucoma Burns when instilled
Action	Anticholinergic action leaves the pupil under unopposed adrenergic influence, causing it to dilate	
Indications	Diagnostic procedures Acute iritis, uveitis	
Adverse effects	Headache Tachycardia Blurred vision Photophobia Dry mouth	
Nursing considerations	Mydriatics cause pupil dilation; cycloplegics paralyze the iris sphincter Watch for signs of glaucoma (increased intraocular pressure, headache, progressive blurring of vision) Apply light pressure on lacrimal sac for 1 minute after instilling medication Avoid hazardous activities until blurring of vision subsides Wear dark glasses	

HEAVY METAL ANTAGONIST MEDICATIONS

MEDICATION	ADVERSE EFFECTS	NURSING CONSIDERATIONS
Deferoxamine mesylate	Pain and induration at injection site Urticaria Hypotension Generalized erythema	Used for acute iron intoxication, chronic iron overload
Dimercaprol	Hypertension Tachycardia Nausea, vomiting Headache	Used for treatment of arsenic, gold, and mercury poisoning; acute lead poisoning when used with edetate calcium disodium Administered as initial dose because of its improved efficiency in removing lead from brain tissue
Edetate calcium disodium (EDTA)		Used for acute and chronic lead poisoning, lead encephalopathy Renal tubular necrosis Multiple deep IM doses or IV Very painful—local anesthetic procaine is injected with the drug (drawn into syringe last, after which the syringe is maintained with needle held slightly down so that it is administered first); rotate sites; provide emotional support and play therapy as outlet for frustration Ensure adequate hydration and monitor I and O and kidney function—$CaNa_2$, EDTA and lead are toxic to kidneys Seizure precautions—initial rapid mobilization of lead may cause an increase in brain lead levels, exacerbating symptoms
Action	Forms stable complexes with metals	
Indications	Poisoning (gold, arsenic) Acute lead encephalopathy	
Adverse effects	Tachycardia Burning sensation in lips, mouth, throat Abdominal pain	
Nursing considerations	Monitor I and O, BUN, EKG Encourage fluids	

IMMUNOSUPPRESSANT MEDICATIONS

MEDICATION	INDICATIONS FOR USE
Azathioprine	Prevent renal transplant rejection Treat severe rheumatoid arthritis not responsive to other treatments
Cyclosporine	Prevent rejection of solid organ (heart, kidney, liver) transplants Prevent graft-versus-host disease in bone marrow transplant

IMMUNOSUPPRESSANT MEDICATIONS *(CONTINUED)*	
MEDICATION	**INDICATIONS FOR USE**
Tacrolimus	Prevent liver, kidney, and heart transplant rejection
Etanercept	Rheumatoid arthritis treatment (acts to reduce the immune response resulting in inflammation and pain)
Infliximab	Treatment of Crohn's disease (inflammatory bowel disease thought to have autoimmune origins)
	Treatment of rheumatoid arthritis
Methotrexate	Treatment of severe rheumatoid arthritis unresponsive to other treatments
Prednisone Prednisolone	Autoimmune disease
Basiliximab Daclizumab	Post transplant surgery

IMMUNOMODULATOR MEDICATIONS	
MEDICATION	**ADVERSE EFFECTS**
Beta interferons Interferon beta-1a Interferon beta-1b	"Flu-like" symptoms
	Liver dysfunction
	Bone marrow depression
	Injection site reactions
	Photosensitivity
Glatiramer acetate Natalizumab	Central nervous system infection (natalizumab)
Action	Modify the immune response
	Decrease the movement of leukocytes into the central nervous system neurons
Indications	Multiple sclerosis
Adverse effects	"Flu-like" symptoms
	Liver dysfunction
	Bone marrow depression
	Injection site reactions
	Photosensitivity
	Central nervous system infection (natalizumab)
Nursing considerations	Monitor liver function tests
	Monitor complete blood count
	Subcutaneous injection: rotate injection sites, apply ice, and then use warm compresses, analgesics for discomfort
	Photosensitivity precautions
	Monitor for signs of depression

IRON PREPARATION MEDICATION

MEDICATION	ADVERSE EFFECTS	NURSING CONSIDERATIONS
Ferrous sulfate	Nausea Constipation Black stools	Food decreases absorption but may be necessary to reduce GI effects Monitor Hgb, Hct Dilute liquid preparations in juice, but not milk or antacids Use straw for liquid to avoid staining teeth
Iron dextran	Nausea Constipation Black stools	IM injections cause pain and skin staining; use the Z-track technique to put med deep into buttock; IV administration is preferred
Action	Iron salts increase availability of iron for hemoglobin	
Indications	Iron-deficiency anemia	
Adverse effects	Constipation, diarrhea Dark stools Tooth enamel stains Seizures Flushing, hypotension Tachycardia	
Nursing considerations	Take iron salts on empty stomach (absorption is reduced by one-third when taken with food) Absorption of iron decreased when administered with tetracyclines, antacids, coffee, tea, milk, eggs (bind to iron) Concurrent use of iron decreases effectiveness of tetracyclines and quinolone antibiotics Vitamin C increases absorption of iron salts Vitamin E delays therapeutic responses to iron salts	

LAXATIVES AND STOOL SOFTENER MEDICATIONS

MEDICATION	ADVERSE EFFECTS	NURSING CONSIDERATIONS
Bisacodyl	Mild cramps, rash, nausea, diarrhea	Stimulant Tablets should not be taken with milk or antacids (causes dissolution of enteric coating and loss of cathartic action) Can cause gastric irritation Effects in 6–12 hours
Mineral oil	Pruritus ani, anorexia, nausea	Lubricant Administer in upright position Prolonged use can cause fat-soluble vitamin malabsorption
Docusate	Few adverse effects Abdominal cramps	Stool softener Contraindicated in atonic bowel, nausea, vomiting, GI pain Effects in 1-3 days

LAXATIVES AND STOOL SOFTENER MEDICATIONS *(CONTINUED)*

MEDICATION	ADVERSE EFFECTS	NURSING CONSIDERATIONS
Milk of Magnesia	Hypermagnesemia, dehydration	Saline agent Na$^+$ salts can exacerbate heart failure
Psyllium hydrophilic mucilloid	Obstruction of GI tract	Take with a full glass of water; do not take dry Report abdominal distention or unusual amount of flatulence
Polyethylene glycol and electrolytes	Nausea and bloating	Large-volume product—allow time to consume it safely
Action	Bulk-forming—absorbs water into stool mass, making stool bulky, thus stimulating peristalsis Lubricants—coat surface of stool and soften fecal mass, allowing for easier passage Osmotic agents and saline laxatives—draw water from plasma by osmosis, increasing bulk of fecal mass, thus promoting peristalsis Stimulants—stimulate peristalsis when they come in contact with intestinal mucosa Stool softeners—soften fecal mass	
Indications	Constipation Preparation for procedures or surgery	
Adverse effects	Diarrhea Dependence	
Nursing considerations	Contraindicated for clients with abdominal pain, nausea and vomiting, fever (acute abdomen) Chronic use may cause hypokalemia	

MINERALS

MEDICATION	ADVERSE EFFECTS	NURSING CONSIDERATIONS
Calcium	Cardiac dysrhythmias Constipation Hypercalcemia Renal calculi	Give 1 hour before meals Give 1/3 dose at bedtime Monitor for urinary stones
Vitamin D	Seizures Impaired renal function Hypercalcemia Renal calculi	Treatment of vitamin D deficiency, rickets, psoriasis, rheumatoid arthritis Check electrolytes Restrict use of antacids containing Mg

MINERALS *(CONTINUED)*		
MEDICATION	**ADVERSE EFFECTS**	**NURSING CONSIDERATIONS**
Sodium fluoride	Bad taste Staining of teeth Nausea, vomiting	Observe for synovitis
Potassium	Nausea, vomiting Cramps, diarrhea	Prevention and treatment of hypokalemia Report hyperkalemia: lethargy, confusion, fainting, decreased urine output Report continued hypokalemia: fatigue, weakness, polyuria, polydipsia, cardiac changes

MUSCULOSKELETAL MEDICATIONS		
MEDICATION	**ADVERSE EFFECTS**	**NURSING CONSIDERATIONS**
Neostigmine	Nausea, vomiting Abdominal cramps Respiratory depression Bronchoconstriction Hypotension Bradycardia	Monitor vital signs frequently Have atropine injection available Observe for improvement in strength, vision, ptosis 45 min after each dose Schedule dose before periods of fatigue (e.g., ac) Take with milk or food Potentiates action of morphine Diagnostic test for myasthenia gravis
Pyridostigmine bromide	Seizures Bradycardia Hypotension Bronchoconstriction	Monitor vital signs frequently Have atropine injection available Take extended-release tablets same time each day at least 6 hours apart Drug of choice for myasthenia gravis to improve muscle strength
Alendronate sodium	Vitamin D deficiency Osteomalacia	Prevents and treats osteoporosis Longer-lasting treatment for Paget's disease Take in AM at least 30 min before other medication, food, water, or other liquids Should sit up for 30 min after taking medication Use sunscreen and wear protective clothing
Glucosamine	Nausea, heartburn, diarrhea	Antirheumatic Contraindicated with shellfish allergy, pregnancy, and lactation May worsen glycemic control Must be taken on regular basis to be effective
Action	Inhibits destruction of acetylcholine released from parasympathetic and somatic efferent nerves	
Indications	Myasthenia gravis Postoperative and postpartum functional urinary retention	

MUSCULOSKELETAL MEDICATIONS *(CONTINUED)*		
MEDICATION	**ADVERSE EFFECTS**	**NURSING CONSIDERATIONS**
Adverse effects	Bronchoconstriction Diarrhea Respiratory paralysis Muscle cramps	
Nursing considerations	Give with milk or food Administer exactly as ordered and on time Doses vary with client's activity level Monitor vital signs, especially respirations	

NITRATES/ANTIANGINAL MEDICATIONS		
MEDICATION	**ADVERSE EFFECTS**	**NURSING CONSIDERATIONS**
Nitroglycerin	Flushing Hypotension Headache Tachycardia Dizziness Blurred vision	Renew supply every 3 months Avoid alcoholic beverages Sublingual dose may be repeated every 5 minutes for 3 doses Protect drug from light Should wet tablet with saliva and place under tongue
Isosorbide	Headache Orthostatic Hypotension	Change position slowly Take between meals Don't discontinue abruptly
Action	Relaxes vascular smooth muscle; decreases venous return; decreases arterial blood pressure; reduces myocardial oxygen consumption	
Indications	Angina Perioperative hypertension CHF associated with MI Raynaud's disease (topical)	

NITRATES/ANTIANGINAL MEDICATIONS *(CONTINUED)*		
MEDICATION	ADVERSE EFFECTS	NURSING CONSIDERATIONS
Adverse effects	Hypotension Tachycardia Headache Dizziness Syncope Rash	
Nursing considerations	Take sublingual tablets under tongue or in buccal pouch; tablet may sting Check expiration date on bottle Discard unused med after 6 months. Take sustained-release tablets with water, don't chew them Administer topically over 6 × 6 inch area using applicator, cover with plastic wrap, rotate sites Administer transdermal to skin free of hair; do not apply to distal extremities; remove before defibrillation or cardioversion Administer transmucosal tablets between lip and gum above the incisors or between cheek and gum; do not swallow or chew Administer translingual spray into oral mucosa; do not inhale Withdraw medication gradually over 4-6 wks Provide rest periods Teach to take medication when chest pain anticipated May take q 5 min × 3 doses Beta-adrenergic blockers and calcium-channel blockers also used for angina	

NONSTEROIDAL ANTI-INFLAMMATORY MEDICATIONS (NSAIDS)		
MEDICATION	ADVERSE EFFECTS	NURSING CONSIDERATIONS
Ibuprofen	GI upset—nausea, vomiting, diarrhea, constipation Skin eruption, dizziness, headache, fluid retention GI bleeding, prolonged bleeding Stevens-Johnson syndrome	Use cautiously with aspirin allergy, asthma or nasal polyps Give with milk Observe for bleeding Observe for skin rash
Indomethacin	Peptic ulcer, ulcerative colitis Headache, dizziness Bone marrow depression	Observe for bleeding tendencies Monitor I and O
Naproxen	Headache, dizziness, epigastric distress	Administer with food Optimal therapeutic response is seen after 2 weeks of treatment Use cautiously in client with history of aspirin allergy, asthma or nasal polyps

NONSTEROIDAL ANTI-INFLAMMATORY MEDICATIONS (NSAIDS) *(CONTINUED)*		
MEDICATION	**ADVERSE EFFECTS**	**NURSING CONSIDERATIONS**
Celecoxib	Fatigue Anxiety, depression, nervousness Nausea, vomiting, anorexia Dry mouth, constipation	COX-2 inhibitor Increasing doses do not appear to increase effectiveness Do not take if allergic to sulfonamides, ASA, or NSAIDs
Ketorolac	Peptic ulcer disease GI bleeding, prolonged bleeding Renal impairment	Dosage is decreased in clients greater than 65 years or with impaired renal function Duration of treatment is less than 5 days
Actions	NSAIDs inhibit prostaglandins COX-2 inhibitors block the enzyme responsible for inflammation without blocking the COX-1 enzyme ASA has antiplatelet activity	
Indications	Pain, fever, arthritis, dysmenorrhea ASA: transient ischemic attacks, prophylaxis of MI, ischemic stroke, angina Ibuprofen: gout, dental pain, musculoskeletal disorders	
Adverse effects	Headache Eye changes Dizziness Somnolence GI disturbances Constipation Bleeding Rash	
Nursing considerations	Take with food or after meals Periodic ophthalmologic exam Monitor liver and renal function Avoid OTC medications; may contain similar medications Also have analgesic and antipyretic actions Postop clients with adequate pain relief have fewer complications and a shorter recovery Pain is the fifth vital sign and needs to be assessed with others	

OPIOID ANALGESIC MEDICATIONS		
MEDICATION	**ADVERSE EFFECTS**	**NURSING CONSIDERATIONS**
Morphine sulfate	Dizziness, weakness Sedation or paradoxic excitement Nausea, flushing, and sweating Respiratory depression, decreased cough reflex Constipation, miosis, hypotension	Give in smallest effective dose Observe for development of dependence Encourage respiratory exercises Use cautiously to prevent respiratory depression Monitor vital signs Monitor I and O, bowel patterns Used for cardiac clients—reduces preload and afterload pressures, decreasing cardiac workload
Codeine	Same as morphine High dose may cause restlessness and excitement Constipation	Less potent and less dependence potential compared with morphine
Methadone	Same as morphine	Observe for dependence, respiratory depression Encourage fluids and high-bulk foods
Hydromorphone	Sedation, hypotension Urine retention	Keep narcotic antagonist (naloxone) available Monitor bowel function
Oxycodone and acetaminophen Oxycodone and aspirin	Lightheadedness, dizziness, sedation, nausea Constipation, pruritus Increased risk bleeding (oxy and ASA)	Administer with milk after meals
Hydrocodone/acetaminophen	Confusion Sedation Hypotension Constipation	Use with extreme caution with MAO inhibitors Additive CNS depression with alcohol, antihistamines, and sedative/hypnotics
Action	Produces analgesia, euphoria, sedation; acts on CNS receptor cells	
Indications	Moderate-to-severe pain Chronic pain Preoperative medication	
Adverse effects	Dizziness Sedation Respiratory depression Cardiac arrest Hypotension	
Nursing considerations	Provide narcotic antagonist if needed Turn, cough, deep breathe Safety precautions (side rails, assist when walking) Avoid alcohol, antihistamines, sedative, tranquilizers, OTC medications Avoid activities requiring mental alertness	

PAGET'S DISEASE MEDICATIONS

MEDICATION	ADVERSE EFFECTS	NURSING CONSIDERATIONS
Calcitonin	Nausea, vomiting, flushing of face Increased urinary frequency	Retards bone resorption Decreases release of calcium from bone Relieves pain Observe for symptoms of tetany Give at bedtime
Etidronate disodium	Diarrhea	Prevents rapid bone turnover Don't give with food, milk, or antacids (reduces absorption) Monitor renal function
Alendronate	Esophagitis	Suppress bone reabsorption Give in morning on an empty stomach, with a full glass of water Remain upright for 30 minutes
Action	Inhibits osteocytic activity	
Indications	Paget's disease	
Adverse effects	Decreased serum calcium Facial flushing	
Nursing considerations	Monitor serum calcium levels Facial flushing and warmth last 1 hour	

THROMBOLYTIC MEDICATIONS

MEDICATION	ADVERSE EFFECTS	NURSING CONSIDERATIONS (SPECIFIC)
Reteplase Alteplase Tissue plasminogen activator	Bleeding	Tissue plasminogen activator is a naturally occurring enzyme Low allergenic risk but high cost Administered as initial bolus followed by 90 minute IV infusion
Tenecteplase	Bleeding	Single IV bolus
Action	Break down plasminogen into plasmin, which dissolves the fibrin network of a clot	
Indications	MIs within the first 6 hours after symptoms, limited arterial thrombosis, thrombotic strokes, occluded shunts, PE (alteplase) MIs (Reteplase and Tenecteplase)	
Nursing considerations (general)	Check for signs of bleeding; minimize number of punctures for inserting IVs; avoid IM injections; apply pressure at least twice as long as usual after any puncture; avoid high dose therapy with anticoagulants and antiplatelet drugs until thrombolytic action has subsided	

VITAMINS		
MEDICATION	ADVERSE EFFECTS	NURSING CONSIDERATIONS
Cyanocobalamin (Vitamin B_{12})	Anaphylaxis Urticaria	Treatment of vitamin B_{12} deficiency, pernicious anemia, hemorrhage, renal and hepatic diseases Monitor reticulocyte count, iron, and folate levels Don't mix with other solutions in syringe Monitor K^+ levels Clients with pernicious anemia need monthly injections
Folic acid	Bronchospasm Malaise	Treatment of anemia, liver disease, alcoholism, intestinal obstruction, pregnancy Don't mix with other meds in syringe
Action	Coenzymes that speed up metabolic processes	
Indications	Vitamin deficiencies	
Adverse effects	Some vitamins are toxic at high levels	
Nursing considerations	Avoid exceeding RDA (recommended daily allowance)	

MEN'S HEALTH MEDICATIONS		
MEDICATION	ADVERSE EFFECTS	NURSING CONSIDERATIONS
Alpha₁-adrenergic blockers		
Terazosin	Dizziness Headache Weakness Nasal congestion Orthostatic hypotension	Used to decrease urinary urgency, hesitancy, nocturia in prostatic hyperplasia Caution to change position slowly Avoid alcohol, CNS depressant, hot showers due to orthostatic hypotension Requires titration Administer at bedtime due to risk orthostatic hypotension Effects may not be noted for 4 weeks
Tamsulosin	Dizziness Headache	Used to decrease urinary urgency, hesitancy, nocturia in prostatic hyperplasia Caution to change position slowly Administer 30 min. after same meal each day
5-alpha-reductase inhibitor		
Finasteride	Decreased libido Impotence	Used to treat benign prostatic hyperplasia by slowing prostatic growth May decrease serum PSA levels 6-12 months therapy required to determine if medication effective May cause harm to male fetus. Pregnant women should not be exposed to semen of partner taking finasteride or they should not handle crushed medication Monitor liver function tests
Dutasteride	Decreased libido Impotence	Used to treat benign prostatic hyperplasia by slowing prostatic growth May cause harm to male fetus. Pregnant women should not be exposed to semen of partner taking finasteride or they should not handle crushed medication Monitor liver function
Anti-impotence agents		
Sildenafil Vardenafil Tadalafil	Headache Flushing Dyspepsia Nasal congestion Mild visual disturbance	Enhances blood flow to the corpus cavernosum to ensure erection to allow sexual intercourse Should not take with nitrates in any form due to dramatic decrease in blood pressure Usually taken 1 hour before sexual activity (sildenafil, vardenafil) Tadalafil has longer duration of action (up to 36 hours) Should not take more than one time per day Notify health care provider if erection lasts longer than 4 hours Avoid grapefruit juice
Saw palmetto	Urinary antiseptic used to treat PBH; may cause false-negative PSA test result	

WOMEN'S HEALTH MEDICATIONS		
MEDICATION	**ADVERSE EFFECTS**	**NURSING CONSIDERATIONS**
Contraceptives, systemic		
Example: Ethinyl Estradiol/norgestrel	Headache Dizziness Nausea Breakthrough bleeding, spotting	Used to prevent pregnancy Use condoms against sexually transmitted diseases Take pill at same time every day No smoking
Contraceptives, systemic		
Levonorgestrel	Breakthrough bleeding, spotting	Prevention of pregnancy for 5 years as a contraceptive implant; emergency contraceptive in oral form when given within 72 hours of unprotected intercourse
Estrogens		
Estradiol Estrogens conjugated	Nausea Gynecomastia Contact lens intolerance	Treatment of menopausal symptoms, some cancers Prevention of osteoporosis Client should contact health care provider if there are breast lumps, vaginal bleeding, edema, jaundice, dark urine, clay-colored stools, dyspnea, blurred vision, numbness or stiffness in leg, chest pain
Progestins		
Medroxyprogestrone acetate	Nausea Contact lens intolerance	Management of abnormal uterine bleeding; prevent endometrial changes of estrogen replacement therapy, some cancers
Actions	Female hormones	
Indications	Contraceptives Treatment of menopausal symptoms Prevention of osteoporosis	
Adverse effects	Nausea Breakthrough bleeding Headache	
Nursing considerations	Client should know when to take medication and what to do for skipped doses Client should know when to contact prescribing health care provider (signs of thrombosis/thromboembolism) Contraindications: smoking, thrombophlebitis, cerebrovascular disease Some oral contraceptives can elevated blood glucose, so monitor, especially in prediabetic or already diagnosed diabetics	
Herbal	Black cohosh—relieves hot flashes; may increase hypotensive effect of antihypertensives; do not take for more than 6 months	

HERBAL SUPPLEMENTS		
SUPPLEMENT	ADVERSE EFFECTS/ CONTRAINDICATIONS	NURSING CONSIDERATIONS
IMMUNE SYSTEM		
Echinacea		
Immunostimulant, anti-inflammatory, antiviral, antibacterial Used to prevent and treat colds, flu, wound healing, urinary tract infections	Immune suppression, tingling sensation and/or unpleasant taste on tongue, nausea, vomiting, allergic reactions	Decreases effectiveness of immunosuppressants Contraindicated in autoimmune diseases Avoid if allergic to ragweed, members of daisy family of plants
Garlic		
Antimicrobial, antilipidemic, antithrombotic, antitumor, anti-inflammatory Used to reduce cholesterol, prevent atherosclerosis, cancer, stroke, and MI; decrease blood pressure, prevent and treat colds and flu	Flatulence, heartburn, halitosis, irritation of mouth, esophagus, stomach, allergic reaction Contraindicated with peptic ulcer, reflux	May potentiate anticoagulant and antiplatelets, antihyper-lipidemics, antihyper-tensives, antidiabetic agents, and herbs with these effects May decrease efficacy of cyclosporine, hormonal contraceptives Avoid if allergic to members of the lily family of plants
Ginseng		
Stimulant and tonic to immune and nervous systems Used to increase stamina, as aphrodisiac, adjunct chemotherapy and radiation therapy	Headache, insomnia, nervousness, palpitations, excitation, diarrhea, vaginal bleeding May cause headache, tremors, irritability, manic episodes if combined with MAOIs or caffeine	May falsely elevate digoxin levels; observe for signs usually associated with high digoxin levels May antagonize warfarin Potentiates antidiabetic agents, steroids, estrogens Caution with cardiovascular disease, hypotension, hypertension, steroid therapy
FEMALE REPRODUCTIVE SYSTEM		
Evening Primrose Oil		
Anti-inflammatory, sedative, astringent Used for premenstrual and menopausal problems, rheumatoid arthritis, elevated serum cholesterol, hypertension, eczema, diabetic neuropathy	Headache, rash, nausea, seizures, inflammation Contraindicated for clients with epilepsy, schizophrenia	May potentiate antiplatelet and anticoagulant meds Increases risk for seizures when taken with phenoth-iazines, antidepressants

HERBAL SUPPLEMENTS *(CONTINUED)*		
SUPPLEMENT	**ADVERSE EFFECTS/ CONTRAINDICATIONS**	**NURSING CONSIDERATIONS**
MUSCULOSKELETAL SYSTEM		
Chondroitin		
Collagen synthesis Used for arthritis for cartilage synthesis (with glucosamine)	Dyspepsia, nausea	May potentiate effects of anticoagulants
Glucosamine		
Collagen synthesis Used for arthritis for cartilage synthesis (with chondroitin)	Dyspepsia, nausea	May impede insulin secretion or increase resistance
NEUROLOGICAL SYSTEM		
Capsicum/Cayenne Pepper		
Analgesia, improves blood circulation Used for arthritis, bowel disorders, nerve pain, PAD, chronic laryngitis, personal self-defense spray	GI discomfort, burning pain in eyes, nose, mouth, blepharospasm and swelling in eyes, skin tissue irritation, cough, bronchospasm Avoid if allergic to ragweed or to chili pepper	May decrease effectiveness of antihypertensives, increases risk of cough with ACE inhibitors May potentiate antiplatelet and anticoagulant meds and herbs May cause hypertensive crisis with MAOIs Increases theophylline absorption
Feverfew		
Analgesic, antipyretic Used for migraine prophylaxis, fever, menstrual problems, arthritis	Mouth ulcers, heartburn, indigestion, dizziness, tachycardia, allergic reactions	Potentiates antiplatelet and anticoagulant meds Do not stop abruptly—causes moderate-to-severe pain with joint and muscle stiffness Caution if allergic to daisy family of plants
GASTROINTESTINAL SYSTEM		
Flaxseed		
Laxative, anticholes-teremic Used for constipation, decrease cholesterol, prevent atherosclerosis, colon disorders	Diarrhea, flatulence, nausea Contraindicated if client has strictures or acute GI inflam-mation	May decrease absorption of oral meds—do not take within 2 hours Immature flax seeds can be very toxic Increase fluids to minimize flatulence

HERBAL SUPPLEMENTS *(CONTINUED)*		
SUPPLEMENT	ADVERSE EFFECTS/ CONTRAINDICATIONS	NURSING CONSIDERATIONS
Ginger		
Antiemetic, antioxidant, digestive aid, anti-inflammatory Used for nausea, vomiting, indigestion, gas, lack of appetite	Minor heartburn, dermatitis Contraindicated with gallstones	May potentiate antiplatelet and anticoagulant meds, antidiabetic meds, herbs that increase bleeding times
Licorice		
Demulcent (soothes), expectorant, anti-inflammatory Used for coughs, colds, stomach pains, ulcers	Hypokalemia, headache, edema, lethargy, hypertension, heart failure (with overdose), cardiac arrest Contraindicated in renal or liver disease, heart disease, hypertension; caution with hormonal contraceptives	Decreases effect of spirono-lactone Avoid use with digoxin, loop diuretics, corticosteroids
GENITOURINARY SYSTEM		
Saw Palmetto		
Mild diuretic, urinary antiseptic Used for BPH, increasing sexual vigor, cystitis	Constipation, diarrhea, nausea, decreased libido, back pain	May interact with hormonal meds such as HRT and oral contraceptives May cause a false-negative PSA test result
PSYCHIATRIC		
Chamomile		
Sedative/hypnotic, anti-inflammatory, antispasmodic, anti-infective Used for stress, anxiety, insomnia, GI disorders	Allergic reactions, contact dermatitis, vomiting, depression	May potentiate sedatives and anticoagulants Avoid if allergic to ragweed, members of daisy family of plants
Kava		
Anti-anxiety, sedative/hypnotic, muscle relaxant Used for anxiety, insomnia, seizure disorders	Hepatotoxicity, psychological dependence, mild euphoria, fatigue, sedation, suicidal thoughts, visual problems, scaly skin reaction Contraindicated in Parkinson's, history of stroke, endogenous depression	May potentiate sedative effects of other sedating meds (benzodiazepines, barbiturates), anticonvulsants, and herbs (chamomile, valerian)
Melatonin		
Hormone from pineal gland Used for insomnia, jet lag	Headache, confusion, sedation, tachycardia	Potentiates CNS depressants May decrease effectiveness of immunosuppressants, Procardia

HERBAL SUPPLEMENTS *(CONTINUED)*		
SUPPLEMENT	**ADVERSE EFFECTS/ CONTRAINDICATIONS**	**NURSING CONSIDERATIONS**
St. John's wort		
Antidepressant, sedative effects, antiviral, antimicrobial Used for mild to moderate depression, sleep disorders, skin and wound healing	Photosensitivity, fatigue, allergic reactions, dry mouth, dizziness, restlessness, nausea Contraindicated for major depression, transplant recipients, clients taking SSRIs (increases risk of serotonin syndrome), MAOIs (increases risk of hypertensive crisis), hormonal contraceptives	Usually decreases effectiveness of (digoxin, antineoplastics, antiviral AIDS medications, anti-rejection medications, theophylline, warfarin, hormonal contraceptives May potentiate medications and herbs with sedative effects Should avoid tyramine in diet, OTC meds
Valerian		
Sedative/hypnotic, antispasmodic Used for insomnia, restlessness, anxiety	Headache, blurred vision, nausea, excitability Contraindicated in liver disease may be hepatotoxic	May potentiate other CNS depressant meds, antihist-amines, and sedating herbs
CARDIOVASCULAR SYSTEM		
Gingko		
Enhances cerebral and peripheral blood circulation; antide-pressive Used for dementia, short-term memory loss, vertigo, PADs, depression, sexual dysfunction (including from SSRIs)	Headache, GI upset, contact dermatitis, dizziness	May potentiate antiplatelet and anticoagulant meds, ASA, NSAIDS, and herbs, which increase bleeding time May potentiate MAOIs May decrease effectiveness of anticonvulsants
Hawthorn		
Antianginal, antiar-rhythmic, vasodilator, antihypertensive, antilipidemic Used for mild to moderate heart failure, hypertension, cholesterol reduction	Nausea, fatigue, sweating	May potentiate or interfere with wide range of cardio-vascular meds used for CHF, angina, arrhythmias, hypertension, vasodilation Potentiates digoxin Potentiates CNS depressants Avoid if allergic to members of the rose family of plants
RESPIRATORY SYSTEM		
Eucalyptus		
Decongestant, anti-inflammatory, antimi-crobial, antifungal Used for coughs, bronchitis, nasal congestion, sore muscles, wounds	Nausea, vomiting, epigastric burning, dizziness, muscle weakness, seizures Contraindicated with liver disease, inflammation of intestinal tract	Potentiates antidiabetic meds and possibly other herbs that cause hypoglycemia May increase metabolism of any medications metabolized in liver

MEDICATION INTERACTIONS WITH GRAPEFRUIT JUICE (INCREASED SERUM DRUG LEVELS)
Anti-anxiety: buspirone, midazolam, triazolam
Anti-dysrhythmic: Amiodarone
Anti-seizure: carmazepine
Calcium channel blockers: amlodipine, diltiazem, felodipine, nicardipine, nifedipine, nimodipine, nisoldipine, verapamil
Erectile dysfunction: sildenafil, tadalafil
Immunosupressants to prevent organ transplant rejection: cyclosporine, sirolimus, tacrolimus
SSRIs: fluoxetine, fluvoxamine, sertraline
Statins: lovastatin, simvastatin
Caffeine (stimulant)
Dextromethorphan(cough supressant)
Pimozide (Tourette's)
Praziquantel (shistosomiasis)

Chapter 17

TERMINOLOGY

Sections

1. Nursing Abbreviations

2. Medication Terminology

3. Terminology Used for Documentation

ABC	airway, breathing, circulation
abd.	abdomen
ABG	arterial blood gas
ABO	system of classifying blood groups
ac	before meals
ACE	angiotensin-converting enzyme
ACS	acute compartment syndrome
ACTH	adrenocorticotrophic hormone
ADL	activities of daily living
ADH	antidiuretic hormone
ad lib	freely, as desired
AFP	alpha-fetoprotein
AIDS	acquired immunodeficiency syndrome
AKA	above-knee amputation
ALL	acute lymphocytic leukemia
ALP	alkaline phosphatase (formerly SGPT)
ALS	amyotrophic lateral sclerosis
ALT	alanine aminotransferase
AMI	antibody-mediated immunity
AML	acute myelogenous leukemia
amt.	amount
ANA	antinuclear antibody
ANS	autonomic nervous system
AP	anteroposterior
A and P	anterior and posterior
APC	atrial premature contraction
aq.	water
ARDS	adult respiratory distress syndrome
ASD	atrial septal defect
ASHD	atherosclerotic heart disease
AST	aspartate aminotransferase (formerly SGOT)
ATP	adenosine triphosphate
AV	atrioventricular
BCG	Bacille Calmette-Guerin
bid	two times a day
BMR	basal metabolic rate

BKA	below-knee amputation
BLS	basic life support
BP	blood pressure
BPH	benign prostatic hyperplasia
bpm	beats per minute
BPR	bathroom privileges
BSA	body surface area
BUN	blood, urea, nitrogen
C and S	culture and sensitivity
C	centigrade, Celsius
$\bar{c}$	with
$\bar{C}a$	calcium
CA	cancer
cal	calorie(s)
CABG	coronary artery bypass graft
CAD	coronary artery disease
caps	capsules
CAPD	continuous ambulatory peritoneal dialysis
CBC	complete blood count
CBI	continuous bladder irrigation
CC	chief complaint
CCU	coronary care unit, critical care unit
CDC	Centers for Disease Control and Prevention
CHF	congestive heart failure
CK	creatine kinase
Cl	chloride
CLL	chronic lymphocytic leukemia
cm	centimeter
CMV	cytomegalovirus infection
CNS	central nervous system
CO	carbon monoxide, cardiac output
CO_2	carbon dioxide
comp	compound
cont	continuous
COPD	chronic obstructive pulmonary disease
CP	cerebral palsy
CPAP	continuous positive airway pressure
CPK	creatine phosphokinase
CPR	cardiopulmonary resuscitation
CRP	C-reactive protein
CSF	cerebrospinal fluid

CT	computerized tomography
CTD	connective tissue disease
CTS	carpal tunnel syndrome
cu	cubic
CVA	costovertebral angle
CVC	central venous catheter
CVP	central venous pressure
D and C	dilation and curettage
DIC	disseminated intravascular coagulation
dil.	dilute
DIFF	differential blood count
DJD	degenerative joint disease
DKA	diabetic ketoacidosis
dL	deciliter (100 mL)
DM	diabetes mellitus
DNA	deoxyribonucleic acid
DNR	do not resuscitate
DO	doctor of osteopathy
DOE	dyspnea on exertion
DTaP	vaccine for diphtheria, pertussis, tetanus
Dr.	doctor
D/W	dextrose in water
Dx	diagnosis
ECF	extracellular fluid
ECG or EKG	electrocardiogram
ECT	electroconvulsive therapy
ED	emergency department
EDD	estimated date of delivery
EEG	electroencephalogram
EMD	electromechanical dissociation
EMG	electromyography
ENT	ear, nose, and throat
ESR	erythrocyte sedimentation rate
ESRD	end-stage renal disease
ET	endotracheal tube
F	Fahrenheit
4 × 4	piece of gauze 4″ by 4″ used for dressings
FBD	fibrocystic breast disease
FDA	Food and Drug Administration
FFP	fresh frozen plasma
FBS	fasting blood sugar

fl	fluid
FHR	fetal heart rate
FM	fetal movement
FSH	follicle-stimulating hormone
ft	foot, feet (unit of measure)
FUO	fever of undetermined origin
g, gm	gram
GB	gall bladder
GFR	glomerular filtration rate
GH	growth hormone
GI	gastrointestinal
gr	grain
GSC	Glasgow coma scale
gtts	drops
GU	genitourinary
GYN	gynecological
(H)	hypodermically
Hb or Hgb	hemoglobin
h or hr	hour(s)
hCG	human chorionic gonadotropin
HCO_3	bicarbonate
Hct	hematocrit
HD	hemodialysis
HDL	high-density lipoproteins
Hg	mercury
Hgb	hemoglobin
HGH	human growth hormone
HHNC	hyperglycemia hyperosmolar nonketotic coma
HIV	human immunodeficiency virus
HLA	human leukocyte antigen
hPL	human placental lactogen
HR	heart rate
hr	hour
H_2O	water
HSV	herpes simplex virus
HTN	hypertension
Hx	history
Hz	hertz (cycles/second)
I and O	intake and output
IAPB	intra-aortic balloon pump
IBS	irritable bowel syndrome

ICF	intracellular fluid
ICP	increased intracranial pressure
ICS	intercostal space
ICU	intensive care unit
ID	intradermal
IDDM	insulin-dependent diabetes mellitus
IgA	immunoglobulin A
IM	intramuscular
in	inch(es)
IOP	increased intraocular pressure
IPG	impedance plethysmogram
IPPB	intermittent positive-pressure breathing
IU	international unit
IUD	intrauterine device
IV	intravenous
IVC	intraventricular catheter
IVP	intravenous pyelogram
JRA	juvenile rheumatoid arthritis
K+	potassium
kcal	kilocalorie (food calorie)
kg	kilogram
KO, KVO	keep vein open
KS	Kaposi's sarcoma
KUB	kidneys, ureters, bladder
L	liter
lab	laboratory
lb	pound
LBBB	left bundle branch block
LDH	lactate dehydrogenase
LDL	low-density lipoproteins
LE	lupus erythematosus
LH	luteinizing hormone
liq	liquid
LLQ	left lower quadrant
LOC	level of consciousness
LP	lumbar puncture
LPN, LVN	licensed practical or vocational nurse
Lt	left
LTC	long-term care
LUQ	left upper quadrant
LV	left ventricle

m	minum, meter, micron
MAO	monoamine oxidase inhibitors
MAST	military antishock trousers
mcg	microgram
MCH	mean corpuscular hemoglobin
MCV	mean corpuscular volume
MD	muscular dystrophy
M.D.	medical doctor
MDI	metered dose inhaler
mEq	milliequivalent
Mg	magnesium
mg	milligram
MG	myasthenia gravis
MI	myocardial infarction
min	minute(s)
mL	milliliter
mm	millimeter
MMR	vaccine for measles, mumps, rubella
mo	month(s)
MRI	magnetic resonance imaging
MS	multiple sclerosis
MRSA	methicillin-resistant *S. aureus*
N	nitrogen, normal (strength of solution)
NIDDM	non-insulin-dependent diabetes mellitus
Na$^+$	sodium
NaCl	sodium chloride
NANDA	North American Nursing Diagnosis Association
NG	nasogastric
NGT	nasogastric tube
NLN	National League for Nursing
noc	at night
NPO	nothing by mouth
NS	normal saline
NSAIDS	nonsteroidal anti-inflammatory drugs
NSNA	National Student Nurses' Association
NST	non-stress test
O$_2$	oxygen
OB-GYN	obstetrics and gynecology
OCT	oxytocin challenge test
OD	right eye
OOB	out of bed

OPC	outpatient clinic
OR	operating room
$\overline{o}\,\overline{s}$	by mouth
OS	left eye
OSHA	Occupational Safety and Health Administration
OT	occupational therapy
OTC	over the counter (drug that can be obtained without a prescription)
OU	both eyes
oz	ounce
$\overline{p}$	after
P	pulse, pressure, phosphorus
PA Chest	posterior-anterior chest x-ray
PAC	premature atrial complexes
$PaCO_2$	partial pressure of carbon dioxide in arterial blood
PaO_2	partial pressure of oxygen in arterial blood
PAD	peripheral artery disease
Pap	Papanicolaou smear
PAT	paroxysmal atrial tachycardia
pc	after meals
PCA	patient-controlled analgesia
PCO_2	partial pressure of carbon dioxide
PCP	*Pneumocystis carinii* pneumonia
PD	peritoneal dialysis
PDA	patent ductus arteriosis
PE	pulmonary embolism
PEEP	positive end-expiratory pressure
PERRLA	pupils equal, round, react to light and accommodation
PET	postural emission tomography
PFT	pulmonary function tests
pH	hydrogen ion concentration
PICC	peripherally inserted central catheter
PID	pelvic inflammatory disease
PIH	pregnancy-induced hypertension
PKD	polycystic disease
PKU	phenylketonuria
PMI	point of maximal impulse
PMS	premenstrual syndrome
PN	parenteral nutrition
PND	paroxysmal nocturnal dyspnea
PO	by mouth

PO$_2$	partial pressure of oxygen
PPD	positive purified protein derivative (of tuberculin)
PPN	partial parenteral nutrition
PRN, prn	as needed, whenever necessary
pro time	prothrombin time
PSA	prostate-specific antigen
psi	pounds per square inch
PT	physical therapy, prothrombin time
PTCA	percutaneous transluminal coronary angioplasty
PTH	parathyroid hormone
PTT	partial thromboplastin time
PUD	peptic ulcer disease
PVC	premature ventricular contraction
$\overline{p}\ \overline{c}$	after meals
PSP	phenol-sulfonphthalein
q	every
QA	quality assurance
q 2 hours	every two hours
q 4 hours	every four hours
qid	four times a day
qs	quantity sufficient
R	rectal temperature, respirations, roentgen
RA	rheumatoid arthritis
RAI	radioactive iodine
RAIU	radioactive iodine uptake
RAS	reticular activating system
RBBB	right bundle branch block
RBC	red blood cell or count
RCA	right coronary artery
RDA	recommended dietary allowance
resp	respirations
RF	rheumatic fever, rheumatoid factor
Rh	antigen on blood cell indicated by + or −
RIND	reversible ischemic neurologic deficit
RLQ	right lower quadrant
RN	registered nurse
RNA	ribonucleic acid
R/O	rule out, to exclude
ROM	range of motion (of joint) or rupture of membranes
Rt	right
RUQ	right upper quadrant

Rx	prescription
s̄	without
s	second(s) (unit of measure)
S. or Sig.	(Signa) to write on label
SA	sinoatrial node
SaO$_2$	systemic arterial oxygen saturation (%)
sat sol	saturated solution
SBE	subacute bacterial endocarditis
SDA	same-day admission
SDS	same-day surgery
sed rate	sedimentation rate
SI	International System of Units
SIADH	syndrome of inappropriate antidiuretic hormone
SIDS	sudden infant death syndrome
SL	sublingual
SLE	systemic lupus erythematosus
SOB	short of breath
sol	solution
SMBG	self-monitoring blood glucose
SMR	submucous resection
spec.	specimen
sp gr	specific gravity
SS	soap suds
SSKI	saturated solution of potassium iodide
stat	immediately
STI	sexually transmitted infection
Syr.	syrup
T	temperature, thoracic (to be followed by the number designating specific thoracic vertebra)
T and A	tonsillectomy and adenoidectomy
tabs	tablets
TB	tuberculosis
T and C	type and cross-match
TED	antiembolitic stockings
temp	temperature
TENS	transcutaneous electrical nerve stimulation
TIA	transient ischemic attack
TIBC	total iron-binding capacity
tid	three times a day
tinct	tincture
TMJ	temporomandibular joint

t-PA	tissue plasminogen activator
TPR	temperature, pulse, respiration
TQM	total quality management
TSE	testicular self-examination
TSH	thyroid-stimulating hormone
tsp	teaspoon
TSS	toxic shock syndrome
TURP	transuretheral prostatectomy
UA	urinalysis
ung	ointment
URI	upper respiratory tract infection
UTI	urinary tract infection
VAD	venous access device
VDRL	Veneral Disease Research Laboratory (test for syphilis)
VF, Vfib	ventricular fibrillation
vol	volume
VPC	ventricular premature complexes
VS	vital signs
VSD	ventricular septal defect
VTE	venous thromboembolism
WBC	white blood cell or count
WHO	World Health Organization
wk	week(s)
wt	weight
y	years(s)

Do not use	Use instead
U, u	unit
Q.D., QD, q.d., qd,	daily
Q.O.D., QOD, q.o.d., qod	every other day
MS, MSO4, MgSO4	morphine or magnesium sulfate
http://www.jointcommission.org/assets/1/18/Do_Not_Use_List.pdf	

Action	Description of the method of how a medication works.
Adverse effects	Actions of a medication other than that for which it was given. Adverse effects may or may not be harmful to the person, and may or may not require a lowering of the dosage or discontinuance of the medication.
Ampoule	Sealed, sterile glass container containing one dose of medication. May be in liquid form or powders that must be diluted.
Aqueous solution	One or more substances dissolved in water or alcohol. Solutions are translucent and do not have to be shaken.
Aqueous suspension	An insoluble drug in hydrated form. Must be shaken before pouring.
Capsules	Gelatin containers for medications which may be plain or enteric coated. Plain capsules dissolve in the stomach. Enteric capsules dissolve in the small intestines.
Disposable plastic syringe	Equipment used for injections consisting of plunger inserted into abarrel, which contains a needle. All parts of the syringe except the outside of the barrel, handle of the plunger, and needle cap are considered sterile.
Elixirs	Aromatic, sweetened beverages containing alcohol used as a flavoring vehicle.
Emulsion	Suspension of fat or oil in water.
Enteric-coated capsules	Tablets that dissolve in the alkaline secretions of the intestines rather than the acid secretions of the stomach. This prevents gastric irritation and protects the medication from being inactivated by stomach acid.
Extracts	Concentrated preparations of vegetable or animal medications that contain the active ingredients of the medication. They can be liquid or pills.
Generic name	Official name of the medication which is never changed and is used in all countries. It relates to the chemical formula and is the name under which the medication is listed in official publications. A medication can have several trade names, but only one generic name.
Lotion	Liquid suspension intended for external use on the skin.
Nursing implications	Actions of the nurse related to the administration of a medication.
Ointment	Semisolid preparation of a medication in a vaseline or lanolin base intended for external use, but may penetrate the skin. They are used for their soothing, astringent, or bacteriostatic effects.
Paste	Ointment-like preparation that tends to absorb secretions. They soften and penetrate the skin less than ointments.
Pills	Globular, oval, or flattened materials containing a mixture of a medication with some cohesive material.
Powders	Fine particles of solid medications.
Route	Method of administration of a medication, i.e. IM (intramuscular), IV (intravenous), SQ or SC (subcutaneous), topical, PO (oral), intradermal, SL (sublingual).
Spansule	Timed release capsule that contains small particles of the medication coated with materials that take varying amounts of time to dissolve. This prolongs action for as long as 24 hours.

Spirits	Concentrated, alcoholic solutions of volatile substances. The dissolved substances may be solid, liquid, or gases.
Suppository	Mixture of a medication in a firm base that is molded so it can be inserted into a body cavity, i.e. rectum, vagina, urethra.
Syrup	Aqueous solution of sucrose or sugar. It is added to a medication to disguise an unpleasant taste, or soothe mucous membranes.
Tablets	Powdered medications that are compressed or molded into shape. When they are scored, i.e., have lines drawn in them, they may be broken along the line, otherwise they must be given whole.
Teaching about medications	Patients should be taught: how to administer the medication, the proper dosage and frequency of the medication, how the medication works, possible adverse effects, and signs of effectiveness of the medication.
Tincture	Alcoholic or hydroalcoholic solutions usually prepared from plants or chemical substances.
Toxic effects	Untoward or severe nontherapeutic effects of the medication, which are dangerous to the person and require the medication to be discontinued immediately or the dosage lowered.
Trade name	Brand name or registered trademark of a medication used by the manufacturer. Medications can have several trade names, depending on which company which manufactures the medication.
Troches or lozenges	Flat, round, or rectangular mediation which are held in the mouth until they dissolve. They are usually used for their local soothing effect, but may cause a systemic effect.
Uses	Medical diagnoses for which a medication is administered.
Vials	Glass containers with rubber stoppers that contain multiple doses of medication. Powders in vials are diluted with either sterile water or sterile saline.

TERMINOLOGY USED FOR DOCUMENTATION

TERM	DEFINITION
abduction	to move away from the midline
abraded	scraped
acetonuria	acetone in the urine
adduction	to move toward the midline
afebrile	without fever
albuminuria	albumin in the urine
ambulatory	walking
amenorrhea	absence of menstruation
amnesia	loss or defective memory
ankyloses	stiff joint
anorexia	loss of appetite
anuria	total suppression of urination
apnea	short periods when breathing has ceased
arthritis	inflammation of joint
asphyxia	suffocation
atrophy	wasting
auscultation, auscultate	to listen for sounds
bradycardia	heartbeat less than 60 beats per minute
Cheyenne-Stokes respirations	increasing dyspnea with periods of apnea
choluria	bile in the urine
clonic tremor	shaking with intervals of rest
conjunctivitis	inflammation of conjunctiva
coryza	watery drainage from nose
cyanotic	bluish in color due to poor oxygenation
defecation	bowel movement
dental caries	decay of the teeth
dentures	false teeth
diarrhea	excessive or frequent defecation
diplopia	double vision
distended	appears swollen
diuresis	large amount of urine voided
dorsal recumbent	lying on back, knees flexed and apart
dysmenorrhea	painful menstruation
dyspnea	difficulty breathing

TERM	DEFINITION
dysrhythmia, arrhythmia	abnormal heart rhythm
dysuria	painful urination
edematous	puffy, swollen
emaciated	thin, underweight
emetic	agent given to produce vomiting
enuresis	bedwetting
epistaxis	nosebleed
eructation	belching
erythema	redness
eupnea	normal breathing
excoriation	raw surface
exophthalmos	abnormal protrusion of eyeball
extension	to straighten
fatigued	tired
feigned	pretended
fetid	foul
fixed	motionless
flaccid	soft, flabby
flatus, flatulence	gas in the digestive tract
flexion	bending
flushed	pink or hot
Fowler position	semi-erect, knee flexed, head of bed elevated 45-60°
gavage	forced feeding through tube passed into stomach
glossy	shiny
glycosuria	glucose in the urine
guaiac	test for occult blood
gustatory	dealing with taste
heliotherapy	using sunlight as a therapeutic agent
hematemesis	blood in vomitus
hematuria	blood in the urine
hemiplegia	paralysis of one side of the body
hemoglobinuria	hemoglobin in the urine
hemoptysis	spitting of blood
horizontal	flat
hydrotherapy	using water as a therapeutic agent
hyperpnea	rapid breathing
hypertonic	concentration greater than body fluids
hypotonic	concentration less than body fluids
infrequent	not often

TERM	DEFINITION
insomnia	inability to sleep
instillation	pouring into a body cavity
intermittent	starting and stopping, not continuous
intradermal	within or through the skin
intramuscular	within or through the muscle
intraspinal	within or through the spinal canal
intravenous	within or through the vein
involuntary, incontinent	unable to control bladder or bowels
isotonic	having the same tonicity or concentration as body fluids
jack-knife position	prone with hips over break in table and feet below level of head
jaundice	yellow color
knee-chest position	in face down position resting on knees and chest
kyphosis	hump back, concavity of spine
labored	difficult, requires an effort
lacerated	torn, broken
lateral position	on the side, knees flexed
lithotomy position	on back, buttocks near edge of table, knees well flexed and separated
lochia	drainage from the vagina after delivery
lordosis	sway back convexity of spine
manipulation, manipulate	to handle
menopause	cessation of menstruation
menorrhagia	profuse menstruation
metrorrhagia	variable amount of uterine bleeding occurring at frequent but irregular intervals
moist	wet
monoplegia	paralysis of one limb
mucopurulent	drainage containing mucus and pus
mydriasis	dilation of pupil
myopia	near-sightedness
myosis	contraction of pupil
nausea	desire to vomit
necrosis	death of tissue
nocturia	frequent voiding at night
obese	overweight
objective	able to document other than by observation
oliguria	scant urination, less than 400 mL in 24 hours
orthopnea	inability to breath or difficulty breathing lying down
palliative	offering temporary relief
pallor	pale

TERM	DEFINITION
palpation, palpate	to feel with hands or fingers
paraplegia	paralysis of legs
paroxysm	spasms or convulsive seizure
paroxysmal	coming in seizures
pediculi, pediculosis	lice
percussion, percuss	to strike
persistent	lasting over a long time
petechia	small rupture of blood vessels
photophobia	sensitive to light
photosensitivity	skin reaction caused by exposure to sunlight
pigmented	containing color
polyuria	increased amount of voiding
profuse, copious	large amount
projectile	ejected or projected some distance
pronation	to turn downward
prone	on abdomen, face turned to one side
prophylactic	preventative
protruding	extends outward
pruritus	itching
ptosis	drooping eyelid
purulent	drainage containing pus
pyrexia	elevated temperature
pyuria	pus in the urine
radiating	spreads to distant areas
radiotherapy	using x-ray or radium as a therapeutic agent
rales, crackles	abnormal breath sounds
rapid	quickly
rotation	to move in circular pattern
sanguineous	bloody drainage
scanty	small amount
semi-Fowler position	semi-erect, head of bed elevated 30-45°
serous	drainage of lymphatic fluid
Sim's position	on left side, left arm behind back, left leg slightly flexed, right leg slightly flexed
sprain	wrenching of joint
stertorous	snoring
stethoscope	instrument used for auscultation
strabismus	squinting
stuporous	partial unconsciousness
subcutaneous	under the skin

TERM	DEFINITION
subjective	observed
sudden onset	started all at once
superficial	on the surface only
supination	to turn upward
suppurating	discharging pus
syncope	fainting
syndrome	group of symptoms
tachycardia	fast heartbeat, greater than 100 beats per minute
tenacious	tough and sticky
thready	barely perceptible
tonic tremor	continuous shaking
Trendelenburg position	flat on back with pelvis higher than head, foot of bed elevated 6 inches
tympanic, tympanites	bell-like, resonant, distention of abdomen due to presence of gas or air in intestine or peritoneal cavity
urticaria	hives or wheals, eruption on skin or mucous membranes
vertigo	dizziness
vesicle	fluid-filled blister
visual acuity	sharpness of vision
void, micturate	to urinate or pass urine

INDEX

A

Abdominal assessment, 14
  liver function testing, 236
  neonates, 464
  preparation, 6
Abdominal hernia, 266
Abdominal respiration, 8, 165
Abdominoperineal resection, 253
Abortion
  history in prenatal assessment, 443
  spontaneous, 468, 469, 470*t*
Abruptio placentae, 470
Abuse
  of persons, 579–581
  of substances (*See* Alcohol abuse; Substance abuse)
Accommodation disorders, 381*t*
ACE. *See* Angiotensin-converting enzyme (ACE) inhibitors
Acetaminophen overdose, 512
Acne vulgaris, 62
Acoustic meatus, 389, 389*f*
Acoustic neuroma, 363
Acquired human immunodeficiency syndrome. *See* AIDS
Acromegaly, 275, 276*t*
Activities of daily living (ADL), guidelines, 28
Activity, physiological need for, 24
Acute drug psychosis, 566
Acute epiglottitis, 177–178
Acute kidney injury, 310
Acute laryngotracheobronchitis, 177
Acute leukemia, 407
Acute otitis media, 391–392
Acute pancreatitis, 247
Acute pulmonary edema, myocardial infarction, 133
Acyanotic heart anomalies, 520*t*, 521
ADC (AIDS-dementia complex), 194
Addiction, management of, 576–577, 578*t*
Addison's disease, 280–281, 285*t*
Adenoma, pituitary, 275
Adenomastectomy, 430

ADHD. *See* Attention deficit hyperactivity disorder
ADH (antidiuretic hormone) deficiencies, 277, 278*t*
ADL (activities of daily living), guidelines, 28
Adolescence
  growth and development in, 493–495, 494*t*
  immunization schedule, 51*t*–52*t*, 503*t*–508*t*
  physical examinations, 501
  pregnancy in, 468
  psychosocial issues, 535, 536*t*
  safety issues, 33
Adrenal gland disorders, 280–286
  Addison's disease, 280–281, 285*t*
  Cushing's disease, 281, 283–284, 285*t*
  medications, 282*t*, 283*t*, 286*t*
Adrenocortical hypofunction, 280
Adrenocortical medications, 588*t*–589*t*
Adulthood (developmental phase), 495–497, 496*t*, 497*t*
Adventitious lung sounds, 12, 165
African-American clients, nutritional intake of, 206
Afterload, cardiac output, 108
Afterpains, 460
AIDS (acquired human immunodeficiency syndrome), 193–196, 196*t*
  medications, 196*t*
  in pregnancy, 468
AIDS-dementia complex (ADC), 194
Airway resistance, 163
Al-Anon, 576
Alcohol abuse, 574–576
  congenital malformations and, 521
  intoxication, 574, 574*t*
  neonatal complications, 475
  withdrawal, 575, 575*t*
Alcoholics Anonymous, 574
Alimentary canal, 203
Alkylating antineoplastic medications, 401*t*

Allergies, 197
  antihistamine medications, 607*t*–608*t*
Alpha-1 adrenergic blockers, 316*t*, 617*t*
Alpha radiation, 398
5-Alpha-reductase inhibitor, 316*t*
Altered thought processes, 565–571, 566*t*
  medications, 568*t*–571*t*
Alternative/complementary therapies
  herbal supplements, 339*t*, 558*t*, 600*t*, 664*t*–667*t*
  menopause, 421
  Parkinson's disease, 374
  perioperative care, 65
  radiation therapy, 398
  seizure management, 353
  skin cancer, 409
Alveolar ventilation, 163
Alzheimer's disease, 377–378
Ambulation, rehabilitation for, 25–29, 26*t*
Amenorrhea, 420
American Cancer Society warning signs, 397
Amino acids, nutrition and, 208
Aminoglycosides, 608*t*
Amniocentesis, 467
Amnion, 437
Amputation, 329–331, 330*t*
Amylase, 236
Amyotrophic lateral sclerosis, 368–369
Analgesia
  labor and delivery, 452, 453, 453*t*
  opioid analgesics, 659*t*
Anal phase of development, 488
Anaphylaxis medications, 150*t*–151*t*, 586*t*–587*t*
Anderson tube, 253
Anemia
  hemolytic, 197, 478
  iron-deficiency anemia, 186–188
  megaloblastic, 189
  pernicious anemia, 212, 218
Anesthesia

intraoperative care, 66, 66*t*
labor and delivery, 452, 453*t*
Angina pectoris, 135–137, 136*f*
medications, 137*t*, 656*t*–657*t*
Angiotensin-converting enzyme
(ACE) inhibitors heart failure,
130
table of, 616*t*–617*t*
Angiotensin-receptor blockers
(ARBs)
heart failure management, 130
table of, 616*t*
Angle of Louis, 13
Anisocytosis, 186
Ankylosing spondylitis, 333
Antacids, 590*t*
Antepartal care, 437–446
Anthropoid pelvis, 420
Antianginals, 137*t*, 656*t*–657*t*
Antianxiety medications,
546*t*–547*t*, 591*t*–592*t*
Antibacterials, 615*t*
Antibiotics, 608*t*
See also Anti-infective
medications
antitumor, 402*t*, 622*t*–623*t*
Antibodies, 197
Anticancer medications
antineoplastic medications,
401*t*–405*t*, 622*t*–627*t*
chemotherapy, 398, 401*t*, 408,
409
side effects, 627*t*
Anticholinergic medications,
592*t*–593*t*
Anticoagulant medications,
138*t*–139*t*, 593*t*–594*t*
Anticonvulsant medications,
349*t*–351*t*, 594*t*–596*t*
Antidepressant medications, 558*t*,
596*t*–600*t*
Antidiabetic medications, 272,
600*t*–602*t*
Antidiarrheal medications, 260*t*,
603*t*
Antidiuretic hormone (ADH)
deficiencies, 277, 278*t*
Antidysrhythmics, 121*t*
Antiemetic medications, 227*t*, 605*t*
Antifungal medications, 606*t*
Antigens, 197
prostate-specific, 433
Antigout medications, 335*t*, 607*t*
Antihistamine medications,
607*t*–608*t*
Antihypertensive medications,
144*t*–145*t*, 616*t*–620*t*
Anti-infective medications,
608*t*–616*t*
Antilipemic medications, 621*t*–622*t*

Antimetabolites, antineoplastic
medications, 401*t*, 622*t*
Antineoplastic medications,
401*t*–405*t*, 622*t*–627*t*
Antiparkinson medications,
627*t*–628*t*
Antiplatelet medications, 629*t*
Antipsychotic medications,
568*t*–569*t*, 630*t*–632*t*
Antipyretic medications, 633*t*
Antiretroviral medications, 195,
196*t*
Antirheumatic medications,
643*t*–644*t*
Antithyroid medications, 634*t*
Antituberculotics medications, 180*t*,
635*t*–636*t*
Antitumor antibiotics, 402*t*,
622*t*–623*t*
Antitussive/expectorant
medications, 636*t*
Antiviral medications, 637*t*–638*t*
Anus
functional assessment, 251
physical assessment, 15
Anxiety, 541–547
assessment of, 541–542
coping mechanisms for, 543*t*,
544*t*
disorders, 543*t*
medications, 546*t*–547*t*
nursing interventions in, 542,
545*t*
Aortic stenosis, 522
Apgar score, 456, 456*t*
Apical rate, neonatal assessment,
463
Apnea
defined, 165
physical assessment, 8
Appendicitis, 261
ARBs. See Angiotensin-receptor
blockers
Arterial blood pressure, intravenous
therapy and, 91
Arterial peripheral vascular disease,
154–155
Arteries, 107
Arthritis
juvenile rheumatoid, 329
medications, 643*t*–644*t*
osteoarthritis, 319, 333–334
rheumatoid, 197, 331–332
Ascending colon, 251
Ascending colostomy, 254, 254*f*
ASD (atrial septal defect), 521
Aspirin, poisoning from, 511–512
Asthma, 171
Athlete's foot, 61
Atria, anatomy, 104
Atrial catheters, 222

Atrial dysrhythmias, 114*f*
Atrial fibrillation, 116, 116*f*
Atrial flutter, 115, 115*f*
Atrial septal defect (ASD), 521
Atrial tachycardia, 114, 114*f*
Atrioventricular (AV) node, 106,
106*f*
Atrioventricular valves, 104
Atrophic vaginitis, 426
Atrophy, skin, 59
Attention deficit hyperactivity
disorder (ADHD), 360
medications, 362*t*, 638*t*–639*t*
Auditory canal, 389, 389*f*
Auricle, anatomy and physiology,
389, 389*f*
Auscultation
pediatric assessment, 500
physical assessment, 7
Autistic thinking, 566
Autoimmune diseases, 197
Autonomic dysreflexia, spinal cord
injury, 366
Autonomic nervous system, cardiac
function, 107–108
Autosomal defects, 497
AV (atrioventricular) node, 106,
106*f*
Avulsion injuries, 322

B

Babinski's sign, 465
Balanced suspension, 324, 326*f*
Ballottement, physical assessment,
6
Barium enema, 219, 252
Barium swallow, 218
Basal cell carcinoma, 409
Basal ganglia, 343*f*, 344
Baths, therapeutic, 53, 54*t*
Battle's sign, 363
Bell's palsy, 361–362
Bend fracture, 529
Benign prostatic hyperplasia/
hypertrophy (BPH), 309, 433
Beriberi, 211
Beta-adrenergic blockers, 130,
617*t*–618*t*
Beta radiation, 398
Biliary atresia, 246
Biliary carcinoma, 246
Biliary tract
anatomy and function, 235
disorders of, 244–247
Billroth I and II surgical procedures,
231
Biophysical profile, fetal
assessment, 467
Biopsies
female reproductive system, 425

liver, 239
testicular, 432
Bipolar disorder, 559–563
    medications, 562*t*, 639*t*–640*t*
Birth asphyxia, 475
Birthmarks, 463
Bisphosphonates, bone-resorption
        inhibitors, 640*t*
Bladder
    anatomy and physiology, 298
    urinary retention, 301
Bleeding, in pregnancy, 469–471
Blindness, 383
Blood components, 94*t*, 183
    in pregnancy, 441
    transfusion reactions, 197
Blood disorders, 185–192
Blood group compatibility, 94*t*
Blood pressure, 9
    cardiac function, 107
    intravenous therapy and, 91
    neonatal assessment, 463
    pediatric assessment, 502
Blood tests
    glucose monitoring, 271
    nutritional assessment, 217, 218*t*
Blood transfusions, 93–95, 197
Blood vessels
    congenital malformations, 475,
        522
    coronary, 104, 104*f*
    medications affecting, 620*t*
    pregnancy, 437
Body structure and function,
        maintenance and promotion,
        23–24
Bone
    diseases, 331–339
    fractures, 321, 322*f*, 529–530
    graft, low back pain, 320
Bone resorption inhibitors, 640*t*
Boredom, prevention of, 30
Boston brace, 531
Bowel disorders, 257–266
    abdominal hernia, 266
    appendicitis, 261
    celiac disease, 260
    constipation, 257, 258*t*
    diarrhea, 259
    diverticular disease, 264
    ileitis, 262
    intestinal obstruction, 265
    malabsorption syndrome, 259
    Meckel's diverticulum, 262
    necrotizing enterocolitis, 480
    neonatal assessment, 464
    peritonitis, 261–262
    postpartum period, 460
    ulcerative colitis, 263–264
Bowel surgery, 253–256, 254*f*

BPH (benign prostatic hyperplasia/
        hypertrophy), 309, 433
Braces, scoliosis, 530
Brachytherapy, 399
Brain
    abscess, 372
    anatomy and function, 343–346,
        345*f*
    organic brain syndrome, 357–359
Brain stem, 345
Breastfeeding, 459, 460*t*
    breast-milk jaundice, 479
Breasts
    anatomy and function, 420
    cancer of, 430
    hypoplasia/hyperplasia, 429
    infections, 430
    physical assessment, 14
    postpartum care, 459–460
    in pregnancy, 440
    problems related to, 426
Breathing patterns
    See also Respiration
    alterations, 165–180
    definitions, 165
    normal, 162
    physical assessment, 8
Breath sounds, 166*t*
Breech presentation, 447
Bronchitis, chronic, 171
Bronchodilators, 173*t*–174*t*, 177,
        640*t*–641*t*
Bronchodilators/mucolytic
        medications, 172
Brudzinski's sign, 371
Buckle fracture, 529
Buck's traction, 324, 324*f*
Bundle branch block, 118
Bundle of His, 106
Burn management, 95–100,
        99*t*–100*t*
    burn classifications, 97*t*
    eyes, 382, 382*t*
Bursitis, 335

C
Calcium
    imbalances, 83–84
    preparations, 337*t*
Calcium channel blockers,
        618*t*–619*t*
Caloric requirements, adult, 217
Cancer, 397–405
    See also specific types of cancer,
        e.g.: Leukemia
    antineoplastic medications,
        401*t*–405*t*, 622*t*–627*t*
    assessment, 397
    chemotherapy, 398, 401*t*, 623*t*
    classifications, 398

etiology, 397–398
    overview, 397–405
Candida albicans
    AIDS clients, 194
    vaginal infection, 425
Cantor tube, 253
Capillaries, 107
Captopril, 130
Caput succedaneum, 464
Carbamazepine, 562*t*
Carbohydrates, 207–208, 217
Carbonic anhydrase inhibitors, 641*t*
Carcinoma, larynx, 415–416
Cardiac arrest, medications for,
        150*t*–151*t*, 586*t*–587*t*
Cardiac conduction system,
        105–106
Cardiac cycle, 106
Cardiac decompensation, 127
Cardiac disease, in pregnancy, 474
Cardiac disturbances, 110–112, 112*f*
Cardiac function
    anatomy of cardiovascular
        system, 103–104, 103*f*
    angina pectoris, 135–137
    basic principles, 105–106
    heart failure, 124–132
    myocardial infarction, 132–135
Cardiac glycosides, 128–129,
        128*t*–129*t*, 642*t*
Cardiac medications, 135*t*
Cardiac output, 108
    alterations, 109–139
    disturbances, 110–112
    rhythm disturbances, 112–124
Cardiac reserve, 106
Cardiac workload, prevention of
        increase in, 30
Cardiogenic shock, 147
Cardiopulmonary arrest, 109–110
Cardiovascular system
    anatomy, 103–104, 103*f*
    cardiac function, 105–106, 106*f*
    postoperative care, 67
    vascular system, 107–108
Cardioversion, 122, 123*t*
Carvedilol, 130
Casting
    fractures, 327
    hip spica cast, 528, 529*f*
    scoliosis, 531
Cataracts, 385
Catatonic schizophrenia, 566, 566*t*
Catheterization
    total parenteral nutrition, 222
    urinary, 303–304, 303*t*
CCT/OCT (contraction/stress test),
        468
Cecum, 251
Celiac disease, 260

Cellular differentiation, cancer and, 397

Centrally-acting alpha-adrenergics, 619*t*

Central nervous system (CNS), 343–346, 344*f*
  alcohol-related disorders, 575*t*

Central venous access devices (CVADs), 92–93

Central venous pressure, fluid volume imbalance, 73, 74*f*

Cephalhematoma, 464

Cephalic/vertex presentation, 447

Cephalosporins, 609*t*

Cerebellum
  anatomy and function, 344*f*, 346
  physical assessment, 14

Cerebral palsy, 525–526

Cerebral spinal fluid (CSF), 345

Cerebrum, 344, 344*f*

Cervical traction (skull tongs), 325, 325*f*

Cervix
  anatomy and function, 419
  biopsy, 425
  infections, 426
  labor and delivery, 450
  in pregnancy, 440
  problems of, 431

Cesium radiation, 399

Chemical digestive process, 204

Chemoreceptors
  cardiac function, 107
  respiration, 164

Chemotherapy
  See also Antineoplastic medications
  cancer, 398, 401*t*
  leukemia, 408
  skin cancer, 409
  tuberculosis, 179

Chest physiotherapy, 172

Chest tubes, 174, 175*f*

Chest x-ray, for tuberculosis, 178

Cheyne-Stokes respirations, 9, 165

Child abuse, 579

Childbearing, 437–446
  labor and delivery, 447–457
  maternal complications, 467–474
  neonatal complications, 475–483
  postpartum care guidelines, 459–461

Child development
  See also Pediatric assessment; *stages of childhood, e.g.:* Infancy, Toddlers, etc.
  nursing management guidelines, 35*t*
  safety factors and, 33
  skin disorders and, 58

Chinese clients, nutritional intake of, 207

Choking, emergency care, 166–167

Cholangiogram, 236

Cholecystectomy, laparoscopic, 245

Cholecystitis, 244

Cholecystokinin, 204

Cholelithiasis, 242, 244

Cholesterol-lowering medications, 621*t*–622*t*

Chorion, 437

Chorionic villus sampling (CVS), 467

Choroid, anatomy and function, 379

Chromosomes, 437, 497

Chronic bronchitis, 171

Chronic kidney disease, 311

Chronic leukemia, 407

Chronic obstructive pulmonary disease (COPD), 171–174

Chronic pancreatitis, 248

Chronic venous insufficiency, 157

Chvostek's sign, 288, 291

Circulatory physiology
  anatomy, 103–104, 103*f*
  intravenous therapy, 90–92
  pregnancy, 438

Circumcision, 466

Cirrhosis, 239–241

Cleft lip and palate, 515–516, 516*f*

Client placement, infection control and, 45

Clitoris, 419

Clonidine suppression test, 279

Closed fracture, 322*f*

Clotting, intravenous therapy, 90

Club foot, 530, 530*f*

CMV. *See* Cytomegalovirus

CNS. *See* Central nervous system

Coagulation disorders, 185

Coarctation of the aorta, 521–522

Cold stress, neonatal, 477

Colic, 516–517

Colon, anatomy and function, 251

Colonoscopy, 251

Colostomies, 254–255, 254*f*, 256*f*

Colostrum, 466

Colposcopy, 424

Coma, assessment, 346, 348*t*

Comminuted fracture, 322

Common bile duct, anatomy and function, 235

Communicable disease
  See also Infection
  assessment, 43
  in children, 509*t*
  common childhood diseases, 509*t*–510*t*
  control protocols, 43

immunizations against (*See* Immunizations)
  management planning and implementation, 44–46

Communication skills, in nurses, 537, 537*t*–538*t*

Community, infection control in, 43

Community-acquired pneumonia, 176

Complementary therapies. *See* Alternative/complementary therapies

Complete fracture, 322*f*

Complete heart block, 118, 120, 120*f*

Concrete operations in growth and development, 488

Concussion, 363

Conductive hearing loss, 390

Conjunctivae, physical assessment, 10

Conjunctivitis of the newborn, 481

Consciousness, levels of, 352, 355

Constipation, 29, 257–258
  medications, 258*t*

Contact transmission, 197

Contraceptive methods, 422*t*–423*t*, 663*t*

Contraction/stress test (CCT/OCT), 468

Contusions, 321, 363

Coombs' test, 479

COPD (chronic obstructive pulmonary disease), 171–174

Coping mechanisms, for anxiety, 544*t*

Cornea, anatomy and function, 379, 379*f*

Corneal reflex, 10

Coronary artery
  anatomy, 136*f*
  bypass surgery, 136–137, 137*t*

Cough
  antitussive/expectorant medications, 636*t*
  coughing techniques, 172
  physical assessment, 9

Cranial meninges, 345

Cranial nerves
  assessment, 347*t*–348*t*
  disorders, 361–363, 364*t*
  physical assessment, 11*t*, 14

Crisis management, 549–553
  assessment, 549
  intervention techniques, 550
  situational crises, 549

Crohn's disease, 262, 263*t*–264*t*

Croup, 177–178

Crutch walking, 28*t*, 29

Cryptococcus neoformans, 194

CSF (cerebral spinal fluid), 345

Culdoscopy, 424
Cultural factors
    nutritional intake, 206–207
    pain awareness, 38
    perioperative care, 64
Cultures, female reproductive
        system, 425
Cushing's disease, 281, 283–284,
        285t
Cutaneous ureterostomy, 303t, 305
CVADs (central venous access
        devices), 92–93
CVS (chorionic villus sampling),
        467
Cyanocobalamin (B12), 212
Cyanosis, 9
Cyanotic heart anomalies, 520t,
        521–523
Cycloplegic eye medications, 650t
Cyclothymic disorder, 559–563
Cystic duct, 235
Cystic fibrosis, 171, 498
Cystitis, 307
Cystocele, 432
Cystoscopy, 432
Cytomegalovirus (CMV), 194, 197
    in pregnancy, 469
Cytoprotective medications, 643t
Cytotoxic agents, 623t
Cytotoxic reactions, 197

D
DDH (cevelopmental dysplasia of
        the hip), 527–529, 528f
Death and dying, handling of, 552,
        553t
Decompression, intestinal tract, 252
Deep tendon reflexes (DTRs), 6, 14,
        210, 291
Defense mechanisms, 542, 544t
Defibrillation, 120, 123t
Degenerative joint disease, 333–334
Delayed hypersensitivity reactions,
        197
Delusions, 565–566
Dementia
    AIDS-dementia complex, 194
    senile dementia, 566
Demographic data, health history, 3
Denver II developmental assessment
        tool, 498
Depressive disorders
    in bipolar disorder, 559
    characteristics and assessment,
        555–556
    medications, 556t–558t
    prevention of, 30
Dermal tissue, 53
Dermatological disorders, 59–62
Descending colon, 251

Desmopressin, 279t
Desmopressina acetate, 240
Developmental dysplasia of the hip
        (DDH), 527–529, 528f
Diabetes insipidus, 277, 278t
medications, 279t
Diabetes mellitus, 197, 272–274
    medications, 273t–274t
    in pregnancy, 471
Dialysis, 311, 312t
Diaphragmatic hernia, 477
Diarrhea, 259
    medications, 260t, 603t
DIC (disseminated intravascular
        coagulation), 470
Diencephalon, 344
Diet
    diabetes management, 272
    elimination and, 252
    post-colostomy, 254
    seizure management, 353
    therapeutic diets, 216t
Digestion
    accessory organs, 235–249
    antacid medications, 590t
    in pregnancy, 441–442
    summary of, 203–205, 203f
Digoxin (digitalis), 128–129,
        128t–129t, 642t
Disaccharides, 208
Disease-modifying antirheumatic
        medications (DMARDs), 643t
Diskectomy, 320
Dislocations, joint, 321, 323
Disorganized schizophrenia, 566,
        566t
Displaced fracture, 323
Disseminated intravascular
        coagulation (DIC), 470
Distributive shock, 147–148
Disulfiram, 574–575
Diuretics, 130, 131t–132t,
        314t–316t, 644t–646t
Divalproex sodium, 562t
Diverticular disease, 264
DMARDs (disease-modifying
        antirheumatic medications),
        643t
DNA topoisomerase, antineoplastic
        medications, 403t
Domestic violence, 581
Down syndrome, 360, 497
Dressings
    postoperative care, 68
    skin integrity and, 54
Drug abuse, 576–578, 578t
DTRs. See Deep tendon reflexes
Duodenal ulcer, 230f, 230t
Duodenum, 203f, 204
Dwyer instrumentation, 531
Dysmenorrhea, 420

Dyspnea, 9, 165
Dysrhythmias, cardiac, 112–124
    antidysrhythmics, 121t
    atrial, 114–117
    cardioversion, 122
    heart block, 118–120
    management, 120–124
    medications, 604t
    myocardial infarction, 133
    ventricular, 116–118
Dysthymic disorder, 555

E
Early adulthood (developmental
        phase), 495–496, 496t
Ears
    anatomy and physiology,
        389–390, 389f
    disorders, 391–393
    functional alterations, 390–391
    infections, 391
    neonatal assessment, 464
    physical assessment, 10
    surgery for, 391
ECF (extracellular fluid), fluid
        volume imbalance, 75
Eclampsia, 472, 472t, 473t
Economic conditions in growth and
        development, 498
ECT (electroconvulsive therapy),
        556, 557t
Ectopic pregnancy, 469
EDD (estimated date of delivery),
        443
EFM (electronic fetal monitor), 467
Ego, psychosocial development and
        anxiety coping mechanisms,
        542, 544t
    Freudian theory, 535
EKG, cardiac output analysis,
        110–112, 111f
Elder abuse, 579
Electroconvulsive therapy (ECT),
        556, 557t
Electrolyte imbalances, 79–86
    calcium, 83–84
    magnesium, 85
    modifiers, 80t, 647t
    potassium, 79
    replacement solutions, 81t, 646t
    sodium, 80
Electronic fetal monitor (EFM), 467
Elimination
    functional assessment, 251
    poison control/prevention, 511
    postpartum period, 460
    promotion of, 252
Embryonic development, 437, 439
Emergency care
    burn management, 96

poison control/prevention, 511
upper airway obstruction, 166–170
Emphysema, 171
Enalapril, 130
Encephalitis, 369–370
Endocrine system
disorders, 271–293
overview, 269, 270*t*
Endometriosis, 432
Endometrium
anatomy and function, 419
biopsy, 425
Endoscopy, 219
lower intestine, 251
variceal ligation, liver, 240
Endotracheal tube, 167*f*
Enteral nutrition, 220–221, 220*t*, 221*t*
Enterogastrone, 204
Environmental factors
growth and development, 498
infection control and, 44
safety and, 34
Epidural anesthesia, labor and delivery, 452
Epiglottitis, acute, 177
Epstein-Barr virus, 198
Erb's point, 13
Erikson growth and development theory, 487, 488*t*, 536, 536*t*
Erosion, skin, 59
Erythematous skin, 463
Erythroblastosis fetalis, 241, 479–480
Erythrocytes (RBCs), 183
abnormalities, 186
in pregnancy, 441
Esophageal atresia, 518, 518*f*
Esophagus, 203*f*, 204
Estimated date of delivery (EDD), 443
Estriol levels, 467
Estrogen
medications using, 663*t*
in pregnancy, 441
replacement therapy, 420
Ethnic influences in growth and development, 498
Eustachian tube, 389, 389*f*
Exercise
physiological need for, 24
therapeutic, 27*t*
Exophthalmos, 287
Expiration, mechanics of, 162
Expiratory reserve volume, 163
External ear, anatomy, 389, 389*f*
Extracellular fluid (ECF), fluid volume imbalance, 75
Extremities, postoperative care, 68
Eye drops, instillation, 381, 382*t*

Eyes
accommodation disorders, 381*t*
anatomy and function, 379–380, 379*f*
disorders of, 384–386, 387*t*
injuries, 382, 382*t*
medications, 387*t*, 649*t*–651*t*
neonatal assessment, 464
neonatal complications, 480–481
physical assessment, 10
problems, signs and symptoms, 381
prophylaxis, neonatal, 466
protection, infection control and, 44
strabismus, 481, 518–519
surgery for, 383–384
treatments for, 380

F

Face shields, infection control and, 44
Facial paralysis, 361
Fallopian tubes, 419
Fat emboli, 323
Fats, 208, 217
alterations in metabolism, 225
Fat-soluble vitamins, 208–210
Fatty acids, 208
Fecal occult blood test (FOBT), 218
Female reproductive system, 419–421
in adolescence, 495
anatomy and function, 419–420
assessment and diagnostic tools, 424–425, 424*t*
contraception methods, 422*t*–423*t*
infertility, 434
neonatal assessment, 464
physiology, 420–421
in pregnancy, 440
problems, 425–432, 427*t*–429*t*
reproductive cycle, 420
sexually transmitted disease, 435–436, 435*t*–436*t*
Fentanyl, 452
Fertilization, 437
Fetal development, 438–439, 439*t*
assessment of, 445
monitoring fetal status, 467
Fetal heart rate (FHR), 446, 467
Fetal membranes, 437
Fetal monitoring, 453–455
Fetal movements (FM), 446, 467
Fetal reference point, labor and delivery, 447
Fever
antipyretic medications, 633*t*
myocardial infarction, 133

Fever blisters, 60
FHR (fetal heart rate), 446, 467
Fiber, dietary, 208
Fibrocystic disease (breast), 426
Fibroids, uterine, 430
"Fight or flight" response, 108
First-degree atrioventricular block, 118, 119*f*
Fluid deficit, 75
Fluid overload, 76
Fluid regulation, 73–77
nutritional requirements, 217
Fluid volume imbalance, 73–77, 73*t*, 77*t*
central venous pressure, 74, 74*f*
shock, 149
Fluoroquinolones, 610*t*
FM (fetal movements), 446, 467
FOBT (fecal occult blood test), 218
Folic acid, 212
Follicle-stimulating hormone (FSH), 420
Fontanelle, 464
Formal operations in growth and development, 488
Fractures
bone, 321–327, 322*f*
in children, 529–530
hip, 327–328, 329*f*
Frank-Starling law, 108
French-American clients, nutritional intake of, 207
Freud, Sigmund, 488, 535, 536*t*
FSH (follicle-stimulating hormone), 420
Fungal infections
AIDS and, 195
antifungal medications, 606*t*

G

Gallbladder, 236, 236*f*
Gamma carboxylation, 210
Gamma radiation, 398
Gastrectomy, 231
Gastric aspiration and analysis, 218
Gastric mucosa, 205
Gastric secretion, 205
Gastric ulcer, 230–233, 230*f*, 230*t*
medications, 231*t*–232*t*, 648*t*
Gastrin, 204
Gastritis, 229
Gastrointestinal tract
hormones, 204
infections, 226, 226*t*
postoperative care, 67
postpartum period, 460
Genetics
cancer and, 398

growth and development and, 497
leukemia risk, 408
Genitalia
See also Female reproductive system; Male reproductive system
physical assessment, 15
Genitourinary tract
congenital malformations, 515
medications, 314t–316t, 647t–648t
neonatal assessment, 464
postoperative care, 67–68
Gerontologic considerations
activity and exercise, 24
autoimmune diseases, 197
brain anatomy, 345
depression, 555
digestion, 205
ears, 389–390
elder abuse, 579
eyes, 380
heart failure, 127
hip fracture, 327, 329f
hypertension, 142, 146
immobility management, 29
immune response, 193
kidney function, 297
musculoskeletal system, 21
pain awareness, 38
respiration, 164
sleep, 23
vascular system, 107
Gestational diabetes, 471
Gestational hypertension, 472
Glasgow coma scale, 348t
Glaucoma, 385–386, 387t
Glial cells, 343
Glomerulonephritis, 197
Gloves, infection control and, 44
Glucagon, pancreatic production of, 236
Glucocorticoids, 282t, 588t
Glucose metabolism, alterations in, 271, 271t
Glucose-6-phosphate deficiency, 210
Glycerol, 208
Glycosylated hemoglobin, 272
Gout, 334
medications, 335t, 607t
Gowns, infection control and, 44
Grapefruit juice, drug interactions with, 668t
Graves' disease, 197, 289t
Greek clients, nutritional intake of, 207
Greenstick fracture, 322, 529
Grief, 551–552, 551t
Groshong catheter, 222

Growth and development, 487–498
adolescence, 493–495, 494t
assessment, 498
early adulthood, 495–496, 496t
genetics and, 497
late adulthood, 496, 497t, 498
middle adulthood, 495–496, 496t
phases of, 487–498
prenatal, neonatal, and infant development, 489
preschool children, 491–492, 492t
psychosocial issues, 535–539, 536t
school-age children, 492–493, 493t
theories of, 487–488, 488t
toddlers, 490–491, 490t
Growth hormone disorders, 275, 276t
Guaiac tests, 218
Guillain-Barré syndrome, 197, 366–367
Gynecoid pelvis, 419
Gynecomastia, 14

H
Hair, physical assessment, 9
Hallucinations, 565
Halo fixation device, 326, 531
Handwashing, infection control and, 44
Harrington rod insertion, 531
HCG (human chorionic gonadotropin), 438, 442
Head
injuries to, 363–364
neonatal assessment, 464
physical assessment, 10
Headaches
hypertension and, 141
migraine, 372–373
Health-care procedures, age-appropriate preparation for, 500t
Health history, 3–4
demographic data, 3
maternal health, neonatal complications and, 475
past history, 3
pediatric assessment, 499, 503f
prenatal assessment, 443
psychosocial processes, 535
Health maintenance, requirements for, 536–537
Hearing
alterations in, 390–391
functional alterations, 390–391
Heart

anatomy, 103–104, 103f, 104f, 136f
congenital anomalies, 520–523, 520t
congenital malformations, 477
pediatric assessment, 502
sounds, physical assessment, 13
Heart block, 118–120, 119f
Heart failure (HF), 124–132
advanced, 126
cardiac glycosides, 128–129, 128t–129t
complications, 127
diuretics, 130
etiology, 126–128, 127t
right-sided, 125
Heavy metal antagonists, 651t
Hematology
blood disorders, 185–192
immune system, 193–200
overview, 183
signs/symptoms of disorders, 183
Hematoma, cranial, 90, 363
Hematopoietic disorders, 185
Hematopoietic medications, 199t
Hemicolectomy, 253
Hemodialysis, 311, 312t
Hemolytic anemia, 197
jaundice, 241
in neonates, 478
Hemolytic disease of newborn, 479–480
Hemophilia, 192
Hemorrhage
cranial, 363
fractures, 323
Hemothorax, 174, 175f
Hepatitis
pathology and etiology, 242–244, 243t–244t
in pregnancy, 469
viruses, 198
Herbal supplements, 339t, 664t–667t
antidepressants, 558t, 600t
Hernia
abdominal, 266
diaphragmatic, 477
hiatal, 229
strangulated, 266
Herniated intervertebral disk, 319, 319f
Herpes simplex 1, 60
Herpes type 2, in pregnancy, 469
Herpesviruses, 198
Herpes zoster, 60, 367
Heterocyclic antidepressants, 558t, 596t, 599t
HF. See Heart failure
Hiatal hernia, 229
Hickman/Biovac catheter, 222

Highly selective C-reactive protein (hsCRP), 43
Hip
developmental dysplasia, 527–529, 528f, 529f
fracture, 327–328, 329f
replacement, 328, 329f
Hispanic clients, nutritional intake of, 206
Histamine test, pheochromocytoma, 278
HIV (human immunodeficiency virus), 193
Hodgkin's lymphoma, 185
Homeostasis, 193
Hormones
See also specific hormones
antineoplastic medications, 402t, 624t
endocrine disorders and, 275–290
gastrointestinal, 204
menstrual cycle, 420
in pregnancy, 441
Hospital-acquired pneumonia, 176
Hospitalized children, interventions for, 515
Hospitals, infection control in, 44
HsCRP (highly selective C-reactive protein), 43
Huber needle, 222
Human chorionic gonadotropin (HCG), 438, 442
Human immunodeficiency virus (HIV), 193
Huntington's disease, 373–374
Hydrocephalus, 519–520, 520f
Hydronephrosis, 309
Hymen, 419
Hyperbilirubinemia, 478
Hypercalcemia, 84, 209
Hyperglycemia, 272
Hyperkalemia, 79
Hypermagnesemia, 86
Hypernatremia, 82
Hyperparathyroidism, 291, 292t, 293
Hyperpnea, 9, 165
Hyperresonance, physical assessment, 7
Hypersensitivity response, 197
antihistamine medications, 607t–608t
Hypertension
medications, 144t–145t
pheochromocytoma, 277–280
pregnancy-induced, 472, 473t
vascular alterations, 141–145
Hyperthyroidism, 287–288
medications, 289t
Hypertonic solution, fluid volume imbalance, 75, 77t

Hyperventilation, 9, 165
Hypocalcemia, 83
in neonates, 476
Hypochondriasis, 565
Hypochromic cells, 186
Hypoglycemia, 272, 274t
medications, 602t
in neonates, 477–478
Hypokalemia, 79
Hypomagnesemia, 85
Hyponatremia, 81
Hypoparathyroidism, 291, 292t
Hypopituitarism (Dwarfism), 275–276, 276t
Hypoprothrombinemia of the newborn, 210
Hypothalamus, 344
Hypothyroidism, 286–287
medications, 289t
Hypotonic solution, fluid volume imbalance, 75, 77t
Hypoventilation, 9, 165
Hypovitaminosis A, 209
Hypovolemic shock, 147
in neonates, 478
Hysterectomy, 430
Hysterosalpingogram/hystogram, 434

I

ICP (intracranial pressure), 348–351
Id, psychosocial development and, 535, 536t
IgE-mediated hypersensitivity reactions, 197
IGIM (Rho(D) immune globulin), 460
IGT (impaired glucose tolerance), 471
Ileal conduit, 305, 305f
Ileitis, 262, 263t
Ileostomy, 255, 264
Ileum, 203f, 204
Immobility
adverse effects, 25, 26t
functional alterations with, 25–31
nursing goals and interventions for, 29–31
predisposing factors, 25
rehabilitation, 25–29, 26t
Immune complex reactions, 197
Immune response, 193, 197
Immune system, 193–200
Immunizations
adolescent schedule, 51t–52t, 503t–508t
adult schedules, 47t–52t
contraindications, 508

nursing considerations for children receiving, 508t
pediatric schedule, 503t–508t
Immunomodulators, 652t
Immunostimulant medications, 199t
Immunosuppressant medications, 200t, 651t–652t
Impacted fracture, 322
Impaired glucose tolerance (IGT), 471
Impetigo, 59
Inborn errors of metabolism, 497–498
Incentive spirometer, 177
Incisions, postoperative care, 68
Incomplete fracture, 322f
Incontinence, urinary, 305
Incubation period, 198
Incus, 389, 389f
Indigestion, myocardial infarction, 133
Infancy
disorders of, 515–524
growth and development in, 489, 489t–490t
physical examinations, 500–501
Infection
AIDS and, 193–196
breasts, 430
defined, 198
ears, 391
female reproductive tract, 425, 427t, 430
gastrointestinal tract, 226, 226t
male reproductive tract, 432
medications, 608t–616t
neonatal complications, 475
in pregnancy, 468
pulmonary disorders, 176
urinary tract, 468
vaginal, 425
Infertility problems, 434–435
Infiltration, intravenous therapy, 89
Informed consent, perioperative care and, 64
Infratentorial intracranial tumors, 411
Injury, prevention of, 24
Inner ear, anatomy, 389
Inspiration, mechanics of, 162
Inspiratory reserve volume, 163
Insulin, 273t, 600t–601t
management of, 272
pancreatic production of, 236
Intellectual delay, 359–360, 360t
Intellectual development, assessment of, 498
Interarticular fracture, 322
Interbody cage fusion, 321
Interferon, 198

Interpersonal factors in growth and development, 498
Intestinal obstruction, 265
Intracranial pressure (ICP), 348–351
Intracranial tumors, 354–356, 411
Intrahepatic jaundice, 242
Intraoperative care, 65–67, 66t–67t
Intrapleural pressure, 162
Intrauterine growth restriction (IUGR), 468
Intravenous anesthesia, 453
Intravenous fluids
  burn management, 96
  fluid volume imbalance, 77t
Intravenous therapy
  blood transfusions, 93–95, 95t
  burn management, 95–100, 99t–100t
  central venous access devices, 92–93
  complications, 89
  equipment, 87–88
  flow rate, 90–92
  nursing guidelines, 87–100
  peripheral IV, 88–90
  procedures, 88–95
  rate calculations, 88t
Intubation, upper airway obstruction, 167, 167f, 168t
Iodine-131 (131I) radiation, 399
Iris, anatomy and function, 379, 379f
Iron-deficiency anemia, 186–188
Iron preparations, 653t
Ischemic pain pattern, 132, 133f
Isoniazid prophylaxis, tuberculosis, 178, 180t
Isotonic fluids, fluid volume imbalance, 75, 77t
Italian clients, nutritional intake of, 207
IUGR (intrauterine growth restriction), 468

J

Japanese clients, nutritional intake of, 207
Jaundice, 241
  in neonates, 478–479
Jejunum, 203f, 204
Jewish clients, nutritional intake of, 206
Joint movement and action
  dislocations, 321, 323
  disorders, 331–339
  normal mobility, 21, 23t
  problems with, 21
Juvenile rheumatoid arthritis (JRA), 332

K

Kaposi's sarcoma, 194
Kernig's sign, 371
Kidneys
  anatomy, 297
  disorders of, 307–313, 312t
Klinefelter's syndrome, 497
Knee replacement, 328, 329f
Kussmaul's respirations, 9, 165
Kwashiorkor, 209
Kyphosis, 21

L

Labia majora, 419
Labia minora, 419
Labor and delivery, 447–457
  assisted delivery, 451
  fetal monitoring, 453–455
  intrapartal management, 455–457
  outside hospital setting, 474
  pharmacological control of, 452–453, 453t
  stages of labor, 455–457, 457t
  true vs. false labor, 450t
  vaginal delivery, 451
Laboratory screening
  pediatric assessment, 502
  prenatal assessment, 444
Lactation, 459, 460t
Laminectomy, 320
Lanugo, 463
Laparoscopy
  cholecystectomy with, 245
  female reproductive system, 425
Laryngeal carcinoma, 415–416
Laryngectomy, 416
Laryngotracheobronchitis, acute, 177
Larynx
  carcinoma, 415–416
  congenital malformations, 477
  structure, 161
Late adulthood (developmental phase), 496, 497t
Latency phase of development, 488
Laxatives, 257, 258t, 653t–654t
Lead toxicity, 512–513
  heavy metal antagonists, 651t
Learning disabilities, 361
Lens, anatomy and function, 379, 379f
Leukemia, 185, 407–408
  assessment, 407
  characteristics and classification, 407
  risk factors, 408
Leukocytes (WBCs), 183
Levin tube, 233, 253
LH (luteinizing hormone), 420

Limbic system, 345
Lincosamides, 610t
Lipase, 236
Lisinopril, 130
Lithium, 562t, 563
Lithotripsy, 308
Liver
  anatomy and function, 235, 236f
  biopsy, 239
  diagnostic testing, 236–239
  digestive system, 203f, 204
  disorders of, 239–243
Liver function studies, 236, 237t–238t
Logan bow, 516, 516f
Longitudinal fracture, 322
Lou Gehrig's disease, 368–369
Lower back pain, 319–321, 319f
Lower intestinal tract, 251–266
  anatomy and function, 251
  diagnostic tests, 251–252
  disorders, 257–266, 263t–264t
  lower GI series, 219
  surgery, 253–256, 254f
Lower respiratory tract, 161
Lumpectomy, 430
Lungs
  capacity, 163
  neonatal complications in, 477, 483
  physical assessment, 12
  respiratory system, 161–164
Luteinizing hormone (LH), 420
Lymphadenopathy, 198
Lymph nodes, 198
Lymphocytes, 198
Lymphoproliferative diseases, 185
Lymphosarcoma, 185

M

Macrocyte abnormalities, 186
Macrolides, 611t
Macrophages, 198
Macule, 58
Magnesium imbalances, 85–86
Major depressive disorder (MDD), 555
Malabsorption syndrome, 259
Male reproductive system
  in adolescence, 495
  anatomy and function, 421, 423
  assessment and diagnostic tools, 432
  contraception methods, 422t–423t
  infertility, 434
  neonatal assessment, 464
  problems, 427t–429t, 432–433

reproductive cycle, 421
sexually transmitted disease, 433–434, 433t–434t
Malignancies, 395
Malignant melanoma, 407
Malleus, 387, 387f
Mammography, 423
Mammoplasty, 427
Mania
    assessment of, 557
    lithium for management of, 561
Manipulative behavior, 571–572
MAO (monoamine oxidase) inhibitors, 556t, 595t, 597t
Marie-Strümpell disease, 333
Masks, for infection control, 44
Maslow's hierarchy of needs, 33, 534
Mastectomy, 428
Mastoiditis, 390–391
MDD (major depressive disorder), 553
Mechanical digestive process, 203
Mechanical ventilation, 168
Meckel's diverticulum, 262
Medications, tables of, 583t–666t
    See also specific medications
Megaloblastic anemias, 189
Ménière's disease, 365–366, 391
Meningitis, 368–369
Meningocele, 522, 522f
Menopause, 418
Menorrhagia, 418
Men's health medications, 316t, 660t
Menstrual cycle, 418
Mental illness
    altered thought processes, 563–569, 564t, 566t–569t
    antipsychotic medications, 566t–567t
    anxiety disorders, 539–545, 541t–545t
    bipolar disorder, 557–561, 560t
    depressive disorders, 553–554, 554t–556t
    treatment modalities, 535, 537t
Mental status assessment, 17–18
Meperidine hydrochloride, 450
Metabolism
    alterations in, 225–228
    inborn errors of metabolism, 495–496
Metal toxicity, heavy metal antagonists, 649t
Metronidazole, 423
MI (myocardial infarction), 132–135
Microcyte abnormalities, 186
Middle adulthood (developmental phase), 493–494, 494t

Middle ear
    anatomy, 387, 387f
    infections, 390
Migraine headache, 370–371
Milia, 461
Miller-Abbott tube, 253
Mineralocorticoids, 283t, 587t
Minerals, 212, 652t–653t
Mini-Mental State Exam (MMSE), 18
Minnesota tube, 240
Miotic eye medications, 647t
Mitral valve, anatomy, 104
Monoamine oxidase (MAO) inhibitors, 556t, 595t, 597t
Monosaccharides, 208
Mons veneris, 417
Mood disorders, 557–561
Moro reflex, 463
Motor function
    growth and development of, 488t, 489
    physical assessment, 14 Mouth
        neonatal assessment, 462
        physical assessment, 12
Mucolytic medications, 173t
Multifactorial cancer development, 395
Multiple sclerosis, 197, 374–375
Muscular dystrophy, 524
Musculoskeletal system
    alterations in, 319–339
    contracture prevention, 29
    developmental disorders, 525–529, 526f, 529f
    developmental structures and functions, 21–22, 22t
    diseases, 331–339
    herbal supplements for, 339t
    immobility in, 25
    medications, 653t–654t
    neonatal assessment, 462, 463
    physical assessment, 15
    in pregnancy, 438
    traumas/injuries/disorders, 319–325
Muslim clients, nutritional intake of, 206
Myasthenia gravis, 197, 373, 374
Mydriatic eye medications, 648t
Myelin sheath, 343
Myelomeningocele, 522, 522f
My Food Plate guidelines, 213, 215t
Myocardial contractility, 108
Myocardial infarction (MI), 132–135
Myometrium, 417
Myxedema, 286, 289t

N
Naegle's rule, 441
Nails, physical assessment, 10
Narcotics, labor and delivery, 450, 451t
NAS (Neonatal Abstinence Syndrome), 478
Native American clients, nutritional intake of, 206
Nausea
    antiemetic medications, 227t, 603t
    etiology and pathology, 226
    in pregnancy, 439, 443, 444t
Neck, physical assessment, 12
Necrotizing enterocolitis, 478, 481
Neonatal Abstinence Syndrome (NAS), 478
Neonates, 461–464
    complications in, 473–481
    growth and development in, 487
    monitoring, 454
    physical assessment, 461–463
    routine care, 464
    vital signs, 8
Neoplasm
    hydrocephalus, 517
    pulmonary disease, 174
    spinal cord injury, 364
Nephron, 298f
Nephrosis (nephrotic syndrome), 310
Nephrostomy, 304
Nervous system
    alterations in, 346–377
    anatomy and physiology, 343–346
    disorders, 353–376
    intravenous therapy and, 91
Neural reflexes, intravenous therapy and, 91
Neural tube defects, 522–523, 522f
Neuroglia, 343
Neurological system alterations, 346–377
    disorders, 354
    mental status assessment, 17
    physical assessment, 14
    tests for, 354
Neurological tests, 354t–355t
Neuromuscular disorders, in children, 522–524
Neuron, 343, 343f
Neuropsychosocial postoperative care, 67
Neutropenic precautions
    infection control, 46
    radiation therapy, 398
Nevus flammeus, 462
Nevus vasculosus, 462
Niacin, 211

Nipple care, postpartum, 457
Nitrates, 654t–655t
Nitrogen balance, negative balance prevention, 29
oxygen, 451
Nodule, skin, 58
Non-Hodgkin's lymphoma, 185
Nonsteroidal anti-inflammatory medications (NSAIDs), 655t–656t
Nonstress test (NST), 465
Nonunion of fractures, 323
Nonverbal communication, 535, 535t
Normal sinus rhythm, 111f
Nose, physical assessment, 10
NSAIDs (nonsteroidal anti-inflammatory medications), 655t–656t
NST (nonstress test), 465
Nursing, in postpartum period, 457, 458t
Nutrition
    alternative nutrition, 220–223, 220t
    assessment, 217, 217t, 218t
    basic concepts, 203–216
    carbohydrates, 207–208
    dietary guidelines, 213, 214f, 215t
    digestive system, 203–205, 203f
    elimination and, 252
    enteral nutrition, 220–221, 220t, 221t
    fats, 208
    food adequacy axioms, 207
    minerals, 212, 213t
    My Food Plate guidelines, 213, 214f, 215t
    neonatal complications, 481
    nutrient absorption, 226
    parameters, 217–219
    parenteral nutrition, 221–223, 222f
    prenatal assessment, 441
    proteins, 208
    sociocultural influences on, 206–207
    status assessment, 9
    therapeutic diets, 216t
    total parenteral nutrition, 223t
    vitamins, 208–212
Nystagmus, 10

O

Oblique fracture, 322
Obstruct (post-hepatic) jaundice, 242
Oligomenorrhea, 418

Oliguria, myocardial infarction and, 133, 134
Open fracture, 322f
Ophthalmoscope exam, 10
Opioid analgesics, 657t
Opportunistic infections, 198
Oral glucose tolerance tests, 271
Oral hypoglycemic medications, 274t
Oral phase of development, 486
Orchitis, 430, 432
Organic brain syndrome, 357
Organ of Corti, 388
Orthopnea, 9, 165
Ossicles, 387, 387f
Osteoarthritis, 319, 333–334
Osteomalacia, 339
Osteomyelitis, 338
Osteoporosis, 336–337, 337t
    prevention, 29
Otitis media, acute, 389–390
Ovarian cancer, 429
Ovaries
    anatomy and function, 417
    problems of, 429
Overflow incontinence, 305
Oviduct, anatomy and function, 417
Ovum
    fertilization, 435
    implantation, 436
Oxygen administration, 149t, 170t
    hazards of, 170t
    neonatal complications, 479–481
    shock management, 148, 149t
    upper airway obstruction, 170t
Oxygen/carbon dioxide exchange, 164

P

PAC (premature atrial contraction), 114, 114f
Pacemakers, 122, 124t
Paget's disease, 335–336
    medications, 658t
Pain
    characteristics of, 37–38
    interventions, 38–40
    ischemic pain pattern, 132, 133f
    labor and delivery, management of, 450, 451t
    low back pain, 319–321, 319f
    medications, 41t
    phases of, 37, 38t
    radiation therapy, 398
    related diagnoses, 38
    types of, 37, 37f
Palpation
    pediatric assessment, 498
    physical assessment, 6
Pancreas

anatomy and function, 236, 236f
    digestive system, 203f, 204
    disorders of, 247–249
Pancreatic cancer, 248–249, 411
Pancreatic enzymes, 236
Pancreatitis, 247–248
Papule, 58
Paracentesis, 239, 241
Paradoxical respirations, 9, 165
Paralytic ileus, 265
Paranoid schizophrenia, 564, 564t
Parasympathetic nervous system, cardiac function, 108
Parathyroid hormone disorders, 291–293, 292t
Parenteral nutrition (PN), 221–223, 223t
Parkinson's disease, 372–374
    medications, 373t–374t, 625t–626t
Paroxysmal atrial tachycardia (PAT), 114–115, 114f
Patent ductus arteriosus (PDA), 519
Pathogens, 198
Pathologic fracture, 322
Pavlik harness, 526f
PCP (pneumocystis carinii pneumonia), 198
PDA (patent ductus arteriosus), 519
Pediatric assessment/wellness, 497–511
    age-appropriate preparation for health care procedures, 498t
    alterations in pediatric health, 513–529
    common childhood problems, 506–511, 507t
    common communicable diseases, 507t–508t
    health history, 497
    immunizations, 500–506, 501t–506t
    infant disorders, 513–522
    interventions for hospitalized children, 513
    musculoskeletal disorders, 525–529
    neuromuscular disorders, 522–524
    physical examinations, 497–500, 498t
    poison control/prevention, 508–511, 508t
Pediculosis, 61
Pellagra, 211
Pelvic inflammatory disease (PID), 424
Pelvis, anatomy and function, 417
Penicillins, 609t
Penis, 419
    neonatal care, 464

Peplau psychosocial development theory, 536
Peptic ulcer disease, 230–233, 230*f*
   medications, 648*t*
Perceptive hearing loss, 390–391
Percussion
   chronic obstructive pulmonary disease, 172
   pediatric assessment, 500
   physical assessment, 6
Percutaneous central catheters, 93
Percutaneous umbilical blood sampling (PUBS), 468
Pericardium, anatomy, 103
Perinatal asphyxia, 476–477
Perineum
   anatomy and function, 419
   postpartum care, 459
Periodic breathing, 9
Perioperative care, 63–65
   fears of surgery and, 63*t*
   teaching and preparation for, 63, 64*t*
Peripheral intravenous therapy, 88–92
Peripherally inserted central catheter (PICC), 92
   parenteral nutrition, 222
Peripheral nervous system (PNS), 343
Peripheral vascular disease, 153–157
   arterial, 154–155
   venous, 155–157
Peripheral vascular system physical assessment, 13
Peristalsis, lower intestine, 251
Peritoneal dialysis, 311, 312*t*
Peritonitis, 261–262
Pernicious anemia, 212, 218
Personal protective equipment (PPE), infection control and, 44
Phallic phase of development, 488
Pharmacology. *See* Medications
Pharynx, physical assessment, 12
Phenylketonuria (PKU), 497
Pheochromocytoma, 277–280
Phlebitis, intravenous therapy, 89
Phototherapy, 478
Phototopia, 10
Physical assessment, 5–15
   findings, 8–15
   neonates, 463–466
   pediatric, 499–502, 500*t*
   prenatal, 442–446, 446*t*
   preparation, 5
   purpose, 5
   techniques, 5–7
   vital signs, 7*t*, 8–9
Physical examination

age-appropriate preparation for, 500*t*
   neonatal, 463–465
   pediatric, 499–502, 500*t*
Piaget's stages of growth and development, 487, 488, 536*t*
Pia mater, 345
PICC. *See* Peripherally inserted central catheter
PID (pelvic inflammatory disease), 426
Pigmentation, neonatal, 463
Pinna
   anatomy and physiology, 389, 389*f*
   neonatal assessment, 464
Pitressin, 240
Pituitary gland
   disorders, 275–276, 276*t*
   menstrual cycle, 420
   in pregnancy, 441
PKU (phenylketonuria), 497
Placenta, 437
Placenta previa, 469
Plasma, 183
Platypelloid pelvis, 420
Play, in growth and development, 490*t*, 491
Pleur-evac procedures, 174, 175*f*
PMI (point of maximal impulse), 13
PN (parenteral nutrition), 221–223, 223*t*
Pneumocystis carinii pneumonia (PCP), 198
Pneumocystis jiroveci pneumonia, 194
Pneumonia, 176, 198
Pneumothorax, 174, 175*f*
PNS (peripheral nervous system), 343
Poikilocytosis, 186
Point of maximal impulse (PMI), 13
Poison control/prevention, 510–513, 510*t*
Polypeptides, 208
Polysaccharides, 208
Port wine stain, 464
Postoperative care, 67–69
Postpartum care guidelines, 459–461
Post-term birth, 475
Postural drainage, 172
Potassium imbalances, 79–81
PPE (personal protective equipment), infection control and, 44
Pre-eclampsia, 472, 472*t*, 473*t*
Pregnancy
   bleeding in, 468–471, 470*t*
   cardiac disease in, 474
   complications, 467–474

diabetes in, 471
   discomforts of, 445, 446*t*
   fetal assessment, 446
   fetal development in, 437–439, 439*t*
   hypertension in, 472–473, 473*t*
   infection in, 468
   labor and delivery, 447–457
   maternal adaptations, 440–442
   postpartum care, 459–461
   prenatal assessment, 442–446, 446*t*
   structures of, 437–438
   testing for, 442
Premature atrial contraction (PAC), 114, 114*f*
Premature birth, 475, 480
Premature ventricular contraction (PVC), 116–117, 117*f*
Prenatal assessment
   growth and development, 442–445
   guidelines for, 442–446, 446*t*
   pregnancy complications, 467–474
Preoperational growth and development, 487
Preschool children
   growth and development in, 491–492, 492*t*
   physical examinations, 501
Pressoreceptors, 107
Pressure ulcers, 30
Proctosigmoidoscopy, 251
Progesterone, 441
   medications using, 663*t*
Prolapse, uterine, 431
Prostate cancer, 433
Prostate gland
   anatomy and function, 421
   disorders of, 309
   health medications, 316*t*
   smear, 432
Prostate-specific antigen (PSA), 432
Prostatic acid phosphatase, 432
Prostatitis, 432
Proteins, 208
   metabolism of, 225, 225*t*
Psoriasis, 61
Psychosocial issues
   adolescents, 494*t*, 495, 535, 536*t*
   alcohol abuse, 574–576, 574*t*, 575*t*
   altered thought processes, 565–571, 566*t*, 568*t*–571*t*
   anxiety, 541–547, 543*t*–547*t*
   basic concepts, 535–539
   bipolar disorder, 559–563, 562*t*
   child abuse, 579
   communication skills in nurses, 537, 537*t*–538*t*

depressive disorders, 555–556, 556*t*–558*t*
domestic violence, 581
drug abuse, 576–578, 578*t*
early-middle adulthood, 496
elder abuse, 579
growth and development, 487–488, 488*t*
health maintenance requirements, 536–537
history, 535–536
labor and delivery, 449
late adulthood, 496
manipulative behavior, 573–574
neonatal complications, 475
postpartum period, 461
in pregnancy, 442
preschool children, 491
psychosocial processes, 535–537
radiation therapy, 400
school age children, 492
sexual abuse, 580–581
situational crises, 549–553, 551*t*, 553*t*
social-interaction disorders, 573–578
stages of development, 536*t*
substance abuse, 576–578, 578*t*
toddlers, 490
treatment modalities, 537, 539*t*
well-being, 535
Ptosis, physical assessment, 10
PUBS (percutaneous umbilical blood sampling), 468
Puerto Rican clients, nutritional intake of, 206
Pulmonary disorders, 171–180
medications, 173*t*–174*t*
Pulmonary hypertension, heart defects and, 521
Pulse
normal, 8
physical assessment, 13
Pupils, physical assessment, 10
Purkinje system, 106
Pustule, 59
PVC (premature ventricular contraction), 116–117, 117*f*
Pyelonephritis, 307–308
Pyloric stenosis
in infants, 517
ulcers and, 233–234
Pyloroplasty, 234
Pyridoxine (B6), 212

Q

Quanti FERON-TB Gold test, tuberculosis, 178

R

RA. *See* Rheumatoid arthritis
Racial factors in growth and development, 498
Radiographic imaging
female reproductive system, 425
liver function, 236
Radiotherapy cancer, 398–399
leukemia risk from, 408
Radium therapy, 399
Rape trauma, 551*t*
RBCs. *See* Erythrocytes
Rectocele, 432
Rectum
anatomy and function, 251
physical assessment, 15
Reflexes, neonatal assessment, 465
Reflex incontinence, 305
Regional block anesthesia, 452
Regitine test, pheochromocytoma, 279
Renal colic, 308
Renal dialysis, 311, 312*t*
Renal failure
acute, 310
chronic, 311
Renal stones, 308
Renal transplantation, 311, 313*f*
Reproductive system, 419–436
See also Female reproductive system; Male reproductive system
Residual schizophrenia, 566*t*, 567
Residual volume, respiration, 163
Resonance, physical assessment, 7
Respiration
See also Breathing patterns; Upper airway obstruction
mechanics of, 162–164
medications, 173*t*–174*t*
neonatal assessment, 463
neonatal complications, 476–477, 482
normal, 8
pediatric assessment, 502
physical assessment, 8
postoperative care, 67
in pregnancy, 441
pulmonary disorders, 171–174
Respiratory distress syndrome, 476
Respiratory system
alterations in airway clearance/breathing patterns, 165–180
breathing patterns, 165–166
breath sounds, 166*t*
overview, 161–164
pulmonary disorders, 171–180
upper airway obstruction, 166–170
Rest, physiological need for, 23

Restrictive pulmonary disease, 174–176
Retina
anatomy and function, 379–380, 379*f*
detached, 384
Retinopathy of prematurity, 480, 482
Retroviruses, 198
Revised Prescreening Developmental Questionnaire (R-PDQ), 498
Rheumatoid arthritis (RA), 197, 331–332
juvenile, 329
Rh incompatibility, 479
Rho(D) Immune globulin (IGIM), 460
Riboflavin (B2), 211
Rickets, 209
Riluzole (Rilutek), 369
Ringworm, 61
Risk factors, for safety, 33–36, 35*t*
Risser-turnbuckle cast, 531
Rubella
congenital malformations and, 521
in pregnancy, 469
vaccine, 460
"Rule of nines," burn management, 96
Russel's traction, 325, 325*f*

S

Saddle block, 452
Safety
adolescents and, 33, 495
elderly and, 33
infants and, 33
poison control/prevention, 510–513, 510*t*
preschoolers and, 33, 492
primary health concerns, 33–36
school-age children and, 33, 493
toddlers and, 33, 491
Salem sump, 233, 253
Salivary glands, 204
Salpingo-oophorectomy, 431
SA (sinoatrial) node, 105, 106*f*
Scabies, 60
Schilling test, 218
Schistocytes, 186
Schizophrenia, 566–567, 566*t*
School-age children
growth and development, 492–493, 493*t*
physical examinations, 501
Sclerae
anatomy and function, 379, 379*f*
physical assessment, 10

Scoliosis, 21, 528–529, 529f
Scrotum, 419
Second-degree atrioventricular block, 119, 119f
Secretary glands, 203
Secretin, 204
Sedatives/hypnotics, labor and delivery, 450, 451t
Sedimentation rate, communicable disease assessment, 43
Seizure disorders, 346, 352t
Selective serotonin-norepinephrine reuptake inhibitors (SSNRI), 556t, 597t
Selective serotonin reuptake inhibitors (SSRIs), 556t, 595t, 597t
Self-care
  nursing assistance for, 29
  safety factors and, 29
Self-esteem, depression and, 553
Semilunar valves, anatomy, 104
Seminiferous tubules, 419
Sengstaken-Blakemore tube, 240, 240f
Senile dementia, 564
Sensorimotor development, 485
Sensorineural hearing loss, 388
Sensory function
  physical assessment, 14
  seizure management, 352
Separation anxiety, 489
Sepsis
  fractures, 323
  in neonates, 476
Serotonin/norepinephrine reuptake inhibitors (SNRIs), 597t
Sex determination, 435
Sex-linked transmission traits, 495
Sexual abuse
  of adults, 578–579
  of children, 577, 578
Sexual activity
  adolescence and, 493
  postpartum period, 459
Sexually transmitted infections (STIs), 433–434, 433t–434t
  in pregnancy, 466
Shingles, 60, 365
  in pregnancy, 467
Shock
  medication for, 584t–585t
  myocardial infarction, 133
  in neonates, 476
  oxygen administration, 148, 149t
  pathophysiology, 147–151
  stages of, 148
  therapeutic medications, 150t–151t

SIADH (syndrome of inappropriate antidiuretic hormone secretion), 278t
Sickle cell disease, 186, 190–191
Side effects
  antineoplastic medications, 402t, 625t
  antipsychotic medications, 630t
  medication interactions with grapefruit juice, 666t
SIDS (sudden infant death syndrome), 521–522
Sigmoid colon, 251
Sigmoid colostomy, 253, 254
Sigmoidoscopy, 251
Sinoatrial (SA) node, 105, 106f
Sinus bradycardia, 113, 113f
Sinuses, physical assessment, 10
Sinus rhythm, normal, 111f
Sinus tachycardia, 113f
Situational/traumatic crises, 547–551, 549t, 551t
Sjögren's syndrome, 197
Skin
  cancer, 407
  disorders, 53, 55–57, 56t–57t
  integrity, maintenance of, 53–62
  medications, 54t
  neonatal assessment, 461
  nursing interventions for, 53–55, 55t
  physical assessment, 9
  in pregnancy, 438
  primary lesions, 58–59
  wound healing and, 54
Skin test, tubercular, 178, 179t
Slate gray nevus (congenital dermal melanocytosis), 461
Sleep, 23
Slow virus infections, 198 Small-for-gestational age infants, 473–474
Small intestine, digestive system, 203f, 204
Smears, vaginal, 423
Smoking
  neonatal complications, 473
  prenatal assessment, 466
Snellen chart, 10
SNRIs (serotonin/norepinephrine reuptake inhibitors), 597t Social interactions, disorders of, 571–576
  alcohol abuse, 572–574, 572t, 573t
  drug abuse, 574–576, 576t
  manipulative behavior, 571–572
Sociocultural influences
  growth and development, 496
  nutritional intake, 206–207
Sodium imbalances, 81–82
Sounds

physical assessment, 7
physiology of, 387
Southeast Asian clients, nutritional intake of, 207
Spherocytes, 186
Sphincter muscles, 203, 203f
Spina bifida, 522–523, 522f
Spinal block, 451
Spinal cord, 346
  injury, 362–364, 363t
Spinal stenosis, 319
Spiral fracture, 323
Spleen, 185, 199
Spontaneous rupture of membranes (SROM), labor and delivery, 448
Squamous cell carcinoma, 407
SSNRI (selective serotonin-norepinephrine reuptake inhibitors), 556t, 597t
SSRIs (selective serotonin reuptake inhibitors), 556t, 595t, 597t
Stapes, 387, 387f
Staphylococcus aureus, 424
Stasis (respiratory), prevention of, 30
Stepping reflex, 463
STIs. See Sexually transmitted infections
Stomach, digestive system, 203f, 204
Stool softeners, 257, 258t, 651t–652t
Stool testing, 218
Stork bites, 461
Strabismus, 10, 516–517
  neonatal assessment, 479
Strains/sprains, 321, 323
Strawberry mark, 462
Stress, toddlers and, 489, 490
Stress fracture, 323
Stress incontinence, 305
Stridor, 9
Stroke, 356–357
Subarachnoid block, 450
Subcutaneous port, 222
Substance abuse, 574–576, 576t
  assessment, 574–576, 576t
  congenital malformations and, 519
  neonatal complications, 478
  prenatal assessment, 466
Suctioning, upper airway obstruction, 167
Sudden infant death syndrome (SIDS), 521–522
Suicide, behavioral cues for, 554, 554t, 555t
Sulfonamides, 610t

Sullivan psychosocial development theory, 536
Superego, psychosocial development and, 535, 536t
Supratentorial intracranial tumors, 411
Surgery
  complications from, 69t–70t
  fear of, 63t
  intraoperative care, 65–67, 66t–67t
  perioperative care, 63–65
  postoperative care, 67–69, 69t–70t
Surgical drains, 68t–69t
Syndrome of inappropriate antidiuretic hormone secretion (SIADH), 278t
Systemic lupus erythematosus, 197

T

Talipes equinovarus (club foot), 530, 530f
Tay-Sachs disease, 498
TCAs (tricyclic antidepressants), 558t, 598t, 599t
Telangiectactic nevi, 463
Temperature
  in neonates, 463
  normal body, 8, 8t
  pediatric assessment, 500
Temporary cecostomy, 253
TENS (transcutaneous electrical nerve stimulation), 320
Tensilon test, 376
Testes
  anatomy and function, 421, 423
  biopsy, 432
  infection, 434
Tetracyclines, 612t–613t
Tetralogy of Fallot, 522
Thalamus, 344
Thalassemia, 188–189
T-helper cells, 199
Therapeutic communication, 537, 538t
Therapeutic exercise, 27t
Thermography, 425
Thiamine (B1), 210
Third-degree atrioventricular block, 120, 120f
Thoracolumbosacral (TLSO) brace, 531
Thorax
  neonatal assessment, 464, 477
  physical assessment, 12
  respiratory system, 161
Thought processes, altered. See Altered thought processes

Thrombocytes (platelets), 183
  antiplatelet medications, 629t
Thrombocytopenia, 191–192
Thrombolytic medications, 139t, 660t
Thrombophlebitis, intravenous therapy, 89
Thrombus formation, prevention, 30
Thymus, 199
Thyroid gland disorders, 286–293, 289t
  medications, 290t, 634t–635t
TIAs (transient ischemic attacks), 356
Tic douloureux, 361
Tidal volume, 163
Tinea, 61
TIPS (transjugular intrahepatic portosystem shunt), 240
Tissue perfusion disorders, 147–151
Tissue-specific hypersensitivity reactions, 197
TLSO (thoracolumbosacral) brace, 531
T lymphocytes, 199
Toddler
  growth and development in, 490–491, 490t
  health assessment of, 503f
  physical examinations, 500–501
Tonicity
  fluid volume imbalance, 75
  neonatal assessment, 465
Topical anti-infectives, 615t–616t
Topoisomerase, 403t, 624t
TORCH test series, 468
Total anomalous venous return, 522–523
Total hip and knee replacement, 328, 329f
Toxic shock syndrome (TSS), 426
Toxoplasmosis, 469
Toys, age-appropriate, 490t
Tracheoesophageal fistula, 518, 518f
Tracheostomy, 168
Traction, 324–327
  childhood fractures, 529
  spinal cord injury, 366
Transcutaneous electrical nerve stimulation (TENS), 320
Transfer activities, 27
Transfusion reactions, 197
  jaundice, 242
Transient ischemic attacks (TIAs), 356
Transjugular intrahepatic portosystem shunt (TIPS), 240

Transmission-based precautions, infection control and, 45–46
Transplant rejection, 197
Transport of clients, infection control and, 45
Transurethral resection of prostate (TURP), 309, 433
Transverse colon, 251
Transverse double-barrel colostomy, 254, 254f
Transverse loop colostomy, 254, 254f
Trauma
  eyes, 382t
  musculoskeletal, 321–327
Traumatic crises. See Situational/ traumatic crises
Trichomonas vaginalis, 426
Tricuspid valve, 104
Tricyclic antidepressants (TCAs), 558t, 598t, 599t
Trigeminal neuralgia, 361
Trisomy 21 (Down syndrome), 360, 497
Tropical sprue, 259
Trousseau's sign
  Graves' disease, 288
  hypocalcemia, 83
  hypoparathyroidism, 291
Truncus arteriosus, 522
Trypsin, 236
TSS (toxic shock syndrome), 426
T4:T8 ratio, 199
Tuberculosis, 178–179
  medications, 180t, 635t–636t
  skin test for, 179t
Turner's syndrome, 497
TURP (transurethral resection of prostate), 309, 433
Tympanic membrane, 389
Tympany sound, 7
Type 1 diabetes, 197
  in pregnancy, 471
Type 2 diabetes, 271
  in pregnancy, 471

U

Ulcer, 230–234, 230f
  common sites for, 229, 230
  duodenal vs. gastric, 230t
  medications, 231t–232t, 648t
  peptic ulcer disease, 230–233, 230f
  skin, 59
  surgical interventions, 231, 233f
Ulcerative colitis, 197, 263–264, 263t
Ultrasound
  fetal status monitoring, 467
  liver, 239

Umbilical cord, 437, 466
Undifferentiated schizophrenia, 566t, 567
Upper airway obstruction, 166–170, 170t
Upper GI series, 218
Upper respiratory system, 161
Ureterosigmoidostomy, 305, 305f
Ureterostomy, 304, 305f
Ureters, 298
Urethra
    female, 419
    male, 421
Urethral stones, 308
Urge incontinence, 305
Urinanalysis, 218
    diabetes testing, 272
    pheochromocytoma, 279
Urinary diversion, 302t
    catheterization, 303–304, 303t
    surgery, 305, 305f
Urinary stasis prevention, 30
Urinary tract
    congenital malformations, 481, 482t
    diagnostic studies, 300t
    disorders, 307–313
    diuretic medications, 314t–315t
    drainage systems, 303–304
    incontinence, 305
    infections, 468
    neonatal assessment, 464
    overview, 297–298, 297f, 300t
    postpartum period, 460
    in pregnancy, 442
    urinary diversion, 302t, 305, 305f
    urinary function, 299–305
    urinary retention management, 301, 302t
Urine, 297
Uterus
    anatomy and function, 419
    cancer of, 431
    contractions, 437
    involution, 459
    labor and delivery, 449
    postpartum changes, 459
    in pregnancy, 440
    problems of, 430–431

V

Vaccinations. See Immunizations
Vagina
    anatomy and function, 419
    infections, 425
    in pregnancy, 440
Vagotomy, 234
Vancomycin, 613t
Varicella-zoster virus (VZV), 199
    in pregnancy, 469
Varicose veins, 157
Vascular system, 107–108
    cholesterol-lowering medications, 621t–622t
    disorders of, 153–157
    hypertension, 141–145
    peripheral vascular disease, 153–157
Vasculitis, 197
vas deferens, 421
Vasodilators, 130, 619t
VEDP (ventricular end-diastolic pressure), cardiac output, 108
Veins, structure, 107
Venous peripheral vascular disease, 155–157
Ventilation
    function, 162
    mechanical, 168–169
Ventricles, 104
Ventricular dilation, 126
Ventricular dysrhythmias, 116–118
Ventricular end-diastolic pressure (VEDP), cardiac output, 108
Ventricular fibrillation, 118, 118f
Ventricular hypertrophy, 126
Ventricular septal defect (VSD), 521
Ventricular system, 345
Ventricular tachycardia, 117, 117f
Ventriculoperitoneal shunt, 520, 520f
Vernix caseosa, 463
Vesicle, 59
Vibration
    chronic obstructive pulmonary disease, 172
    physical assessment, 6, 12, 14
Vinca alkaloids, antineoplastic medications, 403t, 625t
Violent behavior
    and altered thought processes, 571t
    domestic violence, 581
Viral infection medications, 637t–638t
Vision, alterations in, 379–387
Visual fields, physical assessment, 10
Visual function, 380–383
    acuity assessment, 10
    assessment tests, 380t
    disorders of accommodation, 381t
    loss of, 383
Vital signs
    normal signs, 7t
    pediatric assessment, 502
    temperature, 8, 8t
Vitamins, 208–212, 661t
    B vitamins, 210
    vitamin A, 208
    vitamin B12, 212
    vitamin C, 212
    vitamin D, 209, 337t
    vitamin E, 210
    vitamin K, 210, 466
Vocal resonance, physical assessment, 13
Volvulus, 265
Vomiting
    antiemetic medications, 227t, 605t
    etiology and pathology, 228
    in pregnancy, 441, 445, 446t
VSD (ventricular septal defect), 521
Vulva, cancer of, 430
VZV. See Varicella-zoster virus

W

Water soluble vitamins, 208, 210
WBCs (leukocytes), 183
Wet dressings, skin integrity and, 54
Wheal, 59
White blood count (WBC), 43
Withdrawn clients, management of, 567, 570t
Women's health, medications for, 663t
Wounds, postoperative care, 68

X

Xanthines, 174t

Y

Young adulthood (developmental phase), 495–496, 496t